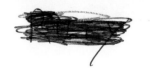

Practical Alimentary Tract Radiology

Edited by

Alexander R. Margulis, M.D.

Professor, Department of Radiology
Associate Chancellor–Special Projects
University of California, San Francisco
San Francisco, California

H. Joachim Burhenne, M.D., FRCP(C), FFRRCSI (Hon.)

Professor, Department of Radiology
University of British Columbia
Vancouver General Hospital
Vancouver, British Columbia, Canada

With **1089** *illustrations*

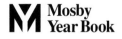 **Mosby Year Book**

St. Louis   Baltimore   Boston   Chicago   London   Philadelphia   Sydney   Toronto

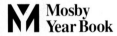

Mosby
Year Book
Dedicated to Publishing Excellence

Publisher: George Stamathis
Editor-in-Chief: Anne S. Patterson
Assistant Editor: Dana Battaglia
Project Manager: Patricia Tannian
Production Editor: Ann E. Rogers
Designer: David Zielinski

Printed in the United States of America

Mosby – Year Book, Inc.
11830 Westline Industrial Drive
St. Louis, Missouri 63146

Library of Congress Cataloging in Publication Data

Practical alimentary tract radiology / edited by Alexander R.
   Margulis, H. Joachim Burhenne.
        p.   cm.
     Based on: Alimentary tract radiology. 4th ed. 1989.
     Includes index.
     ISBN 0-8016-3133-5
     1. Gastrointestinal system—Radiography.   I. Margulis, Alexander
R.   II. Burhenne, H. Joachim (Hans Joachim), 1925-
III. Alimentary tract radiology.
        [DNLM: 1. Digestive System—radiography.   WI 141 P8944]
RC804.R6P73   1992
616.3'307572—dc20
DNLM/DLC   92-18766
   for Library of Congress   CIP

93 94 95 96 97 CL/MV 9 8 7 6 5 4 3 2 1

Contributors

Christoph D. Becker, M.D.
Department of Radiology
University of Bern
Bern, Switzerland

Robert N. Berk, M.D.
Professor, Department of Radiology
University of California, San Diego
Editor-in-Chief, American Journal of Roentgenology
San Diego, California

Douglas P. Boyd, Ph.D.
Professor of Radiology (Physics)
Department of Radiology
University of California, San Francisco
School of Medicine
San Francisco, California

Robert C. Brasch, M.D.
Professor, Department of Radiology and Pediatrics
Director, Contrast Media Laboratory
University of California, San Francisco
School of Medicine
San Francisco, California

Thomas F. Budinger, M.D., Ph.D.
Professor of Radiology
Department of Radiology
University of California, San Francisco
School of Medicine
San Francisco, California
Henry Miller Professor of Bioinstrumentation
Department of Electrical Engineering and Computer
 Science
University of California at Berkeley
Scientist, Research and Radiology Biophysics
Lawrence Berkeley Laboratory
Berkeley, California

**H. Joachim Burhenne, M.D., FRCP(C),
 FFRRCSI (Hon.)**
Professor, Department of Radiology
University of British Columbia
Vancouver General Hospital
Vancouver, British Columbia, Canada

M. Paul Capp, M.D.
Professor and Chairman
Department of Radiology
University of Arizona School of Medicine
Tucson, Arizona

David C. Carter, M.D.
Regius Professor of Clinical Surgery
University of Edinburgh Royal Infirmary
Edinburgh, Scotland

Ronald A. Castellino, M.D.
Professor of Radiology
Cornell University School of Medicine
Chief of Diagnostic Radiology
Memorial Hospital
New York, New York

Arthur R. Clemett, M.D.
Professor of Radiology
New York Medical College
New York University
New York, New York

Ronald A. Cohen, M.D.
Department of Radiology
Children's Hospital Medical Center of Northern
 California
Oakland, California

Michael Collier, Ph.D.
Chief of Clinical Physics
Radiotherapy Service
Lawrence Berkeley Laboratories
Berkeley, California

Peter L. Cooperberg, M.D.
Professor of Radiology
University of British Columbia
Chief, Department of Radiology
St. Paul's Hospital
Vancouver, British Columbia, Canada

Peter B. Cotton, M.D.
Professor of Medicine
Chief of Endoscopy
Division of Gastroenterology
Duke University Medical Center
Durham, North Carolina

Lawrence E. Crooks, Ph.D.
Professor of Electrical Engineering
University of California, San Francisco
San Francisco, California

Peter Dawson, MRCP, FRCR
Senior Lecturer, Department of Diagnostic Radiology
University of London
Royal Postgraduate Medical School
London, England

Barbara E. Demas, M.D.
Clinical Assistant Professor of Radiology
Department of Radiology
University of California, San Francisco
School of Medicine
San Francisco, California

Gerald D. Dodd, M.D.
Olga Keith and Harry Carothers Weiss Professor
    and Head
Division of Diagnostic Imaging
The University of Texas
M.D. Anderson Cancer Center
Houston, Texas

Wylie J. Dodds, M.D.
Professor of Radiology and Medicine
The Medical College of Wisconsin
Milwaukee, Wisconsin

†Martin W. Donner, M.D.
Professor of Radiology and Radiological Science
The Johns Hopkins University School of Medicine
Baltimore, Maryland

J. Scott Dunbar, M.D.
Professor Emeritus
San Francisco, California

Michael P. Federle, M.D.
Professor
Department of Radiology
University of Pittsburgh
Pittsburgh, Pennsylvania

Roy A. Filly, M.D.
Professor of Radiology and Obstetrics, Gynecology,
    and Reproductive Medicine
Chief, Section of Diagnostic Ultrasonography
Department of Radiology
University of California, San Francisco
School of Medicine
San Francisco, California

Harvey V. Fineberg, M.D., Ph.D.
Dean, Harvard School of Public Health
Harvard University
Boston, Massachusetts

Patrick C. Freeny, M.D.
Professor of Radiology
The University of Washington School of Medicine
Seattle, Washington

Barry B. Goldberg, M.D.
Professor of Radiology
Director, Division of Ultrasound
Thomas Jefferson University Hospital
Philadelphia, Pennsylvania

Charles A. Gooding, M.D.
Professor of Radiology and Pediatrics
Executive Vice Chairman
Department of Radiology
University of California, San Francisco
San Francisco, California

Gretchen A. W. Gooding, M.D.
Professor of Radiology
University of California, San Francisco
School of Medicine
Chief, Radiology Service
Veterans Administration Medical Center
San Francisco, California

Peter F. Hahn, M.D., Ph.D.
Assistant in Radiology
Department of Radiology
Massachusetts General Hospital
Boston, Massachusetts

Robert S. Hattner, M.D.
Associate Professor, Nuclear Medicine
Department of Radiology
University of California, San Francisco
San Francisco, California

Hedvig Hricak, M.D.
Professor of Radiology and Urology
University of California, San Francisco
San Francisco, California

Frederick S. Keller, M.D.
Professor and Chairman
Department of Radiology
University of Oregon
Portland, Oregon

Robert Kerlan, M.D.
Assistant Clinical Professor of Radiology
University of California, San Francisco
Radiologist, Scripps Memorial Hospital
La Jolla, California

Robert E. Koehler, M.D.
Professor and Vice Chairman
Department of Radiology
University of Alabama at Birmingham
Birmingham, Alabama

---

† Deceased.

George S. Kossoff
Director, Ultrasonics Institute
Division of Radiophysics
Commonwealth Department of Health
Sydney, Australia

Herbert Y. Kressel, M.D.
Professor of Radiology
Director, David W. Devon Medical Imaging Center
Hospital of the University of Pennsylvania
Department of Radiology
Philadelphia, Pennsylvania

Faye C. Laing, M.D.
Visiting Professor of Radiology
Department of Radiology
Thomas Jefferson University Hospital
Philadelphia, Pennsylvania

Brian C. Lentle, M.D., FRCP(C)
Professor and Head
Department of Radiology
University of British Columbia
Vancouver General Hospital
Vancouver, British Columbia, Canada

George R. Leopold, M.D.
Professor and Chairman
Department of Radiology
University of California, San Diego
San Diego, California

Marc S. Levine, M.D.
Associate Professor, Department of Radiology
Hospital of the University of Pennsylvania
Philadelphia, Pennsylvania

David K. B. Li, M.D., FRCP(C)
Professor, Department of Radiology
University of British Columbia
Vancouver, British Columbia, Canada

Arthur E. Lindner, M.D.
Associate Professor of Medicine and Associate Dean
New York University School of Medicine
New York, New York

Anders Lunderquist, M.D.
Professor
Central Department of Diagnostic Radiology
University of Lund
Lund, Sweden

Pierre H. G. Mahieu, M.D.
Chef de Clinique Associe
Universite Catholique de Louvain
Institut Chirurgical de Bruxelles et Cliniques
    Universitaires
St. Luc, Brussels, Belgium

Daniel Maklansky, M.D.
Associate Clinical Professor
Department of Radiology
Mt. Sinai School of Medicine
The City University of New York
New York, New York

Alexander R. Margulis, M.D.
Professor, Department of Radiology
Associate Chancellor–Special Projects
University of California, San Francisco
San Francisco, California

Masakazu Maruyama, M.D.
Department of Internal Medicine
Cancer Institute Hospital
Emeritus Professor of Montendeo University
Tokyo, Japan

James J. McCort, M.D.
Clinical Professor Emeritus, Department of Radiology
Stanford University School of Medicine
Stanford, California
Chairman, Department of Radiology
Santa Clara Valley Medical Center
San Jose, California

Dieter J. Meyerhoff, Ph.D.
Research Specialist, Magnetic Resonance Unit
Veterans Administration Medical Center
University of California, San Francisco
San Francisco, California

Morton A. Meyers, M.D., FACR
Professor, Department of Radiology
State University of New York at Stony Brook
School of Medicine
Health Sciences Center
Stony Brook, New York

Robert E. Mindelzun, M.D.
Clinical Associate Professor of Radiology
Stanford University School of Medicine
Stanford, California
Chief, Division of Diagnostic Radiology
Santa Clara Medical Center
Santa Clara, California

Albert A. Moss, M.D.
Professor and Chairman
Department of Radiology
University of Washington, School of Medicine
Seattle, Washington

J. Odo Op Den Orth, M.D.
Consultant Radiologist
Department of Radiology
St. Elizabeth's of Groote Gasthuis, Haarlem
The Netherlands

Gary M. Onik, M.D.
Department of Diagnostic Radiology
University of Pittsburgh
Presbyterian University Hospital
Pittsburgh, Pennsylvania

Theron W. Ovitt, M.D.
Professor and Chief
University of Arizona Health Sciences Center
College of Medicine
Tucson, Arizona

Philip E. S. Palmer, M.D., FRCP, FRCR
Professor of Radiology
Department of Radiology
University of California, Davis
School of Medicine
Davis, California

Theodore L. Phillips, M.D.
Professor and Chairman
Department of Radiation Oncology
University of California, San Francisco
School of Medicine
San Francisco, California

David C. Price, M.D.
Professor of Radiology and Medicine
Chief, Section of Nuclear Medicine
University of California, San Francisco
School of Medicine,
San Francisco, California

Jacques Pringot, M.D.
Professor
Department of Diagnostic Radiology
Universite Catholique De Louvian
Cliniques Universitaires
St. Luc, Brussels, Belgium

Maurice M. Reeder, M.D.
Professor and Chairman
Department of Radiology
University of Hawaii School of Medicine
Honolulu, Hawaii

Ernest J. Ring, M.D.
Professor and Head
Interventional Radiology
University of California, San Francisco
School of Medicine
San Francisco, California

Charles A. Rohrmann, Jr., M.D.
Professor and Vice-Chairman
Department of Radiology
University of Washington School of Medicine
Seattle, Washington

Josef Rösch, M.D.
Professor and Head of Interventional Radiology
The Oregon Health Sciences University
Portland, Oregon

Henrietta Kotlus Rosenberg, M.D.
Senior Radiologist and Director
Division of Ultrasound
The Children's Hospital of Philadelphia
Professor of Radiology
University of Pennsylvania
School of Medicine
Philadelphia, Pennsylvania

Leonard Rosenthall, M.D.
Director
Division of Nuclear Medicine
Professor
Department of Radiology
McGill University
Montreal, Quebec, Canada

Pierre Schnyder, M.D.
Professor and Chairman
Department of Radiology
University of Lausanne
Lausanne, Switzerland

Hikoo Shirakabe, M.D.
Honorary Professor of Jutendo University School of
  Medicine
Chairman, Foundation for Detection of Early Gastric
  Carcinoma
Directing Chief of Central Clinic
Tokyo, Japan

Edward B. Singleton, M.D.
Chief and Director of Radiology
St. Luke's Episcopal Hospital and Texas Children's
  Hospital
Professor of Radiology
Baylor College of Medicine
Clinical Professor of Radiology
University of Texas Medical School
Houston, Texas

Jovitas Skucas, M.D.
Professor of Radiology
School of Medicine and Dentistry
University of Rochester
Rochester, New York

Premysl Slezak, M.D., Ph.D.
Associate Professor
Department of Diagnostic Radiology–Endoscopy Unit
Karolinska Hospital
Stockholm, Sweden

Vernon Smith, M.S.C.
Associate Adjunct Professor
Department of Radiation Oncology
University of California, San Francisco
School of Medicine
San Francisco, California

David D. Stark, M.D.
Professor of Radiology
Director of MRI
Department of Radiology
University of Massachusetts Medical Center
Worcester, Massachusetts

David H. Stephens, M.D.
Professor of Radiology
Mayo Medical School
Department of Diagnostic Radiology
Mayo Clinic and Mayo Foundation
Rochester, Minnesota

Giles W. Stevenson, M.D.
Professor and Chairman
Department of Diagnostic Radiology
McMaster University – Head
Department of Radiology
Chedoke-McMaster Hospitals
Hamilton, Ontario, Canada

Edward T. Stewart, M.D.
Professor of Radiology
Chief, Gastrointestinal Radiology
Department of Radiology
Medical College of Wisconsin
Milwaukee, Wisconsin

Hooshang Taybi, M.D., M.Sc.
Clinical Professor of Radiology
University of California, San Francisco
School of Medicine
San Francisco, California
Radiologist
Department of Radiology
Children's Hospital Medical Center
Oakland, California

Ruedi F-L Thoeni, M.D.
Associate Professor
Department of Radiology
Chief, Computed Tomography/Gastrointestinal
    Radiology
University of California, San Francisco
School of Medicine
San Francisco, California

Susan D. Wall, M.D.
Associate Professor
Department of Radiology
University of California, San Francisco
School of Medicine
Assistant Chief, Radiology Service
Veterans Administration Medical Center
San Francisco, California

Michael W. Weiner, M.D.
Professor of Medicine and Radiology
University of California, San Francisco
School of Medicine
Director of Magnetic Resonance Unit
Veterans Administration Medical Center
San Francisco, California

Ralph Weissleder, M.D., Ph.D.
Department of Radiology
Massachusetts General Hospital
Boston, Massachusetts

Werner Wenz, M.D.
Professor and Chairman
Department of Radiology
Klinikum der Albert-Ludwigs-Universität
Freiburg, Germany

Thomas C. Winter
Assistant Professor of Radiology
University of Washington
School of Medicine
Seattle, Washington

Jack Wittenberg, M.D.
Professor
Department of Radiology
Harvard Medical School
Boston, Massachusetts

Preface

Editing *Alimentary Tract Roentgenology* first and then expanding it into *Alimentary Tract Radiology* has been an exhilarating experience over the many years that we worked on the four and one half editions. (The third edition was brought up to date with a third volume dealing with cross sectional imaging.) In this era, when so much knowledge in radiology is accumulated and abdominal radiology is the beneficiary of many of the advances, we thought that an abbreviated text on the practical and clinical aspects of radiology of the alimentary tract is needed. We are basing this book on the fourth edition of *Alimentary Tract Radiology*. We have shortened the chapters, attempted to extract the clinically important substance from each of the authors' contributions, and added new developments with illustrations. The book, in this format, should be easier to read and follow, since it is essentially transformed from an encyclopedic reference text into a practical overview of gastrointestinal radiology.

We hope that the readers will find it informative and worthwhile.

ARM and HJB

**Dedicated to our wives
Hedi and Linda**

Table of Contents

1 GENERAL CONSIDERATIONS, 1

2 GASTROINTESTINAL PHYSIOLOGY, 33

3 ACUTE ABDOMEN, 42
Nontraumatic acute abdomen, 42
Abdominal trauma, 60

4 PHARYNX, 66

5 ESOPHAGUS AND ESOPHAGOGASTRIC
REGION INCLUDING DIAPHRAGM, 78

6 STOMACH AND DUODENUM, 119
Stomach, 119
Nonneoplastic lesions of the stomach, 127
Neoplastic disorders of the stomach, 143
Peptic disease, 152
Duodenum, 161

7 SMALL BOWEL, 172
Technique for examination, 172
Inflammatory diseases of the small bowel, 184
Neoplastic lesions, 205
Malabsorption and immune deficiencies, 216

8 COLON, 221
Radiologic examination of the colon, 221
Defecography, 235
Diverticula, 239
Inflammatory disease of the colon, 246
Polyps, 264
Malignancies, 277

9 PANCREAS, 292
Anatomy, 292
Diagnostic examination, 292
Nonneoplastic lesions of the pancreas, 297
Neoplastic lesions of the pancreas, 308

10 LIVER AND BILIARY TRACT, 319
Jaundice, 319
Trauma, 320
Localized filling defects, 320
Newly developing fields, 321
Diseases of the liver and biliary tract, 323
Liver and biliary tract, 328
Imaging techniques, 337

11 SPLEEN, 365
Imaging of the spleen, 366
Normal spleen, 366
Splenic abnormalities, 367
Interventional radiology, 369
Ultrasonography, 369
Magnetic resonance imaging, 374
Nuclear medicine, 378

12 INFECTIOUS DISEASES, 383

13 POSTOPERATIVE RADIOLOGY, 404

14 RETROPERITONEAL SPACE, 421
Radiologic anatomy and diagnosis, 421

15 PEDIATRIC RADIOLOGY, 438
Disorders of the gastrointestinal tract, 438
Systemic diseases, 444
Disorders associated with pharyngeal
    and esophageal abnormalities, 447
Liver and biliary system, 449
Imaging techniques in pediatric disease, 452

16 SPECIAL PROCEDURES, 459
Angiography of the alimentary tract, 459
Venography, 469

17 INTERVENTIONAL RADIOLOGY, 471
The alimentary canal, 471
The vascular system, 473
The biliary tract, 476
Endoscopic therapies, 485
Percutaneous abdominal biopsy and drainage, 489

18 CLINICAL OVERVIEW, 493
Clinician's perspective on abdominal imaging, 493
Oncology, 496
Cost effectiveness, 497

INDEX, 499

1 *General Considerations*

DP BOYD
ROBERT C BRASCH
TF BUDINGER
M PAUL CAPP
LE CROOKS
PETER DAWSON
GAW GOODING
RS HATTNER
GS KOSSOFF
ALBERT A MOSS
TW OVITT
A JOVITAS SKUCAS
THOMAS C WINTER

INSTRUMENTATION

CONTRAST MEDIA

NUCLEAR MEDICINE

ULTRASONOGRAPHY

INSTRUMENTATION
Radiographic equipment

TW OVITT
M PAUL CAPP

Generator

Factors that must be considered when selecting a generator are the power rating, the phase capability, and the timing control. The *power rating* is an expression of the output or capacity of the generator. It is best expressed in kilowatts (kW), where the kilowatt equals volts × amperes/1000 (or more conveniently in radiologic applications, kilovolts × milliamperes/1000). A generator rated at 1000 milliamperes (mA) *and* 125 kilovolts (kV) does not, as one might assume, produce 1000 mA *at* 125 kV. Rather, the designation means that the generator can be operated at 125 kV (at some unspecified milliamperage) and at up to 1000 mA at some lower (and unspecified) kilovoltage. A 75 to 85 kW, 150 kV, and 600 mA generator is adequate for conventional gastrointestinal studies.

Phase is the second characteristic to be considered. With a full-wave rectified single-phase generator, the voltage applied to the x-ray tube rises from zero voltage to the peak voltage and falls again to zero voltage during each half cycle. As a result, the average voltage impressed on the x-ray tube is only a fraction (approximately 0.7) of the peak voltage, and image-forming photons are generated during only a fraction (approximately 0.35) of the total exposure time. In 3 phase–6

1

pulse equipment, three overlapping patterns of voltage, slightly separated in time, are impressed on the x-ray tube during each half cycle. As the first begins to drop, the second is rising toward the peak value, and as it begins to drop, the third rises toward the peak value. Therefore the average impressed voltage more nearly approaches the peak voltage, and image-forming photons are generated virtually throughout the exposure. As a result, exposure times with 3-phase equipment are significantly shorter than with single-phase equipment. With 3 phase–12 pulse equipment, six patterns of voltage, slightly displaced in time, are impressed on the x-ray tube, further reducing exposure time. Loss of sharpness because of motion may mar studies in certain clinical situations; therefore 3 phase–6 or 12 pulse equipment is strongly recommended despite its cost.

The capability of the *timing control* is the third generator characteristic to be considered. Major manufacturers now offer exposure times ranging from 1 to 3 milliseconds (msec) to 6, 8, or even 10 seconds. Exposure time variations in replicate exposures should not exceed 2% at 100 msec.

X-ray tube

Radiographic/fluoroscopic systems require two x-ray tubes: one mounted above the table for conventional radiography and the other mounted under the table for fluoroscopy and intercurrent recording. The factors to be considered when selecting the x-ray tube include ability to withstand heat, permissible loading, and size of the focal spot.

The heat produced when an x-ray tube is energized is quantified in terms of *heat units* (HU) per second or watts per second (kilovolts x milliamperes/second). Three-phase equipment generates 35% more heat units per second than does single-phase equipment operating at the same exposure factors. In the course of an upper gastrointestinal (GI) series or barium enema, 125,000 to 250,000 HU or more may be generated in the fluoroscopic (under-table) tube.

The *permissible loading,* or *kilowatt rating,* of the tube is calculated as one thousandth of the product of the kilovoltage and milliamperage when the tube is operated for one tenth of a second at 100 kV and the maximum allowable milliamperage. For an under-table tube, minimum values are 25 kW and 50 kW for the small and large focal spots, respectively. For an over-table tube, minimum values are 40 kW and 70 kW, respectively. Anode heat capacity should equal 400,000 HU for a tube that has been recently loaded.

The size of the *focal spot* is of interest to radiologists because it influences image quality. For gastrointestinal studies, nominal 0.6 mm and 1.2 mm focal spots are generally regarded as satisfactory.

Image intensifier tube

There are relatively few options regarding the image intensifier tube. The various performance parameters, however, should be compared. All manufacturers now use cesium iodide input phosphors.

The *conversion factor* is an expression of output phosphor brightness relative to input x-ray dose rate expressed in candela per square meter per milliroentgen per second. Values from 55 for a 7-inch tube to 110 for a 10-inch tube are acceptable. *Resolution* should be on the order of four to six line pairs per millimeter. *Contrast range* is the ratio of the brightness at the center of the output phosphor, when the input phosphor is fully irradiated, to the same measurement when the central portion (10%) of the input phosphor is shielded. The ratio should be at least 10:1. *Lag* is the duration of the continued emission of light photons from the output phosphor after the exciting radiation has been terminated. This value should not exceed 1 msec.

Television viewing system

Television systems consist of three components: (1) the coupling between the image intensifier tube output phosphor and the television camera pickup tube, (2) the television camera pickup tube, and (3) the cathode x-ray tube (kinescope or monitor) on which the image is displayed. As with the image intensifier tube, lag, contrast, and resolution are the performance characteristics governing the choice of components.

The *coupling* makes it possible not only to visualize the video image of the output phosphor of the image intensifier tube, but also to record that image with a photospot camera. This makes an optical coupling much more desirable than a fiberoptic coupling.

The *television camera pickup tube* of choice for radiologic applications is the compact, reliable *vidicon.* The pickup tube measures the amount of current required to recharge each point of the photoconductive surface as a scanning electron beam passes over it. To smooth the image, the electron beam scans every other line in one pass, and the intervening lines on the next; this process is called *interlacing.*

The *monitor* or *kinescope* is dependent on the camera pickup tube, and the characteristics of the monitor are largely determined by the characteristics of the camera pickup tube.

Conventional Bucky radiography

In addition to the generator and x-ray tube, the *geometric relationships* between the overhead tube, the table, and the plane of the Bucky tray (film plane) affect image quality and should be explored. The likelihood of significant loss of geometric sharpness increases with the distance between the tabletop and the film plane.

This distance should not exceed 2.5 inches (assuming a 60-inch target-to-film distance). The *grid* should be a 100-line grid with a ratio of at least 12:1. A high-speed moving grid may provide images free of grid pattern in exposures of 15 msec or longer and, in at least one product, in exposures as short as 2 msec.

Table-tube configurations

The simplest, least expensive, and most commonly used system is a *90-30 table with an overhead fluoroscopy tower*. The radiographic tube is underneath the table and is mechanically coupled to the image intensifier. A second popular configuration is a *90-30 table with an overhead x-ray tube and under-the-table intensifier* mechanically linked to traverse the entire length of the table. These units are designed to be operated by remote control from a radiation-protected booth in or adjacent to the x-ray room. In this configuration the radiologist operates from the control booth, using a microphone to communicate with the patient. The technologist is usually in the room, explaining the procedure and helping to position the patient. One disadvantage of this system is the relatively long time it takes the Bucky tray to come into position when obtaining spot films.

Future instrumentation

Converting GI radiology pictures to digital images should not be difficult. There is evidence that a 2000 × 2000 line matrix system will be ample for the chest examination, and it is unlikely that more than 1000 × 1000 will be needed for any type of GI examination. Satisfactory GI images obviously require a larger intensifier to cover the abdomen. Image intensifiers now being introduced are capable of resolving 2.5 to 3.0 line pairs per millimeter, approaching the equivalent of a 2000 × 2000 matrix.

Another new modality is the x-ray sensitive photostimulable plate, which produces images similar to those of a routine GI examination with the imaging plate substituted for film. A large-field image intensifier will probably be the receptor in the final digital department which, by that time, will be totally electronic.

Future technology

Without question, the greatest impacts in the future of GI radiology will be the elimination of film and the evaluation of total electronic images. By the year 2000, certainly, most major hospitals will have total electronic imaging. The current use of the x-ray sensitive photostimulable plate has already improved portable images and has created a digital image that cannot be lost. The x-ray sensitive imaging plate is a storage phosphor substituted for film. After x-ray exposure, the latent image on the image plate is laser scanned, digitized, and stored on an optical digital disk. One advantage of this system is that it can be incorporated into an existing radiology facility, since the cassettes containing the photostimulable phosphors are the same size as conventional cassettes. The main disadvantage—having to carry the cassette to the cassette tray, make the exposure, and carry it back to the image processor—will be obviated by future development of new devices that will permit "instant" images. Those that are being investigated include large-field intensifiers and charge-coupled slip scanners.

Several major problems must be overcome before the total digital radiology department can exist. At present, connecting different companies' electronics into a single imaging work station is a big problem. The ACR NEMA standards are being developed for this application, but this process will take many years. The networking required to accept, store, and make the images accessible within a few seconds remains an immense problem. This networking is the most formidable task for the future, but technology has progressed significantly. Many companies are developing and evaluating workstations; this is not a major problem. There is now evidence that a 2000 × 2000 × 10 gray levels line matrix system will be ample for the chest examination, and it is unlikely that more than 1000 × 1000 will be needed for any type of GI examination. Many institutions are now evaluating different parts of the total electronic radiology department, and film is slowly being replaced. A total electronic department will be available for any hospital by the year 2000. Those institutions that are involved with the research of picture archival communications systems (PACS) will have developed the technology earlier.

Computed tomography instrumentation
DP BOYD

A modern computed tomography (CT) scanner system consists of a scanning gantry that includes the collimated x-ray source and detectors, the computer data acquisition and reconstruction system, a motorized patient-handling table, and a CT viewing console. The data acquisition and reconstruction system usually consists of one or more minicomputers or microcomputers and related peripheral equipment such as a magnetic tape unit or an optical disk for archival storage, a printer, an operator's keyboard and display, data acquisition electronics, and special processors to speed the reconstruction computations.

Image reconstruction is the process that converts detector readings from hundreds of thousands of data samples into an electronic picture that represents the scanned section. The picture is composed of a matrix of picture elements (pixels), each of which has a density value represented by its CT number. Using the Hounsfield scale of CT number, water is 0, air is −1000, and bone is +1000. Each CT number represents a 0.1% density difference.

The patient-handling table is usually motorized, with horizontal (axial) and vertical drives. The couch is automatically indexed in the horizontal direction, and the computer is used to position a series of adjacent tomographic sections. Laser-produced light beams are used to localize the patient within the gantry. Selection of the scanning volume is usually based on the use of a line-scanned projection image obtained by sweeping the patient horizontally through the stationary x-ray fan beam. The scanning gantry is usually able to tilt ±20 degrees, and in some cases the couch can be tilted or angulated in the horizontal plane.

CT images are usually photographed with multiformat cameras to produce a standard 14 × 17 inch film of multiple sections that is stored in the film file room. Recently introduced laser-based multiformat cameras offer improved image quality and speed over the earlier cathode ray tube (CRT) cameras. Digital image data can also be stored on either magnetic tape or optical disks.

Scanning gantries

Modern CT scanners employ a fan of x-ray beams that are used in combination with a position-sensitive detector array. X-ray fan widths range from 30 degrees to greater than 60 degrees, and detector arrays contain from 300 to more than 4800 discrete detector elements. The more detectors that are simultaneously recording

transmitted x-ray intensities, the faster the scanning sequence may be completed (Fig. 1-1). In addition, larger detector arrays typically permit the size of an individual detector element to be minimized, leading to significant improvements in spatial resolution.

If 300 to 900 detectors are used, it is possible to simultaneously measure all the sample points in a given x-ray fan or profile. Only rotary motion of the detector and source is required, and scanning speeds of 2 seconds or faster can be achieved. Such systems are referred to as *rotate-rotate* systems.

In another type of system, a stationary ring detector array with 1200 to 4800 detectors is arranged in a circle about the patient. Only a fraction of the ring receives x-rays at one time. A rotating fan of x-radiation produces the scan. Such systems are called *rotate-stationary* systems.

Fast CT scanners

The introduction of scanners employing slip rings has significantly reduced scan times. The slip-ring scanners employ continuous rotation by using a slip-ring bearing to deliver power to the x-ray tube through a series of rotating brushes in contact with ring electrodes, allowing continuous rotation at a relatively high speed (Fig. 1-2). Scanners with minimum scan times in the 1-second range are now available.

Ultrafast CT scanners

An alternative approach, using a *scanning electron beam* tube, has a clear advantage for high-speed, mul-

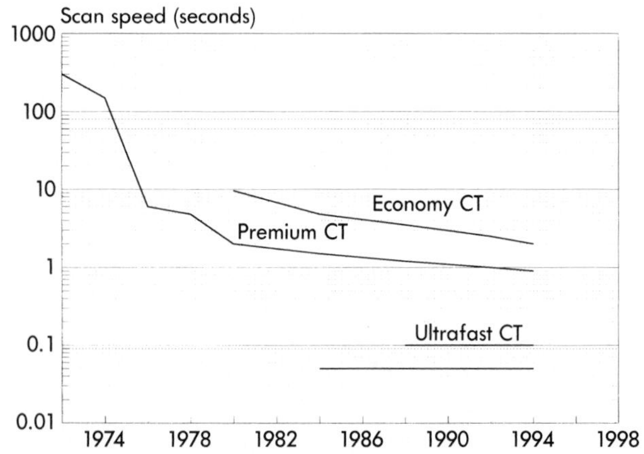

Fig. 1-1 Progressive improvement in scan speeds of CT scanners. Economy scanners and premium scanners all employ a rotating gantry and x-ray tube to achieve scan speeds in the range of 1 to 4 seconds. Ultrafast scanners use a scanning electron beam that sweeps a circular target ring, producing x-ray scans in 50 or 100 msec.

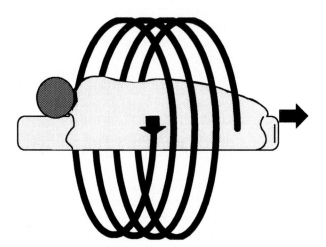

Fig. 1-2 Principle of continuous helical scanning that is used by ultrafast scanners and is being adopted by premium CT scanners that employ slip-rings. The earlier mode of step scanning in 0.5 cm or 1 cm increments is replaced by continuous scanning during smooth couch translation. This mode enables improved slice registration and shorter examination times.

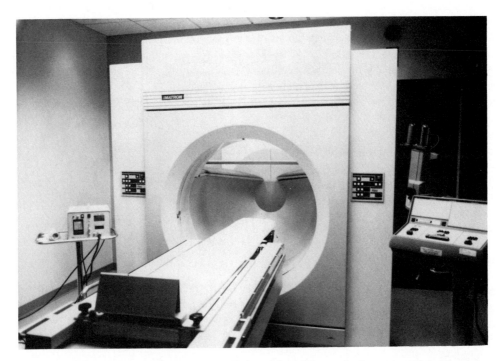

Fig. 1-3 Typical ultrafast CT scanner installation. Most CT examinations are performed using contrast media injected by the programmable power injector at right. Patient table can be angulated and tilted and has provision for bicycle ergometry used in conjunction with cardiac stress studies. ECG monitor is at left.

tislice imaging. In scanning electron beam systems all mechanical motion is replaced with a scanning electron beam, and very large ring tungsten targets, which are directly water cooled. Therefore speed is not restricted by either mechanical considerations or heat-capacity restrictions. Although the ultrafast scanner was originally developed for cardiac imaging, its advantages in speed and resolution have become increasingly important in abdominal imaging (Fig. 1-3).

Ultrasonography instrumentation
GS KOSSOFF

The gray scale of the ultrasound device is distributed between 100 mV (necessary to make an echo visible) and 1 V (which saturates the display) and generally ranges from 16 to 126 shades of gray. With this restricted gray scale range, it is not possible to display the entire range of amplitudes of echoes, and some form of selection and compression must be employed to display the range of magnitude that is considered to be of maximal clinical significance.

Transducer

The electronic and geometric properties of the transducer determine the depth and lateral resolution of sonographic equipment. In general these properties im-

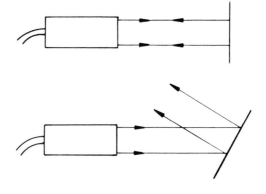

Specular reflection

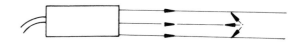

Diffuse reflection

Fig. 1-4 Specular reflection from large interface and diffuse reflection from small interface.

prove as frequency is increased. The *depth resolution* of the transducer is usually significantly better than the *lateral resolution*.

In the simplest case, as in many mechanical sector scanners, lateral resolution is achieved with a single *fixed-focus transducer*. Focusing is achieved by using either a lens in front of a plane or a curved transducer (Fig. 1-4).

Annular array transducers may also be used to electronically focus the beam at different depths. If focusing the beam over a range of distances is desired, several transmit pulses must be employed, reducing the speed of acquisition. In reception, the signal may be kept in focus as it is being received over the entire depth. This feature, known as *dynamic focusing*, significantly improves the lateral resolution. With large-aperture annular array equipment it is possible to employ a small aperture for signals being received from lesser depths and to progressively increase the aperture as echoes from deeper areas are received. This has the effect of keeping the lateral resolution constant over the entire depth (Fig. 1-5).

Linear and *phased array scanners* are the most popular class of equipment used today. In the linear array scanner the ultrasonic beam is generated by energizing

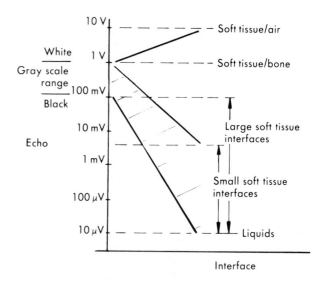

Fig. 1-5 Magnitude of echo received from biologic interfaces and gray-scale range of display unit. Diagonal lines illustrate compression of range of echoes received from small interfaces into major portion of gray-scale range of display unit.

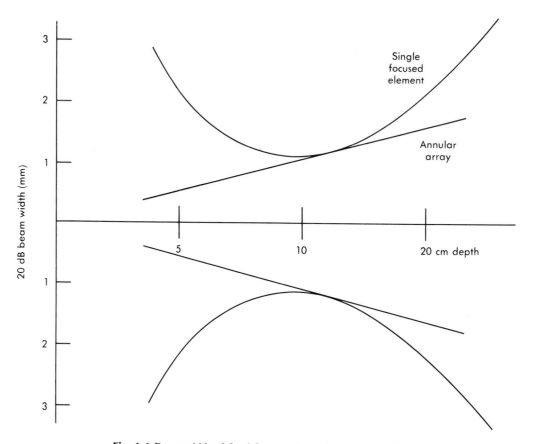

Fig. 1-6 Beam width of fixed focus and annular array transducer.

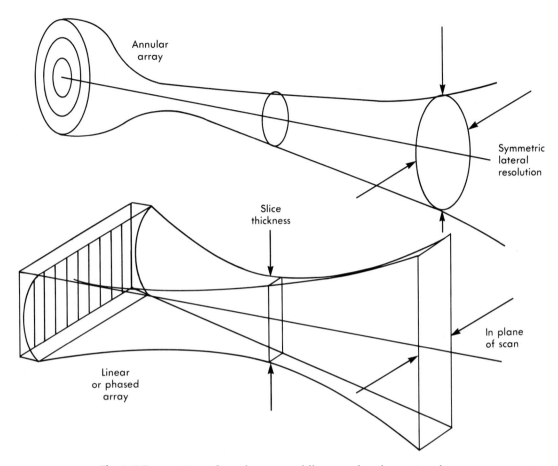

Fig. 1-7 Beam pattern of annular array and linear or phased array transducer.

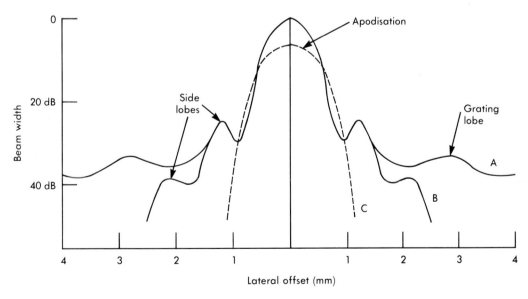

Fig. 1-8 Beam width of transducer made up of, *A*, wide multielements, *B*, narrow multielements, and *C*, narrow multielements with variable amplitude of excitation.

a small group of the elements, and the beam is scanned by sequentially energizing adjacent groups of elements and moving the ultrasonic line of sight correspondingly along the length of the transducer. The image format is thus rectangular, the width being equal to the length of the transducer and the length to the examined depth. In phased array equipment, a small multielement transducer is employed, and a sector image format is obtained by controlling the time sequence with which all of the elements are energized (Figs. 1-6 to 1-8).

Scan converter

The scan converter section restructures the presentation of the sonogram from its natural form (by which echoes are received along the line of sight of the transducer), into a rectangular format for presentation on a television monitor. Digital scan converters, now universally used for this application, store the processed data in the form of gray scale level and pixel number. Some equipment provides a *persistence* feature in which the scan converter is used to average several frames before displaying the image. Although persistence lowers the acquisition frame rate, averaging reduces the flicker effect caused by small tissue movement between frames and also smoothes out the speckled nature of sonographic images.

Nuclear medicine instrumentation
TF BUDINGER

With advances in instrumentation and in the labeling chemistry of biologically active ligands, nuclear medical procedures now play an increasingly important role in the evaluation of diseases of the abdomen and pelvis. Nuclear medicine is of particular use in the detection of normal and pathologic tissue response to therapy, bone metastases, and GI motility (three-dimensional).

Gamma ray–photon production

Gamma rays are produced during radioactive decay when the nucleus of the isotope undergoes a reduction in *nuclear* energy level. These radiations are designated as photons with some stated energy, and the quantity of energy is expressed as electron volts, usually in units of 1000 electron volts (keV). A positron emitter gives off photons with energies of 511 keV.

In *electron emission (b^- emission)* the decay process consists of the transformation of a neutron in the nucleus into a proton and an electron, and the ejection of the electron from the atom. After the electron is released, the new atom is usually left in an excited state, that is, the nucleus energy is greater than that of a stable nucleus having the same atomic electron configuration. To reach a state of lower energy, the nucleus releases one or more photons. For example, ^{131}I decays to a xenon atom, ^{131}Xe, by emission of an electron. The most probable energy state is 364 keV above the ground state, and 87% of the ^{131}I disintegrations lead to this level. Almost immediately, the xenon nucleus goes to the ground state with the emission of a 364 keV photon.

In *positron emission (b^+ emission)* a nuclear proton changes into a positive electron (a positron) and a neutron. The atom maintains its atomic mass but decreases its atomic number by one. The ejected positron combines with an electron almost instantaneously, and these two particles undergo the process of annihilation. The energy associated with the masses of the positron and electron particles is 1.022 MeV. This energy is divided

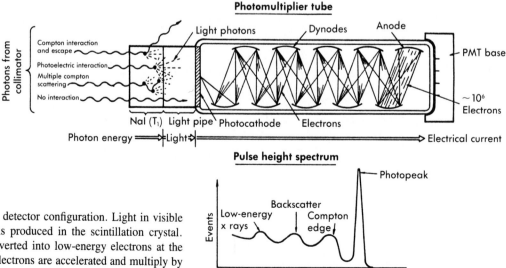

Fig. 1-9 Photoelectron detector configuration. Light in visible or near-visible range is produced in the scintillation crystal. Light photons are converted into low-energy electrons at the photocathode. These electrons are accelerated and multiply by successive interactions with the dynodes.

equally between two photons that fly away from one another at a 180 degree angle. Each photon has an energy of 511 keV, or approximately seven times that of the x-ray photons usually used in radiology.

In *electron capture (EC)* an orbiting electron penetrates and is captured by a nucleus. The capture results in the conversion of a proton to a neutron. The atom decreases in atomic number by one but maintains its mass number. Because the K-shell of planetary electrons is closest to the nucleus, most of the capture events involve electrons from this shell—thus the name *K-capture*.

Detection of photons

Most photon detection instruments employ a sodium iodide crystal doped with thallium, NaI(T1) (Fig. 1-9). When a high-energy photon strikes the NaI(T1) crystals, visual photons are given off with an intensity proportional to the energy of the photon. When a photon of medium energy enters the NaI(T1) crystal, one of three things happens: (1) the photon passes through the crystal without an interaction; (2) the photon collides with an atomic electron and transfers all of its energy (less 29 keV for the binding energy of a K-electron of iodine) to a secondary electron—this is a photoelectric event; or (3) the photon scatters from an electron, giving up only part of its energy to the electron (Compton scattering). The electron energy is subsequently absorbed because it does not travel far in the crystal. The scattered photon, however, can now move through the

crystal and frequently escapes before it is absorbed by the photoelectric phenomenon or is scattered again.

At each interaction of the photon in the crystal, light photons are released. These photons are detected by a *photoelectron multiplier tube (PMT)*. In the PMT, the light photons cause the release of a current of electrons, which gives an electronic signal. The instantaneous signal from the phototube is proportional to the photon energy absorbed in the crystal.

Pulse-height analyzer

This device helps to exclude both pulses corresponding to Compton-scattered radiation in the patient and radiation from radioisotopes other than the one being examined. The readout system consists of both a cathode ray tube, which displays each event as a flash at a position corresponding to the position at which the event occurred in projection from the patient, and a digital storage component of a computer.

Scintillation camera

The Anger camera (Fig. 1-10) consists of a large flat NaI(T1) crystal with from 9 to 91 phototubes closely packed over it. For most cameras in current use, the detection areas are 30 cm or greater in diameter *or* on a side. Whole-body scanning systems have dual detectors 50 cm wide. The photons that interact with the large-camera crystal lose their energy by photoelectric or Compton interactions, or both. The total number of light photons produced is directly proportional to the to-

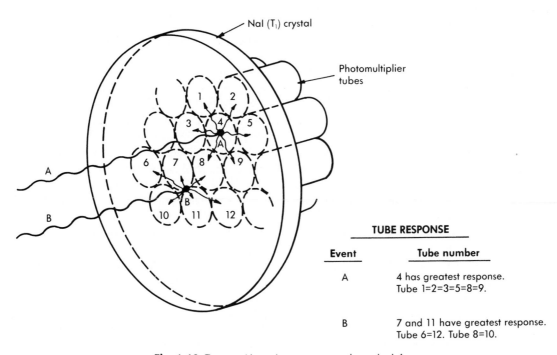

TUBE RESPONSE

Event	Tube number
A	4 has greatest response. Tube 1=2=3=5=8=9.
B	7 and 11 have greatest response. Tube 6=12. Tube 8=10.

Fig. 1-10 Gamma (Anger) camera operating principle.

tal photon energy absorbed by the crystal for each photon-NaI(T1) interaction. The crystal is optically coupled to a series of photomultiplier tubes that are arranged in hexagonal array. Each phototube absorbs the light photons produced within its field of view onto its bi-alkali, photosensitive surface, releasing electrons by a factor of 10^6 or 10^7. This produces an output pulse that is directly proportional to the total energy absorbed within the field of view of the phototube. A computing circuit is used in combination with the phototube array to determine the X-Y scintillations occurring within the crystal on the basis of relative intensity of light seen by each of the phototubes. The circuit determines X and Y positions of the scintillations, and these are the data that make up the image.

Emission tomography

The two major forms of emission tomography are known as single photon-emission tomography (SPECT) and positron emission tomography (PET).

Single photon-emission tomography involves acquisition of multiple projections by rotation of a detector system around a patient (Fig. 1-11). The reconstruction algorithms are similar to those for x-ray computed tomography (CT), except that the SPECT algorithms must incorporate attenuation-compensation methods for accurate data.

Positron-emission tomography involves the class of isotopes known as *positron emitters*. As discussed, these isotopes have a characteristic deficiency in the number of neutrons relative to the number of protons in the nucleus. Such a nucleus is usually produced by bombarding another nucleus with a high-energy proton or deuteron from a cyclotron. For the isotope to return to a stable nonradioactive state, the proton becomes a neutron, and this transition results in the release of the positron. For example, if ^{14}N is bombarded with a deuteron (a hydrogen nucleus with an additional neutron), the result is ^{15}O. In this case the proton is added to the nucleus. Two classes of positron emitters can be used effectively without the need for an on-site cyclotron. These include (1) long-lived isotopes such as ^{18}F, ^{62}Zn, and ^{68}Ga, which can be delivered from cyclotrons geographically remote from the imaging instrument; and (2) generator produced–positron emitters such as ^{68}Ga, ^{82}Rb, and ^{122}I, which are produced as decay daughters from long-lived precursors such as ^{68}Ge, ^{82}Sr, and ^{122}Xe, respectively. In the case of generator-produced nuclides, the precursor is delivered from an accelerator facility and the daughter "milked" from the parent as needed.

Reconstruction of a tomographic image relies on the accurate detection of the two photons that arise from the annihilation of the positron and electron pairs. The de-

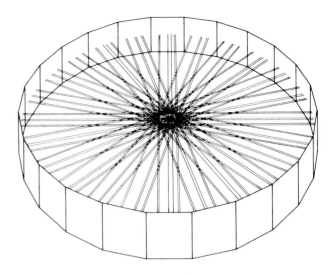

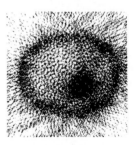

Fig. 1-11 General configurations of tomography devices.

tection is achieved using scintillation crystals that convert the annihilation photons into light, which is then picked up by a photoelectron multiplier tube (phototube) (Fig. 1-12). When two detectors register a signal in time coincidence, the conclusion is that the activity is somewhere along the line between the two detectors. Detection of 300,000 or more annihilation events allows the distribution of activity in a tomographic section to be calculated by procedures somewhat similar to those used in x-ray computed tomography. Resolutions have improved from 17 mm in 1976 to about 5 mm in 1990. Detector configurations have also evolved to simultaneously provide multiple transverse sections for abdominal imaging and metabolic studies.

The valuation of liver metastatic tumors and parenchymal disease using fluorodeoxyglucose and PET has been reported. The finding of increased accumulation of FDG in the injured liver probably indicates a decrease in phosphate activity, and the accumulation of deoxyglucose in liver metastases is probably due to an increase in metabolism.

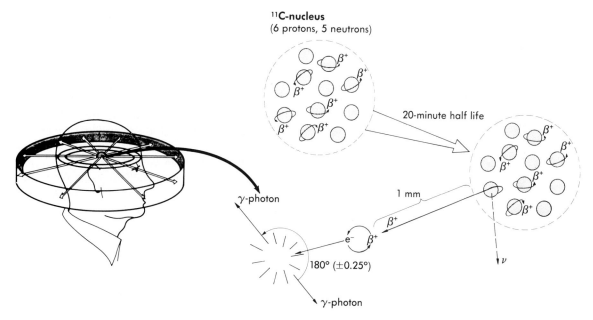

¹¹C-nucleus
(6 protons, 5 neutrons)

20-minute half life

γ-photon

1 mm

180° (±0.25°)

γ-photon

ν

Fig. 1-12 PET involves detection of gamma photons, resulting from annihilation of a positron and electron. Electronic detection of an event in two opposing detectors signals that the radionuclide is somewhere along the line joining the two detectors.

Magnetic resonance imaging instrumentation
LE CROOKS

Magnetic resonance imaging (MRI) uses a basic set of hardware for all imaging techniques. A magnet is used to impose a strong, uniform magnetic field. Gradient coils are used to vary this uniform field in a manner dictated by the pulsing parameters (Figs. 1-13, 1-14).

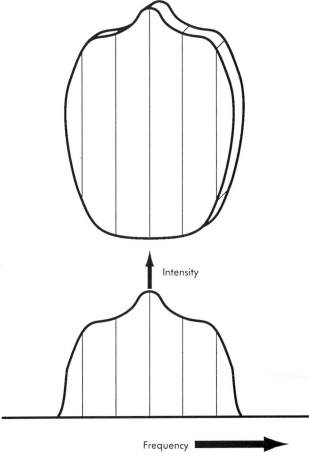

Intensity

Frequency

Fig. 1-14 Spectrum of signal, in presence of gradient, from excited plane is projection of nuclei in that plane onto line. Nuclei in each column through plane have same frequency, so intensity of each frequency in spectrum corresponds to sum of signals from all nucei in column.

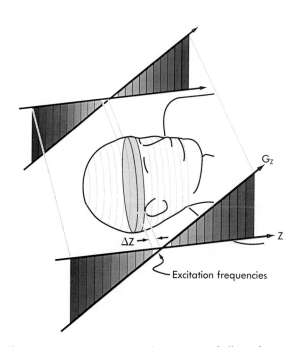

G_z

Z

ΔZ

Excitation frequencies

Fig. 1-13 Selective excitation in presence of slice select gradient G_z.

To induce resonance, a transmitter delivers radiofrequency (RF) power through a coil. The same or another coil also picks up the MRI signals, while a receiver connected to the receiver coil delivers the suitably amplified, demodulated, and filtered signals to digitizing circuitry. Last, a computer system provides for control and data acquisition, processing, storage, and display functions.

Magnets

The static magnetic field is generated by either permanent magnets or electric current through a coil. Coil conductors are either resistive (copper or aluminum wires), in which case a power supply provides a driving current continuously, or superconducting (cooled to extremely low temperatures so that there is practically no electric resistance in the conductor), in which case the power supply can be disconnected once a current has been established (Fig. 1-15).

If iron is not used to shape the field, the configuration of the current-carrying conductors becomes the determining factor in establishing field uniformity. A superconducting magnet with an outside diameter and length of 2 m can have a field uniformity of better than 50 ppm over a 40 cm diameter region. Superconducting magnets offer much higher field strengths (up to 4 tesla [T]) for MRI of hydrogen and other nuclei and for spectroscopy. They permit faster scanning and better signal-to-noise performance with thin slices.

Permanent magnets are attractive for low-field imaging. At 0.065 T an imaging magnet is about 1.6 m wide and deep. Its weight is comparable to a superconducting

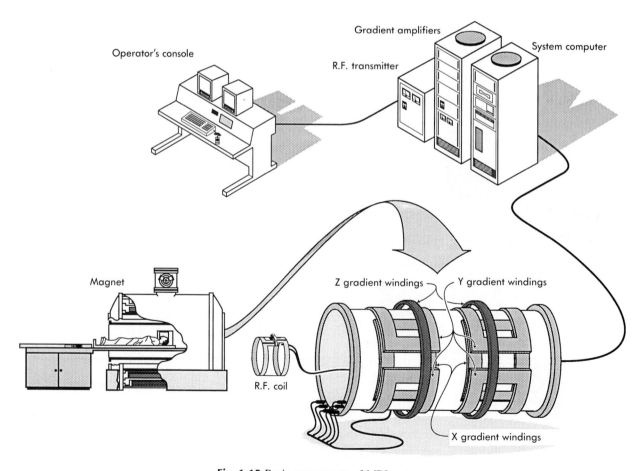

Fig. 1-15 Basic components of MRI system.

magnet, about 12,000 pounds (5500 kg), and the field is provided by commonly available ferrite materials. Field uniformity over the 40 cm diameter imaging volume needs to be only 200 ppm to give the same absolute field variation as a 0.35 T superconducting magnet. The low field strength has a weak attraction for ferromagnetic objects, improving patient safety, and the weaker force on the pulsed gradient coils makes operation almost silent. This, along with the open access between the pole tips, makes the patient more comfortable and reduces claustrophobia. The signal-to-noise performance at the low field is quite good.

The smaller size of a permanent magnet, as well as its small fringe field and lower support requirements, allows it to fit in a small scanner suite. In addition, the reduction in site and equipment costs decreases system cost by more than the reduction in the magnet cost alone (Fig. 1-16).

Magnetic gradients

The linear field gradients needed for imaging are produced by coils mounted within the magnet, which modify the basic uniform field. The on-off switching of the gradients produces distortions that can be corrected by self-shielding the gradients.

Radiofrequency coil, transmitter, and receiver

Excitation and observation of the MRI signal require an antenna that couples RF energy to and from the resonating nuclei. When the RF coil is used for both transmission and reception, it is set up for transmission only during excitation of the nuclei. After excitation, the coil is switched to function as the receiver. Separate transmitter and receiver coils are often used; in this case, the transmitter coil may be large enough for the receiver coil to fit inside it. One coil is detuned when the other is being used. When the organ of interest is near the surface of the body, a surface coil, which couples to only the tissue near the surface, can be used. In this case, the signal comes from the organ of interest and the noise from only this region (Fig. 1-17), yielding an improved signal-to-noise ratio.

The organization and sensitivity of the receiver are similar to those of a shortwave radio. However, unlike a shortwave radio, which covers a broad range of frequencies, the MRI receiver is designed for optimal per-

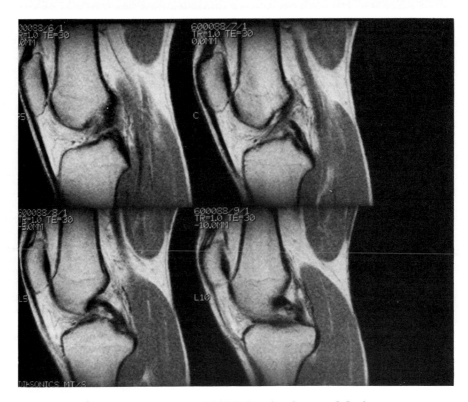

Fig. 1-16 Knee image at 0.065 T. Imaging time was 8.5 minutes.

barium peritonitis, which is associated with significant morbidity and mortality (Fig. 1-19). Mortality rates are related to the amount of contrast media and stool within the peritoneal cavity. Clinically, these patients show signs of acute peritonitis. Eventually the barium sulfate crystals are coated by fibrin, and dense intraperitoneal adhesions develop. The fibrosis can involve not only the small bowel, but also adjacent structures such as the ureter. In subsequent years these patients may experience numerous episodes of small bowel and ureteric obstruction. Surgery is generally difficult because of the extensive adhesions.

Contrast agents for computed tomography
ALBERT A MOSS
THOMAS C WINTER

Oral contrast techniques

To a large extent the sensitivity of computed tomography in diagnosing gastrointestinal pathology depends on adequate bowel opacification and distention. If the GI tract is unopacified and collapsed adjacent to an abnormal organ, the distinction between a pathologic process and a normal segment of the GI tract is often difficult to determine. Collapsed GI tract has a CT attenuation value similar to that of liver, kidney, pancreas, muscle, and nonopacified vascular structures. Therefore, when bowel is not filled with air or fluid, it is often difficult to make the distinction between bowel and an adjacent organ or mass. Because the basic radiopathologic finding in a variety of gastrointestinal diseases is thickening of the intestinal wall, the gut must be distended and filled with a contrast agent that permits the wall of the bowel to be assessed accurately.

Positive contrast material must increase the CT attenuation value of bowel lumen at least 40 Hounsfield units. This can be done by using dilute solutions of water-soluble media or dilute suspensions of barium sulfate. The commercial introduction of dilute 1% to 2% barium sulfate solutions containing special suspending agents has permitted dilute barium to remain homogeneously suspended as it passes through the GI tract (Fig. 1-20).

A solution of 2% to 3% meglumine diatrizoate increases CT attenuation of the gut enough to permit reliable differentiation from surrounding tissues. However, these solutions tend to become diluted as they reach the terminal ileum, and the distal small bowel may be poorly demarcated. Water-soluble contrast agents may precipitate in gastric fluid and produce streak artifacts, which degrade the CT examination.

For most examinations the oral contrast media are administered in two increments: approximately 900 ml 60 minutes before the examination to fill the distal small bowel, and another 250 ml immediately before scanning to ensure that the stomach, duodenum, and proximal small bowel are filled. The esophagus is best marked by using a thick paste that contains 1% barium sulfate.

Uniform bowel opacification is essential to successful CT scan interpretation. Most patients have complete opacification of the small bowel 45 to 60 minutes after ingestion of contrast material. Some authors advocate the routine administration of 10 mg of oral metoclopramide (Reglan) with the first 50 ml of contrast material 60 minutes before the CT study to improve opacification of the ileum and colon. Bedridden patients typi-

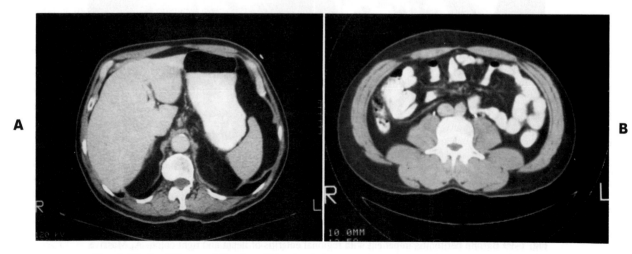

Fig. 1-20 A, CT scan following 250 ml of 2% barium sulfate solution demonstrates well-distended stomach. Note thinness of gastric wall and lack of streak artifacts produced by dilute barium solution. **B,** CT scan at more caudal level reveals small bowel and right colon to be well delineated by 2% barium sulfate. No flocculation is observed.

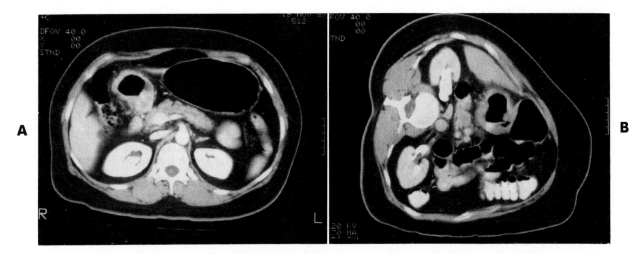

Fig. 1-21 A, Air contrast study: supine CT scan through stomach following administration of effervescent granules, glucagon, and barium. Stomach body is well distended and normal. Antrum wall appears thickened. **B,** Left lateral decubitus position permits better evaluation of antrum and pylorus region. Biopsy revealed edema secondary to benign peptic ulceration.

cally require a longer period of preparation than do ambulatory patients. For bedridden patients, the administration of contrast media several hours before the CT examination with additional oral contrast agents both 45 minutes and immediately before scanning will help ensure adequate bowel opacification.

Air and water are useful contrast agents to distend the stomach and visualize the gastric wall. If gas is to be used as a gastric contrast agent, it is important to allow the patient nothing by mouth (NPO) for 3 to 5 hours before the scan. The supine position is optimal for examining the body of the stomach, the antrum, and the pylorus. The right-side-down decubitus position is ideal for examining the esophageal gastric region, and the left decubitus position provides visual access to the antrum, pylorus, and duodenum (Fig. 1-21).

Water provides similar contrast differentiation between the walls of the stomach and duodenum and intraluminal lipomas. Distention of the stomach with water, followed by a bolus of intravenous contrast material, permits small mural irregularities to be detected that may not be identified by positive contrast methods.

Colorectal contrast techniques

The colon and rectum may be opacified using dilute iodinated solutions (1% to 2%). A 500 ml enema is sufficient to opacify the rectosigmoid colon. Larger amounts may be needed to opacify the entire colon. Colon opacification may also be achieved by having the patient drink oral contrast solution the evening before the CT examination and instructing him not to defecate before the CT study.

Air contrast studies have recently been advocated as the method of choice to evaluate the colon in certain situations. Patients should be given an oral cathartic 12 hours before the CT examination. If a patient cannot be prepared in advance, administration of a 2000 ml tap-water enema can also produce adequate colonic cleansing before air insufflation (Fig. 1-22).

Intravenous contrast techniques

The use of intravenous iodinated contrast material has greatly expanded the diagnostic capabilities of CT body scanning (Fig. 1-23). Most often, 120 to 180 ml of 50% contrast material is administered at a rate of 1.0

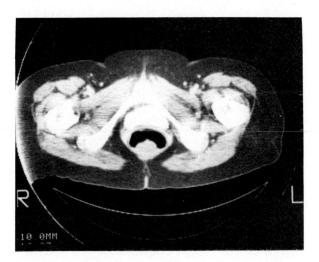

Fig. 1-22 Cloacogenic carcinoma of anus is superbly outlined following insufflation of 300 cc of air.

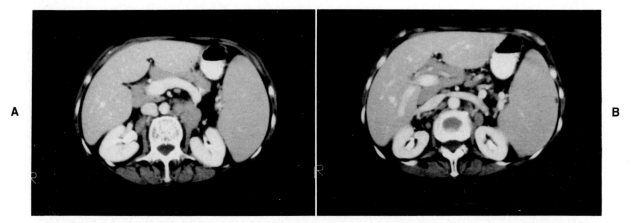

Fig. 1-23 A, Intravenous contrast administered as bolus by mechanical injector produces superb enhancement of splenic vein and its junction with superior mesenteric vein. **B,** Scan 1 cm inferior to that shown in **A.** Left renal vein, inferior vena cava, aorta, and intrahepatic vessels are well delineated. Patient has chronic lymphocytic leukemia, splenomegaly, and retroperitoneal nodal enlargement.

to 1.5 ml per second over 3 minutes. Nonionic contrast agents provide an alternative to conventional iodinated contrast material and also are safer and less painful. Dynamic CT scanning at a particular level permits plotting of the time-density changes that occur within a particular lesion. This has proved useful in demonstrating small vascular tumors in the liver, pancreas, and kidneys.

Detection of highly vascular lesions, arterial venous malformations or fistulas, varices, congenital vascular malformations, intramuscular extensions of tumor, and venous thrombosis is possible by increasing the CT attenuation value of the affected organ by rapid administration of intravenous contrast material. Differentiation of the venous system from the dilated bile ducts is made easier by contrast media administration. Contrast injection can also be employed to identify the splenic vein and to determine whether a hypodense lesion changes in appearance after the injection of contrast media. This differentiation is crucial for evaluating cysts, which do not change in CT value, and solid tumors, which often increase in attenuation value after administration of intravenous contrast material. Bolus injection of contrast media helps to differentiate the inferior vena cava and aorta from retroperitoneal masses, lymph nodes, or tumors. Tumor thrombosis within the inferior vena cava may also be demonstrated by use of contrast injection, and aneurysms of the aorta and other abdominal vessels are clearly delineated.

Contrast agents for vascular and biliary disease
PETER DAWSON

All contrast agents for vascular and biliary disease are iodinated benzene compounds. Relatively small dif-

ferences in chemical structure dictate their distribution and final route of excretion, either by the kidney (nephrotropic or urographic agents) or the liver (hepatotropic or cholangiographic agents).

Nephrotropic agents

The *chemical structures* of all nephrotropic agents are similar. Until recently, all were sodium and/or methyglucamine salts of completely substituted triiodinated benzoic acids (Fig. 1-24). At the iodine concentrations widely used for many clinical purposes (300 to 400 mg/ml), the osmolality of these solutions can be as much as 7 to 8 times that of plasma. However, two new types of compounds, "low-osmolality" agents, have now been introduced. These include non-ionic, monomeric agents (available commercial representatives are iohexol [Omnipaque], iopamidol [Isove], and iopromide [Ultravist]) and monoacid dimeric agents (sodium meglumine ioxaglate [Hexabrix] is the only commercial representative currently available).

Excretion of nephrotropic agents is by passive glomerular filtration with no significant active tubular secretion or reabsorption. Liver uptake and excretion are minimal, unless there is severe impairment of renal function. In this case significant amounts of contrast agent may appear in the bile, occasionally producing a detectable cholecystogram or cholangiogram.

The *toxicity* of nephrotropic agents is mediated by a combination of the hyperosmolality of the solutions and their intrinsic chemotoxicity. The 'low-osmolality' agents are less toxic; in particular the non-ionic types have very low (but not zero) toxicity because they combine low osmolality with low chemotoxicity. Objective adverse effects include damage to vascular endothe-

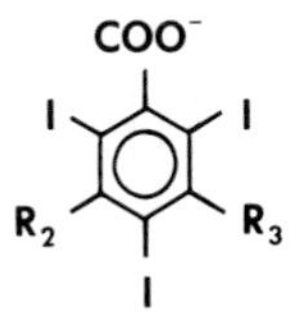

$$COO^-$$

R₂ and R₃ substituent structure on iodinated benzene ring.

R₂	R₃	Proper name	Commercial name
H	NHCOCH₃	Acetrizoate	Urokon, Diaginol
CH₃CONH	NHCOCH₃	Diatrizoate	Urografin, Hypaque
CH₃CONH	CONHCH₃	Iothalamate	Conray
CH₃CONH	NCOCH₃ CH₃	Metrizoate	Isopaque, Triosil

Fig. 1-24 Chemical structures of ionic intravascular contrast agents.

lium, which may predispose to thrombosis; injury to red blood cells; effects on mast cells and basophils with histamine release; interference with the coagulation cascade and platelet function; expansion of plasma volume; activation of complement; and inhibition of enzyme systems.

Major adverse reactions affect only a small minority of patients, with perhaps 1 in 10,000 suffering a life-threatening reaction. Such events are termed *idiosyncratic,* or sometimes *anaphylactoid,* because of their resemblance in many cases to true anaphylactic reactions. Risk factors predisposing to such reactions include ethnic predisposition (Mediterraneans and Asians); previous major adverse reaction to contrast material; allergy to other agent or material; atopy; asthma; cardiac, renal, hepatic, and sickle-cell disease; myeloma or Waldenstrom's macroglobulinemia; pheochromocytoma; age (infants and the elderly); and procedures requiring high doses of contrast agents.

Organ-specific toxicities—neurotoxicity, cardiotoxicity, and nephrotoxicity—are all possibilities with nephrotropic contrast agents. Risk factors for nephrotoxicity include old age, preexisting renal disease, diabetes, high total-dose administration, and prior dehydration, which should always be avoided. Other individuals at risk, and who might benefit from the use of a non-ionic agent, include patients with sickle cell disease who are precipitated into crisis by hyperosmolar media, patients with myeloma and Waldenstrom's macroglobulinemia, and patients with pheochromocytoma who may be precipitated into hypertensive crisis.

Hepatotropic agents

These are based on incompletely substituted iodinated benzenes (Fig. 1-25). Significant intestinal absorption of oral cholecystographic agents requires a degree of water solubility and a high pH, as found in the small intestine. The presence of bile salts enhances absorption by forming micelles around the contrast molecule.

Renal excretion and extravascular distribution are limited by the variable but substantial binding of absorbed contrast agent to albumin, up to 79% in the case of iopanoic acid. Some of the agent however, is temporarily stored in fat, muscle, and other organs.

Hepatic uptake is also affected by albumin binding, although its precise role is unclear. Uptake is a rate-limiting active transport process. In the liver these contrast agents are conjugated to a glucuronide by the action of the microsomal enzyme glucuronyl transferase. Glucuronyl transferase catalyzes the transfer of glucuronic acid from the nucleotide uridine diphosphate glucuronic acid. The conjugated compound is more water soluble and of greater molecular weight, and cannot significantly diffuse back into the liver from the bile canaliculi.

Excretion of oral contrast agents in bile is also an active carrier-mediated transport process. A linear relationship exists between the rate of contrast excretion and the rate of bile salt flow. Contrast agents may also be excreted *heterotopically.* In the case of iopanoic acid, about 65% appears in the feces within 5 days of administration and about 35% in the urine (in the conjugated form leaked back from hepatocytes to blood). Urinary excretion is by passive glomerular filtration. Renal excretion increases as the liver process becomes saturated or when liver function is impaired.

Gallbladder concentration of the conjugated compound is accomplished by water reabsorption. In patients with gallbladder disease the compound may fail to concentrate effectively.

Toxicity of hepatotropic agents is not a major draw-

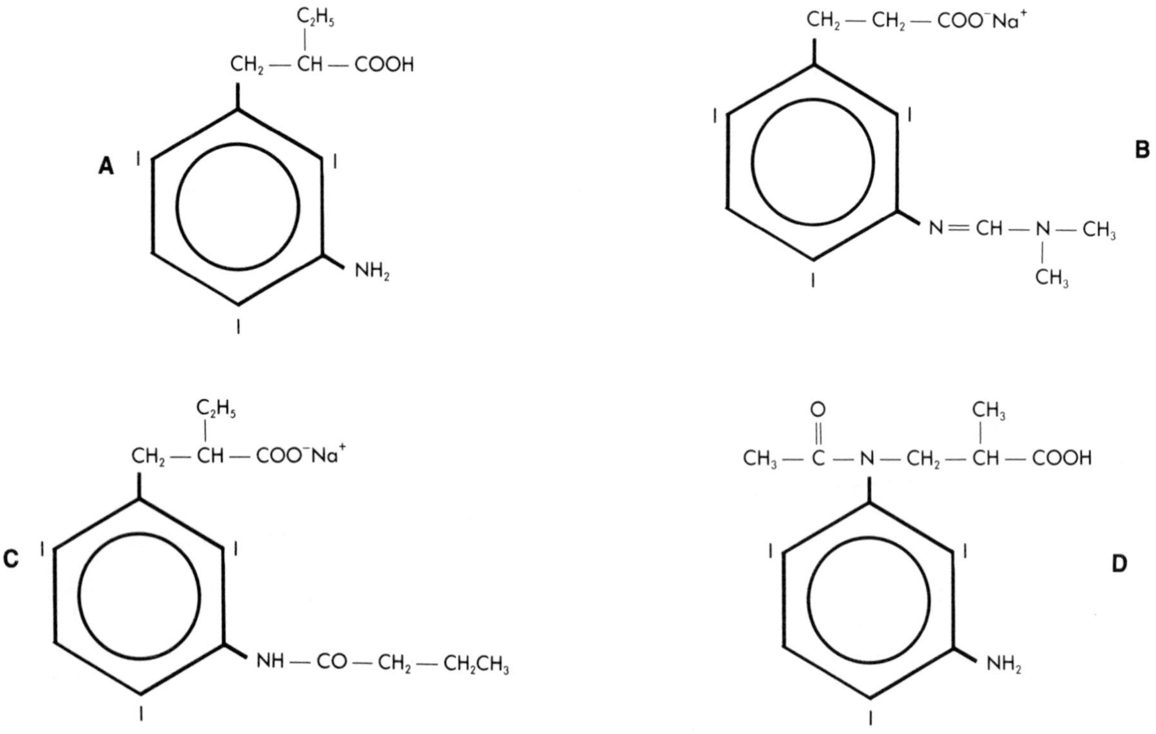

Fig. 1-25 Chemical structures of some oral cholecystographic agents. **A,** Iopanoic acid (Telepaque). **B,** Sodium ipodate (Oragrafin). **C,** Sodium tyropanoate (Bilopaque). **D,** Iocetamic acid (Cholebrin).

back, but mild and transitory side effects occur in as many as 40% of cases; these side effects are usually related to the gastrointestinal tract. Symptoms include nausea, vomiting, abdominal cramps, and diarrhea. Common dermatologic side effects include rash, urticaria, and pruritus. Petechiae caused by thrombocytopenia have also been reported. Mild dysuria, sore throat, heartburn, faintness, and headache are also common.

Major anaphylactoid reactions are rare, but acute coronary insufficiency has been reported. Care should therefore be taken in patients with a history of adverse contrast reaction, even if the episode occurred in entirely different circumstances and with a different type of iodinated agent.

Intravenous cholangiographic agents

These are dimeric compounds (Fig. 1-26), which are highly protein bound and possess pharmacokinetic properties similar to those of the oral agents with active passport uptake by the liver but with virtually no metabolism. The intravenous cholangiographic agents are potent inhibitors of enzymes. Common systemic side effects include flushing, fainting, nausea, vomiting, restlessness, salivation, and headache. Major anaphylactoid reactions occur more frequently with intravenous cholangiographic agents than with nephrotropic agents, and death occurs in approximately 1 of 5000 adminis-

trations. Acute renal failure may also occur, in some cases associated with an obstructive nephropathy. This results from the uricosuric effect of the agents, and is especially likely in hyperuricemic patients. Hepatotoxicity is recognized. Precipitation of contrast agents, both intravascular and urinary, has been reported in patients with myeloma and Waldenstrom's macroglobulinemia.

Contrast media for magnetic resonance imaging
ROBERT C BRASCH

Gastrointestinal contrast agents for magnetic resonance imaging are still being developed. Positive contrast agents for MR imaging include paramagnetic substances such as ferric ammonium citrate or Gd-DTPA, which mix with bowel contents, and oils, which must displace bowel contents (Fig. 1-27). As an alternative, negative contrast agents being evaluated include inert substances such as clay and barium sulfate, gases, perfluorocarbons, and superparamagnetic iron oxide suspensions. The design of gastrointestinal contrast agents requires considerations of the suspending medium, dilutional effects, and potential hyperconcentration.

Contrast enhancement of the liver has been approached with multiple strategies. Solutions of paramagnetic particles or suspensions of superparamagnetic particles are extracted from the blood by hepatocytes,

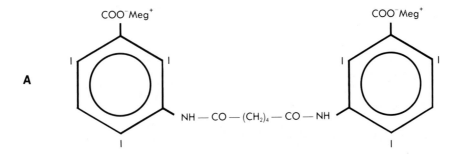

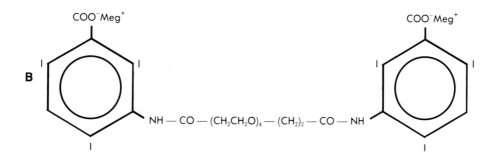

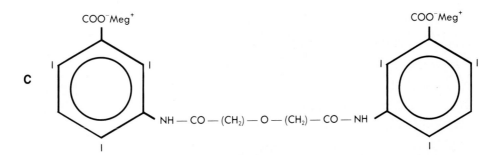

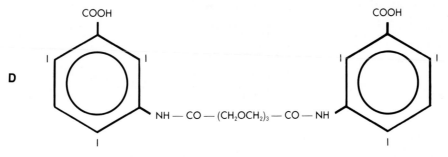

Fig. 1-26 Chemical structures of some intravenous cholangiographic agents. **A,** Iodipamide (Cholografin). **B,** Iodoxamate (Cholevue). **C,** Ioglycamide (Biligram). **D,** Iotroxate (Biliscopin).

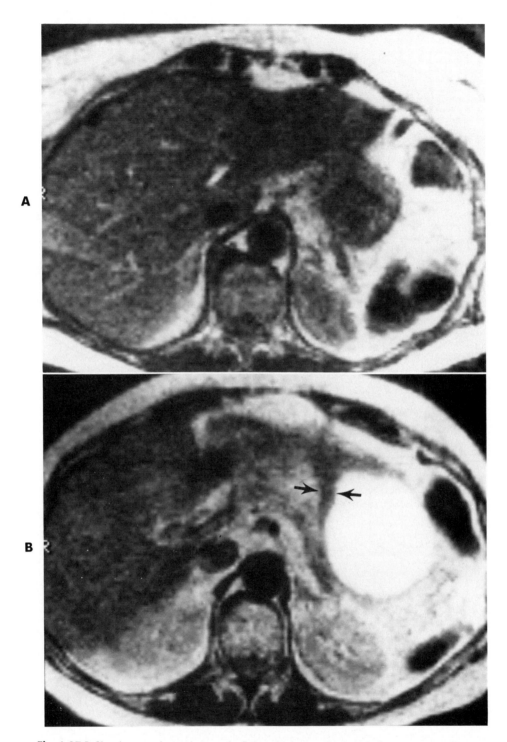

Fig. 1-27 Infiltrating gastric carcinoma. **A,** Spin echo image obtained before contrast medium administration fails to clearly define gastric contour and only vaguely suggests possibility of mural thickening. **B,** Comparison image obtained after oral administration of 1 mmol ferric ammonium citrate shows better distention of stomach with localized mural thickening in antrum, correlating well with surgically demonstrated tumor.

by the reticuloendothelial cells of the liver, or by targeting specific receptors on hepatocytes by combining superparamagnetic particles with receptor-specific polysaccharides. All strategies ultimately produce their effect by changing the signal intensity of the functioning liver. Depending on the choice of contrast agent, the intensity of functioning tissue can be made either higher (with paramagnetic agents) (Fig. 1-28) or lower (with superparamagnetic agents) on spin echo images (Fig. 1-29).

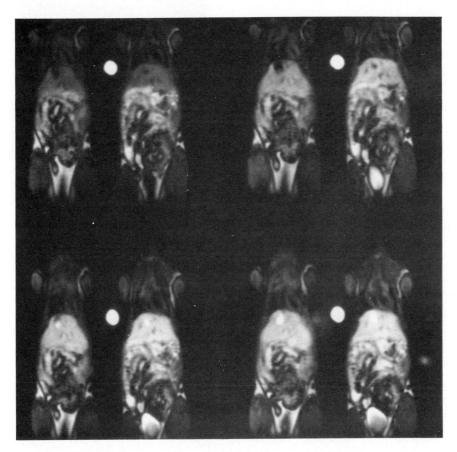

Fig. 1-28 Hepatic and biliary enhancement using Fe-EHPG. Sequential coronal spin echo images in two mice were obtained before contrast administration *(upper left)* and at 5 minutes *(upper right)*, 15 minutes *(lower left)*, and 50 minutes *(lower right)* after intravenous injection of 0.05 mmol/kg Fe-EHPG. Significant liver enhancement persists from 5 to 50 minutes, but enhancement of gallbladder is greatest at 50 minutes. Fe-EHPG is relatively lipophilic, paramagnetic metal complex extracted from serum by functioning hepatocytes and then secreted into biliary system.
(Courtesy David White, PhD, Michael Moseley, PhD, and Barry Englestad, MD.)

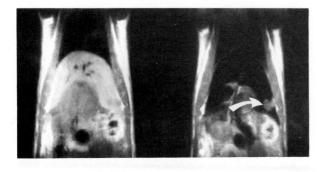

Fig. 1-29 Magnetite hepatic enhancement for demonstration of focal metastases. Precontrast *(left)* and postcontrast *(right)* spin echo images (TR = 360, TE = 17) were obtained in coronal plane using intravenous magnetite suspension, 5 mg Fe/kg. Intrahepatic metastases had been induced previously in rat by percutaneous injection of adenocarcinoma cells. Supraparamagnetic activity of magnetite produces marked shortening of T_2 relaxation times within normally functioning liver, leading to loss of signal intensity. Metastasis *(arrow)* is more clearly identifiable after contrast administration because of induced contrast difference between tumor and normal liver parenchyma.
(Courtesy David White, PhD, Michael Moseley, PhD, and Barry Englestad, MD.)

RECOMMENDED READING

1. Angell G: Use of water as an oral agent for CT study of the stomach, *Am J Roentgenol* 149:1084, 1987.
2. Aronberg DJ: Techniques. In Lee JK et al, editors: *Computed body tomography with MRI correlation,* ed 2, New York, 1989, Raven Press.
3. Balthazar EJ: CT of the gastrointestinal tract: principles and interpretation, *Am J Roentgenol* 156:23, 1991.
4. Dawson P: Contrast agent nephrotoxicity: an appraisal, *Br J Radiol* 58:121, 1985.
5. Dawson P: Iodinated intravascular contrast agents: a review, *J Intervent Radiol* 2:51, 1987.
6. Hahn PF et al: Ferrite particles for bowel contrast in MR imaging: design issues and feasibility studies, *Radiology* 164:37-41, 1987.
7. Hatfield KD et al: Barium sulfate for abdominal computer assisted tomography, *J Comput Assist Tomogr* 4:570, 1980.
8. Katayama H et al: Adverse reactions to ionic and nonionic contrast media, *Radiology* 175:621, 1990.
9. Laniado M et al: MR imaging of the gastrointestinal tract: value of Gd-DTPA, *Am J Roentgenol* 150:817-821, 1988.
10. Lonnemark M et al: Effect of superparamagnetic particles as oral contrast medium at magnetic resonance imaging, *Acta Radiol* 30:193-196, 1989.
11. McClennan BL: Ionic and nonionic iodinated contrast media: evolution and strategies for use, *Am J Roentgenol* 155:225, 1990.
12. Megibow AJ et al: Air contrast techniques in gastrointestinal computed tomography, *Am J Roentgenol* 145:418, 1987.
13. Moss AA: Contrast media in computed tomographic scanning of the abdomen. In Margulis AR, Burhenne HJ, editors: *Alimentary tract radiology,* ed 4, vol 1, St Louis, 1989, Mosby–Year Book.
14. Saini S: Advance in contrast-enhanced MR imaging, *Am J Roentgenol* 156:5-254, 1985.
15. Saini S et al: Ferrite particles: a superparamagnetic MR contrast agent for the reticuloendothelial system, *Radiology* 162:211, 1987.
16. Skucas J, editor: *Radiographic contrast agents,* ed 2, Rockville, MD, 1988, Aspen Publishers.
17. Thoeni RF, Filson RG: Abdominal and pelvic CT: use of oral metoclopramide to enhance bowel opacification, *Radiology* 169:391, 1988.

NUCLEAR MEDICINE
Nuclear medicine of the alimentary tube
ROBERT S HATTNER

Nuclear medicine methods are commonly applied in imaging the gastrointestinal tract, and imaging procedures offer utility in a variety of clinical situations.

Stomach and gastric mucosa

Techniques for evaluating *gastrointestinal propulsion* have been described and used in a variety of applications. In the detection of *gastroesophageal reflux,* gastroesophageal scintiscanning has been found to be the single most accurate predictor of the acid reflux test, with abnormalities detectable in more than 90% of patients. Patients are given an oral preparation of technetium-99m (^{99m}Tc) sulfur colloid, and the gastroesophageal region is imaged sequentially with the gamma camera following increasing abdominal pressure to 100

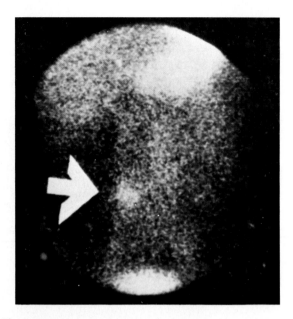

Fig. 1-30 Anterior abdominal scintigraph obtained 30 minutes after administration of TcO_4^- from 5-year-old patient with recurrent lower gastrointestinal hemorrhage. Note gastric uptake superiorly on left, bladder activity inferiorly at midline, and focal abnormality in right lower quadrant. At surgery this proved to be Meckel's diverticulum.

(From Matin P: *Handbook of nuclear medicine,* New York, 1977, Medical Examination Publishing.)

mm Hg using a wide blood pressure cuff. Reflux is easily appreciated in the images.

Gastric emptying can be studied with liquid and solid meals labeled with ^{99m}Tc and In. After a radioactive meal is consumed, the patient's gastric contents are monitored with the scintillation camera, with data acquired by computer. Region-of-interest analysis provides time-activity histograms that yield quantitative parameters of gastric contraction and motility.

Because TcO_4^- accumulates in normal gastric parietal cells, it can be used to locate *anomalous gastric mucosa* and to facilitate the diagnosis of *Meckel's diverticulum,* an uncommon but important cause of gastrointestinal hemorrhage. After administration of TcO_4^-, the scintillation camera is positioned for the best evaluation of the abdomen, from diaphragm to bladder anteriorly. Images are obtained in approximate 10-minute frames for an hour, and follow-up images at 5 to 7 hours and 24 hours may also be acquired. A focal area of activity, usually in the right lower quadrant, is suggestive of Meckel's diverticulum (Fig. 1-30). The same approach has been used to document the presence of gastric mucosa in *Barrett's esophagus* and *enterogenous pulmonary cysts.*

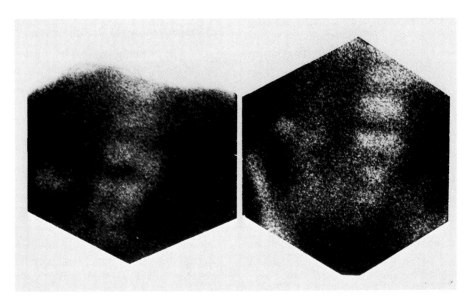

Fig. 1-31 Three days following diversion procedure necessitated by pancreatic carcinoma, 63-year-old man had 3-unit gastrointestinal hemorrhage and negative gastric aspirate. *Left,* Five minutes after administration of 10 mCi ^{99m}Tc-sulfur colloid, image of midabdomen reveals focus of extravasated colloid in right side of midabdomen, adjacent to normal vertebral bone marrow visualization. *Right,* Ten-minute image of lower abdomen shows extravasated colloid has migrated transversely to left. At surgery choledochal anastomosis revealed bleeding artery.

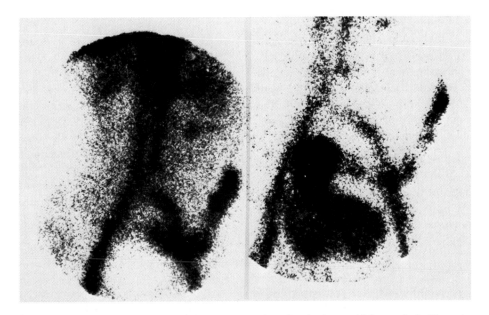

Fig. 1-32 Study of 62-year-old man with five episodes of melena over 24 hours. *Left,* Five minutes after administration of 20 mCi in vitro labeled autologous red blood cells demonstrate blood pools of kidneys and abdominal vasculature, and image of midabdomen reveals blood extravasated into lower descending colon and adjacent sigmoid colon. *Right,* Ten-minute image of lower abdomen demonstrates phenomenon just described, as well as labeled melanotic stool passed during examination. At surgery bleeding diverticulum was found at descending-sigmoid colonic junction.

Bowel infarction

Assessment of gut infarction is achieved by imaging autologous In granulocytes. Granulocytes avidly localize in the mucosa of infarcted bowel, and extent of infarction is readily seen.

Gastrointestinal hemorrhage

If bleeding is intermittent or the rate is less than 0.5 ml/min at the time of evaluation, it may not be possible to localize GI bleeding sites precisely with endoscopy or angiography. Scintigraphic techniques using blood pool tags have demonstrated a remarkable ability to localize occult gastrointestinal bleeding sites, both active and intermittent, at bleeding rates as low as 0.1 ml/min. One such technique involves injecting a bolus of ^{99m}Tc-sulfur colloid and imaging the extravasated colloid. At peak blood concentration, the extravasated colloid can be imaged at a bleeding site with a very low background (Fig. 1-31). The principal drawback of this technique, like that of contrast angiography, is that the patient must be actively bleeding during the relatively short transit time of the material in the blood. In addition, areas of bleeding that might be masked by the subsequently labeled liver and spleen may go unobserved.

^{99m}Tc-labeled red blood cells, which are cleared more slowly, have been used in an attempt to circumvent the problem of the patient who is not actively bleeding. Intact red blood cells continuously circulate, resulting in integration of activity in the region of a bleeding site (Fig. 1-32). With ^{99m}Tc-labeled intact red blood cells, serial images of up to 24 hours can be obtained. Disadvantages of labeled intact red blood cells include loss of the low background achievable with cleared agents and difficulties in the labeling itself. The labeling can be in vitro or in vivo using stannous pyrophosphate, resulting in minimal free pertechnetate localization.

RECOMMENDED READING

1. Berquist TH et al: Specificity of Tc-99m-pertechnetate in scintigraphic diagnosis of Meckel's diverticulum: review of 100 cases, *J Nucl Med* 17:465, 1976.
2. Heading RC et al: Gastric emptying rate measurement in man: double isotope scanning technique for simultaneous study of liquid and solid components of a meal, *Gastroenterology* 71:45, 1976.
3. MacGregor IL, Martin P, Meyer JH: Gastric emptying of solid food in normal man and after sub-total gastrectomy and truncal vagotomy with pyloroplasty, *Gastroenterology* 72:206, 1977.
4. Smith RK, Arterburn G: Detection and localization of gastrointestinal bleeding using Tc-99m-pyrophosphate in vivo labeled red blood cells, *Clin Nucl Med* 5:55, 1980.
5. Som P et al: Detection of gastrointestinal blood loss with ^{99m}Tc-labeled heat-treated red blood cells, *Radiology* 138:207, 1981.
6. Winzelberg GG et al: Evaluation of gastrointestinal bleeding by red blood cells labeled in vivo with technetium-99m, *J Nucl Med* 20:1080, 1979.

ULTRASONOGRAPHY
GAW GOODING

Ultrasonography of the alimentary tube

Despite technical difficulties, ultrasonography is useful in the evaluation of a number of lesions of the bowel.

Bowel gas

Bowel gas severely degrades the ultrasonic image. Given that it is impossible to pass the ultrasonic beam through bowel gas, and that simethicone improves the situation only partially, the remaining alternative is to circumvent bowel gas. Ultrasonographers employ a variety of scanning techniques to avoid the bowel when scanning the abdomen. Distention of the urinary bladder and stomach with fluid provides "windows" to deeper structures. Prone and decubitus scanning (to view the kidneys, spleen, and pancreatic tail) and subcostal scanning of the liver with the patient's breath held in maximal inspiration avoid the bowel and provide organ tissues as windows for viewing various portions of the abdomen. With the patient in the supine position interference from bowel gas may be minimized by specifically angulating the transducer so as to direct the gas shadow away from the area of interest (for example, the pancreas).

Normal bowel

The normal sonographic appearance of bowel depends on its physiologic state at the time of the examination. In addition to the difficulties presented by bowel gas, feces or fluid-filled bowel loops may be mistaken for masses. Normal bowel loops that are filled with fluid and gas occasionally demonstrate an "air-fluid" level. Small bowel loops that are entirely filled with fluid result in a sonogram demonstrating multiple, round, sonolucent, layered structures in close contiguity. Real-time ultrasonography can be extremely valuable in differentiating normal bowel from masses, since observation of the loop may demonstrate peristaltic movement identifying the suspected mass as a portion of bowel. A fluid-filled stomach may also simulate a mass. Having the patient drink freshly run tapwater that contains microbubbles, which act as a contrast agent, can help solve this problem. If all efforts to differentiate between bowel and a mass fail, a repeat examination after a short interval (usually 24 to 48 hours is sufficient) frequently resolves the dilemma. Computed tomography may also be used to solve the problem in difficult cases.

Ascites

Ascitic fluid is largely confined to the flanks and pelvis, and is usually more abundant on the right side of the abdomen. The distinction between ascites and large peritoneal cystic masses is based on the appearance of the bowel. In ascites, which behaves passively, the fluid *surrounds* the bowel and causes it to float centrally (Fig. 1-33). Masses, however, *displace* the bowel. Ascites also insinuates between the right lateral abdominal

wall and the liver and, to a lesser extent, between the left abdominal wall and the spleen.

Abscess

Ultrasonography is of established value in the detection of abdominopelvic abscesses and, when ap-

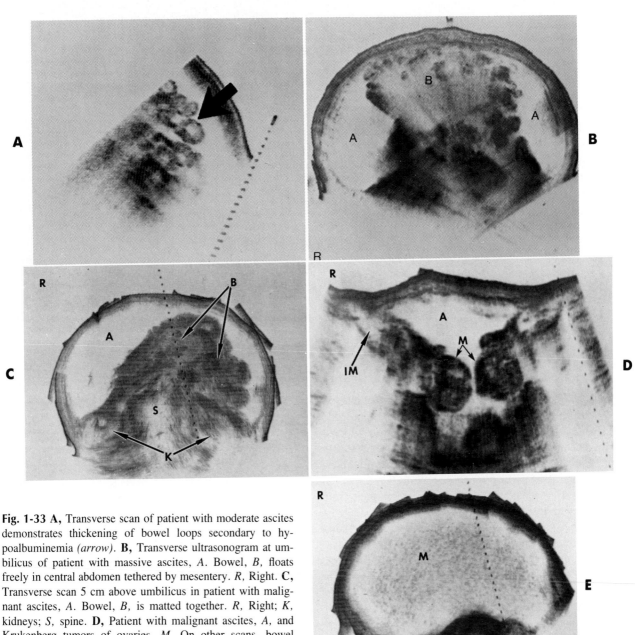

Fig. 1-33 A, Transverse scan of patient with moderate ascites demonstrates thickening of bowel loops secondary to hypoalbuminemia *(arrow).* **B,** Transverse ultrasonogram at umbilicus of patient with massive ascites, *A.* Bowel, *B,* floats freely in central abdomen tethered by mesentery. *R,* Right. **C,** Transverse scan 5 cm above umbilicus in patient with malignant ascites, *A.* Bowel, *B,* is matted together. *R,* Right; *K,* kidneys; *S,* spine. **D,** Patient with malignant ascites, *A,* and Krukenberg tumors of ovaries, *M.* On other scans, bowel floated freely. *R,* Right; *IM,* iliacus muscle. **E,** Transverse scan 2 cm below umbilicus in patient with clinical diagnosis of ascites. Large mass, *M,* was noted that was fluid filled by ultrasonic criteria except for scattered echogenicity (lesion contained large quantities of cholesterol crystals). Note that large fluid-filled masses exclude bowel. *R,* Right; *P,* psoas muscles; *S,* spine.

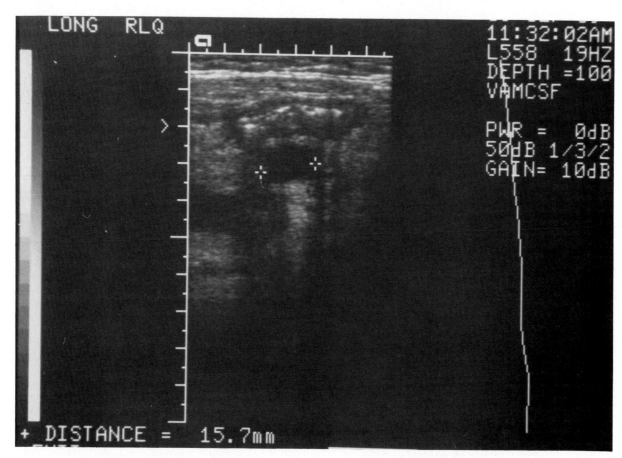

Fig. 1-34 Longitudinal sonogram of right lower quadrant shows an abscess defined by dots as an echo-free mass behind loop of thickened bowel.

proached aggressively, can yield high diagnostic accuracy. Multiple scanning positions should be employed as necessary to avoid interfering gas-filled bowel loops. The echographic appearance of an abscess is classically described as a sonolucent mass with thick irregular margins (Fig. 1-34) and possibly a few scattered internal echoes. The appearance of an abscess may range from that of a simple cyst to that of an extremely echogenic mass. Some abscesses are recognized by the detection of gas in an anatomic position in which no normal gas-containing structure occurs. Retained surgical sponges, usually associated with abdominal abscesses, appear as masses with thin, irregular boundaries and high-amplitude internal echoes.

Omental and mesenteric abnormalities

Mesenteric and omental metastases can be detected when relatively large matted omentum, thickened by tumor, causes a lenticular soft tissue thickening beneath the anterior abdominal wall that posteriorly displaces the bowel echoes (Fig. 1-35). Lymphomatous involvement of the mesentery causes lobulated, relatively so-

Fig. 1-35 A and **B,** Transverse scans of child demonstrate dilation of stomach, *S,* and duodenum, *D.* **C** and **D,** Longitudinal scans of same patient demonstrate greatly dilated duodenum, *D,* and lymphadenopathy, *LN,* elevating superior mesenteric artery, *SMA.* Adenopathy was believed to be etiology of duodenal obstruction as well as ureteric obstruction causing hydronephrosis, *RH,* demonstrated in **C.** *R,* Right; *H,* head; *L,* liver; *PV,* portal vein; *Sp,* spleen; *A,* aorta; *GB,* gallbladder.

Fig. 1-36 Transverse scan 4 cm above umbilicus demonstrates intussusception, *M.* Note echogenic center and sonolucent periphery.

(From Weissberg DL et al: *Radiology* 124:791, 1977.)

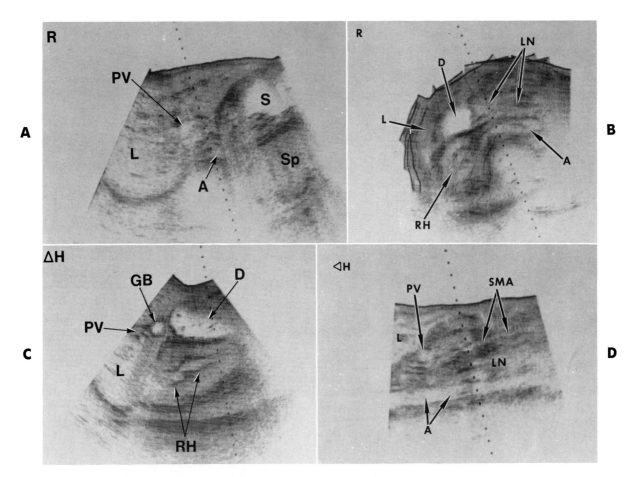

Fig. 1-35 For legend see opposite page.

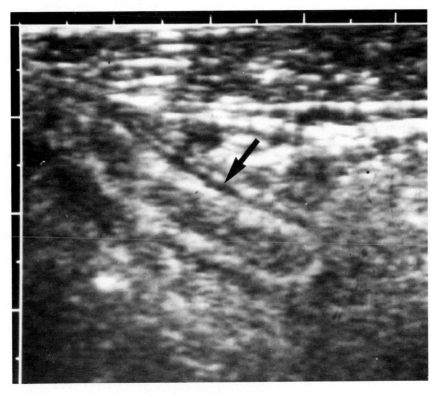

Fig. 1-36 For legend see opposite page.

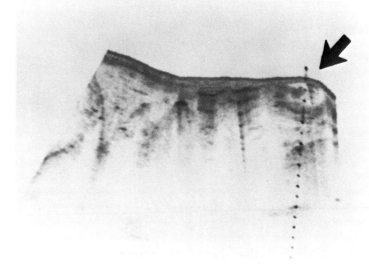

Fig. 1-37 Parasagittal sonogram denotes small ventral hernia in anterior abdominal wall *(arrow)*.

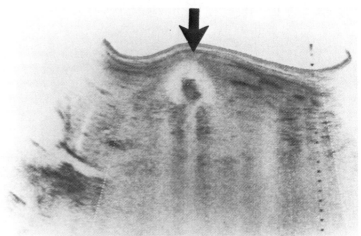

Fig. 1-38 Parasagittal sonogram shows carcinoma of transverse colon *(arrow)* producing thick-walled colon with central echogenic area–mucosal interfaces.

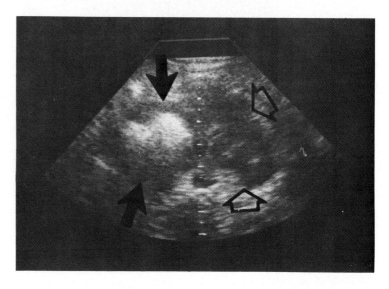

Fig. 1-39 Transverse sonogram shows thick-walled descending colon on right *(arrows)* with large hypoechoic mass extending from it on left *(open arrows)*, all changes secondary to lymphoma.

nolucent, confluent masses that encase and elevate the mesenteric artery and vein.

Bowel obstruction

Ultrasonography is clearly not the diagnostic modality of choice in the evaluation of gut tube obstruction. On occasion, however, obstructed bowel loops may be first detected on an ultrasonogram. In obstruction of the pylorus, duodenum, or proximal jejunum, sonolucent "masses" may be appreciated in the characteristic anatomic location of the stomach and duodenum and a correct diagnosis can be made. Most reports have identified *intussusceptions* as large abdominal masses with sonolucent peripheries and echogenic centers. *Small bowel infarction* usually produces a sonolucent thick-walled bowel with an echogenic center.

Appendicitis

Ultrasound diagnosis of appendicitis requires graded compression to displace or compress overlying bowel and fat to reveal the enlarged, inflamed appendix (Fig. 1-36).

Duplication cyst

On ultrasound scans *intestinal duplication cysts* appear as fluid-containing masses of the gastrointestinal tract. A variety of lesions can mimic the appearance of a duplication cyst, and unless the mass can be localized (Fig. 1-37), the diagnosis remains nonspecific. As in all cysts, hemorrhage or debris within the lesion may produce internal echoes. *Colonic duplication cysts* may be associated with genitourinary tract abnormalities.

Gut tube neoplasms

A multitude of lesions, both malignant and benign, may be seen as masses with sonolucent peripheries and echodense centers. Although nonspecific, this appearance suggests pathologic thickening of the bowel wall (Figs. 1-38, 1-39). Aspiration biopsy under ultrasonic guidance may assist in diagnosis.

The changes of *idiopathic hypertrophic pyloric stenosis* are indicated ultrasonographically by the characteristic elongated and thickened pylorus, and ultrasound is a useful tool for studying infants suspected of having this disorder (Fig. 1-40).

A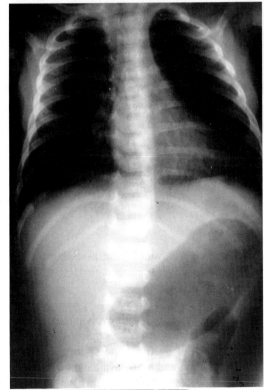

B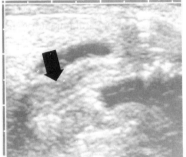

Fig. 1-40 A, Plain film of abdomen demonstrating greatly distended stomach in baby with pyloric stenosis. **B,** Sonogram of same infant demonstrates elongated, thickened pylorus *(arrow)* distal to fluid-filled stomach.

☐ **TABLE 2-1**
Neuropeptides and gut hormones

Neuropeptides	Hormones
Bombesin	Gastrin
Cholecystokinin	Cholecystokinin
Dynorphin	Secretin
Enkephalin	Motilin
Neurotensin	Neurotensin
Neuropeptide Y	Pancreatic polypeptide
Somatostatin	Somatostatin
Substance P	Gastric inhibitory
Vasoactive intestinal	polypeptide
polypeptide	Enteroglucagon
	Peptide YY

gastrin—from tumors, hyperplasia, or retained antrum—produces hypersecretion of acid and hyperplasia of acid-secreting mucosa. Clinical consequences include peptic ulcer disease and diarrhea.

Insulin

Insulin release is stimulated by enteric hormones that are released following ingestion of a meal. Rising blood glucose levels cause further release of insulin and inhibition of glucagon secretion. Insulin lowers blood glucose by trapping it in the liver, for conversion to glycogen, and in the muscle and adipose tissue, where more is stored than is burned. Functioning islet cell tumors are usually insulinomas, which produce clinical effects via hypoglycemia.

Glucagon

Glucagon is best known for its antagonistic action to insulin, that is, raising the blood sugar. It also produces an increase in bile flow from the liver, relaxes the gallbladder and Oddi's sphincter, produces a decrease in gastric and pancreatic secretion, and causes a release of catecholamines from the adrenal medulla. Catecholamine release inhibits the activity of intestinal smooth muscles and produces paralysis, the basis for using glucagon to facilitate cannulation of the bile duct for endoscopy and MR imaging of the abdomen, as well as colon examination in some instances. Catecholamine or insulin release might trigger a crisis in patients with pheochromocytoma or insulinoma, and the use of glucagon is therefore contraindicated in these patients.

Glucagon also relaxes the ileocecal valve, increasing the incidence of coloileal barium reflux from 45% to 75%, relieves painful colonic spasm, and improves the quality of barium enema examinations. True pancreatic glucagonomas cause diabetes (by inhibiting insulin secretion), dermatitis, weight loss, venous thrombosis, and diarrhea (associated with decreased colonic contractility).

Vasoactive intestinal polypeptide

Vasoactive intestinal polypeptide (VIP) is not found in endocrine cells but is present in a wide range of neurons in the gut and elsewhere. Most VIP-producing tumors are either benign (43%) or malignant (37%) islet cell tumors, or islet cell hyperplasia (20%). However, 10% are associated with extrapancreatic ganglioneuromas, adrenal tumors, or bronchogenic carcinomas.

VIP-producing tumors are associated with a syndrome of massive watery diarrhea, with loss of potassium and bicarbonate, and serum hypercalcemia (Verner-Morrison syndrome). VIP may not be the sole peptide involved in this syndrome, since gallbladder dilatation is a frequent unexplained finding and human pancreatic polypeptide (HPP) is the only peptide known to relax the gallbladder and to increase tone in Oddi's sphincter. VIPomas are very rare. The principal functional radiologic feature is the extremely wet intestine and masses of fluid throughout the GI tract, caused by the excess secretion and gut relaxation. The dilated

☐ **TABLE 2-2**
Gut hormone function

Peptide	Main distribution	Actions
Gastrin	Antrum	Acid secretion
Cholecystokinin	Small intestine	Gallbladder contraction; pancreatic hormone secretion
Secretin	Small intestine	Pancreatic bicarbonate secretion
Gastric inhibitory peptide	Small intestine	Insulin secretion
Motilin	Small intestine	Gut motility (including the migrating myoelectric complex)
Neurotensin	Small intestine	Small intestine secretion
Enteroglucagon	Large and small intestines	Trophic to gut mucosa
Pancreatic polypeptide	Pancreas	Pancreatic secretion and gallbladder contraction inhibition

gallbladder serves as a useful clinical clue to the diagnosis.

Somatostatin

Somatostatin is the ultimate inhibitory hormone, exciting nothing and inhibiting virtually all exocrine and endocrine functions. It inhibits release of gastrin, insulin, glucagon, secretin, and cholecystokinin (CCK) in the gut, and of growth hormone from the brain. The somatostatinoma is the rarest of the pancreatic endocrine tumors and is associated clinically with diabetes mellitus, steatorrhea, weight loss, and cholelithiasis.

Although the somatostatinoma is so rare, somatostatin is gaining considerable clinical therapeutic interest. This is because, although the half-life of somatostatin itself is so short (1 to 3 minutes), that it must be continuously infused to have any useful action, a new ocatapeptide called Octreotide has a half-life of 90 minutes and can be given subcutaneously two or three times a day. It is approved for use in treating metastatic carcinoid syndrome and VIPomas, and is very promising for treatment of acromegaly, for reducing diarrhea (for example, in patients with small bowel fistulas in whom the agent may lead to healing of the fistula), and for patients with diabetic retinopathy, since the retinopathy may be related to increased growth hormone activity.

LOCATION OF ENDOCRINE CELLS IN THE GUT

Endocrine cells are scattered throughout the gut, from the cardia to the rectum. In the pylorus, gastrin-containing G cells make up half the endocrine cell population; 30% are serotonin EC cells, and 20% are somatostatin D cells. In the antrum, the acid turn-on (gastrin) and turn-off (somatostatin) cells are both well represented. The upper small intestine has a rich supply of secretin, CCK, gastrointestinal polypeptide (GIP), and motilin cells, as well as serotonin EC cells, somatostatin D cells, and enteroglucagon L cells. There is no cell specific to the large intestine, and most of the endocrine cells of the colon are serotonin EC and enteroglucagon L cells. Four endocrine cell types are found in the pancreas: insulin B cells, glucagon A cells, somatostatin D cells, and pancreatic polypeptide (PP) cells. The only APUD cell found exclusively in the pancreas is the insulin B cell.

PROSTAGLANDINS AND THE GUT

The prostaglandins are compounds that modify inflammation, and their synthesis is blocked by many of the most widely used antiinflammatory agents such as aspirin. Given orally or intravenously, prostaglandins inhibit both basal- and pentagastrin-stimulated gastric acid output by acting intracellularly at an early stage in synthesis. They also cause an increase in gastric mucosal blood flow and may be responsible for the increased blood flow that accompanies acid secretion. The prostaglandins are synthesized in gastric mucosa in response to acid stimulation. They protect the gastric mucosa against damage from aspirin or indomethacin (an effect called *cytoprotection*) and promote ulcer healing.

OROPHARYNX AND SWALLOWING

The digestive functions of the mouth and pharynx are (1) mastication of food, (2) mixing it with the enzymes and lubricants of saliva, and (3) transporting it in manageable boluses past the entrance to the airway and safely into the esophagus. Although 90% of the volume of saliva comes from the major salivary glands, mucus is also secreted by numerous minor polystomatic salivary glands found in the labial, palatine, buccal, lingual, and sublingual mucosal lining.

Swallowing occurs in two distinct phases. In the first the bolus mixed with saliva is transported from the buccal cavity toward the oropharynx by elevation of the tongue and tight closure of the mandible. In the second phase, following a brief inspiratory effort, respiration is suspended and the bolus is moved rapidly backward by the posterior part of the tongue and is immediately ejected from the oropharynx into the esophagus. The second phase is complex and involves forward and upward displacement of the larynx with closure of the nasal, oral, and laryngeal openings to the pharynx. In addition, there is simultaneous relaxation of the upper esophageal sphincter and an extremely rapid peristaltic contraction of the pharyngeal cone of muscles.

Relaxation of the upper sphincter is both passive, as forward movement of the larynx changes the laterally oriented slit into a circular space, and active, as electric activity ceases and the muscle actively relaxes. The actual opening of the closed sphincter, however, is passive as the bolus is pushed through by descending peristalsis. Once the peristaltic wave has passed, the larynx falls back and the cricopharyngeus muscle regains its tone. The entire second phase of swallowing is involuntary once initiated and is centrally controlled by the swallowing center in the reticular formation. Most dysfunction is due to ischemic brainstem disease, local inflammation, or tumor.

ESOPHAGUS, TRANSIT, AND ACID NEUTRALIZATION

Although there is often considerable overlap at the junction between the striated and smooth muscle of the esophagus, the control of peristalsis in each is quite different. In the striated muscle portion the vagal fibers fire in sequence so that motor units are activated from above downward. In the smooth muscle portion, however, a single inhibitory impulse in nonadrenergic noncholinergic fibers is responsible for the entire esophageal peristaltic wave and the relaxation of the lower sphincter.

Although the lower esophageal sphincter is tonically contracted, it undergoes periodic collapses of pressure to zero in all normal individuals. When the individual is supine, or has a full stomach, it is normal for gastroesophageal reflux to occur. This happens several times each night and occasionally during the day. Normally, the refluxed material is cleared into the stomach with the next swallow. Clearance may not occur if peristalsis is defective or if the individual goes rapidly back into deep sleep, when swallowing does not occur. Although peristalsis clears the esophagus of almost the entire volume of fluid, some hydrogen ions become fixed in the "unstirred" layer of esophageal mucus, keeping the pH low. This acidified mucus layer has to be neutralized by the bicarbonate in saliva, and several dry swallows are required before enough saliva has been swallowed to restore the neutral esophageal pH. The process of neutralizing acidified mucus following normal physiologic reflux is probably one of the most important functions of the salivary glands.

PHYSIOLOGY OF THE STOMACH
Gastric secretion

The stomach secretes five types of substances: *hydrochloric acid, pepsin, mucus, intrinsic factor,* and a variety of hormones, principally *gastrin.* Parietal cells secrete acid and intrinsic factor. Chief cells produce pepsinogens that are converted to pepsin by acid, and gastrin is secreted by the G cells of the gastric antrum. Both superficial and neck mucous cells produce mucus. Prostaglandins are secreted by parietal cells and possibly by others as well.

Acid secretion

The three primary stimulants of acid secretion are acetylcholine, gastrin, and histamine. *Acetylcholine,* a vagal neurotransmitter, is responsible for most of the cephalic phase of acid secretion. *Gastrin,* a hormone, is released from antral and duodenal G cells in response to gastric distention. It stimulates acid secretion by the parietal cells. *Histamine,* a paracrine agent, is released from mastlike cells of the lamina propria into the intramucosal extracellular fluid. It then diffuses to the adjacent parietal cell, stimulating acid secretion. Inhibitors, as well as stimulators, participate in the regulation of acid secretion. Acid bathing of the gastric antrum, for example, is a powerful inhibitor to gastrin production.

The parietal cell has three receptors, specific for histamine, gastrin, and acetylcholine, with potentiating interactions. The somatostatin cell has receptors for gastrin (excitatory) and acetylcholine (inhibitory), as well as an excitatory receptor for adrenergic nerve fibers. Thus in the cephalic phase of gastric stimulation, acetylcholine turns on acid production and inhibits somatostatin. Once gastrin and histamine start to respond to a meal, gastrin turns on the regulatory function of somatostatin. The histamine mast cell has several receptors, including one for prostaglandin E2 and an inhibitory receptor for somatostatin.

Three techniques are commonly used to measure gastric secretion of acid: basal, maximal (pentagastrin), and cephalic-stimulated secretion (sham feeding).

Pepsin secretion

Only 1% of pepsinogens, a fundic serum pepsinogen called type 1, is absorbed into the bloodstream; 99% of pepsinogen stays in the stomach, and after conversion to pepsin by acid, initiates protein digestion. The peptides it releases in turn initiate the release of various hormones, including gastrin and CCK.

Mucus secretion

Mucus is a partial barrier to acid and pepsin penetration. Bicarbonate is secreted by the surface mucosal cells into an unstirred mucus layer, where it is trapped and forms a thin but high-concentration barrier. Prostaglandins E and F, administered either systemically or topically, increase the effective thickness of human gastric mucosa gel by stimulating bicarbonate secretion and by causing release of mucin by the mucosa.

Gastric motility
After feeding

After a meal the fundus and upper body of the stomach dilate by two distinct processes. When the throat or esophagus is mechanically distended, the fundal pressure is reduced and the fundus relaxes, an effect that is called *receptive relaxation* and which is abolished by vagotomy. In addition, when material is introduced into the fundus, the intragastric pressure rises only slightly, and relaxation occurs, an effect called *gastric accommodation.* According to one theory, lower esophageal sphincter relaxation is permitted only if gas is present, and gastroesophageal reflux disease is a disorder of belching control.

The introduction of fat into the duodenum produces high-pressure static contractions of the pylorus, which effectively close it and prevent any further pyloric emptying. Although a CCK response occurs at the same time, and the pyloric mucosa is particularly well endowed with CCK receptors, it is not known whether CCK is responsible for the pyloric closure.

During fasting

During fasting, gastric motility is controlled by the migrating myoelectric complex (MMC), which occurs every 90 to 120 minutes. In the longest part of the cycle, phase I, these pacemaker potentials sweep down the stomach but do not produce muscular contractions. Phase I is thus a phase of quiescence. During phase II, contractions begin to appear, and they reach a crescendo in phase III. For 5 to 10 minutes in phase III almost every potential is accompanied by a forceful contraction that sweeps down the stomach, through the antrum, and down the small intestine. In the fasting state there is usually no fat in the gastric contents, and, unlike the situation in the fed state, the pylorus does not close as the peristaltic contraction approaches the antrum. Thus larger fragments of undigested food remaining in the stomach may be passed into the duodenum during phase III. Phase IV is a period of diminishing contractility.

PHYSIOLOGY OF THE DUODENUM AND SMALL INTESTINE
Digestion and absorption

Carbohydrate digestion starts with salivary amylase in the mouth, continues on the inside of food masses in the stomach, and is completed to the level of disaccharides by pancreatic amylase in the duodenum and jejunum. Splitting of disaccharides to monosaccharides for absorption is carried out by brush border enzymes such as lactase, sucrase, and maltases. These brush border enzymes may be temporarily absent after any illness that damages jejunal mucosa, such as gastroenteritis or celiac disease, or as a result of a congenital deficiency. Persistence of the hyperosmolar disaccharides causes diarrhea, a finding that formed the basis of an excellent, highly specific radiologic test for lactase deficiency. Although a plain barium follow-through examination may be normal in a patient with lactase deficiency, mixing 25 g of lactose with the barium produces dilution, dilatation with fluid levels, and rapid transit.

Protein digestion starts with pepsins in the stomach. It is completed in the duodenum, where food causes the release of secretin (which stimulates bicarbonate production by the pancreatic centroacinar cells) and CCK (which makes the acinar cells release enzyme precursor granules). Since the enzyme precursors are inactive at low pH levels, the bicarbonate is necessary to raise the pH level and halt pepsin activity. Enterokinase from the duodenal mucosa converts trypsinogen to trypsin, and the trypsin itself converts the other protease precursors, such as chymotrypsinogen, to their active forms. For the most part protein is hydrolyzed into single amino acids for absorption. Some dipeptides and tripeptides are also absorbed, however, and enhance the amino acid absorption.

Congenital abnormalities of transport of specific amino acids across cell membranes are responsible for several rare disorders. However, pancreatic disease, loss of intestinal mucosa as in celiac disease, and loss of absorptive surface in patients with fistulas or resections are more common causes of nondietary protein deficiency.

Fat, in the form of triglycerides and phospholipids, is emulsified in the stomach by mechanical action. In the duodenum several pancreatic lipases and colipase are secreted in active form, and together they hydrolyze the triglycerides and phospholipids into free fatty acids and monoglycerides. These combine with bile acids to form *micelles,* which render the lipolytic products water soluble. The formation of micelles is crucial in dispersing fatty acids in the aqueous phase of intestinal contents. This increases diffusion across the unstirred layer of mucus to the intestinal mucosal cell by a factor of 100 to 200. After passive diffusion across the cell membrane into the intestinal enterocyte, the fatty acids and monoglycerides have to be resynthesized into triglycerides to be excreted into the lymphatic system. Ninety-five percent of bile acids (but not bilirubin) are reabsorbed from the lower small bowel. This enterohepatic circulation of bile acids facilitates solubilization and transport of fat from the intestinal lumen to the hepatocyte.

Bile acid deficiency and consequent fat malabsorption may result from impaired hepatic synthesis, as in cirrhosis; from loss of functioning ileum, most frequently in Crohn's disease; or from stasis with bacterial overgrowth as the bacteria modify the bile acids, rendering them insoluble. Adults with extensive loss of small bowel usually absorb 75% of ingested fat, however, indicating that some fat absorption still occurs in the absence of bile acids.

Malabsorption

In addition to foods, numerous other essential substances (iron, calcium, magnesium, folate, vitamin B_{12}, and other fat- and water-soluble vitamins) are absorbed from the small intestine. Many are affected by malabsorption states, particularly the fat-soluble vitamins D and K, deficiencies of which cause osteomalacia and impaired coagulation. Hyperoxaluria, which occurs in many small bowel disorders, especially celiac disease, represents a disorder that occurs as a result of substances being absorbed that should not have been.

Motility

The small intestine *transports* about 9 L of fluid and electrolytes a day. Only about 1.5 L of this fluid is from the diet; the rest is derived from the saliva, stomach, pancreas, liver, and the small intestine itself. The small intestine usually *absorbs* 7.5 L a day, but can absorb up to 15 to 20 L of isotonic saline. Two different patterns of motor activity move all this fluid, together with food and the debris from exfoliated cells and mucus, through the small intestine.

Fasting state

In the fasting state most propulsion occurs in phase III of the MMC, when regular peristaltic waves sweep slowly down the entire length of the small intestine. The MMC has been called the intestinal housekeeper, because it sweeps the intestine clear of debris every hour and a half during fasting.

Fed state

In the fed state MMCs are replaced by a more or less continual low level of contractile activity. Antegrade and retrograde movements occur, but antegrade movements predominate. One study on intestinal clearance after feeding demonstrated that 60% of a meal cleared the intestine in the hour and a half before the return of MMCs. After the first MMC, clearance jumped to more than 90%.

Immunology

In the GI tract, lymphocytes are scattered throughout the lamina propria and between the epithelial cells covering the intestinal villi. Twenty-five percent of gut mucosa is composed of lymphoid cells. *B cells* are activated by an antigen and differentiate into plasma cells, which secrete antibodies to bind specifically to the antigen, initiating a variety of elimination responses. *T cells* operate a cellular defense that is especially effective against fungi, parasites, intracellular viruses, and cancer. In addition to these two systems, macrophages and mast cells are important in defense.

Peyer's patches, organized aggregates of lymphoid tissue, are covered with thin M cells that lack villi and rapidly transport antigens (whether intact macromolecules or viral particles) to the interstitial space. In the interstitial space they are processed by the circulating uncommitted B lymphocytes, which then pass through the mesenteric nodes to the thoracic duct, eventually reappearing in the lamina propria of the gut, "homing" to the area where the antigen was first encountered. A few lymphocytes also become dispersed in peripheral lymph nodes.

Peyer's patches are thus the source of activated B cells and plasma cells that populate the lamina propria and produce secretory *immunoglobulin A (IgA)* in response to further antigenic challenge. IgA binds with antigen, preventing its adherence to epithelial cells. If penetration of the epithelium does occur, activation of a systemic antibody response and interaction with mast cells occur. IgA is particularly important in the GI tract. Its function is protective, and it does not initiate any locally destructive processes. Immunoglobulin G (IgG), which is also produced in the bowel, sets a cascade of events in motion when it binds to antigen, and these events may damage the bowel. IgG is elevated in patients with inflammatory bowel disease. *Mast cells,* which are concerned with immediate hypersensitivity, are unique cells involved in antigen recognition. They bind immunoglobulin E (IgE) and release numerous active agents, such as histamine and 5-hydroxytryptamine.

The *lymphoid follicles* are crucial in the defense mechanisms of the GI tract. They are larger in children than in adults, which occasionally causes confusion. The early lesions of Crohn's disease always start on top of lymphoid follicles. In some hypoimmune states, such as common variable hypogammaglobulinemias, the intestinal lymphoid follicles tend to be enlarged. In these patients, infections such as that caused by *Giardia lamblia,* are common.

Intestinal permeability

The intestinal epithelium and its overlying mucus provide a barrier to absorption, particularly to macromolecules. Small amounts do cross the barrier, by intracellular or intercellular routes and through the very thin cell layer at the lymphoid follicle and Peyer's patches. This limited absorption of macromolecules probably represents a sampling mechanism by which the immune system monitors the environment.

PHYSIOLOGY OF THE BILIARY SYSTEM AND LIVER

In addition to synthesis of proteins, bile lipids, and urea and the secretion of proteins and bile, the liver is involved in control of carbohydrate, fat, and protein metabolism. Although the normal liver consists of about 20% to 30% blood by weight, the vascular compartment can contract to expel up to 40% of its blood or can expand so that the liver is 50% blood by weight. The liver is also capable of regeneration, and recovers both size and function within a few months after resection of up to 90% of its mass.

Hepatocytes are the functional unit of the liver, and those nearest the center of the acinus are metabolically the most active (and most oxygenated). Glycogen storage and fat formation occur more peripherally near the central veins. Hepatocytes lie in long chains. Where they abut one another a *bile canaliculus* is trapped and runs at right angles to the chain. *Sinusoids,* which arise from portal venules and empty into hepatic venules, are found adjacent to the two opposite walls of hepatocytes. Terminal hepatic arterioles also enter the sinusoids, so that sinusoidal blood is a mixture of portal and hepatic arterioles, providing both intestinal nutrient and oxygen to the hepatocytes.

An extracellular gap, *Disse's space,* lies between the sinusoids and the chains of hepatocytes beside them. Metabolites in the sinusoids pass freely into Disse's space, which is bathed in nutrients and plasma, highly oxygenated, and in direct contact with hepatocyte microvilli. Disse's space also communicates with the liver lymphatic system. When pressure on the portal veins is high and albumin is low, the lymphatic system is readily overloaded and ascites forms.

The flow of metabolic activity thus starts with the mixing of oxygen and nutrients in the sinusoids. Substances then pass from the sinusoids through Disse's space to the hepatocyte. After modification in the hepatocyte, metabolites leave the cell either by crossing the walls between hepatocytes and into the bile canaliculus, or by crossing the walls through which they entered the cell and back into Disse's space. From there they may either be drained by the lymphatic system or pass back into the sinusoids to travel out of the liver in the hepatic veins.

Synthesis

Numerous crucial proteins are synthesized in the liver, including several concerned with coagulation: fibrinogen; prothrombin; and factors V, VII, IX, and X. All except fibrinogen depend on the fat-soluble vitamin K for synthesis.

Secretion

Albumin plays a major role in the prevention of ascites and maintenance of colloid osmotic pressure. Secretin stimulates secretion of a bicarbonate-rich solution into the larger ducts, and consumption of a meal (which causes secretin release) does the same. CCK produces both gallbladder contraction and a rapid increase in flow of bile into the duodenum. Because CCK relaxes Oddi's sphincter as bile flow increases, the normal physiologic response is for the diameter of the extrahepatic duct to decrease. A 2 mm increase in diameter 45 minutes after stimulation provides good evidence of obstruction.

Since 90% of bile acids are absorbed from the terminal ileum, very little in the ducts is freshly synthesized. Bilirubin, which is produced from heme by the reticuloendothelial cells, is not significantly reabsorbed.

Bile flow

Approximately 600 ml of bile is secreted each day, a little faster during the day than at night, at a pressure of 15 to 25 cm of water, ceasing when the pressure in the common bile duct reaches 35 cm of water. The gallbladder volume varies from individual to individual, but is usually about 60 ml and is rarely more than 100 ml. Morphine and, interestingly, secretin cause sphincter contraction. Secretin thus antagonizes CCK, which causes gallbladder contraction and sphincter relaxation, but it is overwhelmed by the strength of the physiologic response to CCK.

Manometric examination of Oddi's sphincter shows that there is a segment of increased tone (about 5 to 19 mm Hg higher than ductal or duodenal pressures) about 4 to 6 mm long. Superimposed on this are phasic contraction waves three to seven times per minute. Normally the contractions sweep along the sphincter in a downward or antegrade direction; up to 14% may be retrograde. The proportion of retrograde contractions is increased in patients with stones in the bile duct.

The biliary tract is thus a low-pressure, low-flow system in which gallbladder contraction and the hepatic secreting pressure of bile provide the forward pressure and the Oddi's sphincter provides the regulating back pressure. Radiologic aspects of the physiology of the biliary system have recently been summarized by W.J. Dodds. During the fasting state, the phase III MMC is associated with gallbladder contraction. Thus during a meal the gallbladder empties, and once the stomach has emptied (which may take several hours) the gallbladder gradually refills over several more hours in a stepwise manner with intermittent 40% emptying with each MMC until the normal full-fasting volume is reached. This continual filling and partial emptying during fasting probably expels microcalculi into the bile duct and duodenum.

Sphincter of Oddi dysfunction is uncommon but not rare. Disorders include fibrotic stenosis, excessive tone or spasm of the sphincter (relieved by glucagon), tachyoddia or rapid phasic contractions (opiate administration may mimic this condition), paradoxic response to CCK with contraction instead of relaxation, and increased percentage of retrograde contractions (usually in the presence of bile duct stones).

PHYSIOLOGY OF THE PANCREAS

The pancreas is 84% exocrine cells, 10% extracellular matrix, 4% ductules and blood vessels, and 2% endocrine cells.

Endocrine pancreas

There are three types of endocrine cells in the pancreas: an outermost layer of *A cells* that produce glucagon; an intermediate layer of *D cells* that produce somatostatin, gastrin, and pancreatic polypeptide; and an inner layer of *B cells* that produce insulin.

3 *Acute Abdomen*

MICHAEL P FEDERLE
JAMES J McCORT
ROBERT E MINDLEZUN

NONTRAUMATIC ACUTE ABDOMEN
Intraperitoneal air
Intramural air (pneumatosis intestinalis)
Acute inflammatory diseases of the abdomen
Intestinal tract obstruction
Intestinal atony and dilatation

ABDOMINAL TRAUMA
Intrapertioneal bleed
Splenic injuries
Liver injuries
Intestinal injury
Pancreatic trauma

Nontraumatic acute abdomen

Many abdominal diseases have a similar clinical presentation, making the "acute abdomen" one of the most difficult diagnostic problems facing the physician. Differentiation among these entities requires familiarity with their natural histories and with today's imaging modalities. The immediate availability of these sensitive diagnostic probes has markedly reduced the need for exploratory laparotomy.

INTRAPERITONEAL AIR

The decubitus and upright radiographs are most important for demonstrating free air. Cone-down tangential views (at low kilovoltage to enhance the air–soft tissue interface) are recommended for detecting tiny free air collections (Fig. 3-1). In the acutely ill patient, when a decubitus or upright view cannot be obtained, a cross-table lateral radiograph with the patient supine may show air trapped beneath the anterior abdominal wall.

Since the most frequently obtained abdominal radiograph is the supine view, the examiner must recognize the varied signs of free air in this projection. They include (1) Rigler's or the double-wall sign, (2) the football or air-dome sign, (3) the falciform ligament (Fig. 3-2), (4) perihepatic air (free air around the liver may collect between the liver and the anterior peritoneum or it may be trapped beneath the right lobe of the liver as a tapered oblique gas collection), (5) the cupola, (6) the triangle, (7) the inverted V (the lateral umbilical ligaments), (8) Morison's pouch air, (9) the urachus sign (the obliterated tubular canal), and (10) scrotal air in male neonates.

Air enters the peritoneal cavity through the intestinal lumen, the peritoneum, or the female genital tract (see the box on p. 43). The most common cause of pneumoperitoneum is prior surgery, and the air is usually

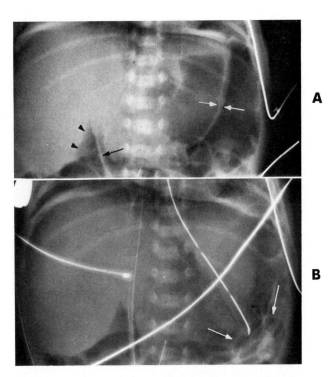

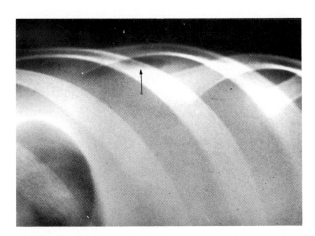

Fig. 3-1 Tiny pneumoperitoneum *(arrow)* that could be identified only on cone-down views of right upper quadrant. Left lateral decubitus projection.

(From McCort JJ, editor: *Abdominal radiology,* © 1981, The Williams & Wilkins Co, Baltimore.)

Fig. 3-2 A, Pneumoperitoneum. Air outlines falciform ligament *(black arrow)* and undersurface of liver *(arrowheads).* Gastric wall *(white arrows)* is outlined by air inside and outside the stomach. **B,** Umbilical vein catheter confirms position of the falciform ligament. Bowel loops are outlined by air *(white arrows).*

(From McCort JJ, editor: *Abdominal radiology,* © 1981, The Williams & Wilkins Co, Baltimore.)

☐ CAUSES OF PNEUMOPERITONEUM ☐

A. Through disruption of the wall of a hollow viscus.
 1. Ulceration
 2. Rupture by blunt or penetrating trauma
 3. Iatrogenic perforation, as in endoscopy, enemas
 4. Neoplasm
 5. Congenital, as in gastric muscular wall defect of infancy
 6. Pneumatosis intestinalis with extension to the peritoneum
 7. Inflammatory bowel disease, diverticulitis, Meckel's diverticulum
 8. Foreign body perforation
 9. Postoperative leakage
 10. Gastric overdistention from endoscopy of effervescent tablets
B. Through the peritoneal surface
 1. Transperitoneal manipulation, as in biopsy, endoscopy, needle placement, catheter drainage
 2. Extension from a retroperitoneal source

 3. Extension from the chest (intubation, positive pressure breathing, pneumomediastinum, bronchopleural fistula, increased intrabronchial and alveolar pressure, anesthesia, surgery)
 4. Manipulation of the bladder with rupture
 5. Penetrating injury
C. Through the genital tract in females
 1. Rubin test, orogenital insufflation, intercourse, knee-chest exercise, douching, postpartum, pelvic examination, water skiing, horseback riding, other strenuous activities (see Fig 13-10)
 2. Manipulation of the uterus or vagina with perforation
 3. Cul-de-sac diagnostic or therapeutic procedures
D. Intraperitoneal
 1. Gas-forming peritonitis or abscess rupture
E. Idiopathic

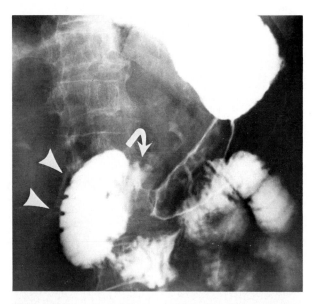

Fig. 3-3 Perforated duodenal ulcer. Water-soluble contrast upper GI study. Patient was first placed in right decubitus position to allow contrast coating of antrum and duodenum. Small perforation *(curved arrow)* allows contrast material to leak into peritoneum *(arrowheads)*.

(From McCort JJ, editor: *Abdominal radiology,* © 1981, The Williams & Wilkins Co, Baltimore.)

absorbed in 1 to 24 days. Body habitus influences the incidence of postoperative pneumoperitoneum. This condition occurs in 80% of asthenic patients, but in only 25% of obese patients. In a child or obese patient, free air that persists after the third postoperative day should be monitored carefully. In the absence of surgical drains, persistent or increasing air suggests an anastomotic leak.

The second most common cause of pneumoperitoneum is a peptic ulcer perforation that concommitantly introduces fluid into the peritoneal cavity. Perforations of the more distal small bowel, and especially of the colon, seldom show large volumes of free-flowing fluid. Local abscess usually follows appendiceal perforation. When confined by retroperitoneal anatomic structures, gas does not move with change in the patient's posture.

In 10% to 35% of patients with intestinal perforation, there is insufficient free air to be detected by plain film examination. In these patients, water-soluble contrast studies can be helpful. After oral administration of 30 to 50 ml of contrast media, the patient is placed on the right side for 10 minutes. This position allows the contrast agent to flow to the duodenum, where 80% of perforations are located (Fig. 3-3). One third of patients with perforation may show a leak in the absence of pneumoperitoneum.

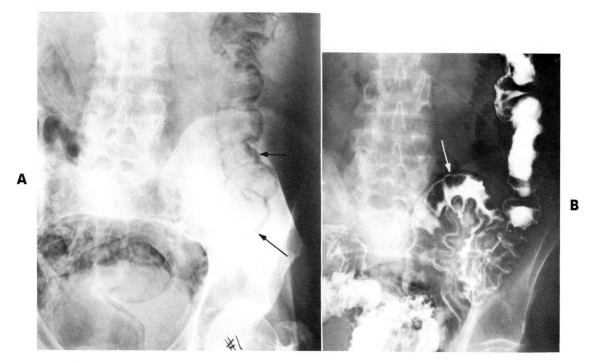

Fig. 3-4 A, Pneumatosis coli. Supine abdomen. Gas is noted in wall of sigmoid and descending colon *(arrows).* **B,** Barium enema.

(From McCort JJ, editor: *Abdominal radiology,* © 1981, The Williams & Wilkins Co, Baltimore.)

INTRAMURAL AIR (PNEUMATOSIS INTESTINALIS)

Pneumatosis intestinalis, or gas collections in the wall of the bowel, can be either primary and idiopathic (usually benign and involving the sigmoid and descending colon) or, as occurs in 85% of cases, secondary (caused by diseases that raise intraluminal pressure and disrupt mucosal integrity). Pneumatosis appears radiographically as gas collections that parallel the bowel wall, usually sparing the rectum (Fig. 3-4). Although these gas collections may narrow the lumen of the bowel, they rarely cause mechanical obstruction. Gas-containing blebs may rupture, causing pneumoperitoneum, but peritonitis is unusual. The neonatal form, which has a soap-bubble appearance, is usually caused by necrotizing enterocolitis. Other causes include intestinal ulceration, intestinal obstruction, pyloric stenosis, arterial or venous compromise, umbilical catheterization, feeding tubes, pneumomediastinum, cystic fibrosis, or imperforate anus.

Abnormal gas collections in the stomach wall (pneumatosis gastrica) are of two types. In the first, the gastric wall is normal and pneumatosis is associated with vomiting, pulmonary emphysema, gastric outlet obstruction, pyloric stenosis, or duodenal obstruction. The second type follows severe inflammation of the gastric mucosa by corrosive agents, gastritis, gastric infarction, or gastroduodenal surgery (Fig. 3-5). Because of the danger of perforation, pneumatosis should always be evaluated with water-soluble contrast agents.

ACUTE INFLAMMATORY DISEASES OF THE ABDOMEN
Appendicitis

Plain films of the abdomen reveal abnormalities in 50% of appendicitis patients. CT can be useful in distinguishing periappendiceal abscess from phlegmon. Ultrasonography by identifying a noncompressible inflamed appendix can establish the diagnosis of appendicitis and exclude other confusing entities such as ectopic pregnancy, pelvic inflammatory disease, or tubal torsion in a young woman (Fig. 3-6).

Radiographic findings in appendicitis include the following (in relative order of importance):

1. Appendiceal calculus (appendicolith, coprolith, or fecalith). These calculi often have a radiolucent center and are usually larger than a phlebolith. On properly exposed radiographs 14% of appendicitis patients demonstrate calculi; 50% of symptomatic patients with an identifiable appendicolith have already developed appendiceal perforation.
2. Appendiceal abscesses. Appendiceal abscesses often contain gas bubbles. They may displace

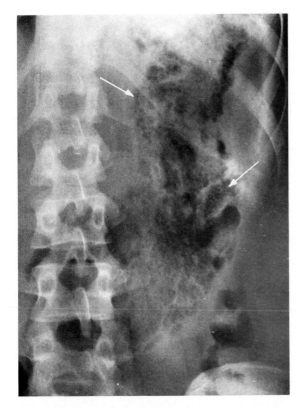

Fig. 3-5 Necrosis of stomach following Drano ingestion. Multiple small collections of gas *(arrows)* outline wall of stomach.

(From McCort JJ, editor: *Abdominal radiology,* © 1981, The Williams & Wilkins Co, Baltimore.)

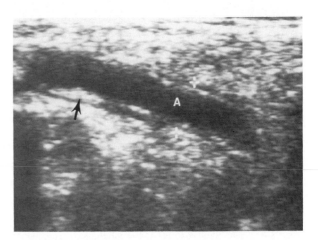

Fig. 3-6 Acute appendicitis. Sagittal plane ultrasound examination shows a distended, fluid-filled appendix, *A,* (between + markers). The echogenic submucosa is irregularly thickened. The examiner was unable to compress the appendix. Diagnosis was confirmed at surgery.

(Courtesy RB Jeffrey, M.D., Stanford University Medical School.)

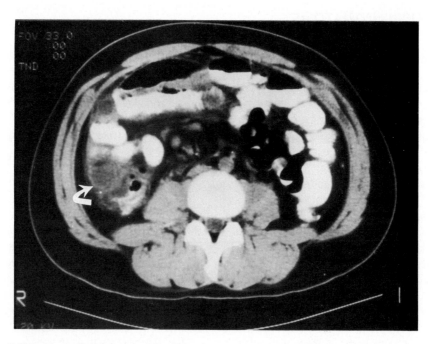

Fig. 3-7 Periappendiceal abscess. Mixed-density mass *(arrow)* containing ectopic gas compresses cecum.

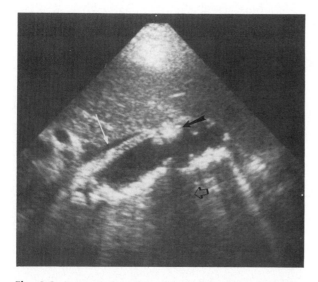

Fig. 3-8 Acute cholecystitis. Ultrasonographic examination shows a distended gallbladder. Multiple calculi *(black arrow)* adjacent to gallbladder wall cause shadowing *(open arrow)*. Gallbladder wall is thickened and shows pericholecystic fluid *(white arrow)*. Surgeon removed an acutely inflamed gallbladder.

(Courtesy RB Jeffrey, M.D., Stanford University Medical School.)

adjacent organs and cause mechanical obstruction as the abscesses enlarge (Fig. 3-7).

3. Periappendiceal soft tissue mass.
4. Separation of the cecum from right extraperitoneal fat planes. In the absence of a colonic malrotation, a right paracolic distance greater than 10 mm suggests a local mass.
5. Abnormal configuration of the cecum and ascending colon. With retroceceal appendicitis, the lateral wall is most often involved.
6. Atony of the cecum and ileum.
7. Intraperitoneal fluid.
8. Effacement of the right extraperitoneal fat line.
9. Pneumoperitoneum and pneumoretroperitoneum. These are relatively rare findings and usually follow rupture of the appendix.
10. Small and large bowel obstruction.
11. Spinal tilt to the right.
12. Gas in the appendix. Gas occurs in a normal appendix especially when it is retrocecal. If it is not retrocecal, then intraappendiceal gas, especially with a fluid level, suggests appendicitis.

Acute cholecystitis

Acute inflammation of the gallbladder may present as acute cholecystitis, hydrops or empyema of the gallbladder, emphysematous cholecystitis, or gallbladder perforation and pericholecystic abscess. In 90% to 95% of patients, acute cholecystitis is associated with gallstones. Important imaging modalities include ultra-

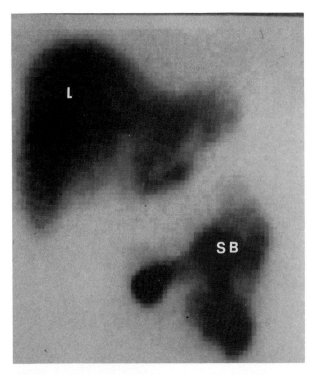

Fig. 3-9 Cystic duct obstruction with acute cholecystitis. At 120 minutes after injection of 5 ml of ^{99m}Technetium disida, isotope is taken up by liver cells *(L)*. Isotope has been excreted and fills small bowel *(SB)*. Cystic duct obstruction indicated by failure of isotope to enter gallbladder. Surgeon found a stone impacted in cystic duct and removed an acutely inflamed gallbladder.

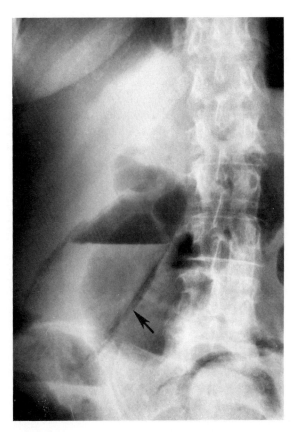

Fig. 3-10 Emphysematous cholecystitis. Gas has entered wall of gallbladder *(arrow)*. Note prominent intraluminal air-fluid level.

sonography and nuclear scanning. Ninety six percent of gallstones can be detected with ultrasound, even those as small as 1 to 2 mm in diameter (Fig. 3-8). Ultrasonography also can show hydrops, intramural edema, pericholecystic abscess, and intraperitoneal fluid when present. Nuclear scanning (^{99m}Tc cholescintigraphy) has a 97% overall accuracy rate for the detection of cystic duct obstruction and gives the earliest evidence of common duct obstruction and gallbladder perforation (Fig. 3-9).

Hydrops and empyema of the gallbladder

In an unscarred gallbladder, obstruction of the cystic or common duct results in marked dilatation (the Courvoisier gallbladder). The condition is called hydrops if the luminal contents remain sterile, and empyema if the fluid is infected.

Emphysematous cholecystitis

Emphysematous cholecystitis is manifested by gas in the gallbladder wall and/or lumen. In 80% of patients it follows obstruction of the cystic duct by stones, but in the other 20% the cystic duct remains patent. Emphysematous cholecystitis occurs more commonly in diabetic patients, and the proposed primary mechanism is gallbladder ischemia. The diagnosis requires a plain film examination, but CT is also diagnostic (Fig. 3-10). The differential diagnosis of a right upper quadrant pear-shaped air collection includes a duodenal diverticulum, an obstructed duodenal bulb, or an intrahepatic or extrahepatic abscess.

Perforation of the gallbladder

The gallbladder may perforate into the peritoneal cavity, resulting in severe peritonitis. If a large stone erodes into the stomach or duodenum, it may produce bowel obstruction at a point of luminal narrowing, such as the distal ileum. This may give rise to radiographic presentation of Rigler's triad of gallstone ileus (gas in the gallbladder or biliary tree, an ectopic calcified gallstone, and partial or complete small bowel obstruction).

Acute acalculous cholecystitis

This condition is most often seen in seriously ill patients following surgery, trauma, hyperalimentation, anesthesia, or transfusions. Gangrene and perforation of the gallbladder are common complications.

Acute pancreatitis

Acute pancreatitis may be caused by alcoholism; cholelithiasis; penetrating peptic ulcer; hereditary diathesis; blunt or penetrating injuries; anomalies of the pancreatic, biliary, and intestinal tracts; surgery; drugs; viral, bacterial, or parasitic agents; iatrogenic manipulation or biopsy; end stage renal disease; or hyperparathyroid states. In some patients no cause is ever established. Pancreatic calculi, usually intraductal, develop with recurrent or chronic inflammation. Alcoholic pancreatitis is the most common cause of pancreatic lithiasis.

Acute pancreatitis leads to pancreatic abscesses in 4% of patients. Two thirds of these abscesses are manifested by ectopic gas collections (Fig. 3-11). Inflammation spreading to adjacent bowel leads to mural edema, paresis, and even necrosis. The stomach is usually distended with fluid and air, and may be displaced anteriorly by a retrogastric fluid collection. Inflammation widens the duodenal sweep and distorts the engorged mucosal folds. The edematous Vater's ampulla projects as a soft tissue mass into the duodenal lumen. Extension along the transverse mesocolon and phrenicocolic ligament leads to local ileus and occasionally to colon obstruction distal to the splenic flexure (the colon cutoff sign).

Pseudocysts—intrapancreatic or extrapancreatic fluid collections—form in 50% of patients with acute pancreatitis. Pancreatic enzymes can dissect almost any tissue in the peritoneal cavity and retroperitoneum, and may even extend to the thorax or lower extremities (Fig. 3-12). Pleural effusions occur in 10% to 15% of patients.

CT is the most cost-effective initial study, and scans demonstrate an inflamed, swollen pancreas surrounded by pancreatic exudates and pseudocysts displacing adjacent viscera and obliterating peripancreatic fat. Calcifications are usually readily seen on plain films, but a larger number are visible on CT.

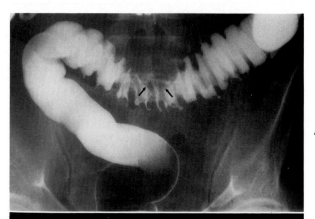

A

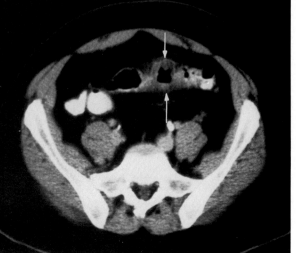

B

Fig. 3-12 Intramural peridiverticular abscess of sigmoid. **A,** Barium enema. Upper segment of sigmoid loop shows multiple diverticula, loss of distensibility, and exaggeration of haustral markings. A smooth mass representing an intramural abscess indents superior margin of involved sigmoid *(arrows)*. **B,** Computed tomogram of the same sigmoid loop reveals more extensive thickening of bowel wall with encroachment on lumen *(arrows)*. Thickening of sigmoid mesentery probably represents spread of inflammatory process. Patient was treated conservatively with recovery.

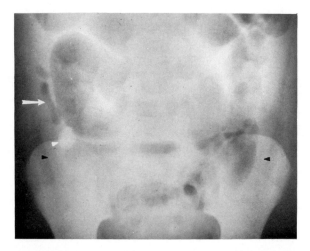

Fig. 3-11 Perforated retrocecal appendicitis. Supine abdomen. Large amounts of pus distend right and left paracolic gutters *(black arrowheads)*. Note air-filled appendix *(arrow)* and coprolith *(white arrowhead)*.

(From McCort JJ, *Emergency radiology syllabus,* Chevy Chase, Md, 1979, American College of Radiology.)

Acute diverticulitis

Acute diverticulitis follows a diverticulum perforation and development of a local abscess. Fifteen percent of patients with diverticulosis will subsequently develop diverticulitis. Three quarters of diverticular perforations spread into the retroperitoneum, leading to subacute symptoms and often delaying diagnosis. Retroperitoneal perforation causes local inflammation, which may seal the perforation, limiting the volume of escaping colonic contents (see Fig. 3-12).

Radiographs reveal a mass with or without an ectopic gas collection adjacent to the colonic wall, suggestive of diverticular perforation. Diverticulitis of the cecum mimics appendicitis. Glucagon given before barium enema reduces spasm and may help differentiate diverticulitis from carcinoma. Suspected colonic perforation should be investigated with water-soluble contrast agents. CT can clearly show the diverticular abscess and secondary involvement of adjoining organs (Fig. 3-13).

Acute ulcerative colitis

Fifteen percent of patients with ulcerative colitis have acute symptoms. The most severe manifestation is "toxic megacolon," which occurs in 2% of patients. The abdominal radiograph usually reveals a thickened mucosa with prominent soft tissue excrescences, representing islands of spared tissue surrounded by a severely ulcerated mucosa (Fig. 3-14). Focal collections of submucosal edema and hemorrhage encroach on the gas-filled intestinal lumen and resemble thumbprints. Ulcerations may contain sufficient gas to be visible on plain film. Correct diagnosis depends on history, sigmoidoscopy, cultures, and biopsy. A gas-distended colon with a transverse diameter of greater than 6.5 cm should be viewed with suspicion, and a barium enema

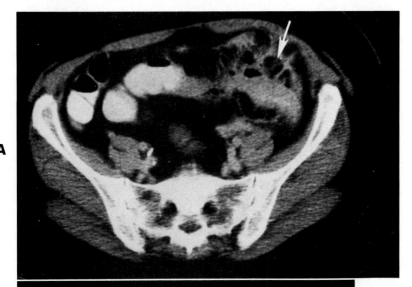

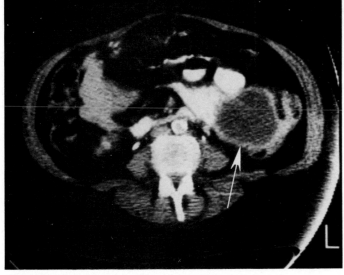

Fig. 3-13 A, Acute diverticulitis. Inflammation of anterior pararenal space *(arrow)* secondary to perforated sigmoid diverticulum. Treatment with antibiotics resulted in complete resolution. **B,** Acute diverticulitis. Localized extracolonic abscess *(arrow)* treated successfully by percutaneous drainage.

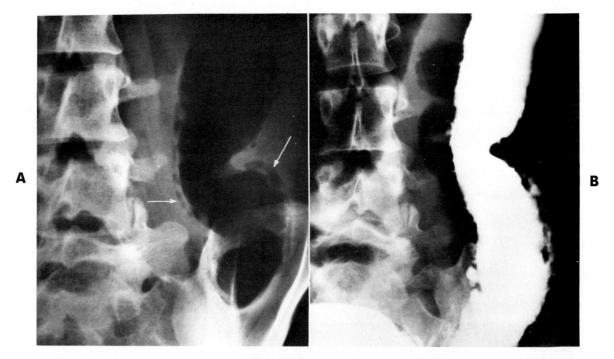

Fig. 3-14 A, Acute colitis. Supine abdomen. Multiple gas collections *(arrows)* parallel wall of descending colon. **B,** Barium enema demonstrates deep ulcerations and parallel fistulas.
(From McCort JJ, editor: *Abdominal radiology,* © 1981, The Williams & Wilkins Co, Baltimore.)

should never be performed when a toxic megacolon is suspected (see also p. 251).

Pseudomembranous enterocolitis

Pseudomembranous enterocolitis is a complication of broad-spectrum antibiotic therapy that permits an intracolic overgrowth of *Clostridium difficile*. The patient complains of watery diarrhea. A gas-distended colon with a markedly thickened bowel wall, coarsened transverse ridges, mucosal nodularity, and widened haustra characterize the abdominal films. CT demonstrates the bowel wall thickening and nodularity with luminal narrowing.

Amebic colitis

The cecum and hepatic flexure are the areas usually involved in amebic colitis. Unlike Crohn's disease, amebiasis usually spares the small intestine.

Acute intestinal ischemia

Acute intestinal ischemia begins with segmental atony, followed by bowel dilatation. The valvulae conniventes swell with edema fluid and develop a corrugated appearance. Mucosal spiculation (picket fence), stretching of the mucosa (stacked coins), and separation of the bowel loops represent successive phases. Submu-

cosal fluid collections cause eccentric intramural protrusions of soft tissue density (thumbprints in the colon and pinky prints in the small bowel). Increasing fluid accumulation effaces the valvulae, and the bowel assumes an amorphous configuration. With loss of mucosal integrity of the bowel wall, intestinal gas may enter (pneumatosis intestinalis). This form of pneumatosis usually has a lineal appearance. Extensive ischemia produces a toxic megacolon pattern and is difficult to differentiate from inflammatory disease.

On CT scans ischemia induces symmetric thickening of the bowel wall, which progresses to effacement of its contour. Infarction leads to the leak of gas into the bowel wall and into the mesenteric and portal veins (Fig. 3-15). Transmural infarction with perforation causes pneumoperitoneum or pneumoretroperitoneum. Ascites frequently accompanies intestinal ischemia.

PERITONITIS

Pneumococcal peritonitis occurs in the malnourished chronic alcoholic. Other causes of peritonitis are bowel perforation, anastomotic leak, and pelvic inflammatory disease. Small and large bowel atony with large accumulation of intraluminal fluid and air (a nonobstructive ileus) is common. Upright and decubitus radiographs show prominent air-fluid levels. The volume of ascitic

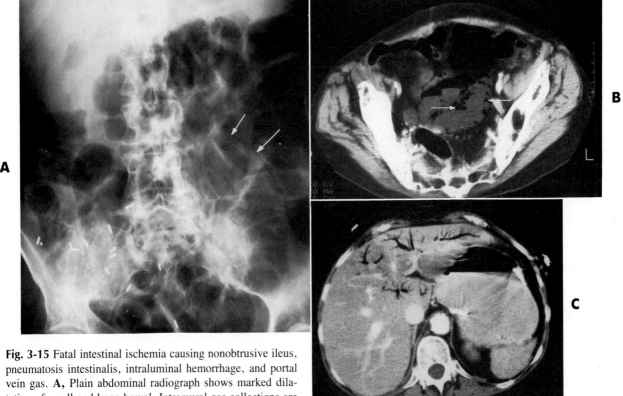

Fig. 3-15 Fatal intestinal ischemia causing nonobtrusive ileus, pneumatosis intestinalis, intraluminal hemorrhage, and portal vein gas. **A,** Plain abdominal radiograph shows marked dilatation of small and large bowel. Intramural gas collections are difficult to appreciate because of extensive ileus *(arrows)*. **B,** CT of lower abdomen shows numerous small bubbles of gas outlining bowel wall *(arrow)*. Fluid fills bowel lumen. **C,** CT of liver. Since patient is supine, gas fills anterior branches of right and left portal veins. At surgery, infarcted bowel was deemed too extensive to be resected; patient expired after surgery.

fluid is variable but may be so large that it dominates the radiographic findings.

INTRAPERITONEAL ABSCESS

The early use of CT and ultrasonography have markedly improved the diagnosis and treatment of intraperitoneal abscesses. For a small abscess, treatment with intravenous antibiotics alone may be effective. In the case of larger abscesses, percutaneous drainage under CT guidance has been successfully employed. Plain film findings, although present in as many as 71% of patients, now play a less important role. Abscesses are three times more frequently in the right subphrenic and subhepatic spaces than on the left.

The radiographic findings include (1) an extramural mass containing gas and/or fluid, (2) a fistulous tract, and (3) loss of normal soft tissue–fat interfaces. Secondary ipsilateral manifestations are (1) generalized or focal elevation of the diaphragm, (2) pleural effusion, (3) basal pneumonitis or atelectasis, (4) diminished diaphragmatic excursion, (5) focal ileus, (6) edema of adjacent bowel, (7) decreased organ mobility, and (8) curvature of the spine toward the inflamed area.

Subphrenic and subhepatic abscess

Perihepatic infections consist of fluid with or without ectopic gas, variable liver displacement, and compression of the hepatic parenchyma (Fig. 3-16). Subphrenic infections cause diaphragmatic paresis, pleural effusions, and pneumonitis.

In plain film evaluation of right subphrenic abscesses, the eleventh rib (the level of the triangular ligament) provides a useful anatomic landmark. Subphrenic abscesses tend to produce abnormal gas collections above the eleventh rib. An abscess in the right anterior subhepatic space displaces the transverse colon

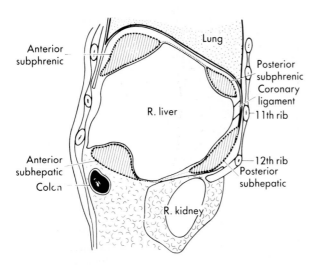

Fig. 3-16 Sagittal section through right lobe of liver. Hatched areas indicate four locations of perihepatic abscesses.
(Modified from Boyd DP. Reprinted by permission of the New England Journal of Medicine 275:911, 1966.)

inferiorly. A mass in the posterior subhepatic space (Morison's pouch) displaces the duodenum inferiorly, medially, and posteriorly.

Left subphrenic abscesses usually remain localized and are unlikely to spill past the phrenicocolic ligament. Displacement of the stomach by the abscess often provides a clue to its anatomic location. Gas in a subphrenic abscess is differentiated from a pneumoperitoneum by its irregular contour, the presence of multiple localized air bubbles, failure of the air to rise to the upper portion of the diaphragm in the erect patient, and air-fluid levels (Fig. 3-17). A liver abscess with or without gas is usually easily detected by CT and ultrasound.

Lesser sac abscess

Use of CT allows earlier diagnosis of lesser sac abscesses. A lesser sac abscess displaces the stomach anteriorly and may widen the gastrocolic space. When located medially in the smaller compartment, the abscess displaces the stomach inferiorly and to the left. A laterally located mass in the larger compartment displaces the stomach superiorly and to the right. The mass often compresses and may displace the spleen laterally and posteriorly.

Pelvic abscesses

The primary radiographic manifestation of a pelvic abscess is a focal or diffuse mass. Gas, as multiple bubbles or one large pocket, can occur within the abscess. Within the rigid pelvic walls, adjoining viscera (especially the sigmoid colon, bladder, and small bowel)

tend to be displaced. The mass effect of the abscess may partially obstruct the bowel or ureters. Evaluation of the suspected pelvic abscesses can be readily performed with ultrasonography. In difficult cases computed tomography or magnetic resonance may be used to clarify the diagnosis.

Retroperitoneal abscess

Clinical suspicion of retroperitoneal sepsis should lead to CT scanning. In pancreatic abscess, CT shows a fluid-filled mass with a high attenuation (Hounsfield) number. The abscess may possess a thickened irregular wall and contain ectopic gas, which is virtually pathognomonic. CT-guided percutaneous aspiration and analysis will identify non–air containing abscesses.

In retroperitoneal colon perforation, plain radiographs often demonstrate a retrocolic soft tissue mass and gas collection. The ipsilateral psoas muscle may be obscured by the soft tissue density, but the properitoneal fat usually remains intact. Colon study with water-soluble contrast material can establish the correct diagnosis. CT provides unique information on possible extension into the pericolic tissues, the adjacent organs, and the peritoneal cavity.

In retroperitoneal duodenal rupture, plain radiographs show an abnormality in only one third of patients. CT demonstrates the ectopic gas and fluid with greater accuracy and speeds diagnosis. A study using oral water-soluble contrast material will localize the tear, which usually occurs at the junction of the second and third duodenal segments.

Gas from rectal perforation usually dissects the soft tissue planes extending into all three retroperitoneal spaces, most commonly the posterior pararenal space.

INTESTINAL TRACT OBSTRUCTION

Mechanical obstruction denotes occlusion or constriction of the bowel lumen, either complete or incomplete. Strangulation, or interruption of the segmental blood supply, may complicate obstruction and lead to mucosal ulceration, bowel necrosis, and perforation. Ileus (adynamic, paralytic, or nonobstructive) is a nonmechanical obstruction of the bowel. Evaluation of the patient with possible obstruction begins with an abdominal series.

Gastric obstruction

Gastric outlet obstruction allows large volumes of gas and fluid to accumulate within the stomach. Even with massive fluid accumulations, a small amount of air persists. On the upright or decubitus radiograph, one or two air-fluid levels characteristically appear. Only after the stomach has been emptied (which may require several days of continuous suction) should a barium diag-

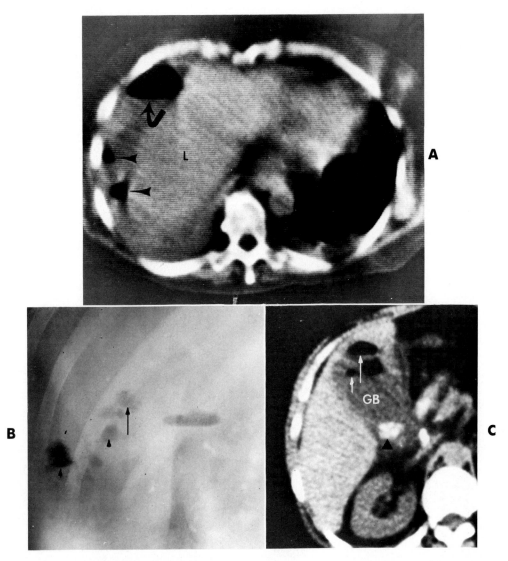

Fig. 3-17 A, Subphrenic abscess. CT scan. Liver *(L)* is displaced medially by anterior *(curved arrow)* and posterior *(arrowheads)* subphrenic collections of pus. **B,** Subphrenic abscess. There are multiple gas-fluid levels *(arrows)* below right eleventh rib. **C,** CT confirms subhepatic pericholecystic abscess *(arrows)*. *GB,* Gallbladder; *black arrowhead,* gallstones.
(From Mindelzun RE, McCort JJ: *Radiol Clin North Am* 18:221, 1980.)

nostic study be undertaken since the presence of intragastric food residues makes an anatomic diagnosis impossible.

Hypertrophic pyloric stenosis

Neonatal gastric obstruction caused by hypertrophic pyloric stenosis may be diagnosed by ultrasonography. Ultrasound scans show the contracted muscle, which has diminished echogenicity, an elongated pylorus, and narrowed lumen. If abdominal distention prevents adequate sonographic study, a barium study with limited fluoroscopy will show the constricted gastric outlet.

Antral web

Congenital antral webs, the likely result of developmental arrest, are an uncommon cause of neonatal gastric obstruction. The larger the web, the earlier the obstruction occurs. Small webs may by asymptomatic.

Carcinoma or ulcer scar

Antral carcinoma or a stricture caused by chronic peptic ulceration may obstruct the stomach. Radiographic differentiation between these two entities may require careful barium study or endoscopy.

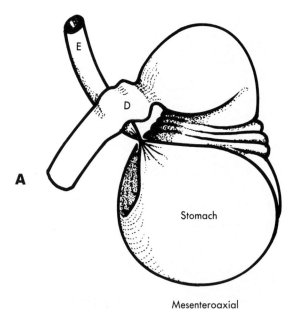

Mesenteroaxial
gastric volvulus

Fig. 3-18 Mesenteroaxial volvulus. **A,** Diagram. Stomach twists about its mesentery, constricting mid body. Fundus remains beneath diaphragm; antrum and pylorus extend above diaphragm. **B,** Posteroanterior chest film. Gastric fundus *(F)* beneath diaphragm. Retrocardiac mass *(arrows)* represents dilated antrum. **C,** Barium study shows twist in body of stomach. *F,* Fundus; *A,* Antrum.

(From McCort JJ, editor: *Abdominal radiology,* © 1981, The Williams & Wilkins Co, Baltimore.)

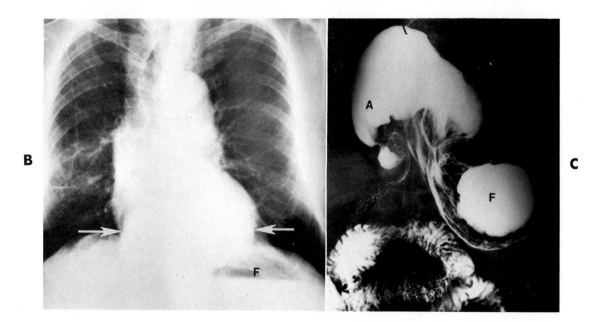

Corrosive gastritis

Corrosive alkaline or acid solutions can destroy the superficial layers of the gastric wall. The antrum is usually involved, and progressive scarring may completely occlude the lumen.

Volvulus

Air-fluid levels of differing heights within a retrocardiac hiatus hernia suggest gastric volvulus. The twist may be organoaxial or mesenteroaxial.

With organoaxial volvulus the stomach twists either anteriorly or posteriorly about its long axis, causing two points of luminal constriction. Organoaxial volvulus can obstruct the stomach but does not usually result in strangulation.

With mesenteroaxial volvulus the stomach twists about its mesentery so that the antrum and pylorus lie above the gastric fundus. The single point of obstruction occurs in the body of the stomach (Fig. 3-18). Mesenteroaxial volvulus can cause complete obstruction and occlude the gastric vessels, leading to strangulation and perforation.

Gastric bezoar

The accretion of hair (trichobezoar) or undigestible vegetable matter (phytobezoar) may cause partial gastric obstruction. Air accumulation in the interstices of the mass gives the bezoar a mottled appearance.

Duodenal obstruction

In duodenal obstruction, gas and fluid distend the stomach and duodenum to produce the double-bubble sign. In the neonate or infant, duodenal obstruction can be due to aberrant pancreas, duodenal atresia or stenosis, duodenal duplication, web, preduodenal portal vein, or peritoneal bands (complicating intestinal malrotation). In the adult, chronic peptic ulceration, primary or metastatic tumor, pancreatic abscess, or massive lymph node enlargement may obstruct the duodenum.

The role played by superior mesenteric vessel compression remains controversial. In patients with extensive burns, in body casts, experiencing rapid weight loss, or at prolonged bed rest, the stomach and duode-num are dilated. Pressure by the superior mesenteric artery and vein on the third portion of the duodenum can cause obstruction often relieved by placing the patient prone.

Jejunal and ilial obstruction

In a healthy adult one or two air-fluid levels may be seen in the small bowel, and the width of the gas-filled bowel lumen rarely exceeds 3 cm. With obstruction, gas and fluid accumulate behind the occluded bowel segment, increasing the number of air-fluid levels. In general, the greater the number of dilated bowel loops, the more distal the level of obstruction. Emptying of the small bowel and colon distal to an obstruction occurs in 12 to 24 hours. The thickness of the bowel wall and valvulae conniventes are accurately depicted on upright or decubitus projections (Figs. 3-19, 3-20). Large amounts of intraluminal fluid with minimal gas produce the appearance of a gasless abdomen (Fig. 3-21). Bowel obstruction at two separate points produces a

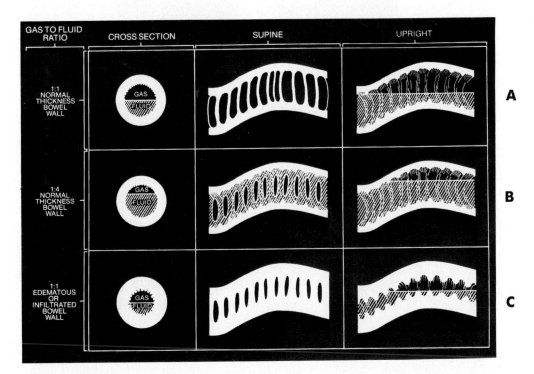

Fig. 3-19 Ratio of intraluminal gas to fluid. **A,** Ratio of gas to fluid greater than 1:1 more accurately portrays bowel wall and valvulae conniventes thickness on both upright and supine radiographs. **B,** Ratio of gas to fluid less than 1:1 gives erroneous impression of bowel wall and valvulae conniventes thickness on supine radiograph. In this situation upright or decubitus projections more correctly depict condition of bowel wall. Intraluminal gas outlines upper margin of bowel and gives more accurate measure of thickness. Free-flowing intraperitoneal fluid (lying between bowel loops) can be differentiated because it will obscure outer wall of bowel and gravitate to dependent intraperitoneal spaces when patient is in erect or decubitus position. **C,** Bowel wall thickened by edema, hemorrhage, or cellular infiltration retains this appearance on supine, decubitus, or upright radiographs regardless of intraluminal fluid content.

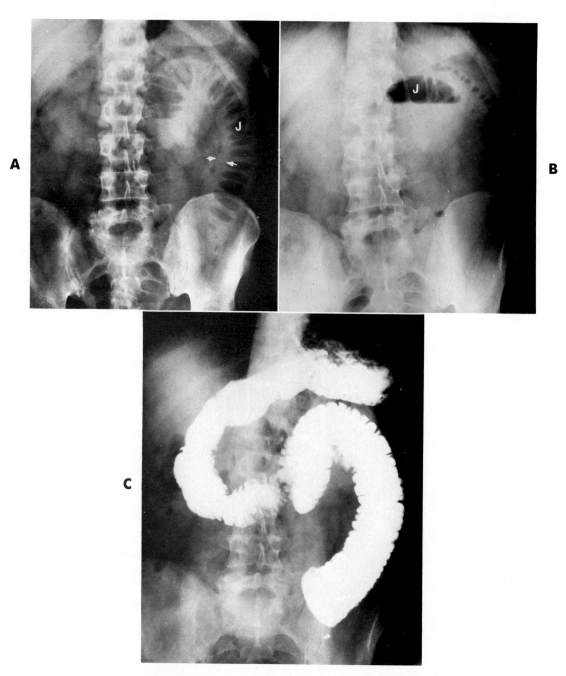

Fig. 3-20 Small bowel obstruction by adhesions (pseudo bowel wall thickening). Ratio of gas to fluid less than 1:1 conveys false impression of bowel wall and valvulae conniventes thickening. **A,** Supine abdominal radiograph. Dilated gas- and fluid-filled loop of jejunum. Bowel wall between arrows appears thickened, as do valvulae conniventes. *J,* Jejunum. **B,** upright abdominal radiograph. Fluid gravitates to dependent portion of jejunum, revealing normal thickness of bowel wall and valvulae conniventes. *J,* Jejunum. **C,** Barium study. Jejunum is markedly dilated because of obstruction by adhesions. Normal thickness of bowel wall and valvulae conniventes is confirmed.

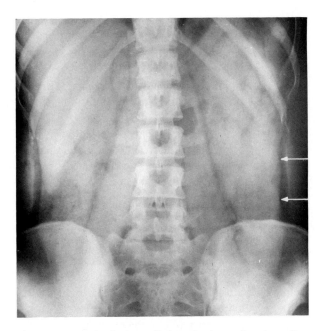

Fig. 3-21 Mechanical small bowel obstruction by adhesions—the gasless abdomen. With minimal gas and large amounts of fluid, distended bowel loops appear as multiple ovoid densities that indent extraperitoneal fat in flanks *(arrows)*. Loops are rarely completely gasless, and small gas bubbles overlying fluid will appear on supine and decubitus radiographs.

closed loop. A gas-filled closed loop may double on itself and assume a U shape, resembling a coffee bean— the coffee bean sign. A closed loop distended with fluid may mimic an intraabdominal tumor (pseudotumor).

In the adult the usual causes of mechanical obstruction are adhesions, incarcerated hernia, obturation, tumor, or inflammatory bowel disease. In the neonate or infant, stenosis, atresia, duplication, meconium plug, mid-gut volvulus, and ileocolic intussusception may obstruct the small bowel (Fig. 3-22).

If the radiographic findings of small bowel obstruction are equivocal and no clinical signs of strangulation, perforation, or peritonitis are elicited, prompt evaluation by oral barium with serial radiographs or by enteroclysis is recommended. The use of water-soluble ionic contrast agents to evaluate small bowel patency is less satisfactory. If the examiner is uncertain whether the obstruction level is in the ileum or right colon, a barium enema is performed first.

In the acutely obstructed patient, bowel wall gas with or without mesenteric portal vein gas or pneumoperitoneum gives clear-cut evidence that strangulation and devitalization; emergency surgery is required.

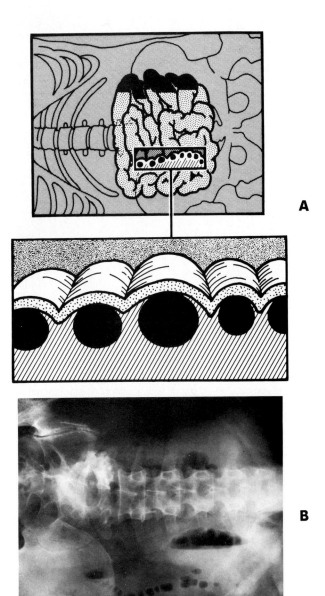

Fig. 3-22 Mechanical small bowel obstruction by adhesions—string of beads sign. **A,** Diagram. On radiographs obtained with horizontal beam, small bubbles of gas are trapped beneath valvulae conniventes in lowermost loops. Meniscus effect of surrounding fluid gives trapped gas an ovoid shape. Note that uppermost bowel loops show fluid levels. **B,** Lateral decubitus abdomen. Uppermost bowel loops show fluid levels. Lowermost bowel loop exhibits string of beads sign. This finding indicates large amounts of intraluminal fluid and is usually associated with mechanical obstruction.

(From McCort JJ, editor: *Abdominal radiology,* © 1981, The Williams & Wilkins Co, Baltimore.)

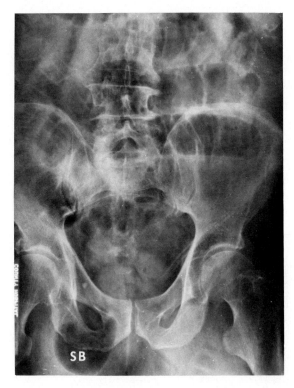

Fig. 3-23 Mechanical small bowel obstruction by right inguinal hernia. Multiple dilated loops of small bowel are present in abdomen, and no gas is seen in colon. Right inguinal hernia contains loop of small bowel *(SB)*.

(From McCort JJ, editor: *Abdominal radiology,* © 1981, The Williams & Wilkins Co, Baltimore.)

Hernias

External hernias are usually indicated by the finding of ectopic gas-filled intestine at sites where hernias usually occur such as the inguinal canal, the femoral canal, or the anterior abdominal wall (Fig. 3-23). Internal hernias are suspected when the bowel remains in a fixed position on different projections or on serial films. Bowel may herniate internally through a congenital, traumatic, or postsurgical mesenteric defect. The herniated bowel lies outside its normal anatomic position and appears encased within a sac.

Mid-gut volvulus

With absent or incomplete fixation the small bowel can twist about its vascular pedicle at the duodenojejunal juncture. Midgut volvulus can rapidly cause bowel infarction with high morbidity and mortality. Oral barium will show an obstruction at the duodenojejunal junction.

Intussusception

Ileocolic intussusception occurs in infants up to 2½ years of age and involves telescoping of the ileum into the ascending colon to produce a masslike density in the right abdomen. On occasion the leading edge of the intussusception bowel (the intussusceptum) can be seen surrounded by gas. In 50% to 60% of patients barium or air enema will reduce the intussusception. Clinical signs of perforation contraindicate barium or air enema reduction and call for immediate surgery.

Jejunojejunal intussusceptions occur following intraabdominal surgery and are transiently seen in patient with sprue. With antegrade small bowel study barium will show a beaklike termination at the point of intussusception. Jejunogastric intussusception can occur following partial gastric resection and gastrojejunostomy. Most often the afferent loop protrudes into the gastric remnant.

Colon obstruction

Regardless of the site of colonic obstruction, the cecum often shows the most marked distention. When the cecal diameter exceeds 10 cm, the probability of perforation increases, and decompression becomes advisable. The patient with suspected large bowel and/or distal ileum obstruction should be further studied with an emergency barium enema of the unprepared colon. A toxic megacolon, pneumatosis intestinalis, and portal vein or extraluminal gas contraindicate enema examination. Sigmoid diverticulitis is the most common obstructing lesion of the colon. Colonic obstruction may be caused by tumors, both primary carcinoma and metastatic lesions, and by inflammatory disease.

Volvulus

In sigmoid volvulus the twisted and obstructed sigmoid becomes markedly distended with gas and fluid. The obstructed sigmoid loop forms two large compartments that share a double wall, terminating at the point of the twist (Fig. 3-24). A barium enema demonstrates a characteristic beaklike termination of the barium column.

With cecal volvulus, twisting of the bowel usually occurs in the ascending colon proximal to the ileocecal valve. An absent or elongated cecal mesentery permits volvulus formation. Viewed from the anterior abdomen, the twist occurs in a clockwise direction. With obstruction, the cecum becomes distended and projects into the left middle or upper abdomen. The colon distal to the twist may be empty. On examination using a barium enema, a beaklike constriction of the barium column in the ascending colon confirms the diagnosis.

Transverse colon volvulus is relatively rare, occurring when the transverse colon twists simultaneously at the hepatic and splenic flexures, resulting in an enormously distended transverse colon. On barium enema the distal twist at the splenic flexure arrests the barium column.

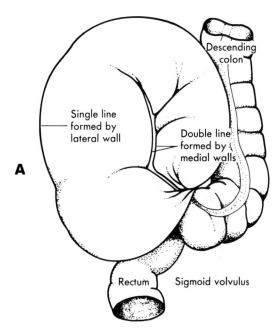

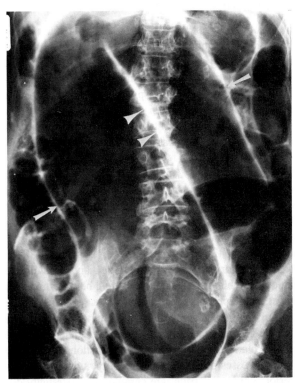

Fig. 3-24 A, Diagrammatic representation of sigmoid volvulus. **B,** Sigmoid volvulus. Distended sigmoid loop extends into right upper abdomen and has convex border superiorly. As sigmoid is bent on itself, it forms two compartments. Hence twisted sigmoid has single out wall *(arrows)* and double central wall *(arrowheads).* Caudally, central double wall terminates at point of twist in sigmoid mesentery.

With compound volvulus, a loop of small bowel wraps around the sigmoid colon, forming an ileosigmoid knot. The proximal small bowel dilates; the constricted sigmoid dilates and remains fixed in the midabdomen.

INTESTINAL ATONY AND DILATATION

In aganglionosis (Hirschsprung's disease), the length of the aganglionic segment varies from a short segment inside the anus to involvement of the entire colon. The aganglionic bowel is narrowed, and the normal proximal colon contains large amounts of gas and stool. A barium enema shows a narrowed aganglionic segment of variable length.

In idiopathic intestinal pseudoobstruction, there is an impaired response to intestinal dilatation and marked bowel distention occurs with minimal symptoms (Fig. 3-25). A special type of pseudoobstruction—Ogilvie's syndrome—involves the elderly and is often seen in patients who come from nursing homes or are immobilized after orthopedic procedures. If the gas can be manipulated into the rectum by first turning the patient to the right decubitus position and then the prone position, a mechanical obstruction is unlikely.

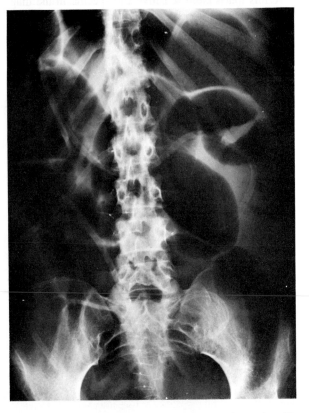

Fig. 3-25 Chronic idiopathic intestinal pseudoobstruction. No cause for intestinal dilatation was discovered on thorough investigation, including exploratory laparotomy.
(Courtesy Dr. H Goldberg.)

4 *Pharynx*

MW DONNER

ANATOMY

NEUROREGULATION OF SWALLOWING

RADIOGRAPHIC EVALUATION OF THE PHARYNX

RADIOGRAPHIC ANATOMY

PHARYNGEAL DISORDERS

ANATOMY

For discussion purposes, the pharynx is divided into three segments. The uppermost segment is the nasopharynx or epipharynx, which is exclusively respiratory in function. The midportion is the oropharynx or mesopharynx, where food and air intermingle, and the lowest segment is the laryngopharynx or hypopharynx.

The *mesopharynx* extends from the free border of the soft palate inferiorly to the level of the tip of the epiglottis. Anteriorly it is continuous with the oral cavity. The mucosa of the lingual surface of the epiglottis and the pharyngoepiglottic and glossoepiglottic folds that bound the valleculae are also included in the mesopharynx.

The *hypopharynx* extends from the level of the hyoid bone to and including the cricopharyngeus muscle. Its superior border is the upper margin of the pharyngoepiglottic fold. The hypopharynx is divided into three main parts: the *pyriform sinus*, the *posterolateral walls*, and the *postcricoid area*. The latter includes the cricopharyngeus muscle and the mucosa covering the posterior surface of the posterior quadrate lamina of the cricoid cartilage. The term *pyriform sinus* is usually used to refer to the region extending from the pharyngoepiglottic fold to the esophageal opening at the level of the lower border of the cricoid cartilage.

The muscular part of the pharynx contains five pairs of voluntary muscles. Three pairs, the superior, middle, and inferior *pharyngeal constrictors,* form an outer circular coat of muscles. An inner or longitudinal layer of muscle is formed by the fibers of the *stylopharyngeus* and *palatopharyngeus muscles.*

The inferior pharyngeal constrictor consists of two parts: an upper oblique portion called the *thyropharyngeus* and a lower horizontal portion known as the *cricopharyngeus.* The fibers of the cricopharyngeus muscle (Fig. 4-1) pass horizontally backward to form a sphincter and diverge from the lower oblique fibers of the inferior pharyngeal constrictor to leave a triangular

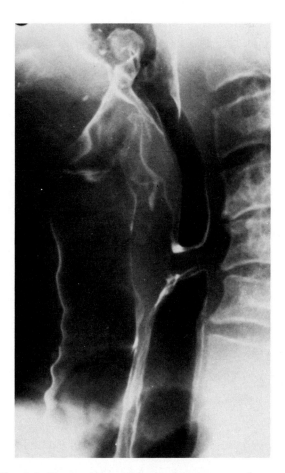

Fig. 4-1 Characteristic position and appearance of normal cricopharyngeus can be observed in this patient because both esophagus and pharynx are air filled. Normal relaxation of cricopharyngeus occurred during deglutition.

area that is relatively devoid of muscle fibers. This potential weak spot, known as *Killian's dehiscence,* is where pulsion or Zenker's pharyngeal diverticula is usually located.

NEUROREGULATION OF SWALLOWING

The preparatory phase of swallowing (mastication and intraoral manipulation) is under voluntary control. Pharyngeal and esophageal phases of deglutition, however, are under involuntary reflexive control. Sensation from the pharynx and larynx that elicits and guides swallowing is conveyed by the glossopharyngeal (IX) and vagus (X) nerves to the nucleus solitarius in the brain stem. The cranial nerve motor nuclei involved in deglutition are the trigeminal (V), facial (VII), glossopharyngeal (IX), vagus (X), and hypoglossal (XII). With the exception of the tensor veli palatini, which is innervated by the trigeminal nerve, the intrinsic muscles of the pharynx, larynx, and soft palate receive motor fibers from the glossopharyngeal and vagus nerves.

RADIOGRAPHIC EVALUATION OF THE PHARYNX

Anatomic variation, presence of disease, and the patient's reaction may make adequate inspection of the pharynx difficult. Radiographic examination not only provides a more physiologic perspective; it can also yield very accurate information on the presence and extent of disease.

Lateral soft tissue radiographs are useful in the detection of radiopaque foreign bodies and increased thickness of the prevertebral soft tissues. Although lateral views yield more diagnostic information than do frontal projections, both films should be obtained during an examination. Exposures should be made while the patient phonates the vowel "e," which permits better visualization of the air-filled pharynx. Some examiners find it helpful to have the patient blow through compressed lips with the nose closed (Jonsson or modified Valsalva maneuver) to maximally distend the hypopharynx (Fig. 4-2). Since most foreign bodies lodge in the region of the cricopharyngeal muscle, the frontal view should include the upper cervical esophagus and should be more heavily exposed than the lateral view. Linear calcification of the quadrate plate of the cricoid cartilage may occasionally simulate a swallowed fishbone or chicken bone.

Since a retropharyngeal abscess or a neoplasm may cause thickening of the prevertebral soft tissues with anterior displacement of the pharyngeal air shadow, the radiograph should be made at the peak of inspiration to ensure that tissue thickness is minimal. In infants it should be about three quarters of the anteroposterior diameter of the body of an adjacent vertebra.

Computed tomography and magnetic resonance imaging

The advantages of *magnetic resonance imaging (MRI)* include multiplanar capability (direct imaging in the sagittal and coronal planes), tissue characterization, and avoidance of both iodine-containing contrast media and ionizing radiation (Fig. 4-3). *Laryngography* has a role in selected cases and can be combined with dynamic recording to document alterations of mobility.

For *computed tomography (CT)* of neck abnormalities, 4 to 5 mm sections are suggested; 2 mm sections are preferable for the glottic region (Fig. 4-4). Sections up to 8 mm may be used for large abnormalities or for overview evaluation. In most cases a window level of 30 to 50 Hounsfield units with a window width of 300 to 400 Hounsfield units is satisfactory. The patient is usually supine, with the head and neck extended to position the long axis of the vocal cords perpendicular to the tabletop. It is very important that the patient not move or swallow during scanning. Most often this can

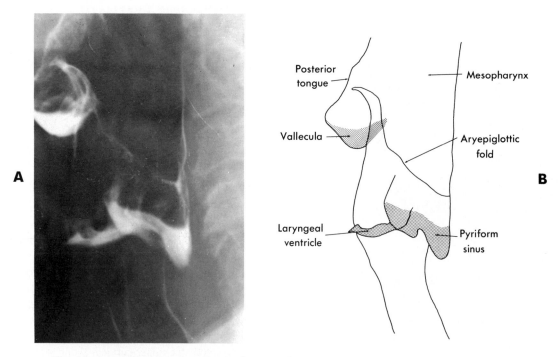

Fig. 4-2 A and **B,** Epiglottis and posterior part of tongue in anterior position during phonation. Act of phonating facilitates visualization by producing increase in anteroposterior dimension of mesopharynx.

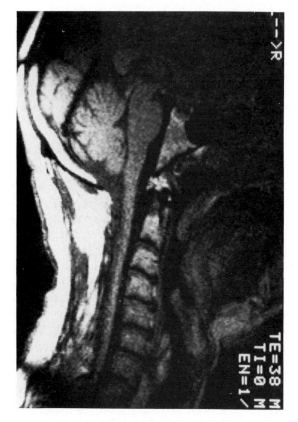

Fig. 4-3 Fifty-one year old man with squamous cancer of epiglottis. MRI demonstrates epiglottic thickening and correctly indicates sparing of preepiglottic space.

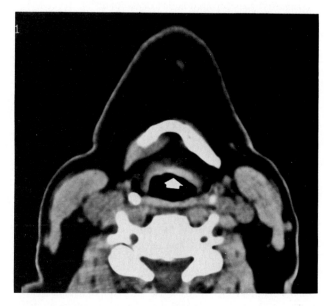

Fig. 4-4 Fifty-one year old man with squamous cancer of epiglottis. CT scan without contrast media shows epiglottic thickening *(arrow)* and correctly indicates sparing of preepiglottic space.

be accomplished by having the patient extend the tongue between the teeth and perform quiet breathing. If the patient moves during quiet breathing, breath holding at the end of a normal expiration usually produces an open airway and is an alternative. The use of contrast media should be individualized; although very useful in distinguishing vessels from lymph nodes, contrast media are is not required in all cases.

Dynamic recording

Dynamic recording of the barium swallow and double-contrast pharyngography are the best techniques for examining the pharynx. Cineradiography and video fluorography use straight frontal and lateral views of the pharynx at frame speeds of 15 to 60 frames per second with the patient in the erect position. It is very important to ensure that the patient is in a true lateral or true frontal position. In sensorimotor disorders, which may impair tight closure of the junction between the mouth and the pharynx, examination in the recumbent position is useful to determine leakage of contrast material from the oral cavity.

Double-contrast pharyngography

Spot film double-contrast radiographs of the pharynx and esophagus are required to complete the routine evaluation of this area. Optimal double-contrast mucosal coating is accomplished with single swallows of high-density barium and various maneuvers (as previously described) are used to distend the pharynx. Anteroposterior, lateral, and occasionally oblique radio-graphs are taken. The cervical esophagus may be included in the examination, since it is functionally closely connected with the pharynx. Lateral pharyngeal pouches, lymphoid hyperplasia, fungus and viral infections affecting the pharyngeal mucosa, and carcinomas of the epiglottis and hypopharynx are well delineated using double-contrast examinations.

RADIOGRAPHIC ANATOMY

When the pharynx is distended with barium, only the pharyngeal margins that are in profile can be seen; intraluminal masses may be hidden by the dense barium column. In the lateral view, the posterior wall is straight and parallel to the spine, although it may be indented by vertebral osteophytes, and the pharyngoesophageal junction is not normally discernible. There are irregularities of the anterior wall, at the level of the valleculae and epiglottis, and of the laryngeal vestibule. Just below the cricoid impression a small indentation that resembles a web (caused by a prolapse of mucosa over submucosal veins) may be observed. It can be distinguished from a true web by its change in shape during swallowing. At times it may simulate a mass lesion (Fig. 4-5).

PHARYNGEAL DISORDERS
Diverticula

Pharyngeal diverticula are usually classified as congenital or acquired and as anterior, lateral, or posterior, according to their anatomic site.

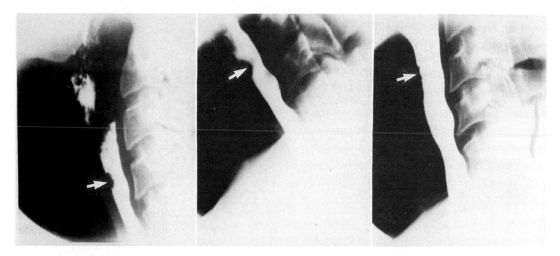

Fig. 4-5 Postcricoid defect simulating mass lesion. Note change in shape and almost complete disappearance on third picture. Surgical exploration was negative.
(Courtesy Dr. JL Clements.)

Anterior diverticula

One form of anterior pharyngeal pouch, which occurs after laryngectomy, is a recess on the anterior of the pharynx at its junction with the base of the tongue. This recess results from separation of the edges of the pharyngeal closure at the point where it joins the base of the tongue.

Lateral diverticula

True lateral pharyngeal diverticula are quite rare, and there is some confusion about terminology with regard to benign or normal variants. Protrusions of the lateral pharyngeal wall may be observed quite frequently on frontal views taken when the pharynx is distended. This occurs in the anterolateral portion of the pyriform sinus at the level of the vallecula. The lateral walls of these recesses are formed by the thyrohyoid membrane, which is relatively weak because it is not supported by cartilage or bone. Although lateral support is afforded by the inferior and middle pharyngeal constrictors and by the thyrohyoid muscle, these muscles fail to overlap completely, and a portion of the thyrohyoid membrane receives no muscular support. Bulges that occur in this anatomic weak spot are more frequent in older patients and have been referred to as *hypopharyngeal pouches, hypopharyngeal ears,* and *pharyngoceles.* They are usually 0.5 to 1.5 cm in diameter, bilaterally symmetric, and of no clinical significance. Lateral bulges that occur in the tonsillar fossa and may be seen to project above the pharyngoepiglottic fold should be considered normal variants.

Congenital lateral pharyngeal diverticula are true branchial cleft cysts and sinuses that connect only with the pharynx internally and end blindly in the neck. The major differential diagnosis is a laryngocele. These pouches are filled with air and never fill with contrast material.

Posterior diverticula

Posterior hypopharyngeal pouches, also known as *Zenker's diverticula, pulsion diverticula,* or *pharyngoesophageal diverticula,* are by far the most common type of pharyngeal diverticula. They always originate in exactly the same place in the midline on the posterior wall (Killian's dehiscence or Laimer's triangle), the result of divergence between the fibers of the cricopharyngeus and the inferior pharyngeal constrictor (Fig. 4-6).

These pouches are thought to be acquired and since all occur above the cricopharyngeus, they are clearly pharyngeal rather than esophageal in location. The posterior hypopharyngeal diverticulum is usually classified as a pulsion type and is thought to arise as a result of pressure from the peristaltic wave sweeping down the pharynx when the cricopharyngeus closes prematurely.

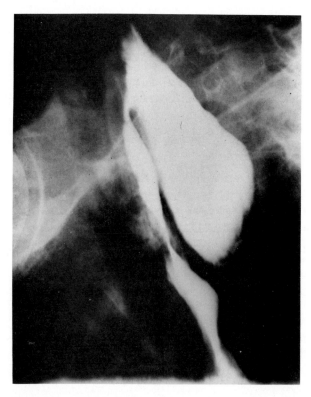

Fig. 4-6 Large Zenker's diverticulum extending inferiorly and compressing esophagus.

The diverticulum begins as a posterior bulge above the cricopharyngeus, and as it enlarges it extends caudally behind and usually to the left of the esophagus. The opening into the sac becomes more dependent than the esophageal opening, which is compressed into a slit as the esophagus itself becomes partially obstructed by the pressure of the sac contents.

Functional disorders

The radiographic examination for studying deglutition should always include evaluation of the mouth, pharynx, and esophagus. It is important to realize that the insidious progression of pharyngeal dysfunction may be accompanied by corresponding adaptations in diet and swallowing, so that the patient may not be aware of the swallowing abnormality.

Normal deglutition

The normal process of swallowing may be divided into oral, pharyngeal, and esophageal stages. The oral stage involves the voluntary transport of a bolus from the oral cavity into the pharynx. The function of both the mesopharynx and the hypopharynx during deglutition is to receive the bolus and convey it to the esophagus. As the bolus is pushed from the oral cavity into the mesopharynx by the elevation and posterior motion of the tongue and its suspension musculature, the reflex portion of deglutition begins. As shown by the abrupt rise of the hyoid and the lateral walls of the pharynx, this phenomenon is a primary elevation of the entire pharyngeal tube, followed by a descending peristaltic wave similar to that used in the engulfing of prey by a snake. At this point the cavity of the mesopharynx is obliterated by the posterior thrust of the tongue, so that in the erect position the posterior pharyngeal wall normally exhibits little motion. When posterior tongue motion is impaired, a striking compensatory anterior movement of the posterior pharynx may be observed. Slight anterior movement of the posterior pharyngeal wall may be seen in normal individuals.

The epiglottis then deflects the bolus into the lateral food channels and bends back and inferiorly to cover the laryngeal vestibule. The role of the epiglottis in preventing aspiration is secondary to the sphincteric action of the supraglottic laryngeal musculature. Food is prevented from returning into the mouth by the continued contraction of those muscles that forced it into the pharynx, and it is prevented from entering the larynx by the supraglottic muscles and the epiglottis. Food is kept out of the epipharynx by contractions of the levator palatini and palatopharyngeus muscles, which close the velo-

pharyngeal portal by elevating the soft palate and approximating it to the posterior pharyngeal wall. There is also medial motion of localized areas of both lateral pharyngeal walls against the edges of the velum to close the lateral aspects of the velopharyngeal portal.

In some patients a localized muscular contraction occasionally produces protrusion of the posterior pharyngeal wall, known as *Passavant's bar*. This bar, originally described in patients with cleft palates, is probably not a normal phenomenon, since it is generally seen only in patients with velopharyngeal incompetence.

Neuromuscular dysfunction

Diseases affecting the pharynx are classified as (1) central nervous system diseases (cerebrovascular occlusive disease; tumors; pseudobulbar palsy; poliomyelitis; trauma; demyelinating disease; extrapyramidal disease; and congenital and degenerative disorders such as hereditary spastic hemiplegia, amyotrophic lateral sclerosis, and familial dysautonomia), (2) muscle disease (polymyositis, dermatomyositis, myotonia dystrophy, and oculomotor myopathy), (3) myoneural junction disease (myasthenia gravis), and (4) peripheral nerve disease (trauma and neuritis). A common radiographic manifestation found in neuromuscular dysfunction is the inability to completely clear the pharynx, so that resid-

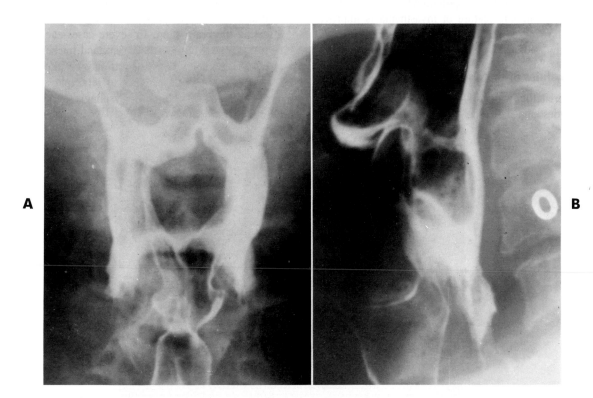

Fig. 4-7 A, Excessive amount of residual barium in pharynx and spillage into larynx and trachea suggest neuromuscular disorder. **B,** Lateral view reveals obstructing carcinoma in distal hypopharynx.

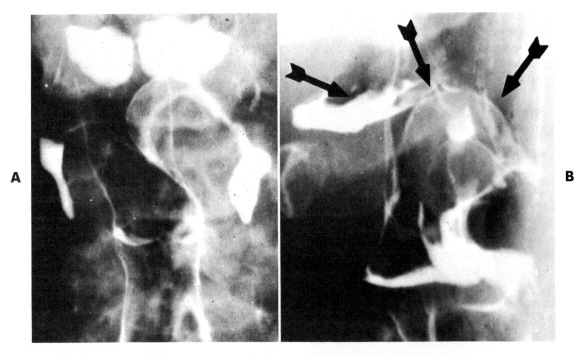

Fig. 4-13 A, Leiomyosarcoma of left aryepiglottic fold bulging into left pyriform sinus and laryngeal vestibule. **B,** Lateral view shows tumor outlined by middle and right arrows. Left arrow at vallecula.

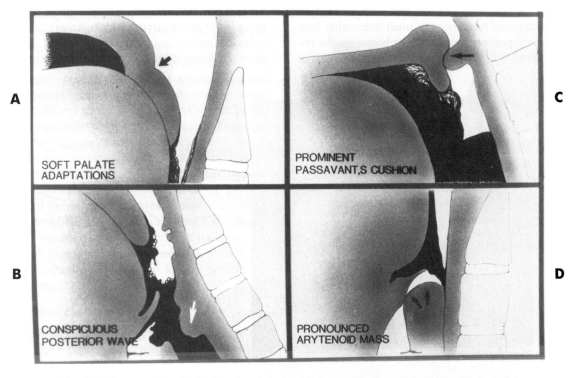

Fig. 4-14 Compensation. **A,** Kinking *(arrow)* of soft palate to "hug" atrophic tongue. **B,** Conspicuous constrictor wall *(arrow)* (displaced anteriorly). **C,** Tonguelike prominence of Passavant's cushion *(arrow)* to meet weak or atrophic palate. **D,** Upward displacement of arytenoids *(arrow)* into larynx to counteract aspiration.

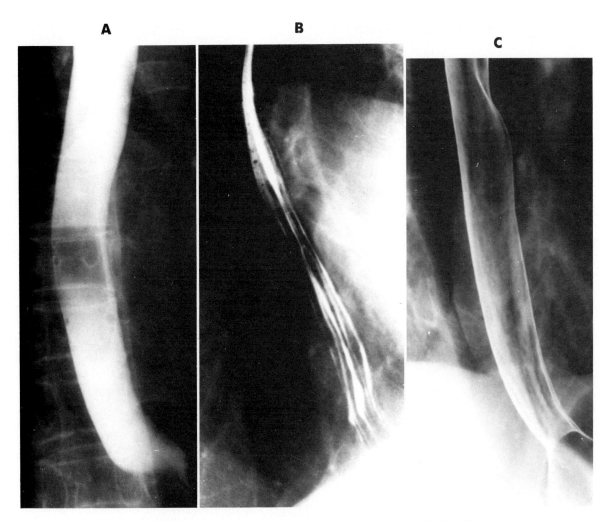

Fig. 5-3 Spot films of esophagus. **A,** Full column. **B,** Mucosal detail. **C,** Double contrast.

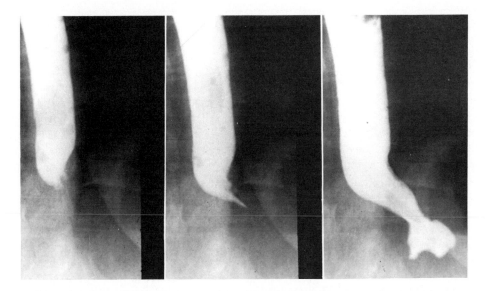

Fig. 5-4 Radiologic appearance of lower esophageal sphincter (LES) opening after barium swallow. With subject upright, three 105 mm films were taken 0.5 seconds apart beginning 1 second after swallowing. As seen in first frame, head of barium column reaches LES before its relaxation. Upper margin of closed sphincter imparts a V- or bullet-shaped configuration to head of column. In middle frame, some barium is seen wedging into unrelaxed sphincter. As sphincter relaxes, it is "blown" open by force of barium column, and barium flows freely into stomach.

□ CLASSIFICATION OF ESOPHAGEAL MOTILITY DISORDERS □

I. Primary
   A. Achalasia
   B. Diffuse esophageal spasm
   C. Intestinal pseudoobstruction
   D. Hypertensive peristalsis
   E. Presbyesophagus
   F. Congenital tracheoesophageal fistula
   G. Chalasia
II. Secondary
   A. Connective tissue
   B. Chemical or physical
      1. Reflux (peptic) esophagitis
      2. Caustic esophagitis
      3. Vagotomy
      4. Radiation
   C. Infection
      1. Fungal: moniliasis
      2. Bacterial: tuberculosis, diphtheria, and so on
      3. Parasitic: Chagas' disease
      4. Viral: herpes simplex, and so on
   D. Metabolic
      1. Diabetes
      2. Alcoholism
      3. Amyloidosis
      4. Serum pH and electrolyte disturbances (possibly)
   E. Endocrine disease
      1. Myxedema
      2. Thyrotoxicosis

   F. Neurologic disease
      1. Parkinsonism
      2. Huntington's chorea
      3. Wilson's disease
      4. Cerebrovascular disease
      5. Multiple sclerosis
      6. Amyotrophic lateral sclerosis
      7. Central nervous system neoplasm
      8. Bulbar poliomyelitis
      9. Pseudobulbar palsy
      10. Friedreich's hereditary spastic ataxia
      11. Familial dysautonomia (Riley-Day syndrome)
      12. Stiff man's syndrome
      13. Ganglioneuromatosis
   G. Muscular disease
      1. Myotonic dystrophy
      2. Muscular dystrophy
      3. Oculopharyngeal dystrophy
      4. Myasthenia gravis (neuromotor end plate)
   H. Vascular
      1. Varices (possibly)
      2. Ischemia (possibly)
   I. Neoplasm
      1. Obstruction
      2. Neural invasion
   J. Pharmacologic
      1. Atropine, propantheline, curare, and so on

ESOPHAGEAL MOTILITY DISORDERS

Esophageal motility disorders are classified as either primary, in which the esophagus is the major organ involved, or secondary, in which the esophageal motor abnormality results from systemic disease or from physical, chemical, or pharmacologic effects (see the box above).

Radiographic evaluation

Examination of esophageal motor function includes a systematic evaluation of motor function in the pharynx, both esophageal sphincters (Fig. 5-5; see Fig. 5-2), and the esophageal body. The patient should be placed in a right-side-down prone oblique position and instructed to take *single* swallows of liquid barium (5 to 10 ml), so that motor events resulting from a single stimulus can be observed. A second swallow taken before the initial peristaltic sequence is completed may inhibit the initial contractile wave, thereby making it appear abnormal.

Rapid, repetitive swallows are used only to distend the esophagus maximally to study morphology.

Because the relaxed LES is more compliant than the esophageal body, the LES segment, when fully distended, often has a bulbous configuration, termed the *phrenic ampulla*. The peristaltic contraction wave is seen as a progressive stripping movement of the inverted V-shaped tail down the esophageal body (see Fig. 5-5). The tail travels fastest in the cervical esophagus and slows distally. In young adults, a normal peristaltic wave generally strips all the barium from the esophagus. In some instances, however, escape of barium may occur at the level of the aortic arch (see Fig. 5-5, *A*). This phenomenon is a normal variation caused by low peristaltic pressure amplitudes in this region. This *escape phenomenon* becomes more prominent with aging. In the LES segment the peristaltic stripping wave generally develops a rounded or flat-top configuration. In many individuals the stripping wave fades out in the

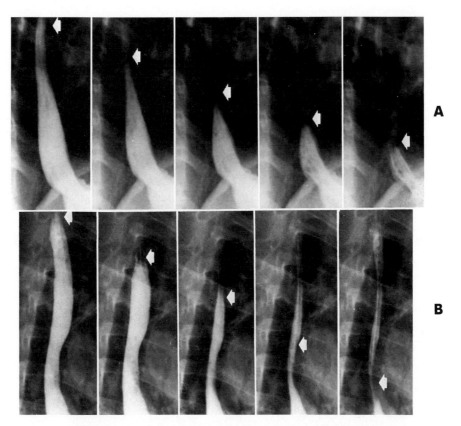

Fig. 5-5 Radiographic appearance of normal primary peristalsis in two recumbent subjects. About 6 to 8 seconds are required for peristaltic contraction wave to traverse entire esophagus. **A,** Complete stripping of swallowed bolus. Peristaltic circular contraction wave *(arrows)* imparts inverted V configuration to tail of barium column. Barium tail often develops flat-top shape in distal esophagus. **B,** Proximal escape of barium. Circular peristaltic contraction wave *(arrows)* does not quite obliterate esophageal lumen at aortic arch level, thereby permitting proximal escape of modest amount of barium. Below aortic arch, peristaltic wave becomes more forceful and obliterates esophageal lumen, and during its continuation sweeps bulk of swallowed barium into stomach.

middle portion of the LES segment, and barium escapes retrogradely into the distal esophageal body. This variation should not be confused with gastroesophageal reflux.

Secondary peristalsis produces the same radiographic appearance as primary peristalsis and is commonly observed after gastroesophageal reflux of barium or primary peristaltic sequence failure, causing sufficient esophageal distention from residual barium to trigger the stretch reflex.

Abnormalities of peristalsis include (1) decreased incidence of peristalsis in response to swallowing, (2) incomplete peristaltic sequences, and (3) aperistalsis. The incidence of nonperistaltic contractions increases in many esophageal motility disorders. A "to-and-fro" or "yo-yo" motion of barium may result from uncoordinated esophageal motor activity. Feeble, repetitive,

non–lumen obliterating, nonperistaltic contractions, often referred to as *tertiary contractions,* may impart a scalloped configuration to the barium column. More forceful non–lumen obliterating contractions may produce a corkscrew appearance, sometimes referred to as *curling* (Fig. 5-6). Lumen-obliterating, nonperistaltic contractions occurring simultaneously at several sites may cause compartmentalization of the barium column, giving it a *rosary bead* or *shish kebab* configuration.

A radiographic *Mecholyl test* may be helpful in selected patients (Fig. 5-7). An abnormal response generally indicates a hypersensitivity response caused by a deficiency of esophageal innervation. The cholinergic drug methacholine is injected subcutaneously, starting with a dose of 5 mg. If a positive response does not occur in 10 minutes, the dose is increased by 2.5 mg increments until a dose of 10 mg is reached. When

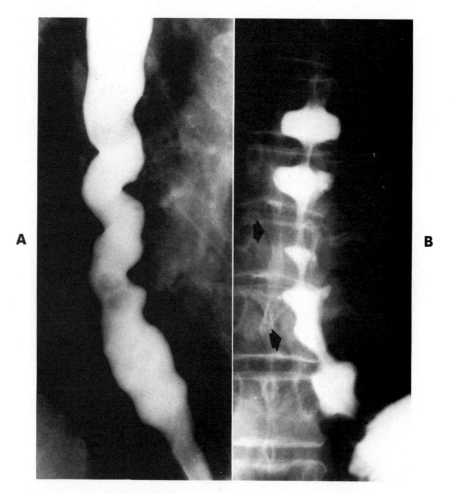

Fig. 5-6 Different types of nonpropulsive esophageal contractions. **A,** Radiographic appearance of "curling" or "corkscrew" esophagus in patient with presbyesophagus. Helix configuration suggests possible shortening of spiral esophageal muscle. **B,** Esophageal segmentation in patient with diffuse esophageal spasm. Nonpropulsive, segmental contractions produce multiple areas of pronounced luminal narrowing alternating with areas of sacculation. This pattern causes transient functional obstruction. Esophageal wall *(arrows)* is thickened by muscle hypertrophy.

present, an abnormal response occurs about 2 to 5 minutes after injection (Fig. 5-7, *A*). On manometry, a positive response consists of a sustained contraction of more than 25 mm Hg. For the radiographic examination the patient is placed in the recumbent position and the esophagus is filled with barium. A positive response is seen as active, nonperistaltic contractions that culminate in a sustained lumen-obliterating contraction in the distal one half to two thirds of the esophagus. Any significant side effects such a chest pain can be rapidly relieved by an intravenous injection of atropine.

Abnormal sphincter function associated with esophageal motility disorders is usually confined to the LES; however, *UES functional abnormalities* may occur. The UES may demonstrate increased or decreased resting pressure or abnormal relaxation. Abnormal UES relaxation or compliance is reflected as incomplete UES opening and abnormal esophageal drainage. Frank UES incompetence is rare and has been observed primarily in a few patients with myotonia congenita. Abnormal UES function is nearly always associated with significant disturbances of pharyngeal motor function.

LES functional abnormalities show four patterns on manometry: (1) absent or incomplete relaxation, (2) low resting pressure (hypotensive sphincter), (3) increased resting pressure (hypertensive sphincter), and (4) abnormal peristaltic contractions. Absent or incomplete LES relaxation is seen as abnormal LES opening on radiographs (Fig. 5-8). In this case barium accumulates above the sphincter until the resting pressure is trans-

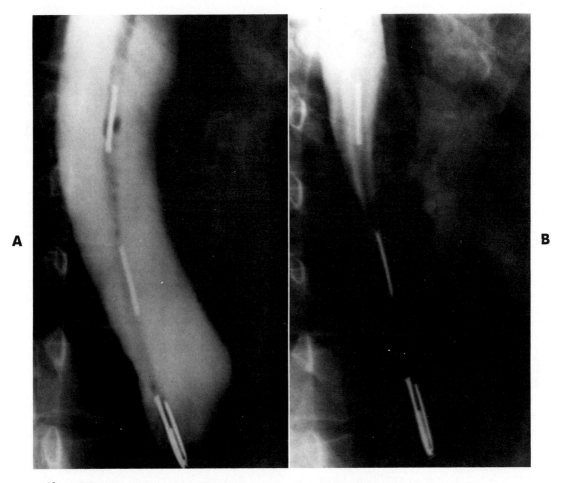

Fig. 5-7 Positive methacholine (Mecholyl) test on radiographic examination. Mercury markers are within monometric tube. Patient is recumbent. **A,** Before methacholine administration, dilated esophagus is filled with barium. **B,** After administration of methacholine, distal esophagus undergoes forceful lumen-obliterating contraction that displaces all of barium from distal esophagus.

mitted to the column by an advancing peristaltic wave or until hydrostatic forces overcome the resistance of the incompletely relaxed sphincter. Barium then wedges the sphincter open slightly and dribbles or squirts into the stomach. In a recumbent patient without normal esophageal body motor activity, swallowed barium often does not traverse the LES, even when the sphincter is relaxed. It is therefore difficult to determine whether a narrowed sphincter lumen is caused by incomplete relaxation, failed relaxation, localized stricture, or tumor infiltration. Testing with the smooth muscle relaxant amyl nitrite may help to distinguish abnormal LES relaxation from mechanical narrowing.

The radiographic examination is a relatively insensitive method for identifying significant gastroesophageal reflux, and negative results may be misleading.

Primary motility disorders
Achalasia

Clinical symptoms of achalasia develop insidiously, usually in patients between 30 and 50 years of age. No sex predilection exists. The predominant symptom is dysphagia, which is often initially intermittent but later becomes persistent. Additional symptoms include foul breath, regurgitation, and aspiration. It is thought that achalasia is caused mainly by an impairment or absence of ganglion cells of Auerbach's plexus. Such findings, however, are not always present, and electron microscopy has shown degenerative vagal nerve changes and decreased cell bodies in the medullary dorsal motor nucleus. The response to Mecholyl is nearly always positive, but a positive response may also occur in some patients with diffuse esophageal spasm, Chagas' disease, pseudoobstruction syndrome, and other entities.

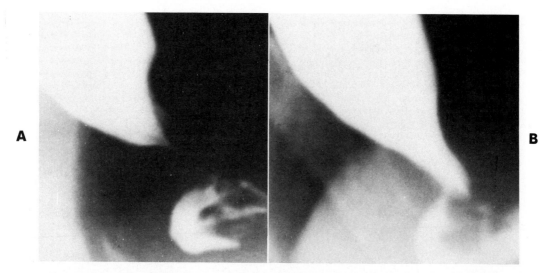

Fig. 5-8 Achalasia. **A,** Failure of normal lower sphincter opening produces persistent V configuration of head of barium column, above sphincter. **B,** Point of V elongates (bird-beak appearance) as barium wedges into sphincter and squirts into stomach.

On radiographic examination, peristalsis is typically absent in the entire esophageal body, but in some patients peristalsis may progress to the aortic arch level. A stripping wave in the proximal few centimeters of the cervical esophagus occurs in about one third of patients who otherwise fulfill all criteria for classic achalasia. Nonperistaltic esophageal body contractions occurring spontaneously, after swallows, or both, may be a predominant finding, especially when esophageal dilatation is mild to moderate. This variation is sometimes termed *vigorous achalasia.* With severe dilatation, or *megaesophagus,* the esophagus is usually atonic (Fig. 5-9).

As mentioned, when the LES does not relax normally, it fails to open normally after a swallow of barium and the barium remains above the closed sphincter until pressure transmitted through the fluid column by esophageal contractions or hydrostatic forces overcomes the resistance of the unrelaxed sphincter. The LES is then wedged open, and barium dribbles or squirts into the stomach through the narrow sphincter lumen (see Fig. 5-8).

A constricting annular carcinoma extending from the gastric fundus may cause motor abnormalities in the esophageal body (caused by high-grade obstruction or tumor infiltration of the esophageal wall, which can damage nerves). This condition *(pseudoachalasia)* so closely simulates achalasia that the true diagnosis is not established until the time of Heller's myotomy. The LES region may take on a bird-beak appearance, mimicking that of achalasia.

Diffuse esophageal spasm

Diffuse esophageal spasm is a clinical syndrome characterized by (1) symptoms of intermittent dysphagia and chest pain; (2) forceful, simultaneous, repetitive contractions on manometry; (3) segmental, lumen-obliterating contractions seen on radiographs (see Fig. 5-6, *B*); and (4) thickening of the esophageal wall. When this syndrome occurs without obvious cause, it is termed idiopathic *diffuse esophageal spasm (DES).* A DES pattern may sometimes result from esophagitis. Dysphagia and pain are characteristically intermittent and are frequently elicited by eating, particularly when swallowing a large bolus.

On radiographic examination peristalsis may occur in the upper esophagus in response to some or all swallows. All nonperistaltic contractions are observed in the smooth-muscle part of the esophagus. Lumen-obliterating nonperistaltic contractions often cause compartmentalization of swallows of barium (see Fig. 5-6, *B*), resulting in a *shish kebab esophageal configuration* and functional obstruction. As the contractions relax, the barium may resume a columnar configuration, only to be disrupted again and again by repetitive contractions. Esophageal wall thickening of 5 mm or more may be seen on radiographs of good quality.

Hypertensive peristalsis

In symptomatic, hypertensive peristalsis, often termed the *nutcracker esophagus,* the fluoroscopic appearance of peristaltic transport of barium appears en-

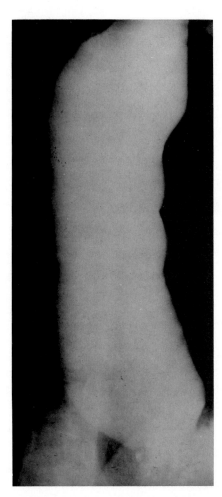

Fig. 5-9 Megaesophagus in patient with achalasia.

esophagus. These findings mimic those of achalasia, and the Mecholyl test gives positive findings.

Presbyesophagus

Presbyesophagus is esophageal motor dysfunction associated with aging. About 20% to 50% of elderly individuals manifest some aberration of esophageal motor function, but these individuals are generally without any esophageal symptoms. The proposed underlying cause is a decreased number of esophageal ganglion cells associated with aging, although some investigators suggest that the primary defect may be muscle atrophy rather than abnormal innervation. Muscle thickness, however, is reported to be normal in the aged.

On radiographic examination a spectrum of abnormalities may be observed. Occasionally no peristaltic activity is identified, and tertiary contractions (see Fig. 5-6, *A*) or other forms of nonperistaltic contractions often involve a long segment of the distal esophagus. Presbyesophagus may mimic achalasia, diffuse esophageal spasm, connective tissue disorders, or other motility disturbances.

Tracheoesophageal fistula

Children with *congenital tracheoesophageal (TE) fistula and esophageal atresia* generally have a primary abnormality of esophageal motor function, and as a result often suffer from aspiration and dysphagia despite successful surgery. Radiographic and manometric studies demonstrate a discontinuity of normal peristaltic function in a 5- to 15-cm esophageal segment that extends above and below the surgical anastomosis. Children with an *H-type TE fistula* commonly have similar abnormal esophageal motor dysfunction.

Chalasia

On radiographic examination some reflux of barium associated with crying or belching is commonly observed in newborn infants. Copious reflux in the newborn, or moderate reflux after 4 to 6 weeks of age, however, is abnormal. Chalasia is a condition in neonates characterized by repetitive episodes of vomiting and cardioesophageal relaxation. Many of these infants have an associated hiatus hernia. Gastroesophageal reflux in such infants is associated with transient relaxation of the LES.

Secondary motility disorders
Connective tissue disorders

The association of esophageal motor dysfunction and connective tissue disease is documented best for *scleroderma (systemic sclerosis),* a condition that affects women three times as often as men. Atrophy of esoph-

tirely normal and the diagnosis must be made by manometry. Some individuals with hypertensive esophageal peristalsis exhibit intermittent findings of DES.

Idiopathic intestinal pseudoobstruction

Chronic idiopathic intestinal pseudoobstruction (CIIP) is a rare syndrome characterized by symptoms and radiographic findings of intestinal obstruction in the absence of a mechanical obstruction or known underlying cause of paralytic ileus. Esophageal motor function abnormalities similar to those of achalasia are commonly present. These heterogeneous abnormalities tend to affect most if not all of the alimentary tract. The condition is commonly hereditary, and patients may be of either sex. Some patients have abnormal peristalsis and feeble nonperistaltic contractions in the smooth-muscle part of the esophagus. Others demonstrate abnormal LES opening caused by incomplete LES relaxation and forceful nonperistaltic contractions in the thoracic

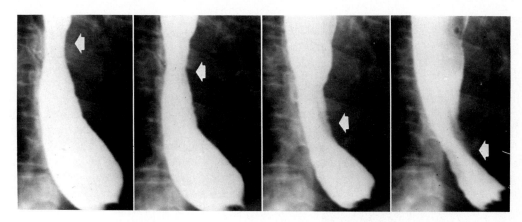

Fig. 5-10 Patient with scleroderma. Feeble, non–lumen obliterating peristaltic contraction wave *(arrows)* is seen to pass through distal esophagus. Esophageal peristalsis was normal above aortic arch level.

ageal smooth muscle is the predominant histologic abnormality. Fibrosis, when present, appears to replace the atrophic smooth muscle. Findings of reflux esophagitis are common. Peristalsis is feeble (Fig. 5-10) or absent in the distal two thirds of the esophagus, and an atonic LES commonly loses it ability to prevent gastroesophageal reflux. When the motility disturbance is mild, the only abnormality is a reduced incidence of primary peristalsis. With moderate impairment the amplitude of peristaltic complexes is low, thereby allowing retrograde escape of barium. On occasion nonperistaltic contractions occur. With severe impairment the thoracic esophagus becomes essentially amotile. Abnormal peristalsis in the proximal, striated muscle portion of the esophageal segment has been reported but is unusual.

On radiographic examination peristalsis nearly always appears normal above the level of the aortic arch, but below this level abnormal function is observed in about 70% of patients. Primary peristalsis may be decreased in incidence, and the contractile wave may appear feeble. The latter finding is seen as a non–lumen obliterating contraction that moves aborally but allows a substantial portion of the barium bolus to escape proximally (see Fig. 5-10). Subtle abnormalities in peristalsis may be unmasked by positioning the patient in a 30- to 50-degree head-down position, which forces peristalsis to work against gravity. When the motor disorder is severe, the amotile distal esophagus may become distended, but esophageal dilatation is generally mild to moderate. Barium pools in the esophagus of the supine patient but readily empties into the stomach when the patient is positioned upright. The LES may be patulous, and free gastroesophageal reflux is often observed. A hiatus hernia and radiographic features of esophagitis are commonly present.

Abnormal esophageal motility may occur with connective tissue diseases other than scleroderma, such a *systemic lupus erythematosus, Raynaud's disease,* or *dermatomyositis.* Disturbed esophageal motility accompanying lupus or Raynaud's disease may be similar in pattern to that of scleroderma. In contrast, dermatomyositis often causes abnormal function of the pharynx or proximal striated muscle part of the esophagus.

Reflux (peptic) esophagitis

Abnormal esophageal motor function is common in patients with reflux esophagitis. Functional abnormalities, generally confined to the smooth muscle portion of the esophagus, include abnormal peristalsis, nonperistaltic contractions, and gastroesophageal reflux. The prevalence of abnormal esophageal motor function correlates with the severity of the esophagitis.

On radiographic examination, motor disturbances include (1) a decreased incidence of peristalsis, (2) breaking of the peristaltic wave in the distal esophagus, (3) nonperistaltic contractions, (4) amotility of the distal esophagus, and (5) gastroesophageal reflux. Motor function of the pharynx, UES, and striated esophageal muscle are almost invariably normal. The most common abnormality is that peristalsis propagates through the proximal esophagus but fails to traverse the entire esophagus. Impaired esophageal function often leads to delayed acid clearance.

Even with the use of vigorous stress maneuvers, fluoroscopic demonstration of gastroesophageal reflux is possible in only about 40% of patients who have endoscopic evidence of reflux esophagitis. Identification of gastroesophageal reflux is increased somewhat by employing the water syphon test, but at the expense of obtaining an unacceptably high incidence of positive findings in normal subjects. Radiographic demonstration of reproducible stress or free gastroesophageal reflux, found in 30% to 40% of patients with esophagitis, indicates a feeble LES.

Postvagotomy syndrome

Postoperative dysphagia is a recognized complication of bilateral vagotomy, particularly transthoracic truncal vagotomy. Swallowing difficulty is generally first noted 1 to 2 weeks after surgery when a diet of solid foods is started. In symptomatic patients radiographic examination generally shows narrowing of the distal esophagus and mild esophageal dilatation, a pattern suggestive of early achalasia. The dysphagia, caused by an esophageal hematoma or vagal denervation, usually remits spontaneously in several weeks to several months. Rarely, distal esophageal narrowing caused by fibrosis may persist and require bougienage or surgery.

Metabolic and endocrine disorders

Metabolic disorders such as *diabetes mellitus* and *chronic alcoholism,* particularly when associated with peripheral neuropathy, may cause abnormal esophageal motor function. On barium swallows the following abnormalities may be observed in either diabetics or alcoholics: (1) decreased incidence of peristalsis, (2) breaking of peristaltic waves in the proximal esophagus, (3) delayed esophageal emptying, and (4) nonpropulsive contractions.

The GI tract is a site of predilection for *amyloidosis.* Esophageal involvement may occur. Amyloid deposits in the esophageal musculature may cause loss of peristalsis and megaesophagus.

Abnormalities of esophageal peristalsis have also been noted in patients with *myxedema* or *hyperthyroidism.* Myxedema causes a decreased incidence of peristalsis. In some cases, thyrotoxicosis causes a pattern of diffuse esophageal spasm and abnormal relaxation of the UES.

Neuromuscular disease

Diseases affecting the *central nervous system* cause significant disturbances of esophageal function when the supranuclear pathways to the medullary brain stem swallow centers are impaired bilaterally. Diseases such as *parkinsonism, Huntington's chorea,* and *Wilson's disease* may also cause abnormal esophageal function. Patients with parkinsonism, for example, may have a decreased incidence of peristalsis, complete loss of peristalsis, or nonperistaltic contractions. Patients with *extrapyramidal diseases* often exhibit difficulty initiating swallowing, as well as unintentional tremors of the tongue that decrease or disappear during swallowing.

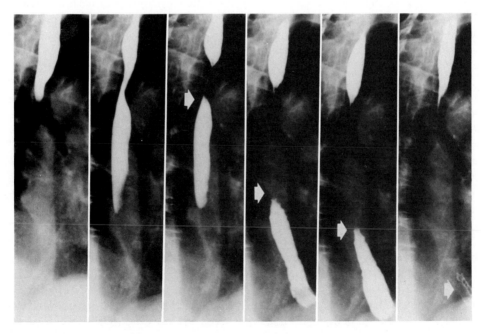

Fig. 5-11 Myasthenia gravis. Patient is supine. After single swallow, barium distributes in proximal two thirds of esophagus *(frames 1 and 2).* No peristalsis occurs in striated muscle esophageal segment; consequently, barium pools in upper esophagus. Secondary peristaltic wave *(arrows),* originating at level of aortic arch *(frame 3),* sweeps barium from arch level into stomach.

Although primary muscle diseases such as *myotonia* and *muscular* and *oculopharyngeal dystrophy* may cause motor dysfunction limited to the proximal, striated-muscle esophageal segment, motor dysfunction may also occur in the distal, smooth-muscle portion of the esophagus. In patients with myotonic dystrophy, the UES may be incompetent. With myotonia, motor function may improve during repetitive swallows. Esophageal dysfunction caused by *myasthenia gravis* is generally limited to the proximal striated-muscle portion of the esophagus (Fig. 5-11). During repeated swallows peristalsis in the upper esophagus often becomes feeble or disappears completely. Myasthenia is the only disease in which esophageal dysfunction may improve with administration of a cholinesterase inhibitor, such as edrophonium chloride (Tensilon test).

Miscellaneous disorders

A characteristic motility disturbance is present only in *Chagas' disease,* which is endemic to areas of South America. The disease, caused by *Trypanosoma cruzi,* damages ganglion cells in the esophageal musculature. The response to Mecholyl is often positive. On barium examination, Chagas' disease and idiopathic achalasia are generally indistinguishable.

Monilial esophagitis is commonly accompanied by loss of peristalsis in most or all of the esophagus. Peristaltic function generally returns after successful treatment, unless an underlying motility disorder is present.

After ingestion of a caustic substance the esophagus often demonstrates motor shock initially, with loss of peristaltic function. Peristalsis may return after several days, only to be subsequently obliterated if substantial fibrosis occurs.

A variety of drugs affect esophageal motor activity. Most general anesthetics nonselectively depress motor function of the entire esophagus. Anticholinergics, such as atropine, diminish or abolish peristalsis in the distal esophagus and decrease resting LES pressure. Glucagon decreases LES pressure but has negligible effect on motor function of the esophageal body, and in this author's opinion does not elicit GE reflux, as has been suggested by some other authors.

Differential diagnosis

Consideration of the predominant motor abnormality may be helpful in approaching the correct cause of an esophageal motility disorder; in addition, evaluation of the entire GI tract may provide clues about the nature of the esophageal motor abnormality. For example, abnormalities of the small bowel or colon are generally observed in scleroderma, idiopathic intestinal pseudoobstruction, Chagas' disease, amyloidosis, and myotonic dystrophy.

Esophageal dilatation

Severe esophageal dilatation (see Fig. 5-9) (megaesophagus) is usually caused by idiopathic achalasia. Other causes include Chagas' disease, idiopathic intestinal pseudoobstruction, amyloidosis, Ehlers-Danlos syndrome, and presbyesophagus. Tumor infiltration or fibrosis of the cardia must also be considered.

Abnormal peristalsis (proximal esophagus)

Focal feeble or absent peristalsis in the proximal esophagus occurs in diseases that predominantly affect striated muscle (myotonic dystrophy, muscular dystrophy, myasthenia gravis, and dermatomyositis), in neurologic disorders involving the brain stem (poliomyelitis and amyotrophic lateral sclerosis), and in tracheoesophageal fistula.

Abnormal peristalsis (distal esophagus)

Feeble or absent peristalsis in the distal two thirds or smooth-muscle part of the esophagus characteristically occurs in scleroderma but may also be found in other connective tissue disorders and in miscellaneous other conditions such as esophagitis, presbyesophagus, alcoholism, diabetes, idiopathic intestinal pseudoobstruction, myxedema, variants of achalasia, and with anticholinergic medication. Motor dysfunction of the distal esophageal body caused by esophagitis is generally accompanied by gastroesophageal reflux, and usually a hiatus hernia is present. Idiopathic intestinal pseudoobstruction syndrome will invariably have abnormal findings of the stomach or intestine.

Nonpropulsive contractions

A large number of esophageal disorders are characterized by infrequent nonpropulsive esophageal contractions, but such contractions may be seen in persons without disorders as well. Vigorous, repetitive, nonpropulsive contractions are clearly abnormal. They occur most commonly in diffuse esophageal spasm; other causes include esophagitis and presbyesophagus, but these contractions may also be found in achalasia, scleroderma, metabolic disorders, neuromuscular diseases, and esophageal obstruction.

Abnormal lower esophageal sphincter opening

Abnormal LES opening may be caused by absent or incomplete LES relaxation (see Fig. 5-8), infiltrating neoplasm, benign stricture, or hematoma. Failure of LES relaxation characteristically occurs in idiopathic achalasia and Chagas' disease.

Gastroesophageal reflux

Copious free reflux is rare in healthy individuals. Free gastroesophageal reflux is usually accompanied by

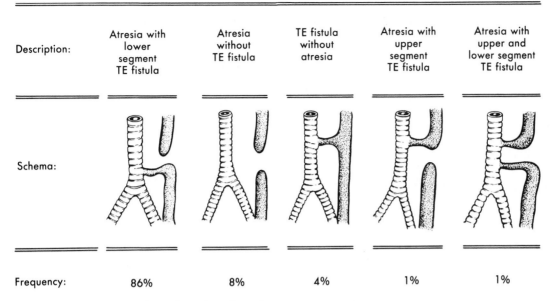

Description:	Atresia with lower segment TE fistula	Atresia without TE fistula	TE fistula without atresia	Atresia with upper segment TE fistula	Atresia with upper and lower segment TE fistula
Schema:					
Frequency:	86%	8%	4%	1%	1%

Fig. 5-12 Types of TE fistulas and esophageal atresia.

a hiatus hernia and, in addition to reflux and peptic esophagitis, is associated with Barrett's esophagus, scleroderma, brain damage, repaired esophageal atresia, and anticholinergic medication.

CONGENITAL ANOMALIES
Atresia and tracheoesophageal fistula

The incidence is about 1 in 2000 live births. Infants with esophageal atresia and TE fistula to the distal esophageal segment often develop gaseous abdominal distention, whereas those with atresia alone or TE fistula to the proximal esophagus have a gasless abdomen (Fig. 5-12). In some cases, an identifiable dilated proximal esophageal pouch may be sufficiently distended with air to compress the trachea. Definitive diagnosis is established by the inability to pass a nasogastric tube into the stomach. If necessary, 0.5 to 1 ml of thin barium can be injected into the pouch for visualization and then aspirated. After resection of the atresia and anastomosis of the esophagus, some children demonstrate subsequent narrowing at the anastomotic site. Peristalsis is invariably absent over a long central esophageal segment or occasionally in the entire esophagus.

H-type TE fistulas (Fig. 5-13) are frequently not diagnosed until late infancy or early childhood. The cardinal feature is recurrent unexplained pneumonia. A clue to the presence of an H-type fistula, however, is absent peristalsis in the proximal half or middle third of the esophagus. For radiographic diagnosis, the esophagus should be intubated with a single-hole catheter and the infant positioned prone or on the side. Dilute barium is injected into the esophagus, beginning just above

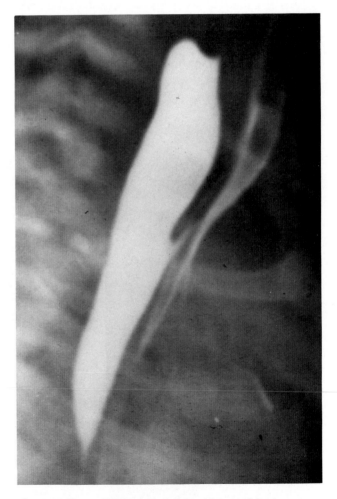

Fig. 5-13 H-type TE fistula in infant with unexplained pneumonia. H-type fistula is seen between proximal esophagus and trachea. Fistula generally takes diagonal course cephalad to join trachea.

the LES and progressing proximally. Most TE fistulas arise from the cervical esophagus and run diagonally cephalad to the trachea (see Fig. 5-13).

Duplication

Esophageal duplication, although rare, may cause either respiratory symptoms in infants (by compressing the trachea or rupturing into the esophageal lumen) or bleeding (by perforation, when it is lined by functional gastric mucosa). Most duplications are segmental and are generally located in the lower posterior mediastinum. There are two types of esophageal duplications: (1) *intramural cyst,* representing a true duplication arising from persistent vacuoles that normally reconstitute the esophageal lumen and (2) *neuroenteric cyst,* representing a foregut anomaly that persists as a remnant of the dorsal part of the notochord. The latter type is often associated with cervical and thoracic spinal abnormalities. On chest films esophageal duplications often appear as a round or oval posterior mediastinal mass. The cystic nature of the lesion is well visualized with CT examination.

Miscellaneous congenital anomalies

Other congenital esophageal malformations include muscle hypertrophy, stenosis, diaphragms, webs, carti-

lage rings, short esophagus, bronchoesophageal fistula, and laryngotracheal esophageal cleft. All these anomalies are rare. Congenital *bronchoesophageal fistulas* usually originate from lobar or segmental bronchi and may be associated with pulmonary sequestration. A unifying concept suggests that intralobar or extralobar pulmonary sequestrations with or without gastroesophageal communication and esophageal bronchogenic duplications are all bronchopulmonary foregut malformations caused by a supernumerary lung bud.

ESOPHAGEAL DIVERTICULA

Esophageal diverticula (Fig. 5-14) are acquired rather than congenital and virtually never occur during childhood. They seldom develop before age 40, after which point the incidence increases in frequency with age. They are more accurately called *pseudodiverticula,* with mucosal eventration or herniation through the muscularis. *Zenker's diverticula* originate just proximal to the UES and are properly classified as *pharyngeal diverticula.* Although diverticula may develop anywhere in the esophagus, they are most common in the middle and distal thirds. Fluoroscopic observations suggest that nearly all esophageal diverticula, regardless of location, are caused by pulsion as opposed to traction forces. Only a small percentage of diverticula in the mid-

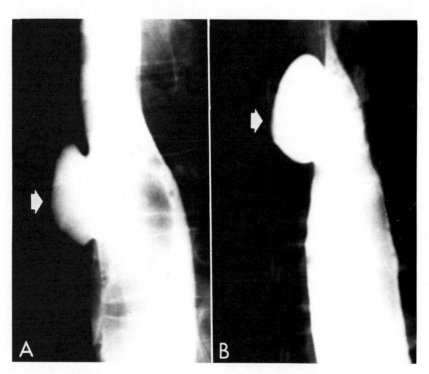

Fig. 5-14 Pulsion diverticulum of midesophagus. **A,** At onset of swallowing, barium demonstrates smooth 2 × 3 cm diverticulum *(arrow)* located near carina. **B,** During esophageal peristalsis, diverticulum makes substantial oral excursion without evidence of distortion caused by traction.

esophagus are conic, have no neck, and may be caused by traction. In addition to normal wear-and-tear processes, underlying motility disorders, such as achalasia, diffuse esophageal spasm, and hypertensive peristalsis may cause esophageal diverticula. On barium swallows, small esophageal diverticula (0.5 to 2 cm in size) are commonly observed as transient outpouchings that develop only during peristalsis. Large diverticula, greater than 4 cm in size, commonly empty only by gravity. *Epiphrenic diverticula,* located just above the LES, generally project to the right, whereas diverticula elsewhere in the esophagus project in any direction except posteriorly. In about 10% to 20% of cases multiple diverticula are present, but they seldom number more than three.

Intramural pseudodiverticulosis

This condition has been detected in all age-groups but usually occurs in persons older than 50 years of age. Originally called *esophageal intramural diverticu-* *losis,* the condition was renamed *pseudodiverticulosis* after studies showed that the outpouchings were dilated glands located interior to the muscularis. The underlying cause is unknown. Although cultured material often yields monilia, this simply represents secondary contamination in areas of stasis.

On esophagrams multiple cystic or flasklike pouches 1 to 3 mm in size are shown in a short esophageal segment (Fig. 5-15, *B*) or in some instances, over the entire length of the esophagus (Fig. 5-15, *A*). Most patients exhibit normal esophageal motor function.

TRAUMATIC LESIONS

Esophageal injury may be caused by an ingested foreign body, endoscopy, dilatation procedures, penetrating wounds, blunt trauma, or surgical procedures.

Foreign bodies

In the esophagus, flat objects such as coins are oriented in the coronal plane, in contrast to the sagittal ori-

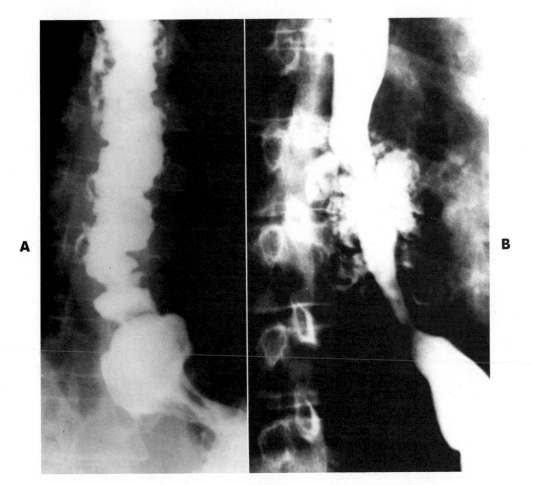

Fig. 5-15 Intramural esophageal pseudodiverticulosis. Numerous sacculations represent dilated esophageal glands. **A,** Diffuse involvement without evidence of stricture. Axial hiatus hernia is present. **B,** Segmental involvement accompanied by esophageal stricture.

entation of flat foreign bodies in the trachea. Cotton balls or marshmallows soaked in barium may be useful to demonstrate a small, hard-to-detect foreign body.

Esophageal perforation

Nearly all esophageal perforations are caused by trauma (Fig. 5-16, *A*). The most common causes are iatrogenic (endoscopy, dilatation procedures, or thoracotomy). Traumatic perforation also results from penetrating injuries such as missile or stab sounds, and occasionally from blunt compression when air is trapped in the esophagus. Even spontaneous esophageal rupture is caused by trauma associated with events such as severe vomiting. Nontraumatic esophageal perforation is generally caused by caustic ingestion or neoplasm. In adults about 75% of esophageal perforations occur during endoscopic examinations. The most frequent sites are adjacent to the cricopharyngeus and the distal esophagus. In infants perforations usually occur in the cervical esophagus and hypopharynx and are generally caused by the passage of tubes.

Spontaneous esophageal rupture, (Fig. 5-16, *B*) described by Boerhaave in 1724 and sometimes called a *Boerhaave rupture,* generally occurs in men and is usually associated with the abrupt onset of chest pain and shock, simulating a heart attack or dissecting aneurysm. The classic triad is vomiting, excruciating chest pain, and subcutaneous emphysema. In 10% to 20% of cases, the clinical onset is insidious and the diagnosis obscure. Neonatal esophageal perforation occurs predominantly

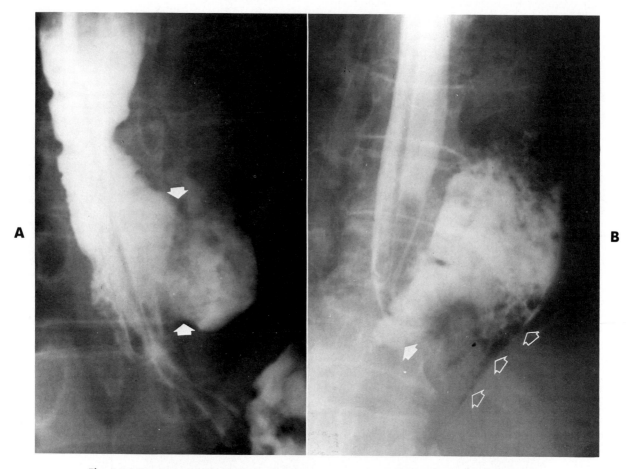

Fig. 5-16 Esophageal perforation. **A,** Achalasia patient immediately following pneumatic dilatation of LES segment. Injection of water-soluble contrast medium through esophageal tube shows perforation, about 4 cm in length *(arrows),* along left lateral wall of distal esophagus. **B,** Spontaneous esophageal rupture caused by vomiting (Boerhaave's syndrome). Injection of water-soluble contrast medium demonstrates characteristic esophageal tear *(closed arrow),* about 2 cm in length, located along left lateral margin of distal esophagus. Contrast medium enters golf ball–size space within lower mediastinum. Air has escaped into mediastinum and dissected beneath parietal pleura of left hemidiaphragm *(open arrows).* This later feature contributes to V sign of Nacleiro.

in girls. Dyspnea and cyanosis associated with a right tension pneumothorax occur shortly after birth.

The inciting incident for a Boerhaave rupture may be forceful vomiting, straining, childbirth, or a blunt blow to the abdomen or thorax. The ruptures are vertical tears 1 to 4 cm long. About 90% occur along the left posterolateral wall of the distal esophagus, where the esophagus is not supported by adjacent mediastinal structures. Abnormal radiographic findings include pneumomediastinum, mediastinal widening, and cervical emphysema. Fluid and gas in the mediastinal pocket may give a soft tissue density that is easily confused with a hiatus hernia or epiphrenic diverticulum. A V-shaped radiolucency seen through the heart (*Nacleiro sign*) represents gas in the left lower mediastinum that dissects under the left diaphragmatic pleura. In neonatal esophageal rupture, pneumomediastinum is relatively uncommon. For direct visualization of the esophagus, a water-soluble contrast medium should be used, followed by barium if gross perforation is not demonstrated initially.

Miscellaneous lesions

Abrupt esophageal distention associated with sudden increases in esophageal pressure may cause incomplete tears limited to the esophageal mucosa *(Mallory-Weiss syndrome)*. Mallory-Weiss tears are rarely demonstrated on an esophagram, but the bleeding site may be shown on selective celiac arteriography. The bleeding usually stops spontaneously, but a vasopressin (Pitressin) infusion is often helpful.

Mucosal tears caused by overdistention, endoscopy, or foreign bodies occasionally give rise to a *double-channel esophagus* (Fig. 5-17).

HIATUS HERNIA

Hiatus hernias are divided into two types: (1) *axial hernia,* in which a loculus of stomach and the gastric cardia pass through the hiatus into the thorax and (2) *periesophageal hernia,* in which a portion of the stomach herniates through the hiatus but the cardia remains normally located. In adults the prevalence of hiatus hernia increases with age. A hiatus hernia as such is seldom accompanied by clinical symptoms unless associated with reflux esophagitis or complicated by bleeding or strangulation.

Radiologic examination is the best method for demonstrating a hiatus hernia. Adequate examination depends on inspection of esophageal function, as well as morphology and obtaining maximal esophageal distention during the examination. Relevant radiologic landmarks include the diaphragmatic hiatus, esophagogastric junction, LES segment, and loculus of herniated stomach (Fig. 5-18). The level of the hiatus should not be judged by the observed level of the left hemidiaphragm. The thin ringlike structure (Fig. 5-18, *A*) often seen at the esophagogastric junction is a passive ring caused by a transverse mucosal fold, whereas the thicker ring (Fig. 5-18, *B*) sometimes present at the upper margin of the sphincter segment is caused by active muscle contraction. These mucosal and muscle rings define the margins of the LES and are recognized by their function, as well as their morphology. Normally the peristaltic stripping wave passes through the area of the muscle ring but stops at the esophagogastric junction. Some axial hernias exhibit a prominent notch caused by the gastric sling fibers looping around the gastroesophageal junction. This appearance should not be mistaken for a paraesophageal hernia.

Paraesophageal hernias are uncommon, usually detected as an incidental finding, and do not have any association with reflux esophagitis.

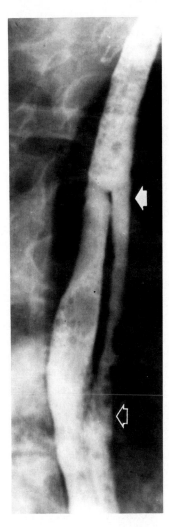

Fig. 5-17 Double-barrel esophagus. False channel *(open arrow)* caused by trauma from endoscopy recommunicates distally *(closed arrow)* to form double-barrel esophagus.

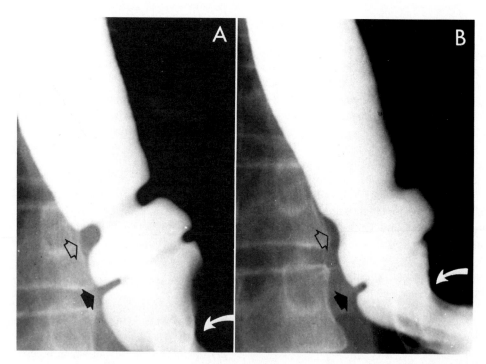

Fig. 5-18 Small axial hiatus hernia. Diaphragmatic hiatus causes mild constriction *(curved arrow)* of portion of stomach within hiatus. Thin mucosal ring *(closed arrow)* is seen at esophagogastric junction, whereas thick muscle ring *(open arrow)* demarcates upper margin of lower esophageal sphincter segment from tubular esophageal body. Muscle ring is contracted in **A,** but relaxes a few seconds later, in **B.** Mucosal fold at esophagogastric junction shows no change. Herniated portion of stomach does not contract as part of esophageal peristaltic sequence.

After surgical repair of an axial hiatus hernia, a *fundoplication defect* (a pseudotumor caused by a fundoplication) may exist in the gastric fundus. This defect is more pronounced for the complete wrap of the Nissen procedure than with the partial wrap of the Belsey procedure. With a split plication the defect may disappear or a complete wrap may slide downward over the stomach *(slipped Nissen),* thereby giving the stomach an hourglass configuration.

ESOPHAGITIS
Gastroesophageal reflux disease

Gastroesophageal reflux disease (GERD) encompasses reflux esophagitis and is characterized histologically by inflammatory cells and reflux changes consisting of epithelial hyperplasia without inflammation.

Heartburn is the most common symptom of gastroesophageal reflux; other symptoms are regurgitation, chest pain, respiratory complaints, and dysphagia. In young children, the predominant reflux symptoms are regurgitation, repetitive vomiting, and failure to thrive. Radiographic assessment of gastroesophageal reflux requires 300 to 500 ml of barium in the stomach. Reflux is sought while the patient rolls from the prone to the supine or from the supine to the right lateral position and during stress maneuvers—such as Trendelenburg, Valsalva, and leg raising—performed with the patient supine. The double-contrast examination for subtle morphologic abnormalities may be done before or after the single-contrast study.

Morphologic findings of peptic esophagitis include irregularity of luminal contour (Fig. 5-19), a granular mucosal pattern, discrete ulcerations, transverse esophageal folds (Fig. 5-20), thickened longitudinal folds, esophageal wall thickening (Fig. 5-21), and segmental narrowing. Although not specific, the finding of transverse esophageal ridging or folds (see Fig. 5-20), known as *felinization,* suggests the presence of esophagitis. Morphologic abnormalities usually are absent in case of mild superficial esophagitis, but are present in 80% to 90% of patients with moderate to severe esophagitis proved on endoscopy.

Even with the use of vigorous stress maneuvers, gastroesophageal reflux is demonstrated in only about 40% of patients. This low sensitivity of the x-ray examination for demonstrating GE reflux is because the under-

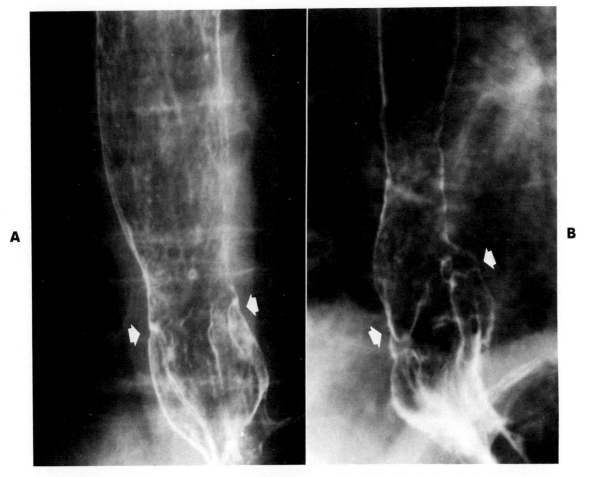

Fig. 5-19 Double-contrast esophagrams in two patients with esophagitis. **A,** Level of esophagogastric junction is indicated by arrows. Small hiatus hernia is present. Esophagitis causes stippled, granular appearance of barium. **B,** Arrows indicate esophagogastric junction. Small hiatus hernia is present. Distal esophagus is narrowed and has irregular contour.

lying mechanism for GE reflux is general transient LES relaxation (Fig. 5-22). Esophageal motor function is abnormal in up to 50% of patients with reflux esophagitis, and a hiatus hernia is present in most patients with severe disease. In a minority of patients, a sliding hiatus hernia may be caused by esophageal shortening. Severe forms of reflux esophagitis may be observed occasionally in association with repeated vomiting, anesthesia, nasogastric intubation, and Zollinger-Ellison syndrome (Fig. 5-23).

Barrett's esophagus

Partial lining of the esophagus by columnar-type epithelium (referred to as *Barrett's esophagus*) reflects an adaptive alteration caused by chronic reflux esophagitis. Many patients have active esophagitis of the squamous epithelium, proximal to the zone of columnar epithelium. The columnar esophageal epithelium has a predilection to develop adenocarcinoma.

Patients with Barrett's esophagus are generally older than 40 years of age and may have heartburn, dysphagia, or upper GI tract bleeding. On radiographic examination, most Barrett's patients demonstrate a hiatus hernia, gastroesophageal reflux, or both. The diagnosis should be suspected when a punched-out esophageal ulcer (Fig. 5-24) that resembles a gastric ulcer in morphology is found, or when an unexplained stricture is observed in the middle esophagus (Fig. 5-25) or proximal esophagus. Most patients with Barrett's esophagus, however, do not have either of these findings. A segmental reticular pattern of the esophageal mucosa is present in some patients. The diagnosis is made more often with the advent of esophagoscopy with biopsy.

Infectious esophagitis

Infectious causes of esophagitis include monilia (Fig. 5-26), herpes simplex, cytomegalic inclusion virus, tuberculosis, lactobacilli, cryptococcoses, blasto-

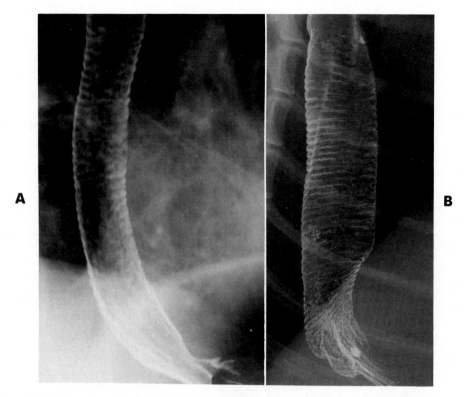

Fig. 5-20 Transverse esophageal folds. **A,** Patient with esophagitis. Well-defined transverse ridges, or folds, are seen in distal half of esophagus. This phenomenon has been termed *felinization* of esophagus. **B,** Cat esophagus demonstrating typical transverse folds present in this species.

mycosis, gram-negative bacteria, streptococci, mixed bacterial infections, and diphtheria. In most cases infectious esophagitis occurs in debilitated individuals; diabetics; immunosuppressed patients; or patients receiving steroids, antibiotics, radiotherapy, or chemotherapy. It is also increasingly more common in immunosuppressed patients and in individuals with impaired T-cell function from acquired immunodeficiency syndrome (AIDS). Typically the initial complaint is odynophagia, or painful swallowing, a symptom rarely encountered with reflux esophagitis.

Moniliasis

Candida albicans infections of the esophagus occur almost exclusively in debilitated patients; diabetics; alcoholics; or patients receiving steroids, immunosuppressants, cytotoxic drugs, or antibiotics. Moniliasis is a frequent companion of esophageal intramural pseudodiverticulosis. About half the patients with esophageal moniliasis also have *oral thrush*. Esophageal involvement generally occurs over a long segment (Fig. 5-26, *A*), and occasionally over the entire esopha-

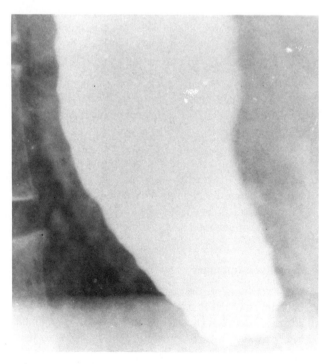

Fig. 5-21 Reflux esophagitis. Luminal contour of distal esophagus is irregular, and esophageal wall is thickened.

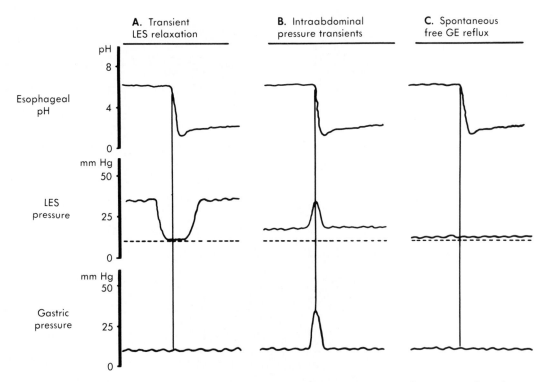

Fig. 5-22 Schematic representation of three general mechanisms responsible for gastroesophageal reflux. Esophageal pH was recorded from distal esophagus by pH electrode. Lower esophageal sphincter (LES) pressure and gastric pressure were recorded concurrently by manometry. Acid gastroesophageal reflux *(vertical line)* may accompany a transient LES relaxation **(A),** develop as stress reflux during transient increase in intraabdominal pressure that overcomes a sphincter with low tone **(B),** or occur as spontaneous free reflux across atonic sphincter **(C).**

(Reprinted by permission of The New England Journal of Medicine, from Dodds WJ et al: *N Engl J Med* 308:1547, 1982.)

gus. The luminal contour may show fine speculations, irregularity, a cobblestone pattern, or bizarre thickened folds simulating varices. Barium may dissect beneath a pseudomembrane, causing a shaggy contour that gives the appearance of ulceration. The esophagus tends to be atonic, and peristalsis may be feeble or incomplete. Because of muscular hypotonia, the esophagus is generally slightly dilated or normal in caliber but may show areas of moderate narrowing. In unusual cases esophageal moniliasis may appear as a solitary ulcer, and on occasion, ulcerated nodular lesions are present in the stomach. Moniliasis may sometimes cause localized masses that simulate carcinoma, segmental strictures, or even narrowing of the entire esophagus. The diagnosis is confirmed by histologic examination or culture of esophageal scrapings. Treatment with nystatin (Mycostatin) gives prompt relief of symptoms.

Viral esophagitis

The most common types of viral esophagitis are *herpes simplex virus type 1 (HSV1)* and *cytomegalovirus*

(CMV). Other types of viral esophagitis include coxsackievirus and retroviruses. HSV1 and CMV esophagitis generally occur as opportunistic infections in compromised patients, but may occur occasionally in otherwise normal individuals. Although odynophagia is the most common clinical symptom, gastrointestinal bleeding may be a prominent feature in hemorrhagic esophagitis.

The viral lesions of herpes esophagitis start initially as vesicles that quickly rupture to form clear punched-out ulcers with raised margins that are sharply marginated from a background of normal-appearing mucosa. The ulcers subsequently coalesce, become covered with debris, and may develop a pseudomembrane similar in appearance to that of moniliasis (see Fig. 5-26).

One to several discrete ulcers are seen against a normal mucosal background on radiographic examination. In an immunocompromised patient with odynophagia, this appearance is nearly pathognomonic for viral esophagitis, generally HSV1 or CMV. A large plaque-like esophageal ulcer in a patient with AIDS suggests

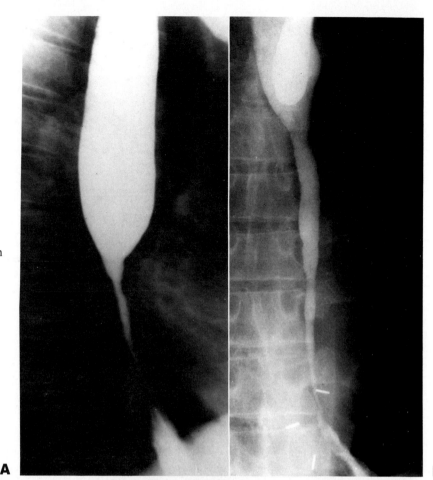

Fig. 5-23 Severe peptic strictures. **A,** Patient with indwelling nasogastric tube for 2 days after abdominal surgery. **B,** Patient with Zollinger-Ellison syndrome. Clips are from truncal vagotomy.

A

B

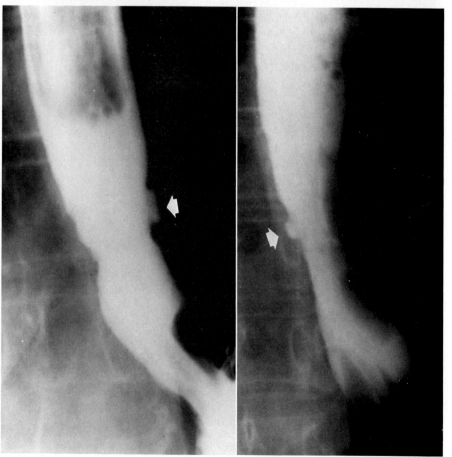

Fig. 5-24 Barrett's columnar-lined esophagus. Two patients with punched-out ulcers *(arrows)* in distal esophagus. Each patient had small hiatus hernia that is not well seen, and columnar epithelium was demonstrated in distal esophagus by biopsy.

A

B

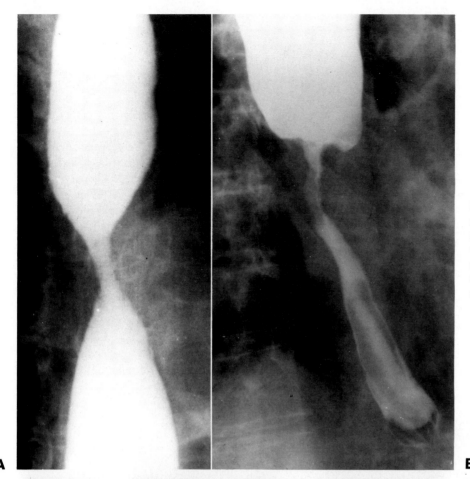

Fig. 5-25 Segmental esophageal narrowing. **A,** Benign stricture at aortic arch level in patient with Barrett's columnar-lined esophagus. **B,** Malignant stricture caused by squamous carcinoma of distal esophagus.

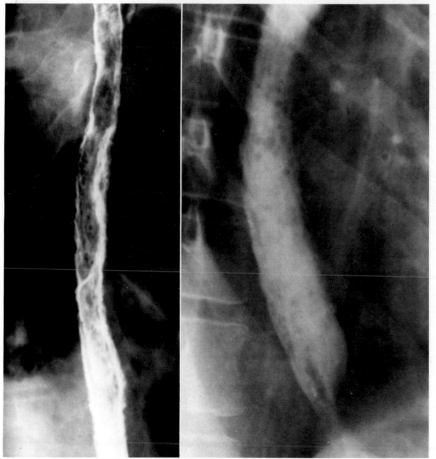

Fig. 5-26 Infectious esophagitis. **A,** Moniliasis. **B,** Herpes simplex. Both patients exhibit diffuse esophagitis of similar radiologic appearance.

the diagnosis of CMV. However, CMV may also appear as a superficial esophagitis with a granular mucosa accompanied by shallow erosions. Viral esophagitis is regional, particularly involving the middle third of the esophagus.

Tuberculosis

Tuberculous esophagitis is rare and is generally accompanied by evidence of tuberculosis in the lungs. Morphologic abnormalities are often eccentric and may show skip areas. Involvement can occur at any level, but the middle third of the esophagus is most commonly affected. The luminal contour may show mild irregularity, large or deep ulcers, and sinus tracts. Fistulas are common. The esophageal wall is generally thickened and the lumen often narrowed, sometimes with a masslike appearance that mimics carcinoma. Enlarged mediastinal nodes may displace or compress the esophagus and widen the mediastinum. A sinus tract accompanied by enlarged mediastinal nodes should suggest the diagnosis, although these findings may also occur with malignancy and less commonly with actinomycosis or syphilis.

Caustic esophagitis

Alkaline agents can produce deep coagulation necrosis in minutes. Necrosis from *acids* tends to be more superficial. In addition to esophageal injury, caustic agents may also produce burns of the pharynx and stomach. Initial clinical symptoms are the rapid onset of chest pain and dysphagia. Acute complications include shock, fever, respiratory distress, mediastinitis, and esophageal perforation. Late complications are related primarily to esophageal fibrosis and stricture, which may cause dysphagia several weeks after the initial injury. Mild injury generally heals without sequelae; moderate injury leads to stricture; severe injury causes acute complications.

The radiographic findings vary depending on the severity and extent of esophageal injury. During the first

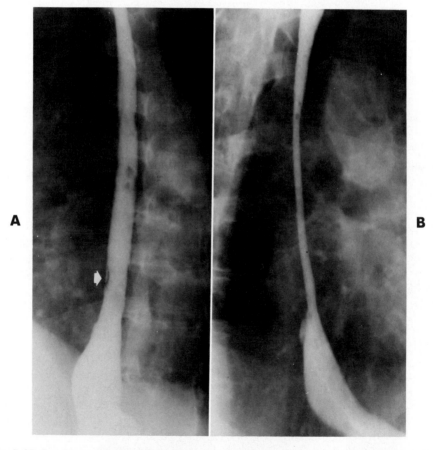

Fig. 5-27 Caustic esophagitis. **A,** Esophagram at 1 week after caustic ingestion shows moderate diffuse esophageal narrowing. In distal esophagus barium has dissected *(arrow)* beneath pseudomembrane. **B,** Esophagram 4 weeks after injury shows severe stricture involving almost entire esophagus.

24 hours the esophagus often appears normal after a mild insult, but with more severe injury may show blurred margins, contour irregularity, ulceration, or thickened folds. Long segments of esophagus are generally involved. Moderate to severe injury usually abolishes peristalsis. The esophagus is hypotonic and may trap air. In the acute stage the examination should be initiated with water-soluble contrast medium to exclude esophageal or gastric perforation; then barium may be used. During the first week an acute inflammatory response develops, and areas of significant injury show frank ulceration on esophagrams. By 2 to 6 weeks healing is well in progress, often accompanied by severe fibrosis (Fig. 5-27). Progressive narrowing of the esophageal lumen is common, heralded by the return or onset of dysphagia. The luminal contour may resume a smooth appearance after epithelial regeneration, but focal areas of submucosal fibrosis usually cause nodular defects or scalloping. Coexisting gastric involvement, primarily in the distal part of the stomach, may cause antral ulceration, pyloric stenosis, or frank gastric outlet obstruction.

Drug-induced esophagitis

Various drugs are reported to cause esophagitis. Antibiotics such as tetracycline and doxycycline are the most common offending agents. Quinidine, antiinflammatory drugs, guanidine, and potassium are additional likely candidates. Drug-induced esophagitis usually involves the proximal or middle esophagus, but occasionally involves the distal esophagus. A typical location is the aortic arch level, where passage of tablets is delayed because of the aortic indentation on the esophagus and the low contractile force of peristalsis. The radiographic findings consist of luminal irregularity, frank ulceration, and luminal narrowing. On occasion the findings may simulate esophageal carcinoma. The disease usually resolves after the offending agent is withdrawn, but in some instances a permanent stricture may develop.

Radiation esophagitis

Patients with radiation esophagitis usually receive 4500 to 6000 rads over a 6- to 8-week period. Patients receiving doxorubicin (Adriamycin), an agent that interferes with tissue repair, may develop symptoms at radiation doses of less than 2000 rads. The most common radiographic finding in symptomatic subjects is normal esophageal morphology; esophageal motor function, however, is generally abnormal. Esophageal peristalsis commonly stops in the proximal esophagus at the upper margin of the radiation field, and below this level it often degenerates into repetitive, nonperistaltic contractions. Morphologic abnormalities from radiation occasionally consist of diffuse ulceration that may cause

pain with swallowing and masquerade as moniliasis. Late findings consist of stricture in the radiation field. Such strictures are generally smooth with tapering margins and rarely show irregularity or ulceration. Mucosal bridging may occasionally occur.

Miscellaneous causes of esophagitis

Bullous dermatoses (including pemphigus, pemphigoid, epidermolysis bullosa dystrophica, toxic epidermal necrolysis, Stevens-Johnson syndrome, and graft-versus-host disease), noninfectious granulomatous disease, Behçet's disease, and ulcerative colitis may all be associated with esophagitis. Esophageal lesions consist of vesicles, bullae, desquamation, and ulcers. The lesions often heal without complication, but their repeated formation may lead to significant fibrosis and stenosis (Fig. 5-28). Whereas pemphigus and pemphigoid are nonhereditary conditions that occur in adults, epidermolysis bullosa dystrophica occurs as an autosomal recessive condition in children. During the acute stage of

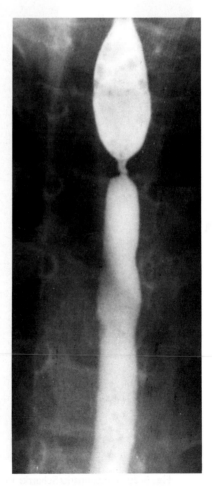

Fig. 5-28 Epidermolysis bullosa dystrophica. Weblike narrowing is seen in proximal esophagus.

ESOPHAGEAL VARICES

Generally, collateral venous flow is "uphill" toward the azygos vein and the superior vena cava. Esophageal varices are caused most commonly by portal hypertension, usually from hepatic cirrhosis. Sometimes varices are caused by prehepatic portal vein obstruction, posthepatic vein obstruction, or congestive heart failure. Varices in the absence of portal hypertension may occur when portal venous flow is increased because of splenic arteriovenous shunting associated with splenic hemangiomatosis or marked splenomegaly. Occasionally, "downhill" esophageal varices exist when the superior vena cava is obstructed distal to the entry of the azygos. *"Hepatofugal" varices* are usually associated with portal hypertension, whereas *"hepatopetal" varices* are present with occlusions of the splenic and/or portal veins. Variceal bleeding is generally abrupt in onset and massive, and small varices are as likely to bleed as large ones.

Standard preparations of liquid barium used for single-contrast esophagrams are often adequate to demonstrate varices. Better esophageal mucosal coating, however, is obtained using high-density liquid barium or barium paste preparations. Films of the barium-coated esophagus should be made with the esophagus collapsed, allowing variceal filling and optimal visualization of the esophageal folds. Because peristalsis transiently squeezes and flattens varices, a minimum of 15 to 20 seconds should elapse after esophageal peristalsis to allow variceal refilling before a radiograph is obtained. Overfilling of the esophagus tends to iron out and obscure the varices.

Multiple spot films should be taken of the collapsed esophagus in several different projections. The prone oblique position is standard. In some patients, however, the upright position enhances variceal filling. No single position or maneuver gives optimal results uniformly. Diagnostic yield is greatest when multiple spot films are

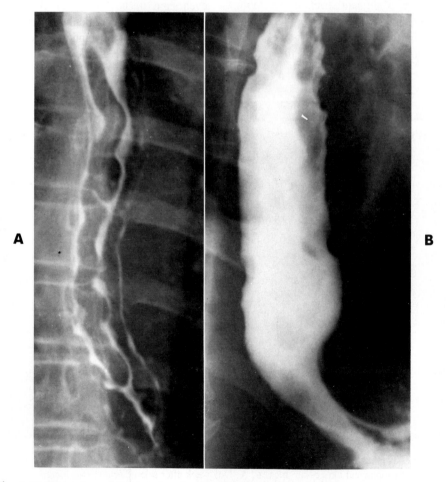

Fig. 5-33 Flagrant esophageal varices in two different patients. **A,** Mucosal view of collapsed esophagus demonstrates varices as serpiginous, slightly nodular filling defects when seen *en face.* **B,** Spot film of barium-filled esophagus. When seen tangentially, varices cause scalloped or modular contour to margin of barium column.

☐ **ESOPHAGEAL TUMORS** ☐

I. Malignant neoplasm
   A. Carcinomas
      1. Squamous
      2. Adenocarcinoma
      3. Carcinoid
   B. Sarcoma
      1. Leiomyosarcoma
      2. Fibrosarcoma
      3. Lymphoma
      4. Others
   C. Metastases

II. Benign neoplasm
   A. Mucosal
      1. Papilloma
      2. Adenoma
   B. Submucosal
      1. Leiomyoma
      2. Neurofibroma
      3. Hemangioma
      4. Fibroma
      5. Lipoma
      6. Myeloblastoma
      7. Hemangiopericytoma

III. Nonneoplastic
   A. Fibrovascular polyp
   B. Inflammatory polyp
   C. Cystic lesions
      1. Retention cyst
      2. Enteric cyst
      3. Duplication
   D. Solitary varix
   E. Focal infection
   F. Ectopic tissue
   G. Hamartoma
   H. Hematoma

---

obtained in several projections and different provocative maneuvers are used. Any fusiform separation of the folds suggests the presence of varices. More definite findings are beaded or serpiginous filling defects (Fig. 5-33) that characteristically change in size during the examination. Occasionally, a varicoid carcinoma may simulate esophageal varices, but varicoid carcinoma shows areas of rigidity and nodular filling defects that do not change in size or show compression by peristalsis.

ESOPHAGEAL TUMORS

Various neoplasms and nonneoplastic conditions cause mass lesions of the esophagus. Masses can be distinguished from an intraluminal foreign body by the fact that on radiographic examination an intraluminal impaction does not show any point of attachment with the esophageal wall. Epithelial lesions such as carcinoma generally have an irregular contour on tangential views, and often have undercut or shelflike margins. In contrast, submucosal tumors generally stretch the esophageal mucosa to form a symmetric, moundlike lesion with exquisitely smooth margins (Fig. 5-34). When seen tangentially, the margins of the lesion taper smoothly to form an obtuse angle with the normal esophageal wall. The estimated center of the mass falls close to or within the projection of the esophageal wall. The extrapolated center of the mass falls outside the esophageal wall.

Malignant esophageal tumors
Esophageal carcinomas

Carcinoma, the most common tumor of the esophagus, makes up about 4% of all GI tract malignancies.

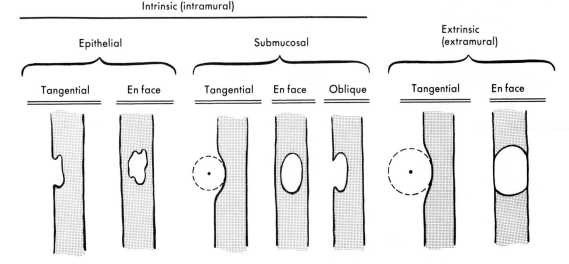

Fig. 5-34 Schematic representation of the three generic categories of polypoid esophageal filling defects.

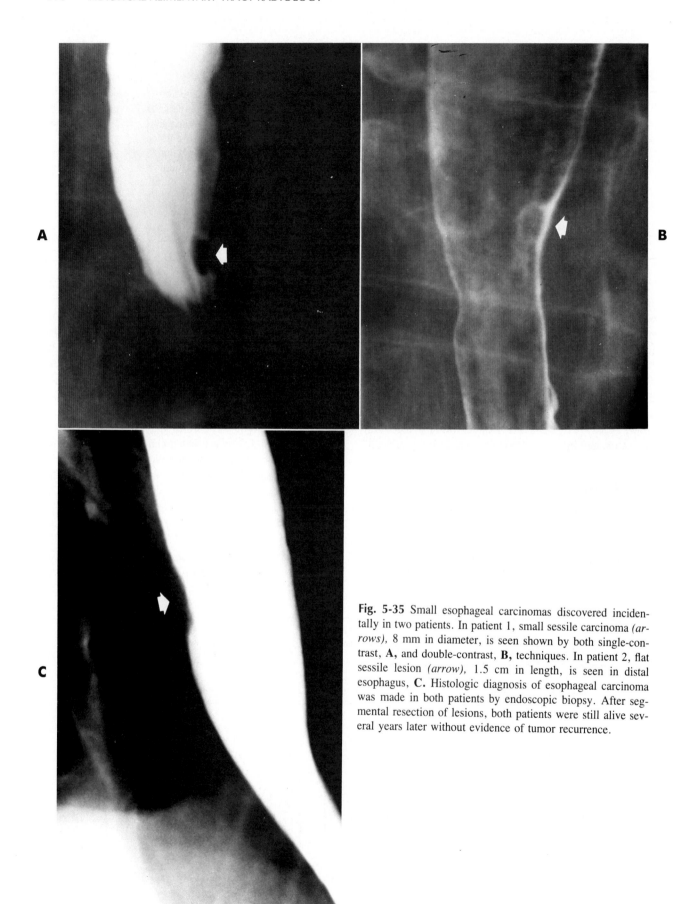

Fig. 5-35 Small esophageal carcinomas discovered incidentally in two patients. In patient 1, small sessile carcinoma *(arrows),* 8 mm in diameter, is seen shown by both single-contrast, **A,** and double-contrast, **B,** techniques. In patient 2, flat sessile lesion *(arrow),* 1.5 cm in length, is seen in distal esophagus, **C.** Histologic diagnosis of esophageal carcinoma was made in both patients by endoscopic biopsy. After segmental resection of lesions, both patients were still alive several years later without evidence of tumor recurrence.

Esophageal carcinoma generally occurs in men older than 50 years of age; patients at increased risk include those with Barrett's esophagus, caustic stricture, radiation stricture, achalasia, sprue, Plummer-Vinson syndrome, previous head or neck tumors, and hereditary tylosis. Other risk factors are alcohol consumption and smoking.

About 90% of esophageal carcinomas are of squamous cell origin. The remainder are adenocarcinomas that arise primarily in the distal esophagus. Although radiographs often show no abnormalities, mediastinal widening, a soft tissue mass, an esophageal gas-fluid level, anterior tracheal bowing, or a thickened retrotracheal stripe may be evident. On esophagrams, esophageal carcinoma presents a variety of morphologic abnormalities (see Fig. 5-31). Advanced tumors may appear as an annular apple-core lesion with overhanging margins, irregular narrowed segment, smooth tapering stricture, bulky endophytic mass, large ulceration, carcinoid infiltrate, or diffuse nodularity. Moderate-sized lesions, 1.5 to 3 cm, generally occur as lobulated sessile lesions that are eccentric and may show evidence of ulceration. Some lesions appear as an area of superficial irregularity or a flattened zone of decreased compliance. Small lesions of less than 1.5 cm (Fig. 5-35) may be seen as moundlike sessile polyps or a patch of mucosal irregularity.

After radiation therapy many esophageal carcinomas shrink rapidly and take on the appearance of a benign esophageal stricture. Fewer than 5% of patients live 5 years, however, reflecting the fact that at initial diagnosis only 25% of patients have a localized potentially curable lesion. When esophageal carcinoma is confined to the mucosa, 75% of cases are without nodal metastases. For patients with lesions less than 1.5 cm in size (Fig. 5-36) the prognosis is excellent.

Single-contrast examination is generally suitable for evaluation of advanced esophageal carcinoma. Small (1 to 2 cm) asymptomatic lesions, however, may be hidden on single-contrast images of the barium-filled esophagus. The double-contrast esophagram is the best method currently available for identifying small esophageal tumors. On single-contrast examination, close observation of several peristaltic sequences offers an opportunity for detecting small esophageal nodules or plaques that are not observed on conventional films of the barium-filled esophagus. Small sessile esophageal polyps that have a smooth innocent appearance should not be assumed to be benign; the morphologic distinction between benign and malignant lesions is highly inaccurate, and biopsy is essential.

Computed tomography

CT scanning has been used extensively to study the esophagus and is helpful in examining the relationships between esophageal lesions and adjacent mediastinal structures. Although CT examination is limited as a screening study for esophageal carcinoma, it is more valuable in staging and showing extent of the lesion. Administration of an oral contrast agent such as a dilute water-soluble contrast medium or barium is occasionally of value in delineating the proximal border of an

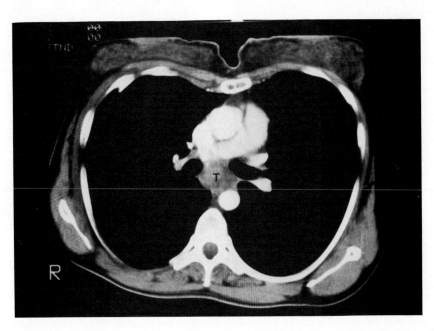

Fig. 5-36 Esophageal tumor *(T)* showing 102-degree contact between tumor and aorta, suggesting aortic invasion. Absence of invasion was proved at surgery.

obstructing esophageal mass. An orally administered dilute barium paste adheres to the esophageal wall and demonstrates the location of the esophageal lumen. CT is most useful in determining recurrent tumor after surgery.

Compared with CT study, conventional esophagography is more accurate in delineating both gastric tumor extension and the craniocaudal length of tumor. In addition, a hiatus hernia and a distal esophageal cancer, which may be confused on CT examination, are easily differentiated with barium esophagography.

CT staging of esophageal carcinoma is still an area of controversy, and there is great variability in reported accuracy for overall staging of esophageal tumors. On CT scans the normal esophageal wall thickness is no more than about 3 mm, depending on the degree of esophageal distention. In small esophageal carcinomas, the only CT finding may be focal or circumferential wall thickening. Tumor invasion through the muscle layer into the mediastinum may manifest as an abnormal soft tissue density in the mediastinal fat. Often, however, mediastinal tumor invasion is microscopic

and not identifiable on a CT scan. Aortic invasion is suggested by CT when the fat plane between the aorta and the esophageal tumor is obliterated over at least 90 degrees of the aortic circumference (see Fig. 5-36). Tracheobronchial invasion can be identified when there is a tracheoesophageal fistula or when tumor tissue is demonstrated within the lumen of the airway.

The majority of patients (68% to 83%) are found at surgery to have T_3 *primary tumors* (that is, tumor extension through the wall into the mediastinal fat). The accuracy of CT for detection of extraluminal spread has been reported to range from 55% to 100%. Invasion of the tracheobronchial tree, although present in only 6% to 20% of proved cases, can be detected with 89% to 100% accuracy (Fig. 5-37). Prior radiation therapy makes CT staging of the primary tumor more difficult

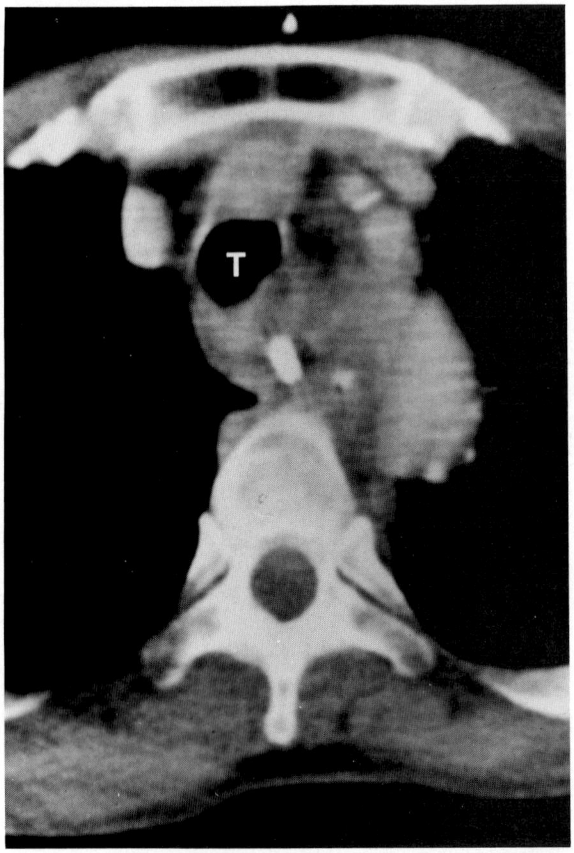

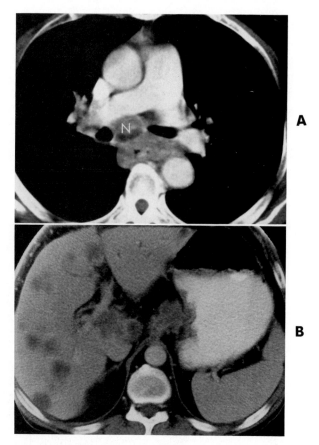

A

B

Fig. 5-38 CT examination of two patients with esophageal carcinoma. **A,** Carcinoma involving middle third of esophagus. Esophageal wall is substantially thickened by tumor, and lesion invades normal fat plane between esophagus and descending aorta. Two-centimeter carinal node *(N)* is present. **B,** Carcinoma involving distal esophagus. Distal esophagus *(arrow)* is seen as irregular mass. Multiple hepatic metastases are present.

Fig. 5-37 True-positive scan for tracheal invasion. Note compression and irregularity of left posterolateral tracheal *(T)* wall.

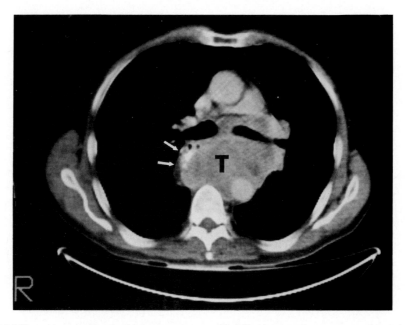

Fig. 5-39 Extensive extraluminal tumor recurrence *(T)* following esophagectomy and gastric pull-through procedure. Stomach *(arrows)* is displaced to right.

because benign fibrotic strictures may cause esophageal wall thickening, suggesting residual tumor.

CT identification of *lymph node involvement* is based on nodal enlargement. Esophageal tumors spread to the paraesophageal lymph nodes and to the celiac and left gastric nodal groups (Fig. 5-38). CT accuracy is affected by microscopic metastases to normal size nodes, which cannot be detected, and lymphadenopathy may be due to benign causes. In some cases it is difficult to distinguish esophageal wall thickening from adjacent enlarged lymph nodes, further decreasing CT accuracy in identification of lymph node spread.

It is generally agreed that CT is highly useful and accurate in detecting distant *metastases* from esophageal carcinoma, for instance, to liver, lung, kidneys, adrenals, and occasionally bone. CT has only limited usefulness, however, in the preoperative assessment of resectability before transhiatal blunt esophagectomy.

In contrast, CT has proved highly efficacious in determining *recurrent tumor* following an esophagectomy and gastric pull-through operation (Fig. 5-39). Tumors usually recur in the mediastinum or the upper abdomen and are generally extramucosal. CT scans generally detect the recurrent disease easily.

Magnetic resonance imaging

Most MRI studies of the esophagus have centered on the evaluation of cancer. Although significant differences have been identified between the T_1 times of tumors and of adjacent normal esophagus, variation in T_1 times among different esophageal cancers or regions of a cancer implies that a measurement of absolute relaxation times has little value in the differential diagnosis of esophageal disease. It seems likely that the value of MRI will relate to its ability to provide anatomic information in all three orthogonal planes rather than relaxation time data.

Because of the current weaknesses in the accurate assessment of local invasion (aortic, tracheobronchial, muscular wall) from esophageal carcinoma coupled with the time-consuming nature and expenses of the examination, MRI is not currently recommended as a routine preoperative imaging test in patients with esophageal cancer. MRI can be used, however, for problem solving or as a guide to radiotherapy planning (Fig. 5-40). As MR technology matures and the use of surface coils plus rapid imaging becomes feasible, a reassessment of MRI for esophageal imaging will become necessary.

Sarcoma

Although esophageal sarcomas are rare, one well-described lesion is *carcinosarcoma*. These lesions have mixed carcinomatous and sarcomatous elements. When metastases occur, they appear as the sarcomatous element of the primary neoplasm. Esophageal carcinosarcomas usually appear as polypoid, nonulcerated tumors in middle-aged or elderly men. Lesions that may have a gross morphology similar to bulky polypoid carcinosarcomas include fibrovascular polyps, adenocarcinomas, occasional squamous carcinomas, leiomyosarcomas, melanomas, and pseudosarcomas. *Pseudosarcomas* dif-

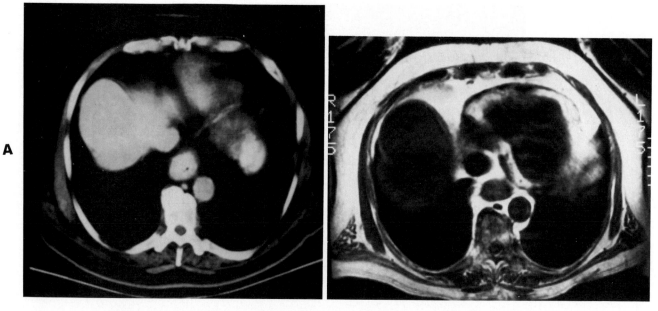

Fig. 5-40 Similar anatomic information provided by MRI and CT. **A,** CT scan shows circumferential esophageal thickening without invasion of mediastinal fat. Note clear fat plane between tumor and aorta. **B,** MR image at slightly more cranial plane (ECG gated spin-echo [SE] image, TR 619 msec, TE 20 msec) shows similar anatomy, with suggestion of strandy tissue extending from right lateral aspect of tumor.

fer from carcinosarcomas in that the carcinomatous and sarcomatous elements are not mixed, and metastases are squamous carcinoma. These tumors predominate in the middle esophagus. The survival prognosis for both pseudosarcoma and carcinosarcoma is better than for common carcinoma. Other rare esophageal sarcomas include chondrosarcoma, believed to develop from malignant degeneration of ectopic tracheobronchial elements; fibrosarcoma; liposarcoma, and myosarcoma. Melanoma of the esophagus may be primary as well as metastatic.

Esophageal *lymphoma* may occur as an isolated lesion or, more commonly, as part of disseminated lymphoma. These lesions generally show contiguous involvement of the distal esophagus and gastric fundus with associated irregularity and narrowing. Morphologically, the lesions are indistinguishable from carcinoma. *Kaposi's sarcoma* may involve the esophagus in patients with AIDS.

Metastatic disease of the esophagus

Metastatic malignant disease of the esophagus may be from (1) direct invasion, (2) involvement from adjacent malignant nodes, and (3) blood-borne metastases (see Fig. 5-30). Characteristically, metastasis of breast carcinoma to the mediastinum elicits an intense fibrotic response that causes smooth, symmetric narrowing of a long esophageal segment resembling a benign stricture[17]

(see Fig. 5-30). The least common form of secondary esophageal involvement is blood-borne metastasis. Metastatic melanoma tends to cause large endophytic lesions that may pedunculate.

BENIGN ESOPHAGEAL TUMORS

Compared with malignant lesions, benign tumors of the esophagus are uncommon.

Leiomyoma

Leiomyoma is by far the most common benign tumor of the esophagus. The mean age of patients is 35 years, about 20 years younger than for esophageal carcinoma. Leiomyomas usually occur as solitary masses in the distal third or, less commonly, in the middle third of the esophagus (Fig. 5-41). About 5% to 10% arise in the proximal esophagus. They develop primarily from the smooth muscle muscularis externa in the distal two thirds of the esophagus. Lesions sometimes appear to arise from the smooth muscle of the muscularis mucosae or blood vessels; this accounts for the occasional development of lesions in the proximal esophagus. The lesions are well encapsulated and on cut section resemble a uterine fibroid. Esophageal symptoms are generally absent, and the tumor is discovered incidentally. Esophageal leiomyomas seldom ulcerate; bleeding is rare.

On chest films leiomyomas are occasionally detected

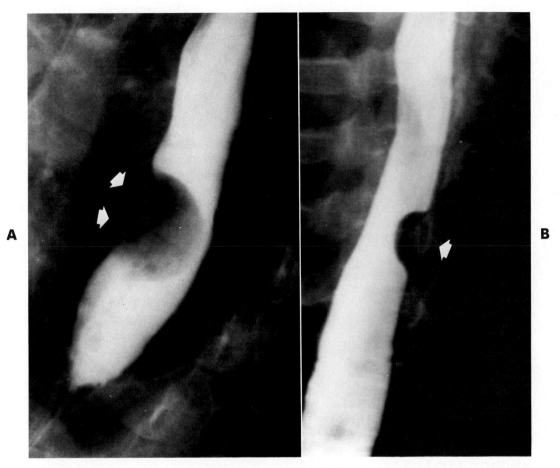

Fig. 5-41 Two patients with esophageal leiomyoma. **A,** Leiomyoma (1.5 cm) *(arrow)* demonstrating smooth contour with tapering margins. **B,** Leiomyoma (2.5 cm) with sharp margins; outer margin *(arrows)* of circular lesion is outlined by adjacent lung.

as a soft tissue mediastinal density, mediastinal widening, or a calcified mass. Esophagrams usually demonstrate a smooth filling defect (see Fig. 5-41). On tangential view a semilunar mass with intact mucosa narrows the barium column. Seen face on, the lesion may cause splitting of the barium column, splaying of the longitudinal folds, and segmental widening of the esophageal diameter. In many cases a soft tissue companion shadow is observed; this is caused by the exophytic component of the lesion. Rarely, leiomyomas may grow into the esophageal lumen, causing a lobulated or pedunculated lesion.

Multiple leiomyomas occasionally develop, but usually no more than two to three lesions are found. Rarely the multiple lesions may be numerous and coalesce. Another rare form is *diffuse esophageal leiomatosis,* which occurs as a segmental nodular narrowing that involves the distal half of the esophagus and may extend into the stomach.

Other benign submucosal neoplasms include neurofi-

broma, fibroma, angioma, lipoma, and granular cell tumor. Granular cell tumors, formerly termed *myelofibromas,* are believed to have a neural origin and are more common in women and blacks.

Fibrovascular polyp

Fibrovascular polyps contain varying amounts of fibrous, vascular, and even adipose tissue. At various times they have been called *fibroma, fibrolipoma, myxofibroma,* and *pedunculated lipoma.* They are more common in males and generally develop in the proximal esophagus. Dysphagia is the prevalent clinical symptom. The lesions appear as small sessile polyps or as large bulky lesions that have a sausagelike intraluminal mass. Pedunculation is common.

Inflammatory polyp

Inflammatory esophageal polyps consist of inflamed granulation and fibrous tissue. They have also been called *inflammatory pseudotumors, fibrous polyps,* and

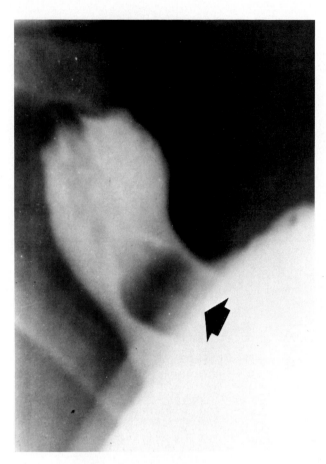

Fig. 5-42 Inflammatory polyp *(arrow)* in distal esophagus. Patient was examined for heartburn.

eosinophilic granuloma. They develop as a response to reflux esophagitis. On radiographic examination they appear as roundish sessile polyps in the distal esophagus, usually 0.5 to 2 cm in diameter (Fig. 5-42). The lesions tend to diminish in size and disappear during effective therapy for esophagitis.

Papillomas

Papillomas are sessile wartlike excrescences that arise from the esophageal squamous mucosa. They generally occur in the distal third of the esophagus and are seen as small plaques 1 to 4 mm in size. They develop most commonly in elderly men and are usually asymptomatic.

Cysts

Esophageal retention cysts are thin-walled, acquired cysts *(mucoceles)* caused by obstruction of an esophageal mucous gland. Multiple retention cysts have been called *esophagitis cystica,* even though little inflammation is present.

Miscellaneous benign tumors

Other tumors affecting the esophagus include solitary varix, focal infection, hamartoma, ectopic tissue, and hematoma. Esophageal hamartomas may occur as isolated lesions or, rarely, in patients with Peutz-Jeghers syndrome.

INDENTATIONS AND DISPLACEMENTS

Adequate esophageal distention is important to demonstrate compression or indentation of the barium column by adjacent masses.

Indentations

Mild indentations are commonly caused by the aortic knob, left main stem bronchus, and diaphragmatic hiatus. A slight posterior arc is also made around the atrial surface of the heart. The descending thoracic aorta indents the esophagus just above the diaphragmatic hiatus and may sometime cause the obstructive symptoms of *dysphagia aortica,* especially when accompanied by cardiomegaly. Left atrial enlargement causes a localized esophageal impression adjacent to the upper half of the posterior cardiac border. Generalized cardiomegaly causes posterior displacement of the distal half of the thoracic esophagus. These relationships are best shown on lateral views.

Other variations of the aortic arch that impress the esophagus are a right-sided aortic arch, cervical aortic arch, double aortic arch, and aortic aneurysm. A *right aortic arch* produces a right-sided indentation slightly higher than the usual indentation of the normal left aortic limb. Two types of right arches occur: (1) an anterior right arch, which is a mirror image of the normal left arch and is commonly associated with cyanotic congenital heart disease, especially tetralogy of Fallot and truncus arteriosus, and (2) a posterior right arch, which is accompanied by an aberrant left subclavian artery that passes behind the esophagus and causes a prominent posterior notch high on the superior part of the thoracic esophagus. These patients seldom have other congenital abnormalities. With a *cervical arch* the ascending aorta passes obliquely upward behind the esophagus, causing a prominent posterior indentation, and forms a palpable pulsatile mass on the right side of the neck. *Double aortic arches* exist with variable patterns of brachycephalic vessels; the descending aorta may be on the right or left. *Aortic coarctation* usually occurs just distal to the takeoff of the left subclavian artery. Poststenotic aortic dilatation commonly impresses the esophagus just below the normal indentation of the aortic knob. These two indentations on the left side of the esophagus create the *reverse-three sign* characteristic of aortic coarctation. The diagnosis may be confirmed by the presence of rib notching.

In children, symptoms from *vascular anomalies* are almost always respiratory, whereas adults usually have esophageal dysphagia. An aberrant right subclavian artery occurs in about 1 in every 200 people. An aberrant left pulmonary artery arises from the right pulmonary artery and forms a sling behind the trachea as it loops back toward the left lung. The vascular sling generally causes a characteristic notch on the anterior wall of the middle esophagus.

Mediastinal masses that indent the esophagus are commonly caused by mediastinal adenopathy, particularly enlarged carinal nodes. The indentations are often subtle and seen only on oblique views. Parathyroid tumors occasionally cause an impression on the cervical esophagus.

Deviation

In the lower mediastinum the esophagus is loosely supported by surrounding structures and may move spontaneously to the right or left of midline *(wandering esophagus)*. Mediastinal shifts that displace the esophagus from the midline may be due to pulmonary atelectasis, pulmonary hypoplasia, unilateral emphysema, pneumonectomy, pneumothorax, or hydrothorax.

DIAPHRAGM

The two major functions of the diaphragm are to separate the abdomen and chest into two distinct cavities with different cavitary pressure and to serve as the major muscle of respiration. Each hemidiaphragm is innervated by an ipsilateral phrenic nerve consisting of nerve bundles from C_3 to C_5.

Anatomy of the diaphragm

The muscle fibers of the diaphragm arise from the xiphoid process, eighth to twelfth ribs, and lumbar spine. They insert into a crescent-shaped central tendon, which corresponds closely to the bare area of the liver, defined by the attachment of the liver suspensory ligaments to the undersurface of the diaphragm. The diaphragm has three normal foramina: (1) the esophageal hiatus, (2) the aortic foramen, and (3) the foramen of the vena cava.

Defects of the diaphragm

Congenital absence of the diaphragm is a rare anomaly that may be detected in utero by ultrasound. This anomaly is usually left sided. The herniated gut fills with gas and compresses intrathoracic structures.

There are three types of *congenital diaphragmatic hernias:* Bochdalek's, Morgagni's, and esophageal diaphragmatic hiatus.

In *Bochdalek's hernia,* a posteromedial diaphragmatic hernia occurs through Bochdalek's foramen, a defect that represents incomplete closure of the pleuroperitoneal membrane. When the defect is large, most of the abdominal contents may herniate into the chest, similar to congenital absence of the diaphragm. When the defect is small, the hernia may be asymptomatic and contain only some retroperitoneal fat or a portion of the spleen or kidney. Most often the lesion is on the left.

In *Morgagni's hernia,* herniation occurs behind the sternum through a persistent diaphragmatic cleft that contains the mammary vessels. Most Morgagni's hernias occur on the right, because the pericardium tends to prevent such herniations on the left. Typically, therefore, Morgagni's hernia presents at the right cardiophrenic angle, although they occasionally occur bilaterally. Usually these hernias are asymptomatic. They generally contain omentum or a portion of transverse colon, but they may also contain small bowel or liver.

Congenital hiatus hernias generally contain only the proximal stomach and appear clinically as excessive reflux and regurgitation.

Acquired diaphragmatic hernias usually are either a sliding hiatus hernia, which is common in the elderly, or an abrupt diaphragmatic rupture from blunt trauma. In many cases the transverse colon enters the hernia because of its connection with the greater curvature of the stomach via the gastrocolic ligament. Such giant hiatus hernias may be encountered incidentally, or the patient may complain of excessive eructation and postprandial symptoms. Occasionally, an obstructed complete gastric volvulus may develop acutely and present as a surgical emergency. A traumatic hernia should be suspected when a diaphragmatic hernia does not involve the esophageal hiatus or any of the usual locations for congenital hernias. About 90% of traumatic hiatus hernias are on the left.

Movement and location of the diaphragm

The hemidiaphragms normally make a synchronous caudal excursion of about 2 to 3 cm during inspiration. Asthenic individuals may show mainly diaphragmatic breathing, with excursion up to 6 to 8 cm. In pulmonary emphysema the diaphragms are low and flat.

The cause of unilateral diaphragmatic elevation is often related to (1) the ipsilateral lung or thorax, (2) the diaphragm ("eventration") or its innervation, or (3) abnormalities in the abdomen. In addition, a subpulmonic effusion may simulate an elevated diaphragm. The sniff test is often useful when searching for paradoxical diaphragmatic movement.

Neoplasms of the diaphragm

Primary neoplasms of the diaphragm are rare. When they do occur, they are generally of mesodermal origin.

An endothelial mesothelioma, however, may be confined to the diaphragm.

RECOMMENDED READING

1. Agha FP: Radiologic diagnosis of Barrett's esophagus: critical analysis of 65 cases, *Gastrointest Radiol* 11:123, 1986.
2. Balthazar EJ et al: Cytomegalovirus esophagitis in AIDS: radiographic features in 16 patients, *Am J Roentgenol* 149:919, 1987.
3. Barrett NR: Chronic peptic ulcer of the oesophagus and oesophagitis, *Br J Surg* 38:175, 1950.
4. Beauchamp JM et al: Esophageal intramural pseudodiverticulosis, *Radiology* 113:273, 1974.
5. Bleshman MH et al: The inflammatory esophagogastric polyp and fold, *Radiology* 128:589, 1978.
6. Cho SR et al: Polypoid carcinoma of the esophagus: a distinct radiological and histopathological entity, *Am J Gastroenterol* 78:476, 1983.
7. Diamant NE, El-Sharkaway TY: Neural control of esophageal peristalsis: a conceptual analysis, *Gastroenterology* 72:546, 1977.
8. Dodds WJ: Cannon lecture: Current concepts of esophageal motor function: clinical implications for radiology, *Am J Roentgenol* 128:549, 1977.
9. Dodds WJ et al: Pathogenesis of reflux esophagitis, *Gastroenterology* 81:376, 1981.
10. Freeny PC, Marks WM: Adenocarcinoma of the gastroesophageal junction: barium and CT examination, *Am J Roentgenol* 138:1077, 1982.
11. Ghahremani GG et al: Esophageal manifestations of Crohn's disease, *Gastrointest Radiol* 7:199, 1982.
12. Haber K, Winfield AC: Multiple leiomyomas of the esophagus, *Am J Dig Dis* 19:678, 1974.
13. Itai Y et al: Superficial esophageal carcinoma: radiological findings in double-contrast studies, *Radiology* 126:597, 1978.
14. Koehler RE et al: Early radiographic manifestations of carcinoma of the esophagus, *Radiology* 119:1, 1976.
15. Lawson TL, Dodds WJ: Infiltrating carcinoma simulating achalasia, *Gastrointest Radiol* 1:245, 1977.
16. Mandelstam P, Lieber A: Cineradiographic evaluation of the esophagus in normal adults: a study of 146 subjects ranging in age from 21 to 90 years. *Gastroenterology* 58:32, 1970.
17. Moss AA et al: Esophageal carcinoma: pretherapy staging by computed tomography, *Am J Roentgenol* 136:1051, 1981.
18. Taylor AJ et al: The esophageal "jet" phenomenon revisited, *Am J Roentgenol* 155:289, 1990.
19. Terrier F et al: CT assessment of operability in carcinoma of the oesophagogastric junction, *Eur J Radiol* 4:114, 1984.
20. Werlin SL et al: Mechanisms of gastroesophageal reflux in children, *J Pediatr* 97:244, 1980.

6 *Stomach and Duodenum*

H JOACHIM BURHENNE
HERBERT Y KRESSEL
MARC S LEVINE
MASAKAZU MARUYAMA
J ODO OP DEN ORTH
CHARLES A ROHRMANN JR
HIKOO SHIRAKABE

STOMACH
Upper Gastrointestinal Radiologic Study

NONNEOPLASTIC LESIONS OF THE STOMACH
Gastric anatomy
Gastritis and gastropathy
Abnormalities of shape and function
Miscellaneous nonneoplastic abnormalities

NEOPLASTIC DISORDERS OF THE STOMACH (GASTRIC CANCER)
Diagnosis
Other malignant and benign tumors

PEPTIC DISEASE
Epidemiology and pathogenesis
Radiographic appearance of peptic ulceration
Location of peptic ulceration
Morphologic features of peptic ulceration
Healing and scar formation
Complications of peptic ulceration
Differential diagnosis of peptic ulcer disease

DUODENUM
Anatomy
Technique of examination
Indentation at aorta and superior mesenteric artery
Benign tumors
Malignant tumors
Enlargement of the major duodenal papilla
Diffuse intrinsic duodenal disease
Congenital stenoses
Miscellaneous radiologic findings

Stomach

UPPER GASTROINTESTINAL RADIOLOGIC STUDY

H JOACHIM BURHENNE

Radiologic examination is the method of choice in the diagnosis of GI tract perforation, and a choice must be made between barium and a water-soluble contrast agent. If no free air can be detected on chest and multiple abdominal radiographs and if there is no clinical evidence of mediastinitis or peritonitis, barium can be used for upper intestinal examinations (Fig. 6-1), even in patients with clinically suspected perforation or fistula formation. Barium provides more detail and is more consistently diagnostic than iodinated contrast materials. If free air is present in the abdomen, if there is a question of early postoperative leakage at the anastomosis site, or if there are clinical signs of peritonitis or mediastinitis, iodinated contrast material is preferred (Fig. 6-2).

Conventional water-soluble media (Gastrografin, for example) are contraindicated in patients known to aspirate. Aspiration of hyperosmotic iodinated contrast material may result in acute pulmonary edema and pneumonitis. The newer non-ionic and isoosmolar contrast agents have recently been shown to be much less dangerous when aspirated than were the older iodinated agents. Because of possible pulmonary complications, patients with gastric outlet obstruction and a history of vomiting or aspiration should have their stomachs intubated after upper GI studies.

Biopsy of the stomach after endoscopy is a relative contraindication to upper GI contrast examination on the same day. Though most biopsies obtained through

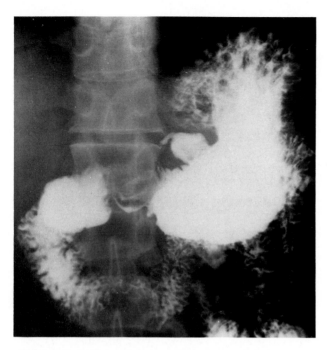

Fig. 6-1 Preliminary film showed no evidence of free air in this patient with suspected visceral perforation. Upper GI study with use of barium sulfate demonstrates deep penetrating lesser curvature peptic ulcer and sealed perforation.

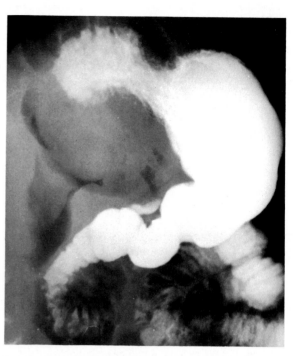

Fig. 6-2 Preliminary film showed air in region of lesser sac. Upper GI study with water-soluble iodinated compound shows point of duodenal ulcer perforation.

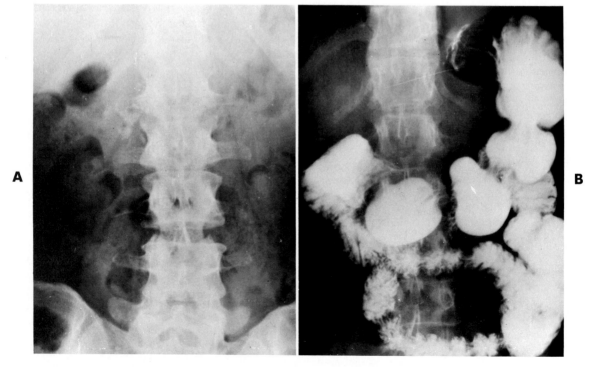

Fig. 6-3 A, Patient with suspected history of chronic pancreatitis shows extensive pancreatic calcification on preliminary radiograph. **B,** Calcification in same patient is hidden after ingestion of contrast material.

the flexible endoscope do not penetrate the mucosa, most radiologists prefer to wait 24 hours after biopsy.

The efficacy of routine preliminary abdominal films before contrast examination of the upper GI tract is in doubt. In specific cases, however—such as patients with a history of vomiting, suspected postoperative leakage, or suspicion of visceral perforation—it is the radiologist's responsibility to obtain plain abdominal films before performing upper GI studies. Preliminary abdominal plain films may also disclose calcifications that otherwise may be hidden by overlying barium (Fig. 6-3).

Patient preparation and instruction

Except in emergency situations, the patient should fast from midnight before the procedure. This includes abstinence from drinking even small amounts of water. The patient should also be cautioned not to smoke before the study. Because the progressive dehydration of barium in the colon may lead to impaction, patients with a history of constipation should routinely receive a mild laxative after an upper GI study.

Techniques

Two questions should be routinely asked of the patient by the examining radiologist: (1) Have you ever had an x-ray examination of your stomach before? and (2) Have you ever had abdominal surgery? In hospitalized patients, the hospital record should accompany the patient to the radiology department.

Single-contrast examination

The term *single-contrast examination* implies that only barium is administered. In fact, a certain amount of normally ingested air is virtually always present in the stomach. However, the thrust of the single-contrast study is to fill the lumen with low-density barium. Any air that might be present provides double-contrast visualization as a fringe benefit. Single-contrast examinations permit good evaluation of disorders of motility, visceral rigidity, spasm, and strictures. However, this technique is inadequate for demonstration of subtle mucosal abnormalities. The large amount of barium present may also obscure small lesions such as gastric polyps.

Single-contrast examination requires the use of barium in a 15% to 25% weight-to-volume mixture and overhead film technique using 120 kV for penetration of the contrast column. A mucosal relief study may be obtained by initially administering a small amount of a higher density barium mixture (150% weight-to-volume), enough to coat the mucosa without pooling in large quantities. Spot films are obtained after the patient is turned in order to coat the entire lumen. Supine right

anterior oblique and prone left posterior oblique projections are used. Approximately 500 ml of the 15% to 25% weight-to-volume barium mixture (enough for adequate distention) is then administered.

The single-contrast examination is acceptable if the patient is unable to cooperate or a limited study is required to answer a specific clinical question. In general, however, a high error rate, both false positive and false negative, has been reported for the single-contrast upper GI study.

Double-contrast examination

The double-contrast technique provides better demonstration of mucosal detail (Fig. 6-4) and therefore should be more accurate in diagnosing small superficial lesions such as erosions. Proponents of the double-contrast examination of the stomach and duodenum recommend routine intravenous use of a hypotonic agent such as glucagon or Buscopan (Boehringer Ingelheim) (0.1 mg). Since additional expense is incurred and the routine use of these agents has not been shown to improve diagnostic accuracy, their use is best restricted to difficult diagnostic problems in the duodenum (Fig. 6-5) or when fluoroscopy is extended and obtaining adequate radiographs of the stomach and duodenum in double contrast may take a long time. Effervescent media for double-contrast examination are available in both granular and tablet form, and a satisfactory agent may also be produced in a hospital pharmacy. Surfactant agents help prevent foaming and artifacts produced by bubbles.

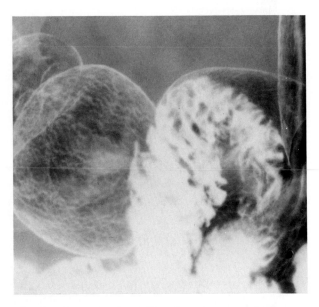

Fig. 6-4 Conventional spot film of gastric antrum showing areae gastricae.

Biphasic routine examination

The goal of the biphasic examination is to have both mucosal delineation in the double-contrast phase and full column distension in the single-contrast phase (Fig. 6-6). The biphasic study can be accomplished in approximately 5 minutes of fluoroscopy time. The sequence of patient positioning (Table 6-1) is designed to start in an erect position and end in a recumbent position, with only one table-tilt maneuver. The double-contrast examination precedes the full-column study.

The routine exam starts with the patient erect. Effer-

vescent granules or tablets are given directly from the single-dose container. The patient is instructed to take these in a single swallow with 15 ml of water provided in a separate small cup. If the effervescent agent does not already contain an antifoaming agent such as simethicone, a few drops of such an agent should be added to the water. The patient is then turned in a shallow right anterior oblique position to throw the esophagus off the spine. At this point, 75 ml of high-density, low-viscosity (250% weight-to-volume ratio) barium sulfate preparation is administered. As the patient is drinking

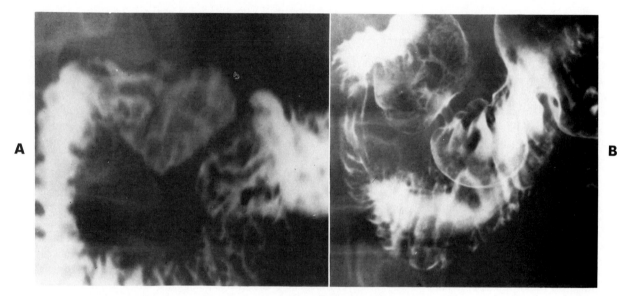

Fig. 6-5 Single- and double-contrast studies of duodenum in patient with ectopic gastric mucosa. **A,** Single contrast shows mucosal fold pattern. **B,** Double contrast demonstrates fine mucosal detail and defines central defect with ectopic mucosa.

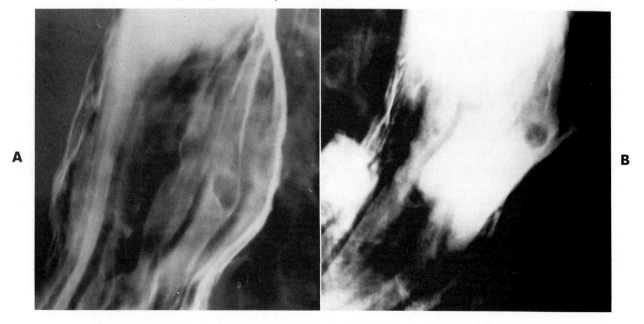

Fig. 6-6 A, Mucosal polyp of stomach seen with double high-density contrast in first phase, and **B,** through thin barium in second phase of examination.

☐ **TABLE 6-1**
Sequence for the routine upper GI study

Patient position	Materials	Patient instruction	Spot films	Remarks
Erect RAO	1 tablespoon of effervescent tablets with 15 ml of water and antifoaming agent followed by 75 ml of 150% weight/volume E-Z-HD	"Place tablets on your tongue, and wash them down with water; do not chew tablets; do not burp. Then take cup in your left hand, and swallow all of the barium."	100 kV split film; distal esophagus and esophagogastric junction; right anterior oblique	Esophagus to the left of spine; work fast; esophageal double contrast usually possible
Tilt table horizontal From erect to left lateral to prone	—	"Turn on your left side and on your stomach as the table goes down. Turn over your left side on your back and again on your stomach, several times."	Double contrast; fundus, body, and antrum of stomach; 100 kV	When turning over left side supine to prone without antral coating, tip patient into oblique to fill antrum but not on right side to fill duodenum yet
Supine RAO	—	"Lie on your right side and then on your back, then raise your right hip."	Double contrast; antrum and entire duodenal bulb and loop; then supine left anterior oblique for face on of lesser curvature	This time patient is turned over right side
GI position Prone LPO	250 ml of 15% weight/volume barium mixture; use plastic tubing (drinking through a straw is too slow for esophageal distention)	"Take tubing in your mouth and swallow rapidly; keep drinking."	Full column; esophagus, antrum, and duodenum	If patient is unable to cooperate, entire upper GI study may be performed in GI position and without preceding double contrast
Supine RAO	—	"Roll on your right side and then on your back; raise your right hip."	Esophagogastric junction; full air contrast film of stomach body, antrum, and duodenum	Check for reflux after turning; do not use unphysiologic maneuvers

the barium, right anterior oblique spot films centered over the midesophagus are obtained. If the film changer on the spot film device can accommodate 11 × 14 films, then a three-way split will usually permit visualization of the entire esophagus on each of the three images. Having the patient drink the barium as quickly as possible immediately after ingestion of the effervescent agent will usually produce good quality double-contrast images with the esophagus adequately distended by gas.

The table is then tilted to the horizontal position. The patient is asked to turn over the left side onto the stomach and then back again to the supine position. This maneuver should be repeated several times to ensure adequate coating. If this amount of turning is not possible for the elderly or debilitated patient, a single supine-to-prone and back again maneuver may have to suffice.

Once mucosal coating of the stomach has occurred, double-contrast films are obtained in both PA and AP projections (patient supine and prone). Ideally, these two films are obtained before filling of the duodenum. Positioning the patient right side down should therefore be avoided at this time. It may be necessary, however, to turn the patient slightly into the left anterior oblique position to adequately fill the gastric antrum.

After the double-contrast views of the stomach have been obtained, the patient is turned into the right-side-down decubitus position to allow barium to enter the duodenum. If there were any previous problems obtaining double-contrast views of the fundus, further views

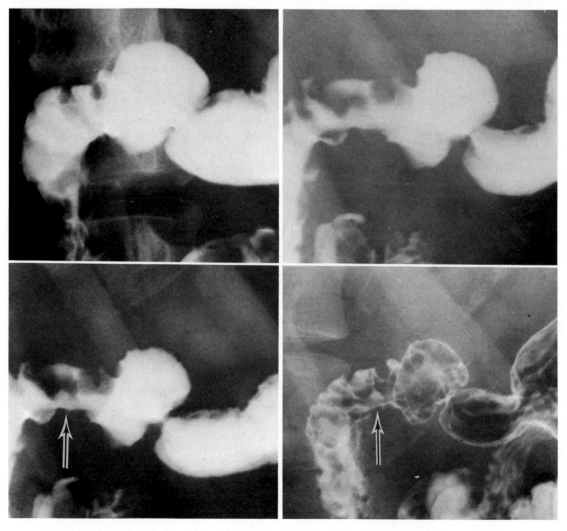

Fig. 6-7 Four spot films of duodenum with patient in recumbent position obtained with full column barium and with double contrast. Double-contrast film shows duodenal ulcer to best advantage.

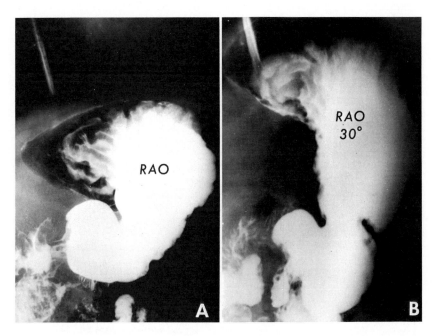

Fig. 6-8 A, Film taken in right anterior oblique position with vertical beam obscures lesser curvature of stomach. **B,** With same patient in same position, 30-degree tube angulation opens up lesser curvature.

of this area may be obtained at this time. Once the barium has opacified the duodenal loop, the patient is turned supine and then into the left-side-down decubitus position to permit air to enter the duodenum for double-contrast views (Fig. 6-7). The ideal position for double-contrast views of the duodenal loop is usually in a fairly steep right anterior oblique projection.

After completion of the double-contrast films of the duodenum, the patient is turned into the prone left posterior oblique GI position and the second, or single-contrast phase, of the examination is initiated by administering 350 ml of 15% to 25% weight-to-volume barium. The patient holds the contrast container in the left hand and drinks the barium rapidly through a large-bore straw made from plastic tubing. This allows full esophageal distention. Full-column spot filming of the esophagus is obtained as the patient drinks the thin barium. With the patient in the GI position, single-contrast spot films of the antrum and duodenum are obtained. The patient is then turned into the supine right anterior oblique position for a large spot film of the stomach with single-contrast views of the body and fundus.

This completes the fluoroscopic and spot-filming portion of the routine examination. Three overhead radiographs are then obtained, all at 120 kV. The first film is an 11 × 14 inch 45-degree right anterior oblique prone view of the stomach and duodenum. The second is a 14 × 17 inch posteroanterior prone projection of the stomach, duodenum, and proximal jejunum. The third is a right lateral 11 × 14 film of the stomach and duodenum. With a horizontal stomach adding a 30 degree tube angulation may be necessary to open up the lesser curvature. In some departments this is a routinely obtained film (Fig. 6-8).

Serial photofluorography and videofluorography

In patients with suspected high esophageal lesions, serial photofluorography, using a 105 mm or similar camera, as well as video recording of the fluorographic images are required. Serial photofluorographic images are generally of higher resolution than video images, though the video images provide uninterrupted visualization of the dynamics of swallowing. Events in the hypopharynx and cervical esophagus occur so rapidly that abnormalities of fluoroscopy may readily be overlooked and timing of spot films becomes impossible. Serial 105 mm images recorded at 4 to 6 frames/second document epiglottic or cricopharyngeal dysfunction, cricopharyngeal achalasia, and cervical esophageal webs.

Functional studies

Gastric emptying is assessed in only the most limited fashion using liquid barium. Gastric emptying time varies for liquids and solids, depending on the temperature of the medium, the amount given, and the type of food material. A mixture of barium with food such as hamburger demonstrates the effect of obstruction more

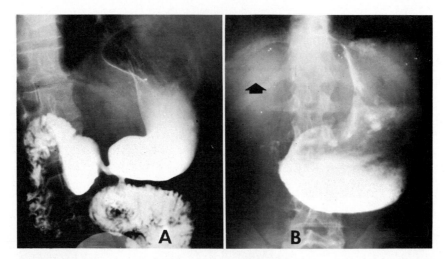

Fig. 6-9 A, With conventional barium mixture, narrowing of pylorus and of gastroenterostomy stoma are demonstrated. Stomach empties well. **B,** With barium-food mixture given on following day, almost complete obstruction is shown on 30-minute upright radiograph. Slight vomiting occurred with physiologic meal.

(From Burhenne HJ: Roentgenologic approach to the physiologic examination of the alimentary tract. In Gamble JR, Wilbur DL, editors: *Current concepts of clinical gastroenterology,* Boston, 1965, Little, Brown.)

clearly (Fig. 6-9). The presence of food along with the contrast medium stimulates intestinal secretion, however, resulting in poor delineation of the mucosal surfaces. Mucosal assessment may be improved by adding a suspending agent to a mixture of Metrecal and barium.

The ingestion of radiodense nondigestable markers followed by serial plain films of the abdomen has been used for assessment of gastric emptying. This is a straightforward and simple way of assessing gastric emptying time for solid nondigestable material. However, *radionuclide labeling* of both solid and liquid components of a standard meal provides a more physiologic way of assessing gastric emptying. Emptying of the stomach can then be followed on a gamma camera with simultaneous measurement of solid and liquid emptying through the use of dual energy detectors.

Emergency studies

Emergency upper GI studies are usually requested for investigation of bleeding or perforation. Endoscopy is best for initial investigation of acute upper GI bleeding, followed by angiography as required. Both of these procedures permit therapeutic, as well as diagnostic, maneuvers. Barium studies may be the first line of investigation if endoscopy is not available or the endoscopic examination is incomplete for technical reasons. It must always be kept in mind, however, that the presence of barium in the GI tract may preclude angiography until the barium has been cleared.

In the investigation of *perforation,* a water-soluble contrast agent should be used, preferably one of the non-ionic low osmolar agents. The minimum amount of contrast material necessary should be used. If the water-soluble contrast study is negative, it should immediately be followed by a barium study, which in a significant proportion of cases will allow detection of abnormalities not seen with the initial water-soluble contrast study.

The second look

All radiographic spot films and overhead films from the upper GI series must be reviewed as soon as they are processed and before the patient leaves the radiology department. This is the time to decide if a second fluoroscopic look or special maneuvers are indicated. Palpation is reserved for special diagnostic problems during a second look. Routine compression films are not necessary.

RECOMMENDED READING

1. Gelfand DW et al: Multiphasic examinations of the stomach: efficacy of individual techniques and combinations of techniques in detecting 153 lesions. *Radiology* 162:829, 1987.
2. Hall FM: Routine upper gastrointestinal examination, *Radiology* 171:283, 1989.
3. Johnsrude IS, Jackson DC: The role of the radiologist in acute gastrointestinal bleeding, *Gastrointest Radiol* 3:357, 1978.
4. Munro TC: A simple model for teaching double-contrast examinations of the gastrointestinal tract, *J Can Assoc Radiol* 10:162, 1989.

5. Nolan Daniel: *The double-contrast barium meal,* HM & M Publishers, Aylesbury, England, Year Book Medical Publishers, Distributors, 1980.
6. Ominsky SH, Margulis AR: Radiographic examination of the upper gastrointestinal tract, *Radiology* 139:11, 1981.

Nonneoplastic lesions of the stomach

CHARLES A ROHRMANN JR

GASTRIC ANATOMY

The *gastric fundus* is that portion of the stomach superior to the plane of the esophagogastric junction. The gastric *body* is that part distal to the fundus. The terminology for the rest of the stomach varies, however, depending on whether the landmarks are based on gross morphology, cellular constituents of the mucosa, or distribution of muscle fibers. A plane passing through the incisura angularis separates the body from the pyloric portion of the stomach, further divided into a proximal component, the *pyloric vestibule,* and a distal component, the *pyloric antrum.* As an alternative, the *antrum* can be considered to be all of the stomach between the incisura angularis and the pyloric canal and to incorporate both the pyloric vestibule and antrum as previously defined.

Histologists and physiologists use terms based on mucosal characteristics and divide the stomach into the fundal and pyloric gland areas. *Fundal epithelium* contains chief, mucous, parietal, and argentaffin cells and encompasses not only the fundus as just defined, but also the entire body and a variable portion of proximal antrum. The *pyloric gland region,* or *antrum* in this concept, is that portion containing mucus- and gastrin-secreting cells. This area includes most of the antral region as defined anatomically. The *pyloric mucosa* is reported to extend along 43% to 56% of the distal lesser curvature and about 15% of the distal greater curvature. Variations are common, and in about 10% of cases the pyloric mucosa may extend almost to the cardia.

Physiologic considerations

Intraluminal manometry has demonstrated a physiologic sphincter at the pylorus, bringing to an end a longstanding controversy over its existence. It is characterized by a zone of high resting pressure that contracts in response to duodenal acidification, thus preventing regurgitation of duodenal contents into the stomach.

Adult pyloric hypertrophy

There are various forms of pyloric hypertrophy. Its pathogenesis is unknown, and in some patients it begins in infancy and persists into adult life. In most, however, symptoms begin in the fifth decade of life. Radiologic diagnostic signs of pyloric hypertrophy include (1) elongation and concentric narrowing of the pyloric canal, (2) a cleft or niche in the mid-portion of the canal, (3) evidence of flexibility or variation in contour of the narrowed distal antrum, and (4) presence of a proximal benign ulcer, usually on the lesser curvature near the incisura. The elongated canal of pyloric hypertrophy is concentric, straight, or slightly curved, and occasionally is funnel shaped. The combination of a lesser curvature benign ulcer near the incisura and concentric nar-

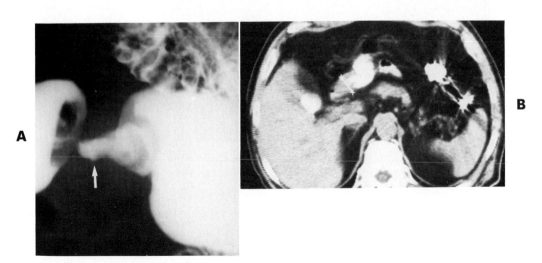

Fig. 6-10 Adult hypertrophic pyloric stenosis. This 73-year-old man was referred for upper gastrointestinal series because of upper abdominal pain and early satiety. **A,** Note antral constriction and inferiorly directed triangular cleft similar to that seen in Fig. 22-5 *(arrow).* **B,** CT image with cursor measuring pyloric thickness of 24 mm.

rowing of the distal antrum points strongly to the diagnosis of pyloric hypertrophy. However, hypertrophy of the pyloric muscle can be present without any radiographic abnormalities (Fig. 6-10).

☐ **CLASSIFICATION OF PYLORIC** ☐
HYPERTROPHY

A. Primary pyloric hypertrophy
   1. Focal form—torus hypertrophy
   2. Diffuse form without proximal lesion
   3. Diffuse form with proximal lesion
      a. Proximal benign ulcer
      b. Proximal cancer
   4. Diffuse form with associated lesions
      a. Gastritis
      b. Gastroenterostomy
      c. Pernicious anemia
B. Secondary pyloric hypertrophy
   1. Associated with a distal obstructive lesion

Antral diaphragm

An antral diaphragm, or *web,* may vary from a crescentic membrane to an almost complete septum perforated only by a 1 mm opening. Histologically it consists of normal gastric mucosa on each side of a central core of submucosa and hypertrophied muscularis mucosa. There is little or no inflammation. Antral webs are usually located about 1 to 1.5 cm proximal to the pylorus but this distance may vary from 7 cm proximal to the pylorus to right at the pylorus.

On radiographs a constant, symmetric, thin, bandlike deformity is seen perpendicular to the long axis of the antrum. The orifice may be central or eccentric, and peristaltic activity is normal (Fig. 6-11). The diaphragm is usually 2 to 3 mm thick. Associated ulcers are found in 30% to 50% of cases.

GASTRITIS AND GASTROPATHY

The term *gastritis* is a convenient label, sanctioned by long usage, to describe a variety of lesions of the gastric mucosa, of which only some are inflammatory in origin.

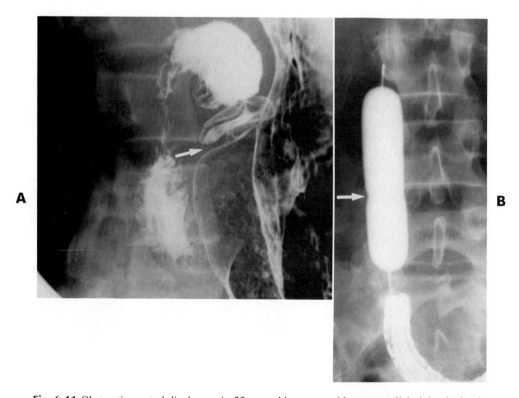

Fig. 6-11 Obstructing antral diaphragm in 22-year-old woman with postprandial abdominal pain, nausea, and vomiting. **A,** Air contrast view of antrum shows constriction 1 cm proximal to pylorus *(arrow)*. This has produced "double-bulb" or "double-pylorus" appearance. **B,** At endoscopy, 3 mm opening was found in constricting antral diaphragm. Transendoscopic wire was threaded through diaphragm and angioplasty-type catheter was used to dilate web. Note waist on balloon *(arrow)* at site of web.

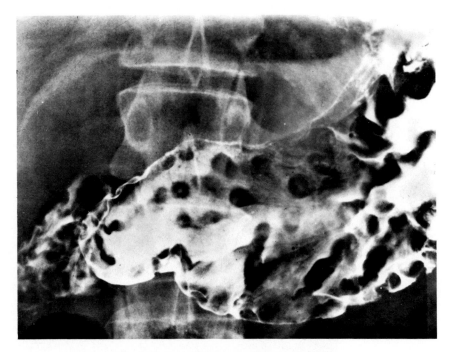

Fig. 6-12 Varioliform type of erosive gastritis.

Acute gastritis

Acute erosive gastritis

In erosive gastritis there are shallow ulcers (erosions) that do not penetrate beyond the muscularis mucosa. The most common radiographic appearance is a varioliform (smallpoxlike) erosion, which is situated centrally on a small mound of edema (Fig. 6-12). Erosions have been observed in Crohn's disease, herpes simplex infections, cytomegalovirus infections, candidiasis, and syphilis. They have also been attributed to alcohol, aspirin, steroids and nonsteroidal antiinflammatory drugs, as well as stress such as that which occurs with burns and trauma. Gastric erosions are often asymptomatic.

Infectious gastritis

A variety of systemic infections may be associated with gastritis.

Gastric tuberculosis may be confused with Crohn's disease, since the histologic picture of the two conditions may be identical. Radiologic manifestations of tuberculosis are similar to those of large, deep benign gastric ulcers. An associated sinus tract or fistula is a typical sign of tuberculosis. It is radiologically indistinguishable from other forms of granulomatous gastritis. The AIDS epidemic has reactivated interest in gastric tuberculosis.

Gastric histoplasmosis is relatively rare, since the stomach is usually spared in disseminated disease. However, gastric ulceration with hemorrhage and masses simulating carcinoma may result from Histoplasma infiltration.

Syphilis of the gastrointestinal tract most commonly involves the stomach. *Secondary syphilis* may manifest as a diffuse, nonspecific gastritis and duodenitis and an inflammatory mass in the stomach with superficial erosions (Fig. 6-13). The rugal folds may be either enlarged or effaced. In *tertiary syphilis* a granulomatous infiltration most commonly involves the antrum. This produces a funnel-shaped narrowing of the antrum with effacement of the mucosal pattern and diminished or absent peristalsis. Pyloric obstruction is rare.

Phlegmonous gastritis

Phlegmonous gastritis is an acute, fulminating, often fatal infection of the stomach with resultant necrosis and marked systemic and local polymorphonuclear leukocytosis. *Alpha-hemolytic streptococci* are the most common causative agent, but *Staphylococcus aureus*, *Escherichia coli*, *Clostridium welchii*, and *Pneumococcus* and *Proteus* species have also been found. At barium examination the gastric wall is markedly thickened and the rugae are swollen, at times to the point of effacement. Intramural penetration of the contrast medium may occur, probably through the multiple sievelike holes that are seen on pathologic examination. CT or ultrasonography may show wall thickening. As healing occurs, marked shrinkage of the stomach results. In *E. coli* or *C. welchii* infections multiple small gas bub-

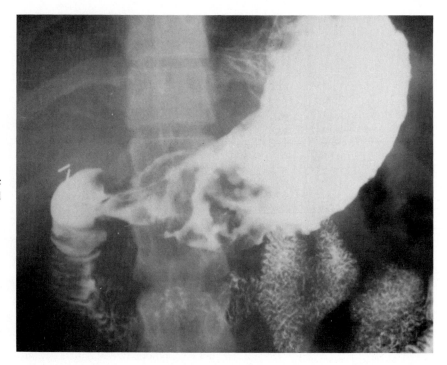

Fig. 6-13 Gastric syphilis. Twenty-seven-year-old woman with secondary syphilis presented with epigastric pain. Antral folds are thickened, and small linear ulcers are seen.

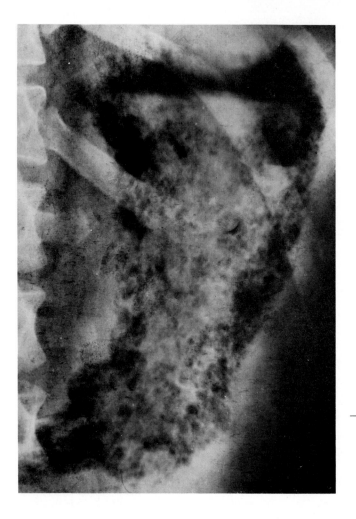

bles may be demonstrated radiographically. The term *emphysematous gastritis* is sometimes applied to patients with intramural gas regardless of the underlying pathogenesis (Fig. 6-14).

Hemorrhagic gastritis

Hemorrhagic gastritis probably represents a group of diseases with different causes but with a similar end result—bleeding mucosa. Acute stress ulceration following hypovolemic shock and sepsis is probably the result of mucosal ischemia caused by shunting of blood away from the mucosa. Conventional radiographic studies are usually negative. If the bleeding is not too severe, superficial erosions may be demonstrated by double-contrast techniques.

Chronic gastritis

Histologically, chronic gastritis is characterized by replacement of the normal epithelial cells by cells that are mainly mucus secreting—a process referred to as *intestinalization* or *intestinal metaplasia*—with the end result of mucosal thinning and atrophy.

Fig. 6-14 Bubbly appearance of stomach caused by intramural gas in patient with emphysematous gastritis.
(From Weens HS: *AJR* 55:589, 1946. © 1946, American Roentgen Ray Society.)

Atrophic gastritis

Criteria for the radiographic diagnosis of atrophic gastritis include the absence of folds on the greater curvature and fundus *(bald fundus)* and a tubular stomach with the greater and lesser curvatures roughly parallel. Loss of the micromucosal pattern, or of areae gastricae, may be a more sensitive index of the presence or absence of mucosal atrophy. In patients with *pernicious*

anemia there is a sharp demarcation between the atrophic mucosa of the body and fundus and the normal mucosa of the antrum.

Chronic erosive gastritis

The characteristic radiologic features of chronic erosive gastritis are best seen with double-contrast upper GI series and include *aphthae* (small ulcers) with sur-

A

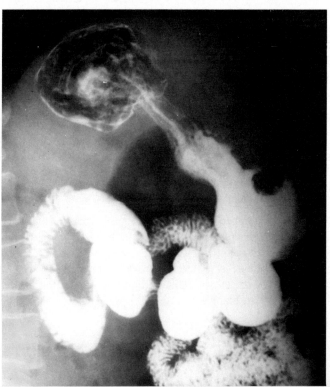

Fig. 6-15 Pseudolymphoma. Forty-five-year-old woman with upper abdominal pain was referred for upper GI series. **A,** Note enlarged fold pattern along greater curvature of fundus and body. Distal stomach is normal. **B,** CT image of stomach shows focal thickening of lateral aspect of gastric wall. Laparotomy revealed gastric wall thickening but was otherwise unremarkable. Full-thickness biopsy showed histologic findings of pseudolymphoma.

B

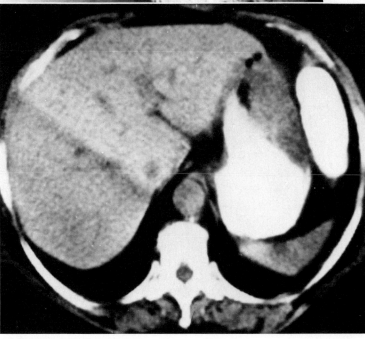

rounding edema clustered or linearly arranged along gastric folds. There is antral predominance of the distribution of these lesions.

Pseudolymphoma

Pseudolymphoma of the stomach is an apt designation since the radiologic and gross appearance of the lesion very closely mimics malignant lymphoma. Pseudolymphoma is an exuberant inflammatory response to chronic gastric ulceration, and most are associated with ulcer disease. Radiographic findings include gastric hyperrugosity, which may be focal; intraluminal masses; and multiple ulcerations (Fig. 6-15). CT findings are similar to those related to gastric lymphoma, except that lymphadenopathy and splenic enlargement are not found.

Granulomatous gastritis

Granulomas are found in conditions in which foreign bodies come into intimate contact with living tissue. Although the conditions are infrequent, the stomach may be involved in a number of infectious and noninfectious granulomatous diseases, including syphilis, tuberculosis, sarcoidosis, histoplasmosis, Crohn's disease, eosinophilic gastritis, and isolated granulomatous gastritis. Regardless of the cause, the radiographic manifestations are similar, consisting of a regular or irregular antral narrowing associated with diminished distensibility;

varying degrees of rigidity; and a granular cobblestone mucosa that replaces the normal rugal pattern. Even microscopic examination may not provide sufficient information for a differential diagnosis.

Crohn's disease

During the acute phases of gastric Crohn's disease, ulceration and fold thickening are the major manifestations. Using air contrast techniques, superficial erosions can be demonstrated in as many as 20% to 40% of cases. These aphthous lesions or erosions represent one of the earliest manifestations of the disease and have been found in asymptomatic patients. The terms *pseudo-Billroth II* and *ram's horn sign* have been applied to the narrowing of the distal stomach that occurs as a late manifestation of the disease involving the antrum. Frequently the adjacent duodenum is also involved (Fig. 6-16). Although the distal stomach is preferentially affected, fundal involvement has also been described.

Injury gastropathy

A number of insults can result in gastric inflammation or necrosis. Hemorrhagic gastritis of varying severity may result from aspirin, nonsteroidal antiinflammatory drugs, and steroids. More severe lesions may be caused by gastric radiation injury and ingestion of corrosive substances.

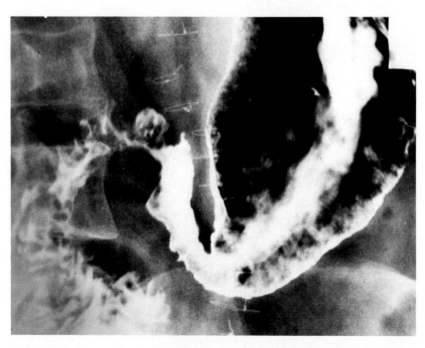

Fig. 6-16 Crohn's disease of antrum and duodenum obliterating normal anatomic landmarks between stomach and duodenum, thus producing "ramshorn" or "pseudoBillroth II" sign.

Corrosive gastropathy

Although it was classically taught that alkalis affect mainly the esophagus and spare the stomach, the ready availability of strong alkali solutions has resulted in more common alkali damage to the stomach. Acids tend to damage mainly the stomach, sparing the esophagus in most cases. The coagulation necrosis produced by these agents may affect only the mucosa and submucosa, or may involve the entire thickness of the gastric wall.

Radiographic studies performed soon after ingestion show striking rugal edema, ulcers, atony, dilatation, intramural gas, sloughing of the mucosa, and perforations (Fig. 6-17). This is followed by cicatrization and varying degrees of gastric outlet obstruction (see Figs. 6-17, 6-18).

Gastric radiation injury

Radiation gastritis, characterized by antral narrowing and mucosal thickening or loss of folds can be observed with dose levels of more than 3500 rads. With doses of 4000 rads or more, ulceration and perforation may occur. On radiologic examination these ulcers are indistinguishable from ordinary peptic ulcers. *Radiation ulcer* with perforation is an acute lesion occurring 1 to 2 months after irradiation. Since the perforation is usually walled off by bowel, adhesions, and inflammatory reactions, it may be confused with inoperable cancer at the time of surgery.

Hypertrophic gastropathy

Four types of hypertrophic gastropathy have been identified. Hypersecretion of gastric acid occurs in three of the four: Zollinger-Ellison syndrome, hypertrophic hypersecretory gastropathy, and hypertrophic hypersecretory gastropathy with protein loss. Ménétrier's disease, the fourth type, is characterized by low acid output and hypoproteinemia because of gastrointestinal protein loss. The hallmark feature of hypertrophic gastropathy is enlargement of gastric folds (hyperrugosity).

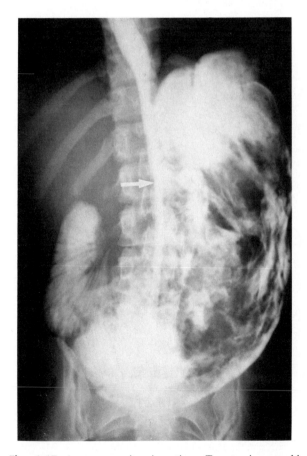

Fig. 6-17 Acute corrosive ingestion. Twenty-six-year-old woman drank concentrated drain cleaner solution. Upper GI series obtained through nasogastric tube *(arrow)* demonstrates diffuse gastric atony and sloughing of mucosa. Necrotic debris fills enlarged stomach. Duodenum was protected by pyloric spasm. Esophagus was severely affected, and resulting esophageal stenosis required bypass.

☐ **BENIGN CAUSES OF HYPERRUGOSTIY** ☐

GASTRITIS

Peptic
Infectious
Pseudolymphoma
Alcoholic
Hypertrophic
Phlegmonous
Parasitic
Granulomatous

INJURY GASTROPATHY

Alcoholic gastritis
Gastric radiation injury
Medication-induced gastritis
Corrosive gastropathy
Freezing gastropathy

HYPERTROPHIC GASTROPATHY

Ménétrier's disease
Zollinger-Ellison syndrome

MISCELLANEOUS GASTROPATHIES

Amyloidosis
Eosinophilic gastritis
Pancreatitis
Varices
Hypoproteinemia
Normal variant

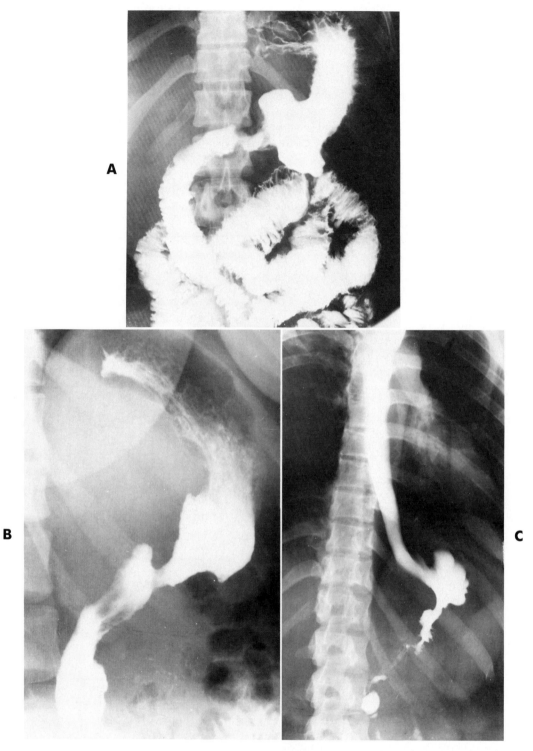

Fig. 6-18 This 32-year-old woman accidentally drank cleaning fluid containing hydrochloric acid. She experienced some burning of the mouth and pharynx but no acute gastrointestinal symptoms. **A,** Initial film taken 24 hours after acid ingestion shows swollen mucosal folds in stomach, duodenum, and proximal jejunum. Note ulcer in distal antrum. There was complete cessation of gastric motor activity. Swollen jejunal folds are similar to those seen in Zollinger-Ellison syndrome. **B,** Two weeks later mucosa has completely sloughed, and there is no mucosal pattern in stomach or duodenum. **C,** Five weeks after initial examination; note striking stenosis of stomach and duodenum and absence of esophageal involvement.

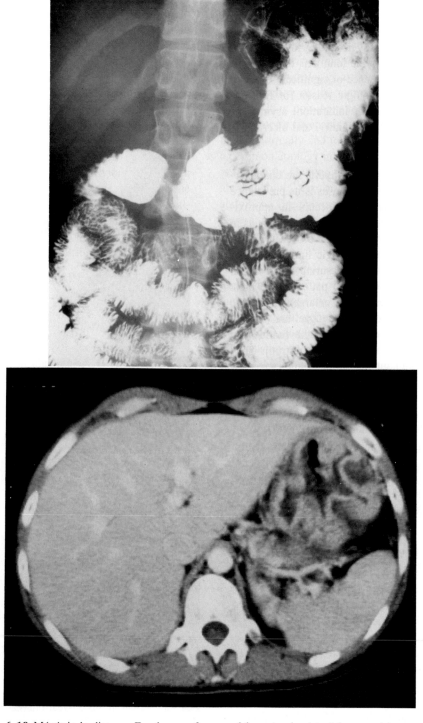

Fig. 6-19 Ménétrier's disease. Focal area of mucosal hypertrophy *(straight arrow)* is separated from second separate area *(curved arrow)* on lesser curvature near esophagogastric junction.
(Courtesy Drs. Peter Huzyk and Harold Shulman.)

volvulus with obstruction. As much as 180 degrees of twisting may occur without obstruction or strangulation of the blood supply. Twisting beyond 180 degrees usually produces complete obstruction with clinical manifestations of an acute condition within the abdomen. When rotation is around a line extending from the cardia to the pylorus along the longitudinal axis of the stomach it is classified as an *organoaxial volvulus*. When rotation occurs around an axis running transversely across the stomach at right angles to the lesser and greater curvatures it is designated as a *mesenteroaxial volvulus*. Mixed types are also seen.

Abnormalities of the four suspensory ligaments of the stomach (hepatic, splenic, colic, and phrenic) are probably the most frequent causes of volvulus. Most reported cases have been associated with diaphragmatic abnormalities, such as eventration or hiatus hernia. About one third of cases are associated with large paraesophageal hernia.

The large, distended stomach resulting from volvulus is easily recognized in an abdominal radiograph. It may extend up into the chest because of diaphragmatic eventration or hernia. This may result in mucosal ischemia with areas of focal necrosis that permit gas to dissect into the gastric wall producing *intramural emphysema* (Fig. 6-26). A barium examination may demonstrate the area of twist and show an inability of barium to enter the stomach.

MISCELLANEOUS NONNEOPLASTIC ABNORMALITIES
Intramural pneumatosis

The presence of gas within the wall of the stomach has been termed *emphysematous gastritis, gastric pneumatosis,* and *interstitial gastric emphysema*. The gas may enter from outside (gastric emphysema), or be the result of intramural gas–forming organisms (emphysematous gastritis). Causes of gastric emphysema are in-

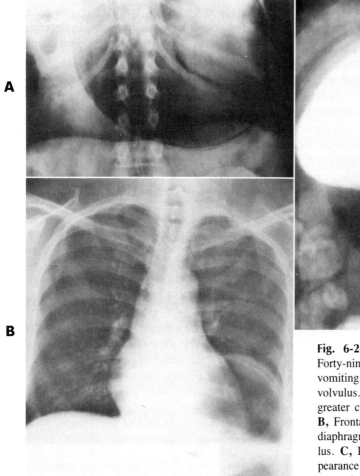

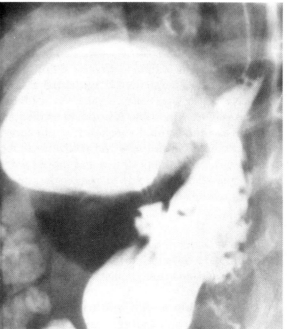

Fig. 6-26 Gastric volvulus with intramural pneumatosis. Forty-nine-year-old woman with 10-day history of nausea and vomiting. **A,** Large, gas-distended stomach is result of gastric volvulus. Note double radiolucent lines within gastric wall on greater curvature caused by submucosal and subserosal gas. **B,** Frontal radiograph of chest illustrating eventration of left diaphragm, which is frequently associated with gastric volvulus. **C,** Barium study done several days later reveals disappearance of obstruction but persistence of marked torsion of stomach.

(**B** from Seaman WB, Fleming RJ: *AJR* 101:431, 1967. © 1967 American Roentgen Ray Society.)

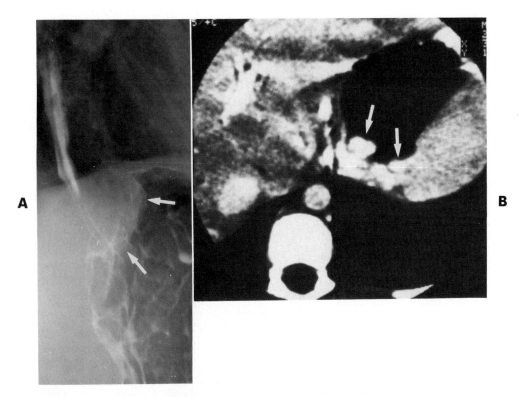

Fig. 6-27 Gastric varix. **A,** Fifteen-year-old boy with congenital hepatic fibrosis was evaluated for anemia. There is lobular mass at esophagogastric junction *(arrows).* No varices were seen in esophagus. **B,** CT image following contrast bolus infusion shows enhancing lobular masses in and about gastric fundus *(arrows)* confirming presence of gastric varices.

creased intraluminal pressure (such as may occur with obstruction), severe vomiting, volvulus, and overinflation during gastroscopy. Trauma, focal areas of ischemic necrosis resulting from distention, or both, may permit intramural dissection of air. Extensive loss of mucosa, as seen following ingestion of a corrosive substance, or ischemic necrosis subsequent to vascular occlusion may also be accompanied by intramural gas. Emphysematous gastritis is a variant of phlegmonous gastritis in which infection in the gastric wall is caused by gas-forming organisms. Gas from intramural gastric pneumatosis may migrate into the portal venous system and be seen in the liver.

Varices

Varices are the most common vascular abnormality of the stomach. Although usually located in the fundus and proximal gastric body, they may also be found in the gastric antrum. They are usually associated with esophageal varices. The radiographic appearance of smooth lobulated filling defects in the fundus or antrum should suggest gastric varices. The diagnosis is more difficult when there are no esophageal varices, as may occur when the splenic vein is obstructed distal to a

patent, normotensive left coronary vein. CT with bolus injection of contrast material may show well-defined rounded or tubular densities that enhance to distinguish them from the gastric wall (Fig. 6-27).

Ectopic pancreas

Most heterotopic pancreatic rests are asymptomatic and are incidental findings. When located in strategic locations such as about the pyloric channel, however, they may cause obstruction. All the pathologic changes that may occur in the pancreas proper have also been observed in ectopic rests, including pancreatitis, carcinoma, and hyperinsulinism.

Ectopic pancreas typically occurs as an umbilicated submucosal nodule, 1 to 2 cm in diameter, 3 to 6 cm from the pylorus, and on the greater curvature of the stomach (Fig. 6-28). The characteristic central depression or umbilication is present in 40% to 60% of cases. The depression is covered by normal-appearing epithelium, although rudimentary ducts may empty into this central pit.

The radiographic appearance is of a sessile, submucosal mass that is indistinguishable from a leiomyoma unless an umbilication is present. Precise, reliable iden-

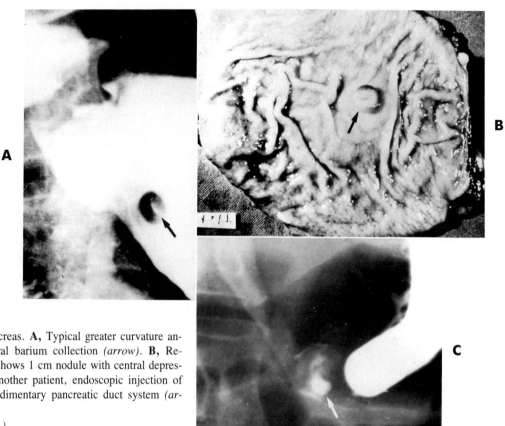

Fig. 6-28 Ectopic pancreas. **A,** Typical greater curvature antral nodule with central barium collection *(arrow).* **B,** Resected gastric antrum shows 1 cm nodule with central depression *(arrow).* **C,** In another patient, endoscopic injection of umbilication shows rudimentary pancreatic duct system *(arrow).*

(Courtesy Dr. Sidney Nelson.)

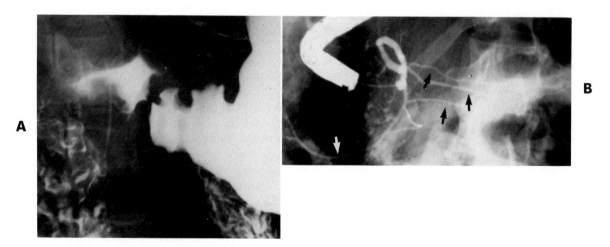

Fig. 6-29 Ectopic pancreas. Thirty-three-year-old woman had persistent pain following cholecystectomy and operative sphincteroplasty. **A,** Marked fold thickening about the gastric antrum. Contrast reflux into common bile duct is caused by prior sphincteroplasty. **B,** Injection of pancreatic duct system shows annular duct around duodenum *(white arrow)* and anomalous ducts in wall of gastric antrum *(black arrows).*

(Courtesy Martin Green, MD.)

tification can be made if ducts are demonstrated by reflux of barium or by endoscopic injection of the rudimentary ducts with contrast medium (Fig. 6-29).

RECOMMENDED READING

1. Ariyama J et al: Gastro-duodenal erosions in Crohn's disease, *Gastrointest Radiol* 5:121, 1980.
2. Balthazar EJ et al: Computed tomographic recognition of gastric varices, *Am J Roentgenol* 142:1121, 1984.
3. Brody JM et al: Gastric tuberculosis, a manifestation of acquired immunodeficiency syndrome, *Radiology* 159:347, 1986.
4. Carlson HC, Breen JF: Amyloidosis and plasma cell dyscrasias: gastrointestinal involvement, *Semin Roentgenol* 21:128, 1986.
5. Carter R et al: Acute gastric volvulus. *Am J Surg* 140:99, 1980.
6. Chiles JT, Platz CE: The radiographic manifestations of pseudolymphoma of the stomach, *Radiology* 116:551, 1975.
7. DeBakey M, Ochsner A: Bezoars and concretions: a comprehensive review of the literature with an analysis of 303 collected cases, *Surgery* 4:934, 1938.
8. Laufer I et al: Demonstration of superficial gastric erosions by double contrast radiography, *Gastroenterology* 68:387, 1975.
9. Meyers H, Parker J: Emphysematous gastritis, *Radiology* 89:426, 1967.
10. Rohrmann CA et al: Radiologic and histologic differentiation of neuromuscular disorders of the gastrointestinal tract: visceral myopathies, visceral neuropathies, and progressive systemic sclerosis, *Am J Roentgenol* 143:933, 1981.
11. Scharschmidt BF: The natural history of hypertrophic gastropathy (Menetrier's disease): report of a case with 16 year follow-up and review of 120 cases from the literature, *Am J Med* 63:644, 1977.
12. Thoeni RF, Gedgaudas RK: Ectopic pancreas: usual and unusual features, *Gastrointest Radiol* 5:37, 1980.

Neoplastic disorders of the stomach (gastric cancer)

HIKOO SHIRAKABE
MASAKAZU MARUYAMA

DIAGNOSIS

Unless there is a palpable mass in the abdomen, radiographic or endoscopic examination is usually the first procedure performed in the diagnosis of cancer. When there is a palpable mass, CT or ultrasound may be the first choice. The architecture of the gastric wall, including evaluation of a cancerous lesion and its relation to neighboring structures, may be accurately assessed by endoscopic ultrasonography (EUS). CT is useful for visualizing the thickness of the affected gastric wall and its relation to the neighboring structures and for detection of lymph node and liver metastases. Liver metastases may also be evaluated with ultrasound.

Role of computed tomography

A system for classifying and correlating CT findings and staging of gastric adenocarcinoma with surgical and pathologic findings is summarized as follows:

Stage I: Intraluminal mass without gastric wall thickening (gastric wall less than 1 cm thick); no metastases or tumor extension
Stage II: Thickening of the gastric wall to greater than 1 cm, but no evidence of metastatic disease or direct tumor extension
Stage III: Thickening of the gastric wall with direct extension of tumor into adjacent organs, but without evidence of distant metastatic disease (Fig. 6-30)
Stage IV: Thickening of the gastric wall with evidence of metastatic disease; direct extension of tumor into adjacent organs possible.

With CT, lymph node metastasis is judged on the basis of lymphadenopathy alone, and a lymph node measuring more than 1 cm is considered positive. Since metastatic nodes may be less than 1 cm, and since inflammatory processes may cause lymph node enlargement, CT is not a reliable modality for determining lymph node metastasis.

Early gastric cancer
Definition and classification

Early gastric cancer has been defined as "carcinoma in which invasion was limited to the mucosa and submucosa, regardless of lymph nodes and distant metastases." The following classification can be applied to endoscopic and radiographic findings:

Type I: Polypoid (> 0.5 cm in height)
Type II: Superficial
    Type IIa: Elevated (> 0.5 cm in height)
    Type IIb: Flat (minimal or no alteration in height of mucosa)
    Type IIc: Depressed (superficial erosion, usually not extending beyond the muscularis mucosae)
Type III: Excavated (prominent depression, usually caused by ulceration)

When an early cancer reveals different morphologic patterns, the two or more types are described together. The predominant pattern precedes the other, for example, a lesion might be described as type IIc + III or type I + IIa.

Radiographic diagnosis and correlation with endoscopy

In the diagnosis of gastric cancer, including early and advanced cancers, only a minor difference exists in the sensitivity and specificity between radiology and endoscopy. Maruyama's studies have shown that the sensitivity of the initial radiographic examination is 97.1%, specificity is 32.3%, and accuracy is 33.8%. With endoscopy, sensitivity is 99.8%, specificity is 39.7%, and accuracy is 46.2%. It is important to be aware that panendoscopy with a forward-view endoscope gives much

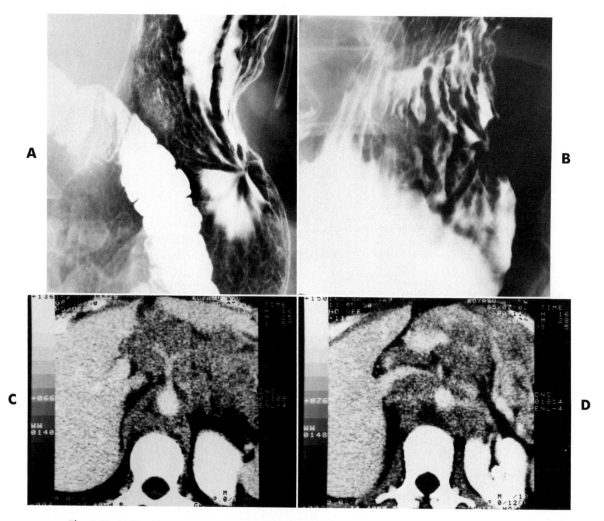

Fig. 6-30 A, Double-contrast radiograph of advanced cancer simulating type IIc. **B,** Compression film of same patient showing a tumor formation that was not detected by CT. **C** and **D,** CT showing conglomerated mass consisting of metastatic lymph nodes and lesser omentum. Direct invasion to liver has occurred.

(**B,** Courtesy Dr. Y. Masijda; **C** and **D** courtesy Dr. M Hori.)

less information about the diagnosis than do other types of endoscopy.

Conventional and endoscopic ultrasonography

On endoscopic ultrasound studies the normal gastric wall is visualized as a five-layer structure. Described from the inside out, the gastric wall consists of (1) a slightly hyperechoic layer corresponding histologically to the foveolar gastric glands, (2) a hypoechoic thin layer corresponding histologically to the propria gastric glands, (3) a hyperechoic thick layer corresponding histologically to the submucosa, (4) a hypoechoic thick layer corresponding histologically to the propria muscle, and (5) a hyperechoic layer on the outside corresponding histologically to the serosa.

Recognition of abnormalities in each layer leads to estimation of the invasive depth of the cancer and to the differential diagnosis between benign and malignant submucosal tumors. Ultrasonography also provides information on the condition of the extragastric space and on the relation of the stomach to the neighboring structures and organs. The layer examination is used to answer questions that other methods cannot and helps to determine the treatment modality and to assess the clinical course before and after treatment.

Endoscopic ultrasonography is used for the same purpose as conventional ultrasound and is especially important in the assessment of the depth of cancer. EUS, because it provides substantial evidence of cancer-induced alterations in each layer of the gastric wall

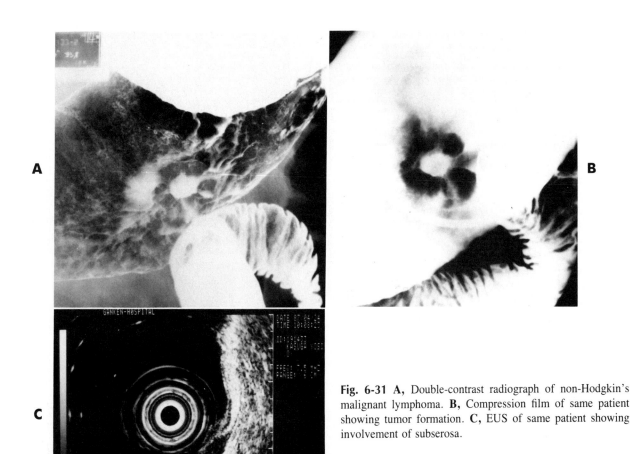

Fig. 6-31 A, Double-contrast radiograph of non-Hodgkin's malignant lymphoma. **B,** Compression film of same patient showing tumor formation. **C,** EUS of same patient showing involvement of subserosa.

(Fig. 6-31), is more accurate than traditional ultrasound in the estimation of the invasive depth of cancer, particularly that of early cancer.

Early polypoid cancer

Diagnosis of early polypoid cancers begins with recognition of the size, form, and surface pattern of these lesions. Their largest diameter typically ranges from 1 to 4 cm. Height, which is estimated on a compression or double-contrast image, provides a rough distinction between type I and type IIa lesions. Most important for the differentiation between malignant and benign lesions, however, is the surface pattern of the lesion. Malignant lesions smaller than 1 cm usually have a granular or lobular surface pattern, which is characteristic of early cancer. The contours of these lesions are also notched. The granular or lobular pattern, although irregular and enlarged, is similar to that of the surrounding mucosa that bears the lesion. For example, a tendency to imitate the pattern of the areae gastricae is preserved in a polypoid cancer with invasion limited to the submucosal layer. Double-contrast radiography is best suited for visualizing a background where polypoid cancer has developed.

As the cancer infiltrates beyond the submucosal layer, the similarity of surface pattern disappears and is usually replaced by erosion or ulceration. In contrast, even a large polypoid cancer preserves its similarity to the surrounding mucosa as long as the invasive depth is limited to the submucosa.

The *gross appearance* of gastric polypoid lesions is described as pedunculated, subpedunculated, or sessile. The sessile lesion is further divided into two subtypes, one with constriction at the base and the other with gradual sloping. Most type IIa lesions have a constriction at the base, whereas benign lesions, including epithelial and submucosal lesions, show a gradual sloping.

Adenoma

Adenomas, or *adenomatous polyps* as they are sometimes called, are classified histologically as *"tubular adenoma of small intestinal type."* They occur most frequently in patients older than 50 years of age, and the incidence is highest in patients 60 years of age. The gross appearance is that of a flat, mucosal elevation or polypoid lesion, usually no larger than 2 cm, and often (in approximately 50% of cases), only 1 cm. The gastric antrum is the most common site, and adenomas are seen only rarely in the upper portion of the stomach. Malignant transformation is uncommon, occurring in not more than 0.4% of cases.

Types I and IIA

Early polyploid cancer (types I and IIa) is most frequently seen in older patients, usually 60 to 70 years of age. Type I is less common than type IIa, and its gross appearance is usually sessile, with an irregular surface pattern that simulates the areae gastricae. Rarely the lesion is pedunculated. Most type I lesions measure more than 2 cm.

Most pedunculated lesions are *benign hyperplastic polyps* with a surface pattern that is nearly always smooth, as opposed to the granular surface and lobulation of early polypoid cancers.

Type IIa lesions have a flat mucosal elevation not higher than 0.5 cm and a constriction at the base. They are usually larger than 2 cm with a surface pattern of somewhat irregular granularity (Fig. 6-32).

Double-contrast radiography is indispensable for comparison of the lesion's surface pattern with the surrounding areae gastricae.

Type IIa + IIc gastric cancer

The gross appearance of a type IIa + IIc lesion is that of a flat mucosal elevation with a recognizable central depression. Although lesions usually range from 1 to 3 cm in diameter, they are sometimes larger than 3 cm. The central depression is usually irregular, and its size and depth are closely related to the invasive depth of the cancer. The larger and deeper the depression, the deeper is the estimated invasive depth and the greater the likelihood of lymph node and liver metastases. The depression is not always in the center of a polypoid lesion. A type IIa + IIc lesion is best delineated with the compression method, which is particularly well suited for the demonstration of the exact form of the central depression.

Early depressed gastric cancer

The radiographic diagnosis of early depressed cancer is based on the analysis of the depression and converging folds. The depression is assessed in terms of its outline, surface, and depth. The depression in cancer is usually irregular and has a serrated or spiculated margin, whereas a benign ulcer has a sharp, straight margin. The extent of early depressed cancer is difficult to

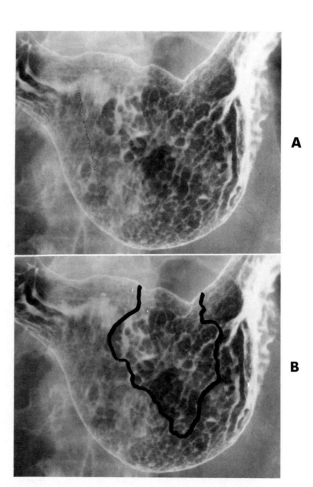

Fig. 6-32 A, Double-contrast radiograph of type IIa early cancer limited to mucosal membrane. **B,** Diagram of same cancer showing limit of lesion.

define. In most cases the surface of the depression is uneven because of an irregular proliferation of cancerous tissue. Sometimes an islandlike nodule remains in the depression and is more prominent than the unevenness of the cancer depression. The converging folds reveal characteristic changes, such as tapering, clubbing, interruption, and fusion. The fusion of the folds is called the *V deformity* (Fig. 6-33).

Type IIc, type IIc + III, and type III gastric cancer

The difference between type IIc and type III lesions is recognized radiographically by the thickness of the collected contrast medium in a depression. A relatively thick collection of contrast medium, approximately the same as found in a peptic ulcer, indicates a type III lesion. A thinner collection indicates a type IIc depression. A combination of the two is termed *type IIc + III* or *type III + IIc*. Usually the deeper part (type III) is in

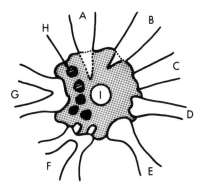

Fig. 6-33 Various appearances of converging folds and unevenness in early depressed cancer. *A,* Gradual tapering; *B,* abrupt tapering; *C,* abrupt interruption; *D* and *E,* clubbing; *F,* fusion with abrupt tapering; *G,* fusion (V-shaped deformity); *H,* unevenness; *I,* regenerative epithelium.

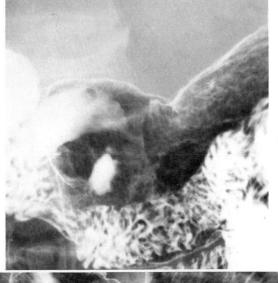

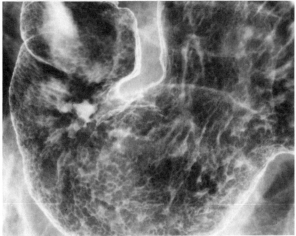

Fig. 6-34 A, Double-contrast radiograph of type III early cancer. **B,** Double-contrast radiograph of same patient taken 2 months later. Ulceration (type III) was replaced by type IIc lesion limited to mucosa.

the center of the depression surrounded by the more shallow part. An ulcer scar may sometimes be seen as a slight depression, as may an erosion or a healing peptic ulcer. In these cases, however, the depression is fainter than that seen in a type IIc lesion, and the density of the contrast medium is homogeneous.

Type IIc lesions are best demonstrated with double-contrast examinations. A profile niche without any irregularity should be closely examined. In type III + IIc lesions the profile niche is so prominent that the surrounding type IIc lesion may be missed and a benign peptic ulcer diagnosed. During follow-up studies the niche in a type III lesion may decrease in size, and the surrounding type IIc lesion may increase and be recognized clearly. The niche finally disappears and a fairly large type IIc lesion then becomes evident. This phenomenon is sometimes called the *malignant cycle* (Fig. 6-34).

Early gastric cancer smaller than 1 cm

Lesions with a largest diameter of less than 0.5 cm (*microcarcinomas*) may be too small for the radiographic criteria of malignancy to be applied, and endoscopy may be more effective for their detection. *Type IIb lesions* are sometimes referred to as cancerous lesions in an incipient phase. A simulated type IIb appearance has also been identified in which a subtle difference between the elevation or depression and the normal surrounding mucosa can be seen. Consequently the border of these lesions is not clearly defined and they are sometimes called *type IIb-like lesions.*

Superficial spreading carcinoma

Type II early carcinomas are frequently referred to as superficial spreading carcinomas. The radiographic

diagnosis is simple, except for differentiation from the type IIb-like lesions already described. A typical type IIa or type IIc lesion with surface dimensions of 25 to 36 cm^2 is easily diagnosed by double-contrast radiography. Lesions greater than 36 cm are difficult to identify because the area of affected mucosa is so large in comparison with a relatively small part of normal mucosa.

Advanced gastric cancer
Classification

Advanced cancer is defined as a lesion that involves at least the muscularis propria layer or the deeper layer of the gastric wall (subserosa and serosa). The Borrmann classification (Fig. 6-35), based on gross alterations, will be used as the basis for this discussion.

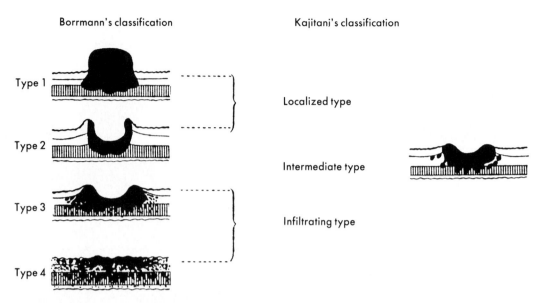

Fig. 6-35 Gross classification of advanced cancer.

Borrmann types 1 and 2

A *Borrmann type 1* lesion (Fig. 6-36) is a large polypoid lesion, usually exceeding 3 cm in its greatest diameter, with large irregular lobulation. Sometimes a slight surface depression is present. On barium examinations the *Borrmann type 2* lesion is visible as a localized filling defect of the gastric wall. On compression studies with contrast medium it appears as an irregular crater with a greatly raised margin sharply circumscribed from the normal surrounding mucosa. Its size usually exceeds 3 cm in its greatest diameter. The smaller Borrmann type is difficult to distinguish from early cancer type IIa + IIc with involvement of the submucosa.

Borrmann type 3

Usually the Borrmann type 3 lesion is larger than Borrmann type 2. Radiographs after barium filling reveal a filling defect and stiffening of the gastric wall. Compression radiographs show a large, irregular crater and the surrounding radiolucent defect, which is not as well defined as that of the Borrmann type 2 lesion. Double-contrast radiographs best demonstrate the whole aspect of the Borrmann type 3 lesion. Sometimes a component of type IIc may surround the crater; in this case a greater or lesser deformity of the stomach resulting from extensive cancerous infiltration may be revealed.

Borrmann type 4

On barium radiographs the Borrmann type 4 lesion, also known as *diffuse infiltrative carcinoma,* is seen as a deformity of the stomach. The greatly narrowed gastric antrum is the typical site of involvement. Direct invasion to the pancreas can be assessed by CT and/or MRI.

Linitis plastica

In a broad classification linitis plastica is a Borrmann type 4 lesion (Fig. 6-37). Many efforts have been made

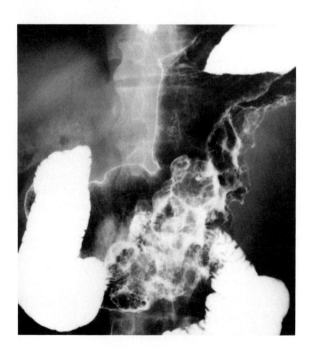

Fig. 6-36 Double-contrast radiograph of Borrmann type 1 lesion consisting of huge mass involving serosa and neighboring structures.

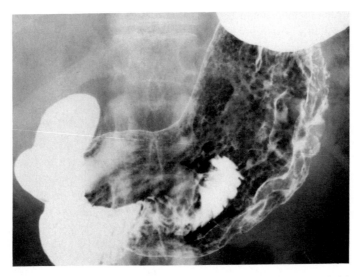

Fig. 6-37 Double-contrast radiograph of linitis plastica type of cancer without shrinkage of stomach.

(Courtesy Dr. H Shimizu.)

to detect the early phase of linitis plastica. Indeed, it is the only problem that remains unsettled in the diagnosis of gastric cancer. A stomach that has been judged normal on routine radiographic examinations may change into a *"leather bottle"* structure within a few months.

Differentiation of advanced and type IIc cancer

Advanced cancer consistently reveals a filling defect, a surrounding raised margin, and shrinkage of the affected portion or of the entire thickness of the stomach (Fig. 6-38). In addition, ultrasound and CT are indispensable in the assessment of the thickness of the affected gastric wall and lymph node metastases. If available, EUS provides the best information on the architecture of the invasive pattern.

Carcinoma of the gastric stump after gastrectomy

Cancer of the gastric stump or gastric remnant is grossly divided into two groups: (1) cancer arising after an initial gastrectomy for a benign lesion and (2) cancer arising after an initial gastrectomy for cancer. At present, double-contrast radiography is able to detect early cancer of the gastric stump after gastrectomy for benign lesions.

Remaining and recurrent cancer of the gastric stump

Remaining cancer refers to a stomal cancer in the cut end of the resected stomach. Improvements in surgical technique have minimized the incidence of remaining cancer. *Recurrent cancer* refers to a cancer that involves the gastric stump and may result from intragastric metastases. Peritoneal dissemination or direct invasion of the gastric stump from metastatic lymph nodes is common in cases of recurrent cancer of the stomach. Ascites and a recurrent mass in the abdomen, including lymph node metastases, are best assessed by CT. However, peritoneal dissemination without ascites is difficult to detect by CT.

Multiple cancers

Late recurrence of a remaining cancer of the stump may be seen several years after the initial gastrectomy and may be difficult to distinguish from synchronous multiple cancers near the stoma. For radiographic diag-

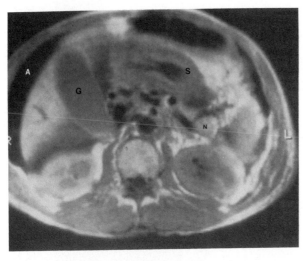

Fig. 6-38 T_1 weighted image of a scirrhous carcinoma of the stomach *(S)*. A large gallbladder *(G)* is seen. Multiple nodes are seen around celiac artery and a very large node *(N)* is seen next to the spleen. Varices are seen posterior to the stomach. *A*, ascites.

nosis, as much compression as possible should be employed to the stoma and its vicinity. Appropriate double-contrast studies facilitate the diagnosis not only of advanced cancer, but also of early cancer of the gastric stump. Endoscopy and biopsy, however, are indispensable when an abnormality is suspected on the basis of radiographic results.

Malignant lymphoma

Malignant lymphoma is grossly divided into two groups: non-Hodgkin's malignant lymphoma and Hodgkin's disease. The most common sites of malignant lymphomas of the stomach are the lower and middle thirds.

Classification

Several classifications for malignant lymphoma have been proposed. One based on gross appearance divides the lesions into four types:

Polypoid type: localized protuberance into the gastric lumen

Ulcerating type: localized ulceration with prominent and circumscribed margin

Intermediate type: ulceration with less prominent and circumscribed margin

Infiltrating type: (1) giant rugae or nodular tumor formation or (2) lesions simulating superficial, depressed type IIc early cancer.

A classification for *early* lesions has also been proposed and again consists of four types: *superficial depressed, polypoid, ulceropolypoid,* and *giant rugal.* In this classification the superficial depressed type is most common and most important in the differential diagnosis with type IIc early cancer.

Radiographic features

The radiographic features of both early and advanced malignant lymphomas consist of two basic components: (1) a mucosal elevation that suggests a submucosal origin and (2) multiple erosions or ulcerations (Figs. 6-39, 6-40). The lesion may develop into a large mass consisting of giant rugal folds with ulcerations that simulate the linitis plastica type of cancer. In cases of early malignant lymphoma the combination of the two components is recognized by a meticulous examination with compression and double-contrast radiographs. In the depressed type, resembling a type IIc early cancer (Fig. 6-41), a partially raised margin may reveal a submucosal origin. Large lymphomas sometimes decrease in size during a short period preceding the follow-up study. An early malignant lymphoma may be reduced in size by ulceration.

OTHER MALIGNANT AND BENIGN TUMORS

Leiomyosarcomas are the only important smooth muscle malignant tumors except for malignant lympho-

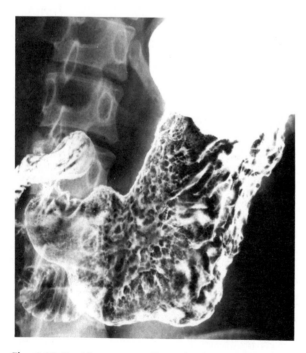

Fig. 6-39 Double-contrast radiograph of non-Hodgkin's malignant lymphoma involving muscularis propria layer.

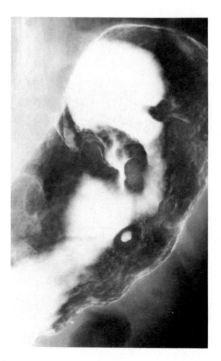

Fig. 6-40 Double-contrast radiograph of advanced non-Hodgkin's malignant lymphoma. Multiple lesions are noted.

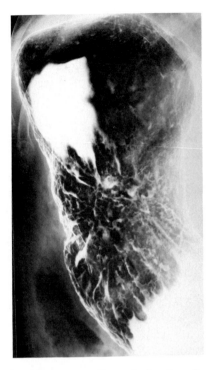

Fig. 6-41 Double-contrast radiograph of early malignant lymphoma. Non-Hodgkin's malignant lymphoma involves submucosa.

(Courtesy Dr. Y Baba.)

mas. Gastric carcinoid tumors also deserve mention because of their metastasizing potential. Soft tumors such as lipomas and glomus tumors, which change shape with compression, are also important. Radiographic signs of submucosal tumors, such as the gradual sloping of the tumor and a bridging fold, are seen in almost all cases.

Leiomyosarcomas and leiomyomas

Leiomyosarcomas and leiomyomas are the most common submucosal tumors of the stomach, and although they occur most often in the upper portion, they may appear in any part. They vary in size from 2 to 8 cm, and many measure 3 to 4 cm.

Leiomyomas and leiomyosarcomas appear on radiograph as round, hemispheric tumor shadows, frequently showing a central depression or ulceration (Fig. 6-42). The surface of the tumor is usually smooth, and the central depression sometimes becomes so deep that it appears to be a diverticulum. A large ulceration that appears to be a Borrmann type 2 advanced cancer may be seen in cases of leiomyosarcoma.

Leiomyomas and leiomyosarcomas may be difficult to differentiate by radiography and endoscopy, but double-contrast and compression radiographs are effective. Double-contrast radiography is the only method by which tumors located in the upper portion and fornix of the stomach can be discerned.

Carcinoid tumors

Carcinoid tumors rarely appear in the stomach. They arise from the deeper portions of the gastric mucosa and

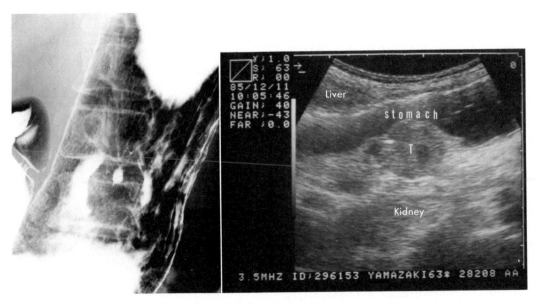

Fig. 6-42 Double-contrast radiograph of leiomyosarcoma. Ultrasonograph of same patient.

(Courtesy Dr. H Matsue.)

are similar to a submucosal tumor in an early phase. As the lesion enlarges, an erosion appears on the central surface, and finally an ulceration develops. Endoscopic biopsy is a decisive factor in diagnosis.

Neurogenic tumors

Neurogenic tumors show essentially the same radiographic features as myogenic tumors.

Metastatic tumors

The incidence of metastases to the stomach is reported to be low (2.3% according to the Japanese literature and 0.2% to 0.4% in the Western literature). Esophageal cancer, especially malignant melanoma, and breast cancer are the two most common primaries. The *bull's eye sign* was first considered characteristic of a gastric metastasis from malignant melanoma. However, this sign is also seen in metastatic growths from cancer of the lungs, pancreas, and colon. Metastatic neoplasms usually appear radiographically as multiple, sharply delineated filling defects with a wide base.

RECOMMENDED READING

1. Maruyama M: Early gastric cancer. In Laufer I: *Double contrast gastrointestinal radiology with endoscopic correlation,* Philadelphia, 1979, WB Saunders.
2. Matsue H: Ultrasonographic examination and diagnosis of stomach diseases. In Maruyama M, Kimura K, editors: *Review of clinical research in gastroenterology,* Tokyo, 1988, Igaku-Shoin.
3. Nishizawa M, Maruyama M: Radiographic diagnosis of depth of invasion of gastric cancer. In Shirakaba H et al, editors: *Atlas of x-ray diagnosis of early gastric cancer,* ed. 2, Tokyo. 1981, Igaku-Shoin.
4. Pomeranz H, Margolin HN: Metastases to the gastrointestinal tract from malignant melanoma, *Am J Roentgenol* 88:712, 1962.
5. Sakita T et al: Observations on the healing of ulcerations in early gastric cancer: the life cycle of the malignant ulcer, *Gastroenterology* 60:835, 1971.
6. Yarita T, Baba Y: Radiographic diagnosis of cancer smaller than 10 mm. In Shirakabe H et al, editors: *Atlas of x-ray diagnosis of early gastric cancer,* Tokyo, 1982, Igaku-Shoin.

Peptic disease
HERBERT Y KRESSEL
MARC S LEVINE

EPIDEMIOLOGY AND PATHOGENESIS

Duodenal ulcers are generally accepted to be clinically three or four times more common than gastric ulcers, yet at autopsy the incidence of the two diseases is more nearly equal. In general, duodenal ulcers are associated with increased acid production, whereas gastric ulcers commonly occur in patients with decreased acid production. The two groups overlap, however, and gastric and duodenal ulcer disease often coexist. Prostaglandins that are produced throughout the GI tract appear to be important in maintaining normal cytoprotec-

tion. There appears to exist a decrease in endogenous prostaglandin production in the gastric mucosa of patients with peptic ulceration, implicating prostaglandins in the complex pathogenesis of peptic ulceration. A substantial body of evidence demonstrates an association between peptic ulcer disease and cigarette smoking and long-term aspirin use.

RADIOGRAPHIC APPEARANCE OF PEPTIC ULCERATION

Understanding the basic terms used to describe pathologic changes in peptic ulcer disease is helpful in assessing the radiographic appearance. An *erosion* is a localized loss of less than the full thickness of the mucosa. An *ulcer* is a localized loss of the full thickness of the mucosa that may extend into deeper layers of the stomach, for example, the submucosa or muscularis propria.

The diagnostic hallmark of peptic ulceration is the identifiable presence of a fixed niche or collection that is unchanging in size or location. With conventional single-contrast examination, ulcers are generally identified as barium collections that may be radiographed *en face,* obliquely, or in profile. With double-contrast examination, the coated ulcer may be radiographed either filled or empty, further altering its appearance.

The site of peptic ulceration and its relation to the barium pool also affect its radiographic appearance. When ulcers on the dependent surface (that is, the posterior wall) are filled with barium and viewed *en face,* they appear as barium collections that may have associated radiating folds or a mass effect. When the ulcer is emptied of barium during the course of the examination, the emptied but coated ulcer crater appears as a ring shadow. Similarly, when ulcers on the nondependent surface (that is, the anterior wall), are seen *en face,* they appear as ring shadows on double-contrast views; they fill with barium on prone compression views (Fig. 6-43). Ulcer craters on the nondependent surface with gradually sloping margins may not be visualized on routine double-contrast views, and both upright and prone compression films are helpful in the search for ulcers in this location. When viewed in profile, barium-filled peptic ulcers are seen as unchanging barium collections that typically project beyond the lumen. Viewed in profile, the coated but air-filled ulcer crater is somewhat confusing, appearing as a fixed curving line that extends beyond the expected lumen. When seen obliquely, a coated air-filled ulcer may appear merely as an unexplained curving line.

En face appearance

Typically, the radiating folds are smooth and symmetric; clubbing, nodularity, fusion, or penciling of radiating folds should suggest the possibility of a neo-

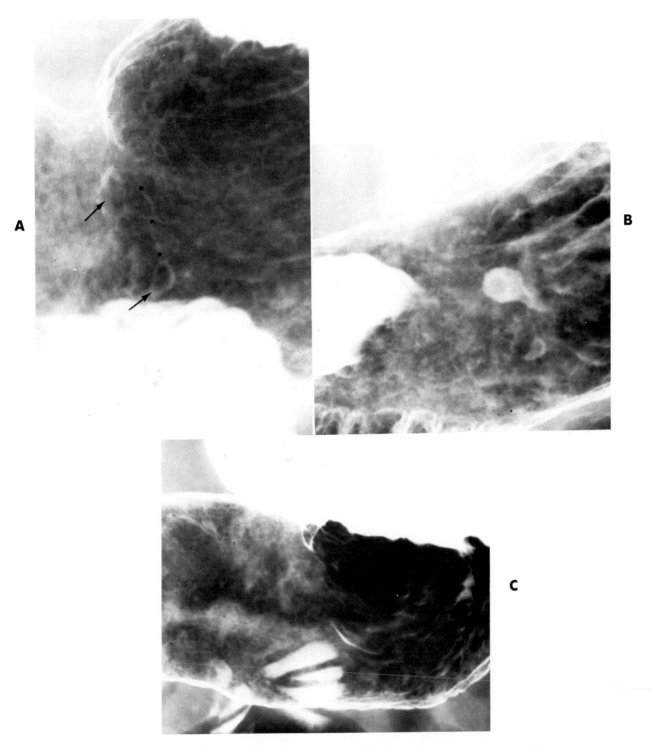

Fig. 6-43 Filled vs. empty ulcer craters. **A,** When additional barium covers dependent surface, flame-shaped ulcers fill with barium and are more readily discerned. **B,** Cone-down RPO view of body of stomach in patient with abdominal pain. Two ring shadows *(arrows)* and connecting linear grooves *(dots)* are noted. **C,** Follow-up examination 4 weeks later shows ulcer healing without evidence of scar formation.

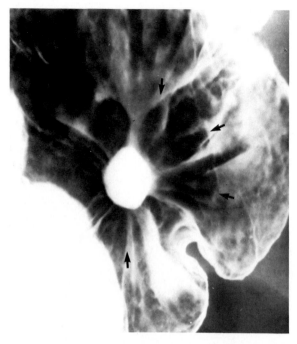

Fig. 6-44 *En face* view of gastric ulcer. Note prominent radiating folds that extend directly to ulcer. There is lucency around ulcer *(arrows)* that reflects inflammatory mass effect.

plasm and the need for a biopsy. Depending on the stage of ulceration, the folds radiate to the ulcer bed (Fig. 6-44). In ulcers with little residual inflammatory reaction, folds may reach the ulcer crater. In ulcers with significant inflammatory reaction, an *ulcer collar* or *mound* is present and the radiating folds seem to originate not at the ulcer margin but more peripherally, at the edges of the associated mound or collar of edema. If normal areae gastricae are identified at the edges of the ulcer crater, the lesion is unlikely to harbor a malignant change.

Profile appearance

In the profile view, three features are associated with benign peptic ulceration: (1) the Hampton line, (2) the ulcer collar, and (3) the ulcer mound (Fig. 6-45).

The *Hampton line* is a thin, sharply delineated lucency with straight parallel margins. The line traverses the orifice of the ulcer niche and is usually approximately 1 mm in width. It represents the edge of overhanging gastric mucosa at the orifice of an undermined benign gastric ulcer. Generally this finding is best visualized on spot films obtained with compression.

Ulcer collar is the term used to describe a thicker lucent band interposed between the ulcer niche and the lumen of the stomach. This band generally indicates a mild or moderate extent of edema and inflammatory re-

action surrounding the ulcer crater. If the inflammatory reaction associated with an ulcer is more severe, an *ulcer mound* may be identified in the profile view. The mound of edema should be smooth and sharply delineated, and the ulcer should arise centrally within it. The margins should form a smooth obtuse angle where they join with the adjacent normal gastric wall.

LOCATION OF PEPTIC ULCERATION

If an ulcer is identified in the duodenal bulb, the assessment of malignant potential is of minimal concern because duodenal ulceration rarely heralds malignant disease. In the stomach, however, identification of the small subgroup of ulcerations that represent malignant disease is of the utmost importance.

Gastric ulcers

The majority of ulcers occur along the lesser curvature or the antrum or body of the stomach. Double-contrast radiographs, as well as prone or upright compression films, should be obtained to carefully evaluate the tangential appearance of *lesser curvature ulcers* for features of benign or malignant disease. When high lesser curvature ulcers are encountered, however, a double-contrast right posterior oblique view with the table semiupright at 45 degrees is preferred.

If not on the lesser curvature, most benign ulcers in the antrum or body of the stomach are located on the *posterior wall*. The *en face* appearance of these lesions should be evaluated for features of benign or malignant disease. Benign gastric lesions occasionally are located on the anterior wall. Double-contrast examination should be supplemented by prone compression views to avoid missing these lesions.

Although benign gastric ulcers are rarely found on the proximal half of the greater curvature, they are often found in the distal half of the stomach and are usually caused by aspirin or aspirin-containing compounds. Unlike ulcers on the lesser curvature or posterior wall, *greater curvature ulcers* tend to be associated with considerable mass effect and may have an apparent intraluminal location on profile views, erroneously suggesting an ulcerated malignancy (Fig. 6-46). Furthermore, the edges of the associated mass effect may be shouldered, and the borders of the mound of edema surrounding the edema may be scalloped and irregular. The latter findings relate to the extensive circular muscle spasm associated with these lesions, as well as the profile appearance of radiating gastric rugae on the greater curvature.

The term *juxtapyloric ulcer* has been introduced to include the morphologic pyloric channel and the immediate prepyloric region. Approximately 25% of gastric ulcers are pyloric or prepyloric in location. The overwhelming majority of ulcers in this location are benign.

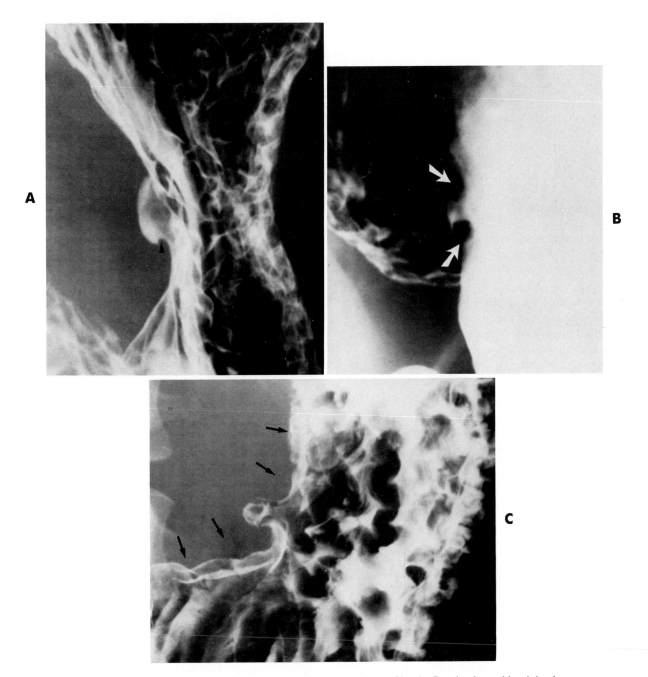

Fig. 6-45 Variation of inflammatory mass effect as seen in profile. **A,** Gastric ulcer with minimal mass effect. Note Hampton line *(arrow)* that represents edge of overhanging gastric mucosa. **B,** Gastric ulcer with greater inflammatory mass effect. Ulcer collar is identified *(arrows).* **C,** Lesser curvature gastric ulcer with smooth symmetric mound of edema *(arrows).*

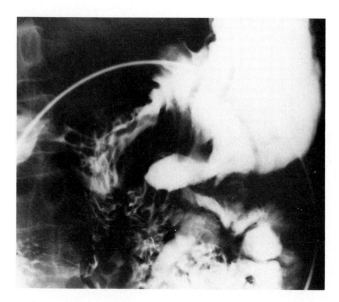

Fig. 6-46 Benign greater curvature antral ulcer. Note excessive mass effect and nodularity.

Juxtapyloric ulcers tend to be small and are typically less than 4 mm in diameter. On occasion, shallow pyloric channel ulcers may appear as ring shadows on double-contrast views so that prone or upright compression films should be obtained to better delineate these lesions.

Duodenal ulcers

Duodenal ulcers overwhelmingly tend to occur proximally in the duodenal bulb *(bulbar ulcers)* (Fig. 6-47). Whereas peptic ulcerations of the stomach occur predominantly on the posterior wall, duodenal ulcers commonly involve the anterior wall, making a detailed search for anterior wall duodenal ulcers an essential part of the examination of the duodenum. Although supine left posterior oblique double-contrast views probably demonstrate three fourths of duodenal ulcers, prone oblique compression views that provide information about the anterior wall are essential. In one study 12% of duodenal ulcers were demonstrated solely on prone compression spot films. Prone films are also helpful in demonstrating the barium-filled ulcer crater. Duodenal ulcers are seen as fixed barium collections or rings that may be associated with radiating folds and deformity. Often the associated deformity and convergence of mucosal folds are readily apparent and suggest the location of active ulceration. However, it is important to remember that the deformity and convergence of the folds alone are not sufficient for the diagnosis of active peptic ulcer; rather the actual crater must be visualized. Severe peptic scarring may render the duodenal bulb so deformed that precise identification of an ulcer is no longer possible. Sometimes, however, duodenal ulcers occur with minimal or no deformity and in an apparently pliable duodenal bulb.

Because duodenal ulcer disease is characterized by episodes of recurrent ulceration, morphologic analysis is important. The overwhelming majority of duodenal ulcers are less than 1 cm in diameter. Less common are large, or so-called *giant duodenal ulcers,* defined as those measuring greater than 2 cm in diameter. The hallmark for radiographic identification is the constant size and shape of the lesion throughout the examination. Therefore it is important to pay attention to the pliability of the bulb and changes in its shape during the course of the examination. Nodularity in the ulcer base or associated filling defects may also be noted. A marked narrowing of the pyloric canal or the immediate postbulbar region is present in nearly all cases.

Postbulbar ulceration in the duodenum is another source of difficulty in the radiographic diagnosis. Postbulbar ulcerations probably account for fewer than 5% of ulcers in the duodenum. These lesions are commonly obscured by extensive fold thickening and spasm. Over time, untreated lesions may progress to a characteristic ring stricture that may simulate the appearance of an annular pancreas.

MORPHOLOGIC FEATURES OF PEPTIC ULCERATION
Shape

Ulcers occurring in either the stomach or the duodenum are typically round or oval. Shape may vary, however, especially with shallow ulcers. Because shallow ulcers are more easily evaluated with double-contrast examinations, a wide variety of ulcer shapes is more likely to be encountered with these techniques. Though irregularly shaped ulcers should suggest the possibility of neoplasm and the need for biopsy, (Fig. 6-48) irregular or unusual shapes occur commonly in benign disease as well.

Linear ulceration is relatively frequent in Japan (where it makes up approximately 20% of all gastric ulcers), and is being more commonly identified in the West as the application of double-contrast techniques becomes more popular. Long linear ulcers tend to be associated with marked shortening and deformity of the lesser curve, whereas shorter linear ulcers tend to be associated with less deformity. Radiologic recognition of linear ulcers is important because (1) these lesions may be difficult to identify endoscopically, (2) they may be resistant to therapy, and (3) they serve as the site for recurrent larger peptic ulcerations. Four criteria useful in identifying these lesions and in differentiating them from barium trapped between folds are (1) a contour deformity that may be U-shaped in the duodenum, (2) a

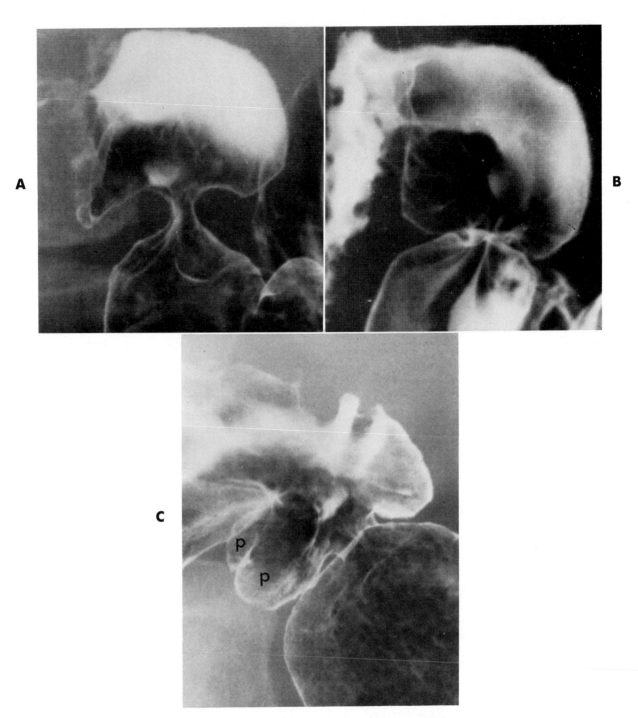

Fig. 6-47 Duodenal ulcer. **A,** Duodenal ulcer at base of duodenal bulb. Note absence of radiating folds and deformity. **B,** Duodenal ulcer with radiating folds. **C,** Duodenal ulcer with radiating folds and deformity. Note pseudodiverticula *(p)* formation.

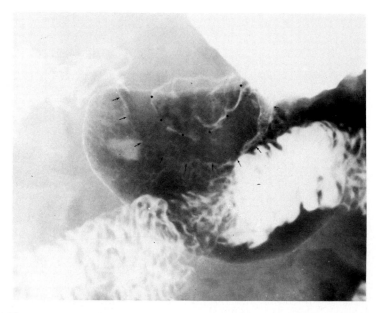

Fig. 6-48 Ulcerated gastric carcinoma. Note nodular mass effect *(arrows)* and irregularity of ulcer crater *(dots)*.

niche projection in the profile view, (3) a fuzziness or irregularity of the linear collection representing the ulcer, and (4) the identification of folds radiating to a line. Some reports have indicated that most linear ulcers in the duodenum have a transverse orientation in relation to the bulb.

Multiple ulcers

The occurrence of multiple ulcers in the stomach or duodenum is reported to be as high as 17% to 30% in surgical or autopsy series. Radiologic identification of multiple gastric lesions is more common with double-contrast techniques than with single-contrast examination. Multiple ulcers characteristically occur in patients with benign disease and do not appear to be more common in patients with a history of salicylate ingestion. An analysis of the morphology of each individual ulcerating lesion may assist in the identification of a malignant lesion in patients with multiple ulcers.

Multiple duodenal ulcers may be identified in 10% to 15% of cases. When these lesions occur separately on the anterior and posterior walls of the duodenum, they are called *kissing ulcers*. The presence of multiple ulcers in the postbulbar duodenum suggests *Zollinger-Ellison syndrome*. In one study nearly 42% of patients with a gastric ulcer had a coexisting duodenal ulceration, suggesting that the finding of a gastric or duodenal ulcer should stimulate a vigorous search for an associated ulcer.

HEALING AND SCAR FORMATION
Medical therapy

The introduction of H_2 *histamine receptor antagonists* such as cimetidine has had a major impact on the treatment of peptic ulcer disease. These agents block the stimulation of acid secretion by other secretagogues such as gastrin and acetylcholine. Cimetidine has been shown to be remarkably effective in inhibiting gastric acid secretion, and long-term prophylactic cimetidine therapy has been reported to dramatically reduce the typical 50% recurrence rate of duodenal ulcers. Cimetidine is also effective in the treatment of gastric ulcer. Similar results have been achieved with ranitidine.

Mucosal cytoprotective agents (such as sucralfate, misoprotol, and enprostol), which are synthetic prostaglandins, have been recently introduced and are also effective in the treatment of gastric and duodenal ulcers.

Radiographic appearance of healing
Gastric ulcers

Keller and co-workers have described the characteristic sequence of gastric ulcer healing and scar formation. Initially there is a diminution in crater size and a reduction or disappearance of the associated ulcer mound or collar. As the associated inflammatory changes regress, the radiating folds become more apparent and may extend directly to the ulcer crater. Some tapering or bridging of the radiating folds may be

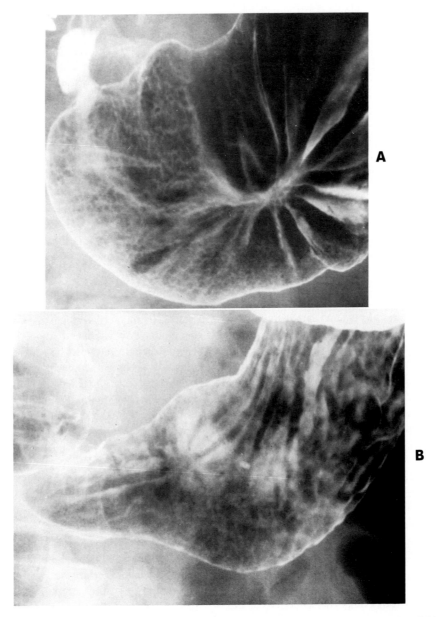

Fig. 6-49 Gastric ulcer scars. **A,** Depressed greater curvature scar. Note normal radiating folds and normal areae gastricae in depression. **B,** Flat gastric ulcer scar.

present. During healing, the areae gastricae pattern, which may be focally lost near a region of ulceration, may once again become apparent. With re-epithelialization of the mucosa, healing is complete. The re-epithelialized surface may be flat with associated radiating folds or retracted with resultant focal depression or dimpling. Most gastric ulcers heal completely in 6 to 8 weeks, and even large gastric ulcers usually heal within 12 weeks.

Radiologic manifestation of ulcer healing includes not only a decrease in the size of the ulcer, but also a change in its shape. Healing ulcers often have an asymmetric or linear appearance and occasionally may undergo splitting. Some researchers have suggested that linear ulcers represent a stage of ulcer healing. Double-contrast technique is extremely helpful in demonstrating these lesions, because linear ulcers are difficult to detect on conventional single-contrast examinations.

Between 50% and 90% of healed gastric ulcers produce visible ulcer scars on double-contrast examinations. These scars are characterized by a central pit or depression, radiating folds, and/or retraction of the adjacent gastric wall. The central depression may be round, linear, or rod shaped. The lack of discrete edges in a depression or niche, and the identification of areae gastricae within the apparent depression with radiating folds may serve to differentiate such a depression from a shallow active ulcer.

The location of ulceration affects the radiographic appearance of the resultant ulcer scar. *Greater curvature ulcer scars* commonly have a stellate, well-defined radiating fold pattern (Fig 6-49), whereas *lesser curvature ulcer scars* tend to have a less well-defined radiating fold and are accompanied by a flattening or decreased distensibility along the lesser curvature.

Duodenal ulcers

The process of healing and scar formation of duodenal ulcer is much the same as that in the stomach. Duodenal ulcers, like gastric ulcers, may heal without any evidence of scar formation. Scarring in the duodenum may lead to a variety of characteristic radiographic appearances and is commonly accompanied by the formation of pseudodiverticula. *Pseudodiverticula* are somewhat pliable outpouchings between regions of scarring and retraction. Because they may fill with barium and appear as outpouchings, they can be easily confused with active duodenal ulcers. In general, pseudodiverticula can be distinguished from ulcers because folds do not radiate to these outpouchings but appear around them. In addition, pseudodiverticula are usually pliable and may change shape during the course of an examination. The healing and scar formation of a centrally located duodenal ulcer may result in a characteristic *cloverleaf deformity*.

COMPLICATIONS OF PEPTIC ULCERATION

The major complications of peptic ulceration in the stomach or duodenum are bleeding, obstruction, and perforation.

Bleeding

Bleeding appears to occur somewhat more commonly in the duodenum (17%) than in the stomach (15%). Patients with low-grade chronic bleeding may have unexplained fatigue, anemia, or evidence of gastrointestinal blood loss in Hemocult testing of the stool. More brisk bleeding may cause melena, hematemesis, or even hematochezia. The diagnostic evaluation of patients with acute upper gastrointestinal blood loss usually relies on endoscopic examination to determine the site of bleeding. If endoscopy is not readily available, double-contrast examination may be used. Findings include

1. *Halo sign:* nonopaque blood around the ulcer crater
2. *Lava flow pattern:* nonopaque blood mixed with barium flowing from the bleeding site
3. A *filling defect* in an ulcer crater that may represent a clot or bleeding vessel.

Obstruction

Gastric outlet obstructions are a less common complication than bleeding, probably occurring in less than 5% of cases of peptic ulcer disease. Obstructions may be caused by (1) scarring and stenosis about the pylorus, (2) an inflammatory reaction around an active ulcer near the pylorus, or (3) a combination of both factors. The role of radiology in these patients is twofold: (1) to confirm the presence of an outlet obstruction and (2) to examine the morphology at the site of the obstruction to determine its cause. The excess fluid in the obstructed stomach and the associated debris severely limit the quality of mucosal coating that may be obtained with the double-contrast examination. Because a gastric outlet obstruction may also be secondary to a carcinoma, lymphoma, benign neoplasm, ring stricture, or acquired pyloric stenosis, a detailed study of the mucosal surface in the obstructed region is important. Gastric lavage before the examination commonly helps remove the associated debris and thus improves the quality of the examination.

Perforation

Both duodenal and gastric ulceration may extend through the serosa into a free abdominal space or into adjacent organs or structures. Perforation probably occurs in 5% to 11% of cases and is more common with duodenal than with gastric ulcers. Most duodenal perforations occur anteriorly in the proximal duodenum, whereas most gastric perforations occur in lesser curvature ulcers. In cases of free intraperitoneal perforation, abdominal radiographs often reveal evidence of pneumoperitoneum. However, free intraperitoneal air is not detected radiographically in as many as 25% to 35% of patients with perforated duodenal ulcers. Patients with a suspected gastric or duodenal perforation should be examined with water-soluble contrast materials to avoid barium extravasation into the peritoneal cavity and resultant *barium peritonitis*.

Penetration

Penetration is the extension of ulcers beyond the serosa into adjacent structures. The most common site of penetration is the pancreas, but penetration into the omentum, biliary tract, liver, mesocolon, and colon may also occur. In addition to the duodenal ulcer, thickening of duodenal folds in the second portion of the duodenum and evidence of a mass effect on the duodenal sweep may be demonstrated on barium examination of such patients.

Ulcer penetration into adjacent hollow organs is somewhat less common than penetration into the pancreas. Benign aspirin-induced gastric ulcers arising on the greater curvature may penetrate through the gastrocolic ligament into the colon, resulting in gastrocolic fistulas. In today's pill-oriented society, these benign greater curvature ulcers are a more common cause of gastrocolic fistulas than gastric carcinomas or colonic carcinomas. Ulcers that result in gastrocolic fistulas tend to occur on the posterior gastric wall near the greater curvature.

The *double pylorus,* once thought to be a congenital disorder, has now been demonstrated to be an acquired lesion secondary to peptic ulcer disease. It is most commonly caused by the penetration of a lesser curvature prepyloric ulcer into the base of the duodenal bulb with a resultant gastroduodenal fistula, but it may also occur as a result of the penetration of duodenal or greater curvature gastric ulcers with resultant fistula formation.

DIFFERENTIAL DIAGNOSIS OF PEPTIC ULCER DISEASE

A variety of nonneoplastic diseases may be seen with ulcerative gastric lesions. In patients with *Zollinger-Ellison syndrome* the ulcers are peptic in nature, but result from gastrin-secreting tumors that usually arise in the pancreas. Radiologic features suggesting this diagnosis include thick gastric folds, the enlargement of small intestinal folds, and increased intestinal fluid in the small bowel examination in association with a peptic ulcer. Of the ulcers in patients with Zollinger-Ellison syndrome, 75% occur in the duodenal bulb or stomach and are nonspecific. Nevertheless, the identification of multiple postbulbar ulcers is suggestive of this syndrome.

Granulomatous diseases such as Crohn's disease, tuberculosis, or syphilis may also manifest as ulcerative gastric or duodenal lesions. In these diseases the involvement is commonly segmental and may be associated with considerable mass effect and deformity.

RECOMMENDED READING

1. Amaral NM: Radiographic diagnosis of shallow gastric ulcers: a comparative study of techniques, *Radiology* 129:597, 1978.
2. Braver JM et al: Roentgen diagnosis of linear ulcers, *Radiology* 132:29, 1979.
3. de Roos A, Op den Orth JO: Linear niches in the duodenal bulb, *Am J Roentgenol* 140:941, 1983.
4. Eisenberg RL et al: Giant duodenal ulcers, *Gastrointest Radiol* 2:347, 1978.
5. Gelfand DW et al: The location and size of gastric ulcers: radiologic and endoscopic evaluation, *Am J Roentgenol* 143:755, 1984.
6. Oi M, Sakurai Y: Location of duodenal ulcer, *Gastroenterology* 36:60, 1959.
7. Zboralske FF, Amberg JR: Detection of Zollinger-Ellison syndrome: the radiologist's responsibility, *Am J Roentgenol* 104:529, 1968.

Duodenum
J ODO OP DEN ORTH

ANATOMY

The duodenum is the first part of the small bowel. It extends from the pylorus to the duodenojejunal flexure, about the breadth of 12 fingers (25 to 30 cm). For the radiologist, it is practical to consider the duodenum as being divided into three parts. The first, or superior, part begins at the pylorus and extends toward the right posteriorly to the superior duodenal flexure. This part is freely movable because of its intraperitoneal position. In radiology, this part of the duodenum, which often extends to the superior flexure, is commonly called the *duodenal bulb.*

The second, or descending, part of the duodenum has a dorsal retroperitoneal position and is therefore relatively fixed. It extends in a nearly vertical direction from the superior to the inferior duodenal flexure.

The *major duodenal papilla (Vater's papilla)* is usually located on the posteromedial wall of the descending part of the duodenum (Fig. 6-50). This papilla may occasionally be found on the superior aspect of the inferior duodenal flexure or even on the proximal third part of the duodenum. In most instances Vater's papilla appears as a round or oval filling defect on double-contrast hypotonic duodenograms. The average major papilla is 8 to 10 mm in length; the upper limit of a normal major papilla is generally considered to be 1.5 cm, although normal papillae of larger size have been reported.

The *minor duodenal papilla (accessory papilla* or *Santorini's papilla)* is a constant finding in macroscopic examinations of the descending duodenum. It is a flat protrusion, measuring several millimeters in diameter with or without a central excavation. It is best visualized by double-contrast hypotonic duodenography in *en face* films with the patient in the prone position (Fig. 6-51). At times, profile visualization with the patient in the supine left posterior oblique position may be obtained. The average distance between the major and minor papillae is 18 to 20 mm.

The third part of the duodenum extends upward and to the left from the inferior flexure and anteriorly to the duodenojejunal flexure.

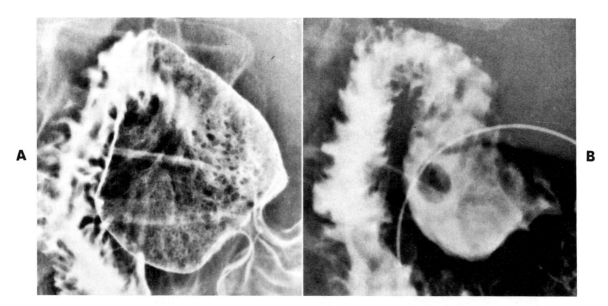

Fig. 6-53 Elevated lesions caused by heterotopic gastric mucosa. **A,** Supine left posterior oblique film shows multiple elevated lesions of differing individual forms and diameters. Some of defects have somewhat angular form. Lesions are predominantly in juxtapyloric region. Characteristic radiologic appearance of elevated lesions caused by heterotopic gastric mucosa was also observed at endoscopy. Biopsy confirmed diagnosis. **B,** Erect left posterior oblique film. Double-contrast study (not shown) of this patient demonstrated appearance characteristic of multiple elevated lesions caused by heterotopic gastric mucosa. This film shows spherical polyp. Biopsies from this polyp and the small lesions demonstrated heterotopic gastric epithelium. Appearance in **A** is characteristic of elevated lesions caused by heterotopic gastric epithelium. Spherical polyp in **B** might be caused by any benign duodenal tumor.

(From Langkemper R et al: *Radiology* 137:621, 1980.)

contrast (monophasic) examination of the descending part of the duodenum reveals the complete lining of the first and second part of the viscus with high resolution, noticeably improving the imaging of the duodenum. Both the minor papilla and elevated lesions in the duodenal bulb caused by heterotopic gastric mucosa can be visualized with this technique (Fig. 6-53; see Fig. 6-50). Drug-induced hypotony further facilitates the diagnosis of small niches in the duodenal bulb, especially linear ones.

The third part of the duodenum—interposed between the first and second parts, with their frequent specific pathologic conditions—as well as the rest of the small bowel, is in danger of being neglected in studies of the duodenum. Tubeless hypotonic duodenography is not usually effective beyond the inferior duodenal flexure.

Detailed examination of the duodenal bulb and the descending duodenum

The examination of the duodenal bulb and the descending duodenum usually takes place after the bipha-

sic contrast gastric examination, when sufficient quantities of barium and gas are still available in the stomach. Immediately before the gastric examination a premedication of glucagon, 0.1 mg, is injected intravenously. Four spot films are made with the patient in (1) the right procubitus position with a compression paddle between the table and the patient (Fig. 6-54), (2) left posterior oblique and (3) right posterior oblique compression studies with the patient erect (Fig. 6-54, *B,C*), and (4) a left posterior oblique double-contrast study of the duodenal bulb with the patient supine (Fig. 6-54, *D*). If the effect of the glucagon has worn off by the time of the duodenal examination, the patient is turned on the right side, and when barium is seen in the duodenum, a vein is punctured and another dose of 0.1 mg glucagon is injected when a peristaltic wave is seen to progress to the pylorus. This dose is usually sufficient to obtain optimal distention of the duodenal bulb. If, however, a detailed hypotonic study of the descending duodenum is required, a dose of 0.3 mg of glucagon is recommended. Immediately after the needle has been withdrawn (the pylorus not yet having closed), the patient is turned to

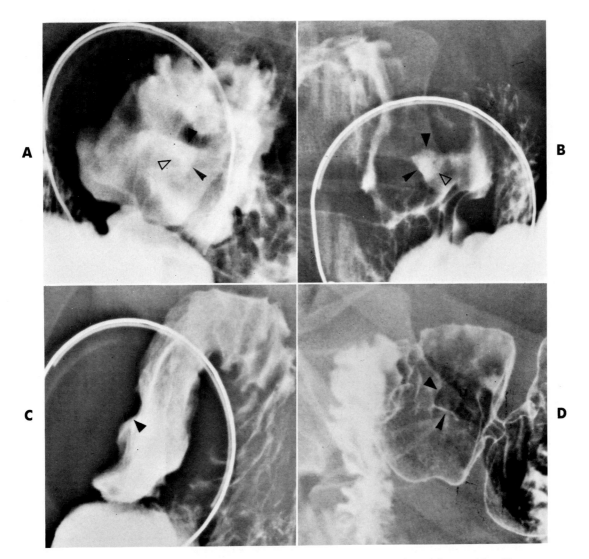

Fig. 6-54 Biphasic duodenal bulb series. **A,** Positive contrast compression, right procubitus film. **B,** Positive contrast compression, erect left posterior oblique film. **C,** Positive contrast compression, erect right posterior oblique film. **D,** Double-contrast left posterior oblique film. **A** and **B** demonstrate niche with surrounding swelling. **C** shows that niche is in anterior wall. In **D** niche is barely visualized, and only inferior border of niche is sharply demarcated by linear shadow. Analysis of anterior wall niche: (1) shape is roughly triangular; (2) one side (▶) is abrupt, which is perfectly demonstrated in **A, B,** and **D;** (3) one side (▶) is slightly sloping, which is visualized in **A, B,** and **C,** but barely in **D;** and (4) third side (▷) is sloping, as is visualized in **A** and **B** but not in **D.**

the left posterior oblique position to allow gas to pass into the duodenum. If fluoroscopic control shows that this does not occur instantaneously—because the pylorus has already closed or there is extensive duodenal scarring—the patient is asked to cough vigorously, which nearly always results in gaseous distention of the duodenum. To provide a good mucosal coating, the patient is turned approximately 135 degrees from the supine left posterior oblique position to the prone position

and back again. If necessary, this procedure can be repeated several times. Films are then made with the patient in the supine left posterior oblique and the prone positions. In most instances a compression cone or paddle between the patient and the table is necessary in the prone position to eliminate the troublesome superimposition of the barium-filled antrum and the duodenal loop filled with the double-contrast medium (Fig. 6-55).

If this technique is not successful, usually because of

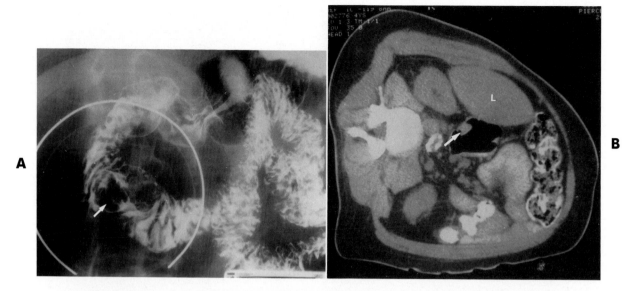

Fig. 6-55 A, Barium study spot film with compression showing a large duodenal adenomatous polyp *(arrow)*. **B,** Left lateral decubitus computed tomogram showing the large adenomatous polyp *(arrow)* in air distended duodenum. *L,* liver.

persistent pyloric spasm or a deviant position of the descending duodenum, duodenal intubation and repeat double-contrast hypotonic duodenography are necessary. This procedure is usually scheduled for a second session. After a tube has been advanced to the inferior duodenal flexure, 0.5 mg of glucagon is injected intravenously. Approximately 100 ml of barium suspension is introduced while the patient lies on the right side. The patient then turns back to the supine left posterior oblique position, and 150 ml of air is introduced. Supine left posterior oblique and prone films can be made even after the tube has been withdrawn, thus preventing the troublesome superimposition of the tube and the descending duodenum.

Hypotonic agent

The total dose of glucagon, even if two injections are needed, rarely exceeds 0.4 mg. This amount only very seldom has side effects, which are mainly nausea and vomiting. Relative contraindications are pheochromocytoma and insulinoma.

Barium suspension

With a medium-density barium suspension, both the double-contrast and the single-contrast techniques can be used during a biphasic examination. When a high-density barium suspension for double-contrast radiographs is used, a biphasic examination can be obtained by administering a low-density barium suspension after the double-contrast radiographs have been obtained.

INDENTATION AT AORTA AND SUPERIOR MESENTERIC ARTERY

An indentation is frequently seen where the third part of the duodenum passes between the aorta and superior mesenteric artery. In cases of *superior mesenteric artery syndrome* or *arteriomesenterial occlusion syndrome,* there is partial obstruction of the contrast flow at this point and dilatation of the duodenum orally to the obstruction, sometimes with to-and-fro duodenal movements. The condition often occurs in extremely thin females suffering from anorexia nervosa. Acute superior mesenteric artery syndrome may occur in patients with severe burns and subsequent marked weight loss, acute pancreatitis, or severe trauma. It also occurs in association with the application of a plaster hip spica case or body jacket *(body cast syndrome)* and in patients subjected to traction for correction of scoliosis. Congenital extrinsic duodenal bands *(Ladd's bands)* may play a role in the pathogenesis. Other causes of intrinsic or extrinsic obstruction have to be excluded before the diagnosis of this still debated condition is made. Ultrasonography, CT, and MRI are often included in the evaluation. One of the conditions most frequently causing this appearance is scleroderma.

BENIGN TUMORS

Benign tumors of the duodenum include tumorlike lesions such as elevated lesions caused by heterotopic gastric mucosa, hyperplasia of Brunner's glands, benign lymphoid hyperplasia, and heterotopic pancreatic tissue. Benign duodenal tumors are rare, and when they do occur tend to be located in the proximal part of the duodenum. The most commonly seen benign tumors are adenomas (adenomatous polyps and villous adenomas), leiomyomas, and lipomas. Neurogenic tumors and lymphangiomas are sporadically reported in the literature. In patients with neurofibromatosis, the duodenum is one of the more common gastrointestinal sites of involvement.

Adenomatous polyps are usually small and may be pedunculated or sessile. They progress to carcinomas in many instances. Multiple adenomatous polyps occur in cases of familial adenomatous gastrointestinal polyposis and Gardner's syndrome. *Villous adenomas* of the duodenum have a characteristic cauliflower or soap bubble appearance (Fig. 6-56). As with cases in the colon,

there is a high incidence of malignant degeneration. *Leiomyomas* occur as an extraluminal, intramural, or endoluminal mass. Ulceration is frequent with endoluminal leiomyomas. *Lipomas* may grow to a large size; they are soft tumors that at times can be appreciated during the radiologic examination if they are molded by the wall of the bowel. In most cases of benign tumors the radiologic appearance alone does not permit definite diagnosis. Endoscopy and biopsy are commonly indicated.

Lesions such as elevated lesions caused by heterotopic gastric mucosa, hyperplasia of Brunner's glands, benign lymphoid hyperplasia, and heterotopic pancreatic tissue are considered benign tumors. The first three conditions generally appear as multiple filling defects, sometimes with a characteristic appearance that facilitates a radiologic diagnosis in many cases.

Heterotopic gastric mucosa commonly occurs in the duodenal bulb and sometimes causes elevated lesions that are macroscopically visible. They are scattered over the surface of the bulb in one or more clusters, predominantly in the juxtapyloric region (see Fig. 6-53). The prevalence of peptic ulceration in patients with these characteristic nodules in the duodenal bulb is very low. Rarely, heterotopic gastric mucosa is present as a solitary spherical or multilobulated polyp that cannot be differentiated from other tumors of the duodenum without biopsy (see Fig. 6-53).

Brunner's gland "adenoma" is usually a small protuberant lesion covered by duodenal mucosa, although lesions with a diameter of several centimeters have been

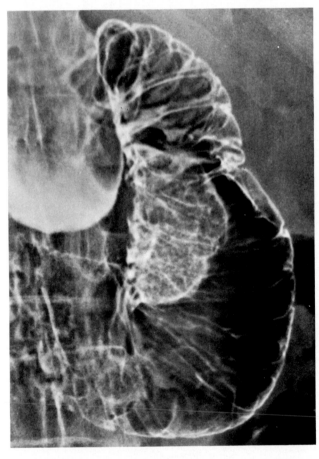

Fig. 6-56 Villous adenoma. Prone film shows on medial aspect of descending duodenum huge filling defect with cauliflower or soap bubble appearance that was also seen at endoscopy. Histologic examination of resected specimen detected villous adenoma. Note indentation on lateral aspect of descending duodenum, probably caused by right kidney.

(From Op den Orth JO: *The standard biphasic-contrast examination of the stomach and duodenum: methods, results and radiological atlas*, The Hague, 1979, Martinus Nijhoff Publishers BV.)

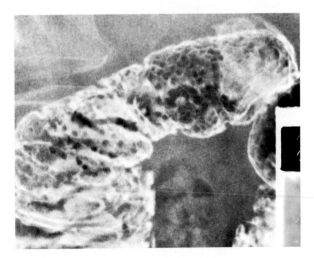

Fig. 6-57 Benign lymphoid hyperplasia. Supine left posterior oblique film shows multiple roundish elevations evenly spread over duodenal surface. There is no great variation in size, and lesions are not restricted to bulb. Biopsy proved this was benign lymphoid hyperplasia.

(From Langkemper R et al: *Radiology* 137:621, 1980.)

reported. Some consider the lesion to be a hamartoma, others a hyperplasia. If multiple lesions occur, the condition is generally called *hyperplasia of Brunner's glands,* which is a fairly common condition. It causes roundish, rather smoothly demarcated filling defects with a diameter varying from several millimeters to approximately 1 cm (cobblestone appearance). There is no predilection for the juxtapyloric region, and the lesions often extend into the second part of the duodenum.

In *benign lymphoid hyperplasia,* multiple roundish elevations with a uniform diameter of about 1 to 2 mm are evenly scattered on the surface of the duodenum (Fig. 6-57). These elevations are more sharply demarcated than those occurring in hyperplasia of Brunner's glands.

Heterotopic pancreatic tissue usually occurs as a single submucosal nodule with central umbilication. A definite radiologic diagnosis is usually impossible.

MALIGNANT TUMORS

Primary malignancies, which have a low incidence in the small intestine, are encountered relatively frequently in the duodenum. The sites of predilection of malignant tumors are the periampullary and infraampullary parts of the duodenum.

Adenocarcinoma and *leiomyosarcoma* are the first and second most common malignant duodenal tumors. Adenocarcinomas in the duodenum are usually seen as polypoid, stenosing, or ulcerating lesions. A leiomyosarcoma usually cannot be differentiated from a leiomyoma, although it may mimic a polypoid adenocarcinoma. The presence of a sinus or fistula suggests a leiomyosarcoma.

Malignant lymphomas of the duodenum may show growth patterns similar to those occurring in the distal part of the small bowel. Nodularity, together with thickened folds or with a constrictive lesion in the duodenum, may suggest a malignant lymphoma, but this appearance also occurs in cases of Crohn's disease.

Villous adenoma and *carcinoid tumors* or *carcinoid islet cell tumors* have a variably malignant potential. The former can usually be recognized by its typical cauliflower or soap bubble appearance (see Fig. 6-56). The latter are usually smooth-surface tumors with a predilection for the duodenal bulb. The radiologic appearance may vary from a benign-appearing intramural mass to a large, bulky, ulcerating lesion. Carcinoid islet cell tumors of the duodenum have features of both foregut carcinoid tumors and islet cell tumors of the pancreas, and are often ulcerogenic.

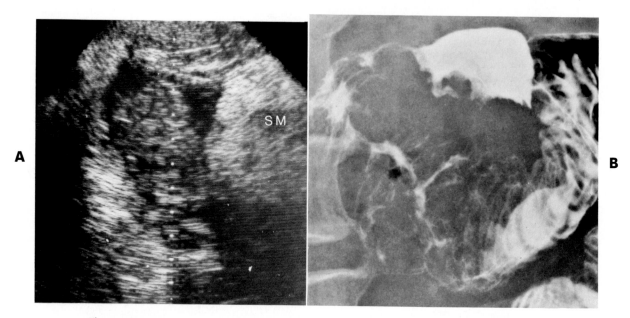

Fig. 6-58 Contiguous cancer of duodenum. **A,** Transverse right lateral decubitus scan after oral water administration with intravenous injection of 0.3 mg of glucagon. Pancreatic scanning was done because duodenoscopic findings were compatible with adenocarcinoma of pancreatic head infiltrating duodenum. Irregular echogenic mass fills duodenum, but pancreatic neoplasm is not identified. **B,** Supine left posterior oblique hypotonic duodenogram also shows intraluminal mass. Autopsy demonstrated tumor mass in duodenal lumen, which appeared to be contiguous cancer originating from adenocarcinoma of hepatic flexure of colon. *SM,* superior mesenteric vein.

Whenever a mass lesion in the duodenum is seen, the possibility of a *secondary cancer* must be considered. A secondary cancer may be a metastasis or a contiguous cancer originating from an adjacent organ (Fig. 6-58) such as the pancreas, distal biliary tract or gallbladder, stomach, colon, or right kidney.

ENLARGEMENT OF THE MAJOR DUODENAL PAPILLA

Although a normal major duodenal papilla may be as long as 3 cm, it is usually regarded as abnormal if it is longer than 1.5 cm. Papillary enlargement may be the result of edema (Fig. 6-59, *A*) or neoplastic infiltration. Edema can be caused by a stone in the distal common bile duct, pancreatitis, or a peptic ulcer. To differentiate between an impacted stone (the most common cause of a smooth-surface enlargement of the major duodenal papilla) and these other conditions, endoscopic retrograde pancreaticocholangiography or percutaneous transhepatic cholangiography are of great help.

An irregular surface filling defect in the region of Vater's papilla strongly suggests an adenocarcinoma arising from Vater's papilla or the adjacent duodenal mucosa, Vater's ampulla, the distal parts of the pancreatic duct and common bile duct, or the head of the pancreas. They are usually designated as *periampullary carcinomas* (Fig. 6-59, *B*).

DIFFUSE INTRINSIC DUODENAL DISEASE
Erosions

An erosion can be defined as a mucosal defect that does not penetrate the muscularis mucosae and that may or may not involve an elevation of the surrounding mucosa. A defect with a surrounding mucosal elevation (a *varioliform, complete,* or *aphthoid erosion*) may occur with or without similar changes in the stomach. Multiple varioliform erosions in the duodenal bulb usually reflect nonspecific duodenitis but are also found in patients suffering from Crohn's disease elsewhere in the GI tract.

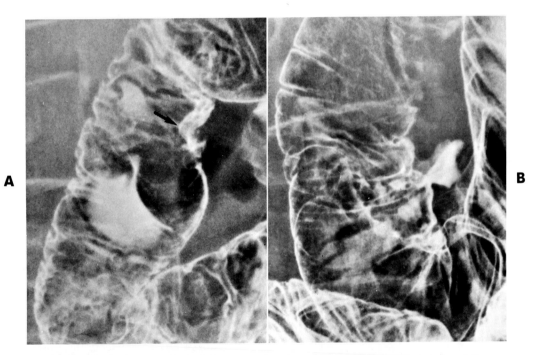

Fig. 6-59 Benign and malignant enlargement of major papilla. **A,** Supine left posterior oblique film shows smooth-surface filling defect on medial aspect of descending duodenum, compatible with edema of major papilla, which was seen also at endoscopy. Endoscopic retrograde pancreaticocholangiography demonstrated stones in distal common bile duct that were considered cause of edema of major papilla. Superior to edematous major papilla is filling defect *(arrow)* probably caused by minor papilla. **B,** Supine left posterior oblique film shows irregular-surface filling defect at site where major papilla can be expected. Reflux of contrast material in ampulla and smoothly demarcated indentation on inner aspect of superior second duodenum are revealed. Further examination and surgery demonstrated small periampullary adenocarcinoma as cause of irregular filling defect and mass resulting from chronic pancreatitis as cause of smoothly demarcated indentation.

7 *Small Bowel*

ROBERT KOEHLER
ARTHUR E LINDNER
DANIEL MAKLANSKY
JACQUES PRINGOT
RUEDI F-L THOENI

TECHNIQUE FOR EXAMINATION
    Anatomy of the small bowel
    Radiologic examination of the small bowel
INFLAMMATORY DISEASES OF THE SMALL BOWEL
    Crohn's disease
    Miscellaneous nonspecific inflammatory diseases
    Infectious diseases
    Segmental ischemia
    Radiation enteritis
    Drug-associated disorders
    Eosinophilic gastroenteritis
NEOPLASTIC LESIONS
    Benign tumors
    Carcinoid tumors
    Lymphomas
    Adenocarcinomas
    Sarcomas
    Metastatic tumors
MALABSORPTION AND IMMUNE DEFICIENCIES
    Diseases associated with malabsorption
    Immune deficiencies

Technique for examination

RUEDI F-L THOENI

ANATOMY OF THE SMALL BOWEL

The small intestine consists of the *jejunum* and *ileum;* its total length varies from 300 to 600 cm. In most people the jejunum is located in the left upper quadrant and the ileum is located in the right pelvis. The location of small bowel loops can vary because of malrotation, changes in patient position, or palpation. The nondistended jejunum shows a typical feathery pattern on radiographs. This pattern is caused by collapsed bowel walls and *valvulae conniventes.* These valvulae conniventes are best visualized if the small bowel is distended.

The mucosa consists of crypts and villi. The *villi* increase the total mucosal surface but cannot normally be seen on conventional radiographs unless their number is decreased from atrophy. The villi, fingerlike protrusions 0.5 to 1 mm long, are visible on macroscopic inspection of small bowel specimens, and normally range in number from 10 to 40 per mm^2 in the jejunum. These villi are visible on magnification radiographs.

RADIOLOGIC EXAMINATION OF THE SMALL BOWEL

Barium studies are still the mainstay for evaluating patients with suspected small bowel abnormalities. The following describes and compares the different radiographic methods for examining the small bowel with barium, including small bowel follow-through (SBFT), dedicated SBFT, enteroclysis, peroral pneumocolon (PPC), and retrograde small bowel examination.

Agents affecting transit time through the small bowel
Accelerating agents

Passage of food through the pylorus influences transit through the small bowel and is accelerated if the patient is placed on the right side. Rate of transit can also be increased by larger amounts of fluid, or by administration of cold fluids. Drugs that speed up transit time *(accelerating, cholinergic, or parasympathomimetic agents)* also can be used. Such drugs include neostigmine (Prostigmin), a synthetic anticholinesterase injected intramuscularly, and acetyl betamethycholin (Mecholyl). Cholecystokinin or cholecystokinin-like substances also induce bowel peristalsis, but they delay gastric emptying. Therefore the latter drugs should be given intravenously after a large amount of barium has entered the duodenum. Metoclopramide (Reglan), given orally or intravenously, speeds passage time of barium through the stomach and through the small bowel. Metoclopramide is the most frequently used of these agents.

Transit-delaying agents

Any *anticholinergic drug,* such as propantheline bromide (Pro-Banthine), hyoscine butylbromide (Buscopan), and oxyphenonium bromide (Antrenyl), delays transit through the small bowel. Morphine, codeine, and atropine also produce small bowel atony and should be discontinued at least 6 hours before radiographic examination of the small bowel, or even earlier if these agents were used over an extended period. *Sedatives* or *tranquilizers* should also be avoided for at least 24 hours before a study. Interpreting a radiographic small bowel examination in patients under the effect of sedative or anticholinergic drugs is difficult not only because of delayed passage of barium through the small bowel, but also because of the resulting bizarre contractions and flaccid loops.

Glucagon diminishes or completely eliminates peristalsis and produces hypotonicity or atonicity, depending on the dosage. The effect of glucagon is shorter when given intravenously than when injected subcutaneously or intramuscularly. It is used only rarely for small bowel barium examinations, and then is usually given as a 1 mg dose.

Preliminary plain radiographs of the abdomen

Plain films of the abdomen taken before performing radiologic examination of the small bowel are useful for determining whether a patient is adequately prepared and for excluding the presence of barium remaining from a previous barium examination. Plain films are also helpful in deciding the best radiographic method for evaluating patients with suspected small bowel disease. For example, a patient with distention of only proximal small bowel loops would be best examined with enteroclysis, whereas a patient with distention of the entire small bowel may benefit from a retrograde examination. In addition, the presence of a large

amount of fluid (which must be aspirated before a radiographic small bowel examination) can be assessed on an upright film. However, fluid content in the stomach and small bowel can also be visualized during initial fluoroscopy, as can free intraperitoneal air, displacement of bowel loops by a mass, calcifications, or abnormality other than distention of bowel loops.

Barium examinations
Small bowel follow-through (SBFT) examination

In many radiology departments in the United States, SBFT is performed after an upper GI series in patients who have fasted from midnight on the day before the examination. First the esophagus, stomach, and duodenum are carefully evaluated, in most instances by double-contrast examination. High-density barium (for example, 150 ml E-Z-hd) and effervescent agents (E-Z-gas II, [both from E-Z-EM, Inc, Westbury, NY]) or similar products are recommended for this purpose. In many institutions a single-contrast phase (using 450 ml Barosperse [Mallinckrodt, Inc, St Louis, MO]) follows the double-contrast study in the upper GI tract. However, for optimal radiographic results in the small bowel, the examination of the small bowel should be separated from the upper GI series.

The initial 200 ml of barium given for SBFT should be more dilute (about 20% to 24% weight to volume [w/v]) to decrease the high-density effect from the double-contrast study of the upper GI study. The remaining barium is given as a 40% to 45% w/v suspension. A series of overhead radiographs is then obtained for evaluating the small bowel (Fig. 7-1). The series is usually obtained at half-hourly or hourly intervals until the terminal ileum is reached. At that point compression views are taken. Additional compression views are obtained whenever an overhead radiograph shows an area of abnormality.

Dedicated small bowel follow-through (Dedicated SBFT) examination

Dedicated SBFT is a barium examination of the small bowel that is completely separate from upper GI evaluations. The patient is again asked to fast after midnight on the day before the examination.

For *single-contrast SFBT,* barium (approximately 600 to 900 ml Barosperse or a similar type of barium) is administered orally, and the patient is brought to the fluoroscopy room, where compression views are immediately obtained to visualize the proximal jejunal loops. The patient is then placed on the right side to encourage emptying of the stomach, and more spot films are taken in the area of the middle and distal jejunum. Overhead radiographs are generally taken at 15 minutes, 30 min-

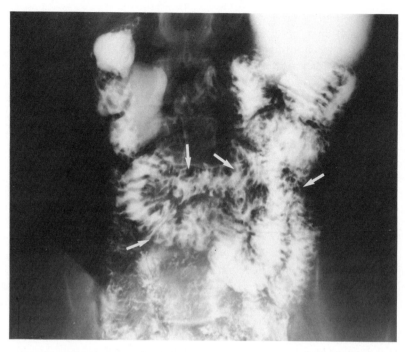

Fig. 7-1 Fifteen-minute overhead film during SBFT shows markedly thickened folds in jejunum with some nodularity *(arrows)*. Patient suffered from giardiasis.

utes, 1 hour, 1½ hours, and 2 hours. Delayed films are taken at hourly intervals thereafter until the terminal ileum is reached. Frequent fluoroscopy is performed to assess progression of the barium column and to adjust the time of delayed filming. Compression spot films are obtained in the entire small bowel with particular attention to any abnormal loop and the terminal ileum. If the transit time of barium through the small bowel is slow, an accelerating agent such as metoclopromide can be given. In some instances a large amount of barium, ice water, or the addition of meglumine diatrizoate to the barium is used to achieve a similar goal.

A *double-contrast SBFT* can be performed by introducing an effervescent agent that produces approximately 750 to 1000 ml of gas once the barium has reached the cecum. After administration of the effervescent agent, the patient is placed in the left lateral or left oblique and Trendelenburg position, so that gas can enter the duodenum and small bowel. In most instances gas reaches the distal ileum in 5 to 10 minutes. Radiographs with slight compression in the different areas of the small bowel can then be obtained. In one published series this procedure produced good double-contrast images in 43% of patients, with good distention of the small bowel loops achieved in 96% and separation of loops in 85% of patients.

Enteroclysis, or small bowel enema

The patient who is to undergo enteroclysis may be subjected to a colonic preparation similar to that for co-

lonic barium examination, particularly if the terminal ileum must be assessed. Drugs such as tranquilizers, sedatives, and antispasmodic agents that have been prescribed for a long time should be discontinued for several days, and the patient should be subjected to 2 days of liquid diet before enteroclysis is performed.

Preferred *tube placement* for enteroclysis is through the nasal route into the stomach and into the proximal jejunum beyond the ligament of Treitz. The tube can also be placed through the mouth. A special nasogastric tube (Maglinte-Enteroclysis Catheter [Lafayette Pharmacal, Inc., Lafayette, IN]) is recommended for this purpose. This 10F tube has an inflatable balloon near its distal end and several distal side holes for infusion of barium and methylcellulose. Administration of 20 mg of metoclopromide (Reglan) intravenously immediately before placement of the tube facilitates these maneuvers and permits fast infusion rates of barium and methylcellulose. For patient comfort, lidocaine 2% jelly (5 cc) is introduced into the nostril through which the tube is placed. Topical anesthesia of the throat is achieved with a spray. Overanesthetization of the pharyngeal area should be avoided, so that the patient can swallow normally during the intubation process. A mild short-acting sedative may be used to minimize discomfort of anxious patients. The enteroclysis tube is then inserted through one of the nostrils. Care must be taken not to force the tube against resistance, and fluoroscopy should be performed if breathing difficulty or resistance is experienced. When 5 to 7 cm of the enteroclysis tube

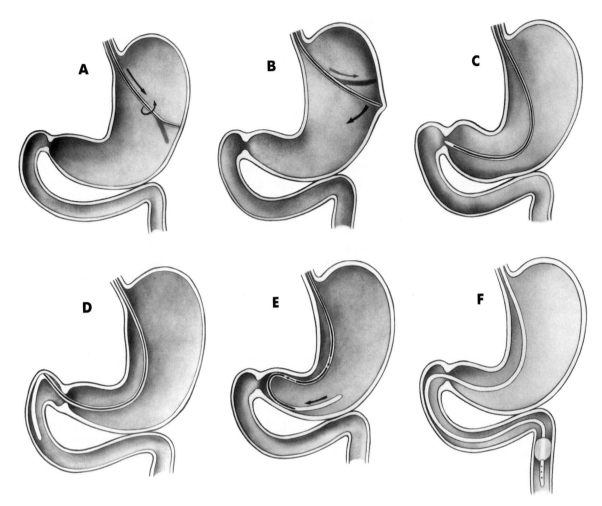

Fig. 7-2 Maneuvers for enteroclysis tube placement. **A,** If the enteroclysis tube is projecting into greater curvature and cannot be moved, angled tip of guidewire and torque maneuver can be used to advance tube into stomach distally. **B,** Placing patient on right side enables gravity to move tube away from greater curvature, which also advances tube into stomach distally. **C,** Placement of tube through pylorus into duodenum is facilitated by placing patient on left side so that air can rise and distend antrum and duodenum. **D,** Care must be taken not to allow guidewire to go beyond sharp turn between duodenal bulb and second portion of duodenum so that wire can be removed for administration of barium. **E,** Double-back maneuver. Tube is coiled up in fundus and pushed in toto into antrum. Then it is slowly removed while wire is advanced. **F,** Enteroclysis tube is optimally placed if tip and inflated balloon are beyond ligament of Treitz.

is introduced, the patient's neck is slightly flexed and the tube is further advanced while the patient swallows. All these maneuvers are best performed with the patient sitting upright on the fluoroscopy table or in a chair placed against a wall, so that he or she cannot easily move away from the advancing tube. In patients who cannot sit up, the tube can be placed with the patient on the fluoroscopy table in a right lateral position (Fig. 7-2).

Once two thirds of the enteroclysis tube has been placed through the nose, the patient is moved to the fluoroscopy table and asked to lie down. The tube, the tip

of which should be located in the stomach at this time, is further advanced and guided into the distal antrum and duodenum. For this purpose the guidewire is introduced further into the tube, leaving only 1 cm at the distal end free. In most instances the tube easily enters the pylorus and duodenum and can be progressively advanced into the duodenal sweep and through the ligament of Treitz. At the end of the procedure the tip should be approximately 4 to 5 cm distal to the ligament of Treitz. This placement prevents reflux of barium or methylcellulose into the proximal duodenum and stomach, as does inflating the balloon with 15 to 20 ml of air. Such reflux can cause patients to become nauseated and vomit because of the distention of the stomach with barium or methylcellulose, and must be avoided. Coiling up the tube end with the tip pointing toward the duodenal bulb should be avoided for the same reason. During infusion of barium or methylcellulose, some reflux can be reduced if the patient is placed in a left posterior oblique and semiupright position.

In patients with a deformed stomach or scarred pylorus, tube placement may be difficult. Also, placement in patients with large sliding hiatus hernias can be problematic. Adequate intubation is not always possible in these instances, but some special maneuvers can be used to facilitate tube placement. If the tube tends to turn to the left and get held up against the greater curvature, the wire can be torqued away from the greater curvature, particularly if the angled end is used (loop torque maneuver). As an alternative, the patient can be placed on the right side, which permits the tube to fall away from the greater curvature because of gravity. If the tube cannot be easily manipulated into the pylorus, the patient can be placed on the left side so that air rises into the antrum and duodenum and distends these areas. Once the tube has reached the apex of the duodenal bulb, it should be further advanced through the duodenal sweep, but the guidewire should be withdrawn to the apex of the bulb before each further advancement. Failure to do so may render the guidewire irretrievable from the tube in patients with sharp angulation of the duodenal bulb and sweep.

The *double-back maneuver* can be used if the tube cannot be easily advanced into the antrum. When the tube starts to curl up in the fundus, it should be further advanced so that the curved part is in the antrum. Once this is accomplished, the tube is withdrawn and the guidewire simultaneously advanced, which flips the end of the tube into the distal antrum.

Once the tube is correctly placed, it is taped to the nose. The optimal location of the tip of the tube is in the proximal jejunum, with the balloon inflated distal to the ligament of Treitz. The enteroclysis tube is then hooked up to the connecting tube, which passes through an electric motor-driven infusion pump (such as RS-7800 Minipump [Renal Systems, Inc, Minneapolis MN]), and the proximal portion of the connecting tube is taped to the fluoroscopy table to avoid dislodgement during the procedure. The pump permits infusion at predetermined rates that can be set manually. The connecting tube is attached to a plastic bag filled with barium for the single-contrast examination and through a Y connector to one bag of barium and one bag of methylcellulose for the biphasic examination (Fig. 7-3).

Enteroclysis can be a *single, double, or biphasic* examination. In all three the infusion rate must be carefully monitored. Very high infusion rates at the beginning of the study result in reflux into the stomach, and rates of more than 125 ml/min may produce an adynamic ileus, preventing adequate administration of barium throughout the small bowel. If the duodenum also must be evaluated, the tube is withdrawn slowly while a

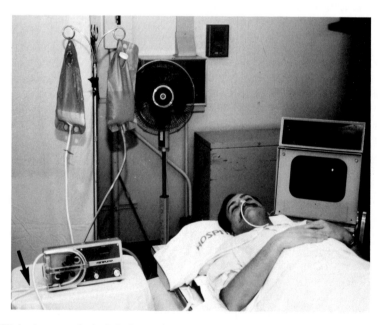

Fig. 7-3 Biphasic enteroclysis. Infusion pump and bags containing barium and methylcellulose are near fluoroscopy table. Tube is taped to table to avoid inadvertent removal of tube during procedure when table is elevated (*arrow* shows Y connector).

small amount of barium and methylcellulose is infused. Several spot films are then obtained during careful compression in the area of the duodenal sweep. In patients with complete or near-complete obstruction, barium and methylcellulose are aspirated at the end of the examination, and the tube may be flushed with water to eliminate the barium in the tube. The tube may be left in place for decompression with intermittent suction or exchanged for a larger bore tube.

Biphasic enteroclysis, using 250 ml of barium (Entrobar [E-Z-EM, Inc, Westbury, NY], undiluted, or similar 50% w/v products) infused at 70 to 90 ml/min

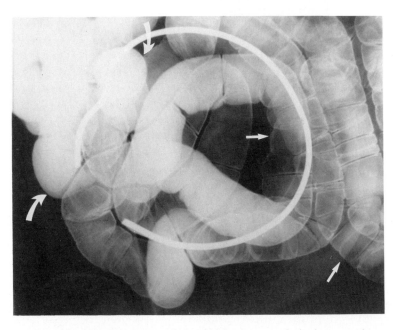

Fig. 7-4 Spot film during double-contrast phase of biphasic enteroclysis shows good separation of jejunal loops. Double-contrast phase is seen on right *(straight arrows)* and single-contrast phase is seen in ileum on the left *(curved arrows)*.

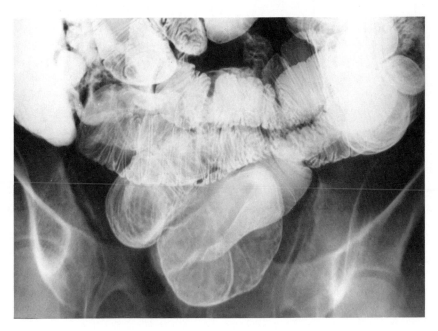

Fig. 7-5 Prone-angled distal overhead film allows separation of even distal small bowel loops in lower pelvis. Note the excellent see-through effect of biphasic method.

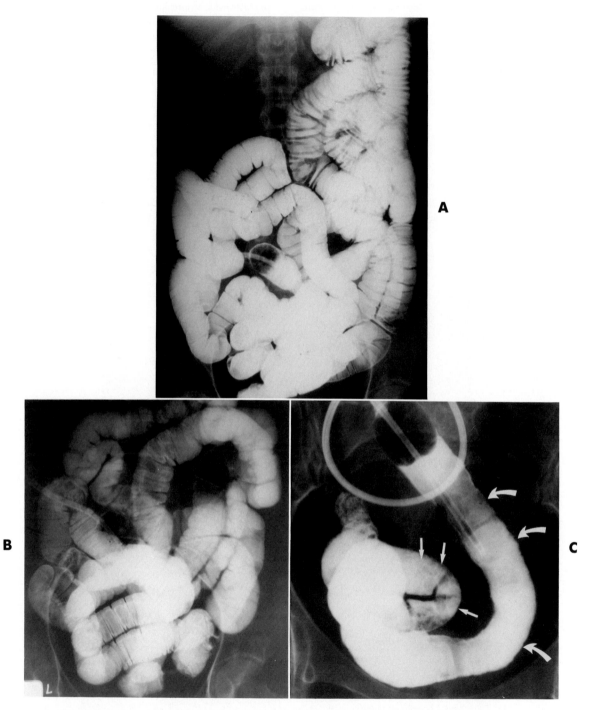

Fig. 7-6 A, Retrograde ileostomy study with modified tube shows abnormality of ileum immediately proximal to stoma and markedly thickened folds in jejunum. Patient suffered from recurrent Crohn's disease. **B,** In retrograde ileostomy study obtained 6 months after tetracycline and steroid therapy, jejunum is completely unremarkable. **C,** Ileostomy study using special tube with inflatable balloon shows slight irregularity of ileal margins *(curved arrows)* caused by Crohn's disease. These findings are remarkably improved from 6 months before. Filling defects *(straight arrows)* represent food particles.

followed by 1000 to 1500 ml of 0.5% methylcellulose infused at 100 to 115 ml/min is the preferred method. This option provides the advantages of a single-contrast phase combined with the double-contrast visualization of the fold pattern and mucosal detail, which is particularly useful in the pelvis, where multiple overlapping loops frequently cause interpretive problems. The single-contrast phase is initially carefully observed in the proximal small bowel, and spot films are taken once barium has reached the middle pelvis. Thereafter, infusion of methylcellulose produces the double-contrast phase proximally, while barium is simultaneously pushed distally, and the single-contrast phase of the distal small bowel can be assessed. Spot films are taken first of the single-contrast phase of the distal small bowel and then of the double-contrast phase in the proximal small bowel. This is followed by the double-contrast phase of the distal segments, which is also photographed (Fig. 7-4). At all times the radiologist watches the flow of barium and records any abnormality of bowel contour, fold pattern, mucosal detail, or motility. Two overhead films (prone and prone-angled) are obtained at the end of the examination (Fig. 7-5). *Retrograde enteroclysis,* through an ileostomy, can also be performed using a modified short tube with an inflatable balloon (Fig. 7-6).

Peroral pneumocolon (PPC)

The PPC is used for evaluating the distal ileum. Prior to the study the patient undergoes a colonic preparation similar to that for a barium enema, and barium is administered orally. When barium has reached the right and proximal transverse colon, air is insufflated into the rectum and refluxed into the distal small bowel. Glucagon can be used for relaxing the ileocecal valve. Multiple spot films of the terminal ileum and distal ileal loops are obtained. PPC frequently is employed at the end of SBFT, or even after enteroclysis, if the appearance of the terminal ileum is suspicious and needs clarification.

Retrograde small bowel examination

Today retrograde small bowel examination has been largely replaced by enteroclysis. As with enteroclysis and PPC, the patient scheduled for retrograde small bowel examination should undergo a colonic preparation to permit adequate examination of the small bowel. Barium (approximately 2000 ml of 20% w/v suspension) is administered to the rectum, and the entire colon is filled. Slightly more than 2000 ml of water is then introduced into the rectum and the barium is refluxed into the small bowel. The small bowel loops are distended individually, and the process is aided by the intravenous injection of glucagon. The examination is terminated when barium reaches the distal duodenum or when an area of obstruction is reached.

Indications for barium examination

Enteroclysis should be used as the primary method in most instances, particularly for intermittent or partial small bowel obstruction and for Crohn's disease if surgery is planned or the full extent of the disease must be assessed (Figs. 7-7, 7-8). It should always be the first modality for suspected Meckel's diverticulum (Fig. 7-9); malabsorption; tumors (Figs. 7-10, 7-11); occult GI bleeding if an upper GI series, barium enema, and an upper and lower endoscopy were negative (Figs. 7-12, 7-13); and in any patient who had pelvic surgery. After an equivocal result with dedicated SBFT, or in any patient who has negative SBFT but exhibits strong clinical suggestion of small bowel disease, enteroclysis is the best modality to unequivocally ascertain normality or pathologic changes (Fig. 7-14).

Water-soluble contrast material for small bowel examination

In young patients, the obvious benefits of enteroclysis must be weighed against disadvantages such as invasiveness and high radiation.

Because water-soluble contrast materials are hyperosmolar, they draw intestinal fluid across the intestinal mucosa into the lumen. Therefore the volume of bowel contents in the jejunum and ileum increases, which

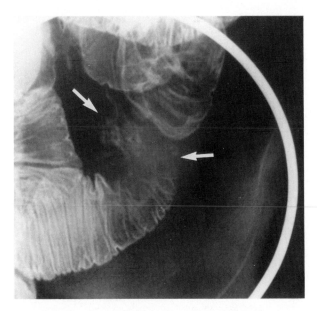

Fig. 7-7 Spot film during double-contrast phase of biphasic enteroclysis. Irregular narrowing of jejunum is noted over lengths of 3 inches in patient with Crohn's disease *(arrows)*. This finding was not identified on SBFT.

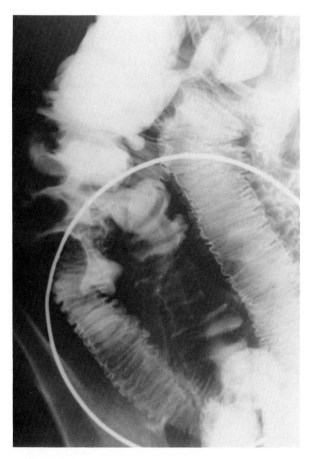

Fig. 7-8 Spot film of terminal ileum during biphasic enteroclysis shows marked thickening of folds and irregular margins in patient with terminal ileitis of Crohn's disease.

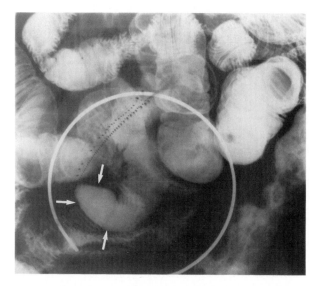

Fig. 7-9 Biphasic examination of enteroclysis shows a Meckel diverticulum *(arrows)* in this 35-year-old patient with a history of recurrent partial small bowel obstruction. A previous small bowel follow-through examination had been normal.

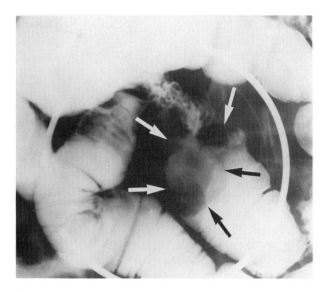

Fig. 7-10 Biphasic enteroclysis demonstrates an irregular mass *(arrows)* in distal jejeunum. During surgery, a large lymphocytic lymphoma was found.

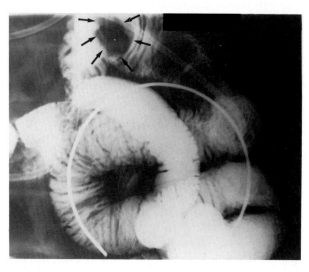

Fig. 7-11 A round mass with a corrugated surface *(arrows)* is shown by enteroclysis in area of ligament of Treitz. Patient suffered from occult blood loss, and at surgery, an infiltrating adenocarcinoma was found.

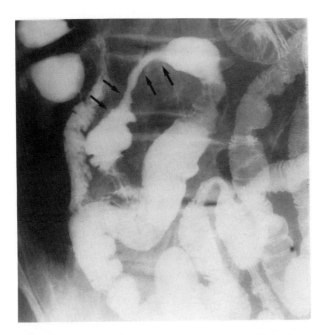

Fig. 7-12 A stricture *(arrows)* is well demonstrated by entero-clysis in this elderly patient with severe ischemic changes in area of terminal ileum.

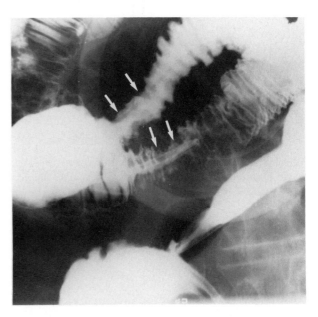

Fig. 7-13 In this patient with known hemophilia, the single-contrast phase of enteroclysis shows thickened straight folds in the proximal ileum with some mass impression *(arrows)* on lumen, indicative of intramural hemorrhage.

stimulates peristaltic activity. Although passage of the contrast material is increased, the diluting effect prevents specific diagnoses beyond the mere conclusion that a partial or complete small bowel obstruction is present. Non-ionic, water-soluble contrast material can be used to avoid this dilution effect and facilitate clear visualization of the cause of obstruction. When a partial small bowel obstruction is combined with a postoperative ileus, water-soluble contrast material could be therapeutic.

Water-soluble contrast material is indicated for patients with a suspected leak in the small bowel, for those in whom a colon obstruction has been demonstrated, and for those in whom a synchronous small bowel obstruction (for example, cancer with metastases of the small bowel) is suspected. Closed-loop small bowel obstruction is better examined by enteroclysis or computed tomography than by SBFT with iodinated contrast material.

Computed tomography for small bowel examination

In large part the success of computed tomography (CT) of the small bowel depends on the degree to which the small bowel is filled with contrast material (Figs. 7-15, 7-16). To ensure optimal filling, patients are asked to drink 400 to 600 ml of a 1% to 2% solution of contrast medium 45 minutes before the examination, a second cup with the same amount at 30 minutes, and an additional 250 ml 5 to 10 minutes before the CT scan. Administration of the contrast material in distinct phases helps ensure that the proximal and distal small intestine will be filled with contrast material when the CT scans are performed. Dilute meglumine diatrizoate can be employed, but a dilute mixture of barium sulfate (such as E-Z-CAT) has also proved satisfactory.

If a lesion is suspected in the terminal ileum, pelvis, or right colon, additional time is allowed before the CT scan is obtained to ensure than the region in question contains sufficient contrast material. It is preferred that contrast medium be given several hours before CT scanning and then again 30 to 45 minutes before the study. Rectal contrast material is given as an enema just before a pelvic CT study.

Another method is to use drugs to propel the contrast material into the distal small bowel. A 10 mg tablet of metoclopromide is given with the first cup of contrast material at 45 minutes, followed by the same amount of contrast medium at 30 minutes. Because of the rapid emptying from the stomach and proximal small bowel caused by the metoclopromide, a large cup of oral contrast material must be administered 5 to 10 minutes before the examination to ensure filling of the stomach, duodenum, and proximal small bowel loops.

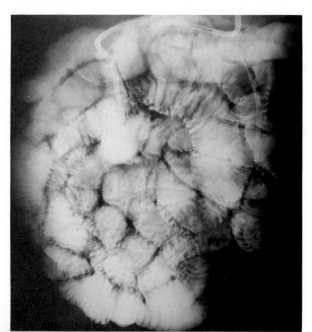

A

Fig. 7-14 A, Biphasic enteroclysis demonstrates diffusely thickened folds throughout small bowel. Previous SBFT was completely normal. **B,** CT shows thickened walls and valvulae conniventes *(arrows)* in jejunum because of surgically proved leukemic infiltrates in same patient.

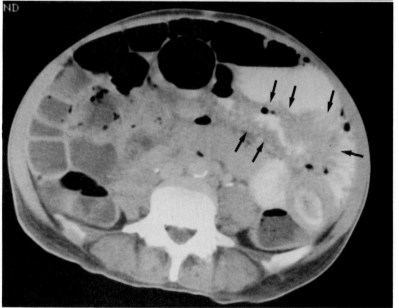

B

Magnetic resonance imaging for small bowel examination

At present, the small bowel is not well evaluated by magnetic resonance imaging (MRI). This is due partially to respiratory and peristaltic artifacts and partially to the lack of a good contrast material. Fast scanning techniques such as echo-planar imaging and new oral contrast material will improve the diagnostic quality of MRI of the small bowel. As these technical problems are resolved, the role of MRI in small bowel examination will need to be reevaluated.

RECOMMENDED READING

1. Abu-Yousef MM et al: Enteroclysis aided by an electric pump, *Radiology* 147:268, 1983.
2. Dehn TC, Nolan DJ: Enteroclysis in the diagnosis of intestinal obstruction in the early postoperative period, *Gastrointest Radiol* 14:15, 1989.
3. Herlinger H: A modified technique for the double-contrast small-bowel enema, *Gastrointest Radiol* 3:201, 1978.
4. Kressel HY et al: The peroral pneumocolon examination: technique and indications, *Radiology* 144:414, 1982.
5. Lappas JC, Maglinte DT: Enteroclysis edges in on follow-through methods, *Diagn Imaging* 56:88, 1987.
6. McGovern R, Barkin JS: Enteroscopy and enteroclysis: an im-

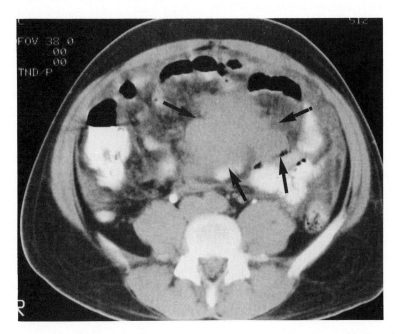

Fig. 7-15 CT of small bowel. Large Burkitt's lymphoma is seen in mesentery with direct invasion of jejunum *(arrows)*.

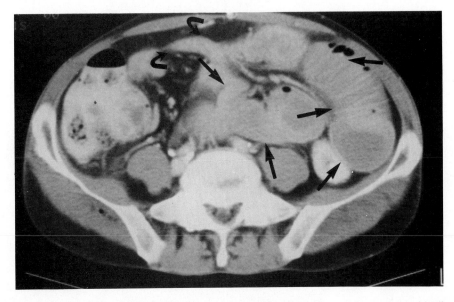

Fig. 7-16 CT of small bowel. Dilated loops of jejunum are seen *(straight arrows)* with distal loops *(curved arrows)* not distended. The actual cause of obstruction is not visualized but was due to adhesions.

proved method for combined procedure, *Gastrointest Radiol* 15:327, 1990.

7. Richards DG, Stevens GW: Laxatives prior to small bowel follow-through: are they necessary for rapid and good-quality examination? *Gastrointest Radiol* 15:66, 1990.

8. Thoeni RF, Gould RG: Enteroclysis and small bowel series: comparison of radiation dose and examination time, *Radiology* 178:659, 1991.

Inflammatory diseases of the small bowel

JACQUES PRINGOT

CROHN'S DISEASE

Crohn's disease is the most common nonspecific inflammatory disease of the small bowel. It is currently defined as a chronic inflammatory disease of unknown cause that may involve any segment of the digestive tract from the oral cavity to the anus. Classic Crohn's disease is found predominantly in the terminal ileum. The specific character of the disease is an inflammation, most often of a granulomatous nature, submucosal in the beginning and transmural when fully developed. It is characterized macroscopically by edema, ulceration, and fibrosis. The chronic evolution of the lesions toward stenosis, fistulization, and recurrence after surgical excision is an important characteristic. Ileal involvement has been reported to occur in 85% of granulomatous colitis, the remaining 15% being cases of isolated colitis. Appendicitis may be associated with concurrent inflammation in the distal ileum or cecum or in both, or it may occur as primary Crohn's disease of the appendix.

Patients with Crohn's disease may have an associated lesion of the anus at some time during the course of the disease. This anal lesion is either an ulceration, or more commonly, a sinus or fistula. In patients with involvement of the terminal ileum, 25% have an anal lesion; as many as 75% have anal lesions when the colon is involved. Extraenteric manifestations of Crohn's disease may occur in the joints, skin, mouth, and eyes, and may, clinically at least, precede intestinal involve-

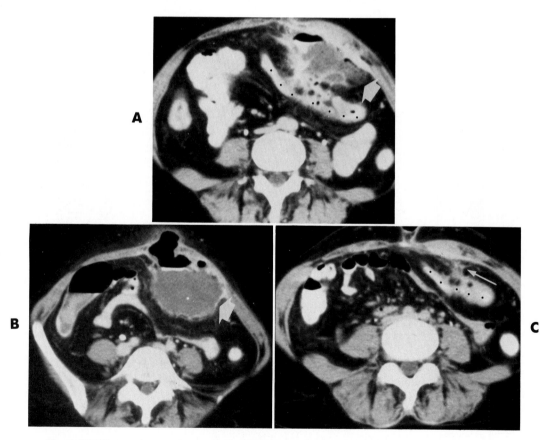

Fig. 7-17 CT scan demonstrates complicated abscess, **A,** *(broad arrow),* with fistula to adjacent bowel *(dots).* Abscess opacified by oral contrast extends through abdominal wall, **B.** After percutaneous drainage of abscess, **C,** there is formation of fibrotic scar *(small arrow),* and extraintestinal contrast is no longer detected by CT scanning.

ment. It has been shown that patients with regional enteritis positive for HLA-B27 develop ankylosing spondylitis. It is also generally admitted that the risk of cancer is slightly increased in Crohn's disease.

Computed tomography is the most accurate radiologic modality for detection of enterovesical fistulas. It is less sensitive than contrast radiography of the detection of subtle mucosal lesions but has proved to be superior to ultrasonography in the evaluation of abscesses (Fig. 7-17) and can be used for guidance of drainage. CT is challenged by MR, which is technologically more advanced than CT and can demonstrate the extra intestinal changes associated with Crohn's disease, as well as fistulas and sinus tracts. Magnetic resonance imaging has many advantages over other imaging modalities in the accurate demonstration of pelvic abscesses (Figs. 7-18, 7-19). Because of long scanning times, MRI is not useful for examinations of the mesenteric bowel. With gallium and ^{99m}Tc (or more recently ^{111}In) *white-blood cell scintigraphy,* it has been found that isotopic scanning can not only detect abscesses, but it can also identify sites of disease activity in inflammatory bowel disease, particularly in the colon.

Radiologic features

The radiologic features of basic lesions in Crohn's disease include the following.

Fine granular pattern: Radiographic studies of surgical specimens in correlation with visual studies have shown that a granular appearance of the mucosal surface is usually observed over a variable length of intestine and in the transitional zone between normal intestine and the main lesions. This pattern is believed to correspond to slight mucosal and submucosal edema. With peroral pneumocolon techniques mucosal granularity is demonstrated in the small bowel in a majority of patients with Crohn's disease in the small bowel or in the colon. This pattern is nonspecific, reflecting an alteration in villous structure, and corresponds on histologic specimens to villous hypertrophy and bridging resulting from edema or vascular congestion of the lamina propria or both.

Thickening of the folds: Along with associated functional disorders, thickening of the folds may be the first manifestation of the disease or its recurrence. Because of submucosal edema and the moist surface, the folds appear blurred, swollen, straightened, irregular, and on occasion, fused or nodular (Fig. 7-20).

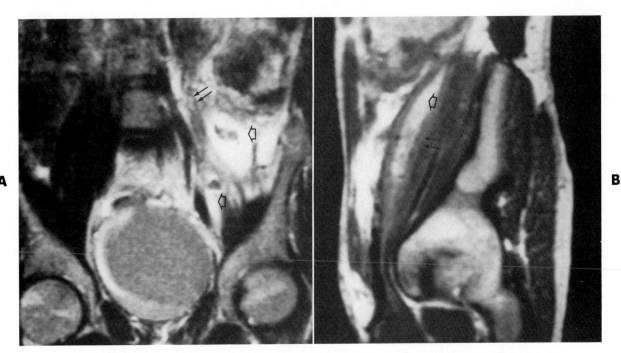

A   B

Fig. 7-18 Abscess of left psoas muscle complicating Crohn's disease **A,** Coronal T_2-weighted image showing extraintestinal fluid collections *(arrows)* and inflammatory changes in left psoas muscle *(double arrow),* which appears brighter than right psoas muscle. **B,** Sagittal T_1-weighted image of left psoas and iliac muscles delineating extension of fluid collection *(arrow)* in inflammated psoas muscle *(double arrow).*

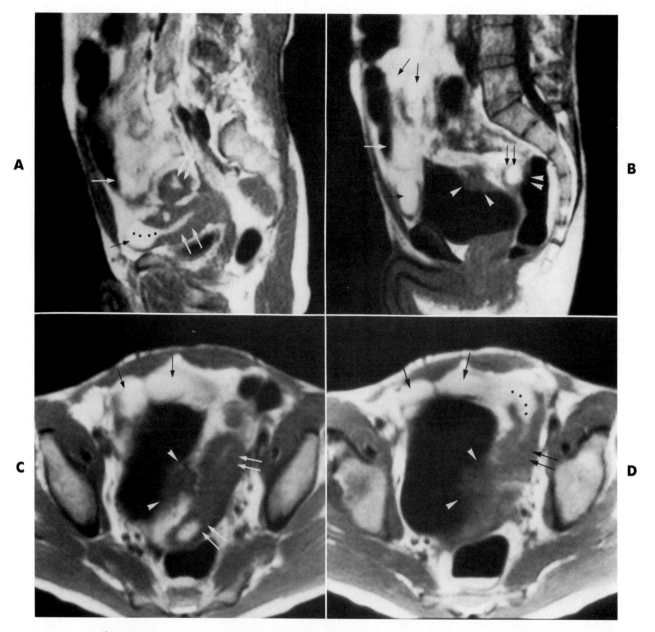

Fig. 7-19 Crohn's disease extending to sigmoid colon and urinary bladder imaged with spin-echo technique after oral intake of Gadolinium DTPA as positive contrast agent. **A,** Medial, and **B,** left paramedial sagittal T_1-weighted images of abdomen and pelvis, and **C, D,** axial T_1-weighted images of pelvis show normal *(arrows)* and diseased *(double arrows)* small bowel, as well as bladder *(arrowheads)* and rectosigmoid *(double arrowhead)* involvement. Both normal and thickened small bowel walls appear hypointense to surrounding fat and to contrasted intestine. Note the transition *(dots)* between normal and thickened small bowel on **A** and **D,** and sinus tracts appearing as low signal intensity structures extending from one bowel segment to another on **A** and from bowel to bladder wall on **C.**

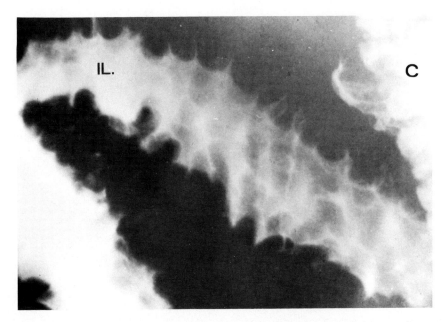

Fig. 7-20 Thickening of ileal folds occurs proximal to ileocolic anastomosis in case of recurrent Crohn's disease. *C,* Colon; *IL,* ileum.

Nodular pattern: The nodular pattern may also be seen in cases of submucosal edema and inflammation.

Ulceronodular pattern: As the lesions progress, ulceration between the nodules becomes evident. The cobblestone pattern results from a combination of longitudinal and transverse ulcerations with residual islands of mucosa in between (Figs 7-21 to 7-23).

String sign: The string sign characterizes the tubular narrowing of the intestinal lumen. When caused mainly by edema and accentuated by spasm, the degree of narrowing is not constant. The diameter of the lumen does remain constant, however, when a marked fibrous thickening of the intestinal wall is present. When the disease stabilizes, the mucosa may be restored, but the epithelium is scarred and atrophied. In this case the outline of the lumen is smooth, and pseudopolyps may occasionally be observed.

Ulcerations: Aphthous ulcers are considered to be early lesions of Crohn's disease and correspond to erosions of the intestinal mucosa overlying hyperplastic lymphoid follicles in which granulomas may be found (Fig. 7-24). An aphthous ulcer presents the *en face* appearance of a pinpoint fleck of barium in the center of a round filling defect or nodule. If the ulcer is larger than a few millimeters, the central barium fleck may be round, oval, or stellate (Figs. 7-25, 7-26). In profile the nodular elevations of the mucosa in which ulcers occur appear as smooth, convex, marginal defects. The ulcer crater is often seen at its top as a distinct barium collection. The mucosa between the ulcers is normal or slightly granular. Aphthous ulcers are usually multiple and sometimes diffuse. Although they may be found as isolated lesions, they are most often associated with large ulcers or more extensive lesions or both. These ulcers are commonly observed in the initial stages of primary or recurrent lesions, as well as in the proximal segment of the main lesion. They may even be found at some distance from this main lesion. Large ulcers may be found near or at some distance from the main lesions, and in the latter case appear separated from them by macroscopically normal segments. Annular ulcers are often multiple and are most commonly seen as skip lesions in the proximal ileum and in the jejunum.

In many cases a long, deep, longitudinal ulcer is observed along the mesenteric attachment of the small intestine in continuity with the main lesion.

Filiform polyposis: Filiform pseudopolyps are thin, elongated, fingerlike mucosal lesions of inflammatory origin. They are found most often in the colon, less frequently in the stomach, and very rarely in the small bowel.

Fistulas and sinuses: Fistulas and sinuses originate in intramural fissures or in deep longitudinal furrowed ulcers. They are characteristic of the advanced stages of Crohn's disease and occur with strictures (Fig. 7-27), with a tendency to arise proximal to the point of maximal stricture.

Thickening and retraction of the mesentery: Thickening of the mesentery is a constant phenomenon reported by all authors. The mesentery opposite the intes-

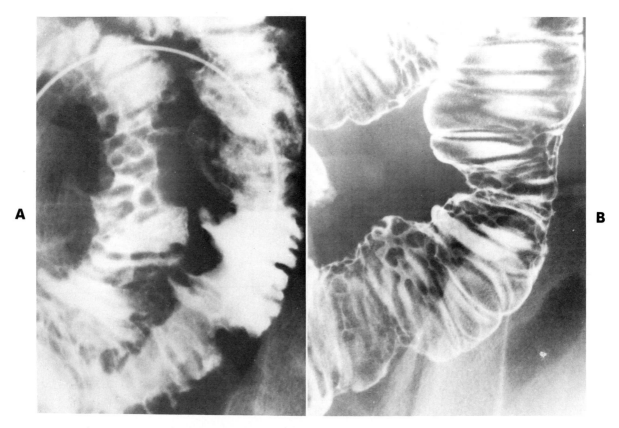

Fig. 7-21 In case of Crohn's jejunoileitis, close-up views in single, **A,** and double (following dental intubation) **B,** contrasts show cobblestoning as well as asymmetric and discontinuous involvement.

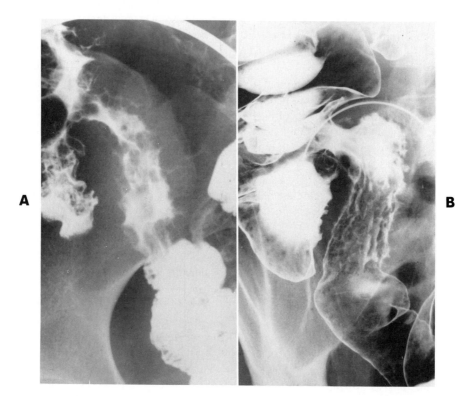

Fig. 7-22 Comparative views of terminal ileum in case of Crohn's ileitis show ulceronodular pattern in single, **A,** and double, **B,** contrast (peroral pneumocolon). Latter view demonstrates extent of lesions more precisely.

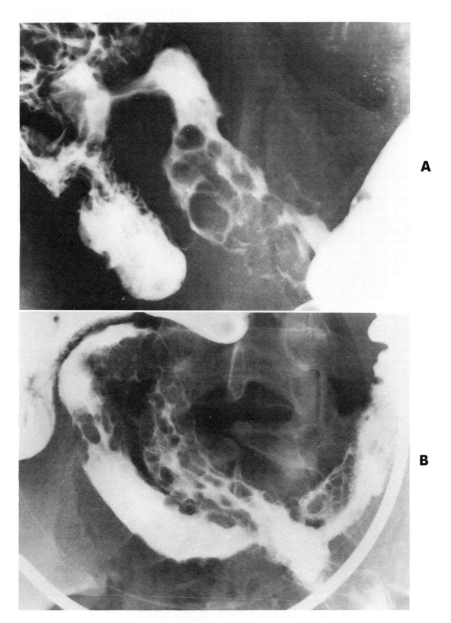

Fig. 7-23 Typical ulceronodular pattern (cobblestone pattern) is seen in terminal ileum, **A,** as well as in long segment of preterminal ileum, **B.**

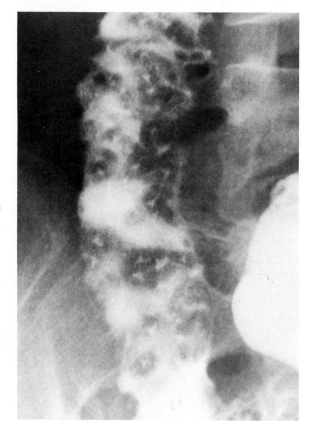

Fig. 7-24 Numerous aphthoid ulcers, mainly of stellate type, are seen along with diffuse granular appearance of mucosal surface.

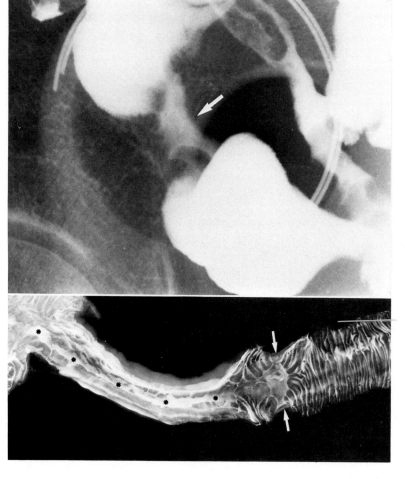

Fig. 7-25 A, Diamond-shaped ulcer *(arrow)* is seen short distance from main distal lesions located on mesenteric border of loop, which is asymmetrically narrowed because of retraction of its opposite border. Ulcer *(arrows)* in barium-coated surgical specimen is seen in face-on, **B,** and profile, **C,** views. Note typical cobblestone appearance of main lesions where deeper longitudinal ulcer *(arrow)* follows mesenteric border, as well as granular appearance of mucosal surface surrounding "isolated" ulcer.

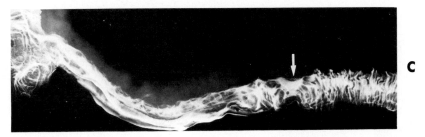

Fig 7-25, cont'd For legend see opposite page.

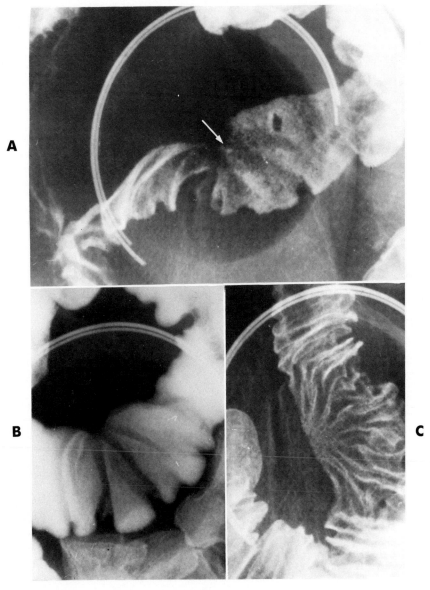

Fig. 7-26 A, Small ulcer *(arrow)* associated with converging folds. **B** and **C,** Ulcer scar. Note scalloping of opposite border.

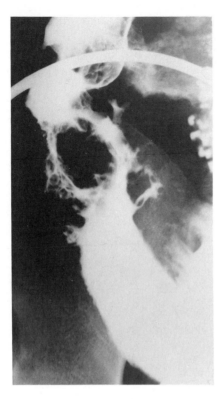

Fig. 7-27 Stricture and dilatation of terminal ileum. Numerous sinuses are opacified; most of them are proximal to point of most severe narrowing.

tinal lesion is thick and infiltrated, and the mesenteric fat spreads over the loop, progressing until it joins the antimesenteric border in places where intestinal lesions and, especially, ulcerations of the mucosa are most pronounced. Regional lymph nodes in the diseased area are consistently enlarged. If the mesentery becomes sclerotic, certain intestinal loops may take on the shape of the Greek letter *omega* (Fig. 7-28). This appearance is not specific to regional enteritis and may be observed in all types of mesenteric infiltration, particularly in cases of peritoneal carcinomatosis or carcinoid tumors.

The *spatial arrangement* of lesions is important in the diagnosis of Crohn's disease. Two fundamental characteristics are independent of the basic pattern of the lesion, and, when present, are decisive factors in diagnosis.

The existence of a gradation in the severity of lesions within the involved intestinal loop and the mesentery is one of the most characteristic features of Crohn's disease (Fig. 7-29). The occurrence of *skip lesions,* a classic characteristic of the disease, is in agreement with the concept of a gradation in severity of the lesions.

The second characteristic is the tendency for lesions to appear preferentially on the mesenteric side of the intestine and to show an asymmetric distribution or sacculation. CT with contrast media–opacified intestine is an excellent way of studying bowel wall and mesenteric

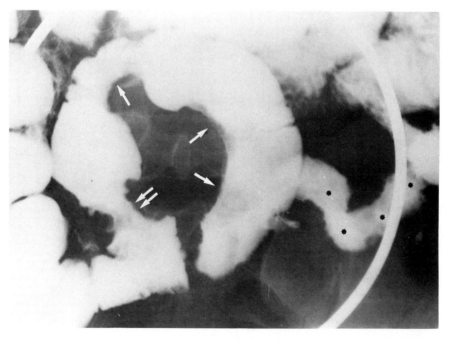

Fig. 7-28 Omega sign associated with concentric lesions *(asterisks).* Note focal narrowing *(double arrows)* as well as two areas in which mesenteric border is curvilinear and rigid *(arrows).*

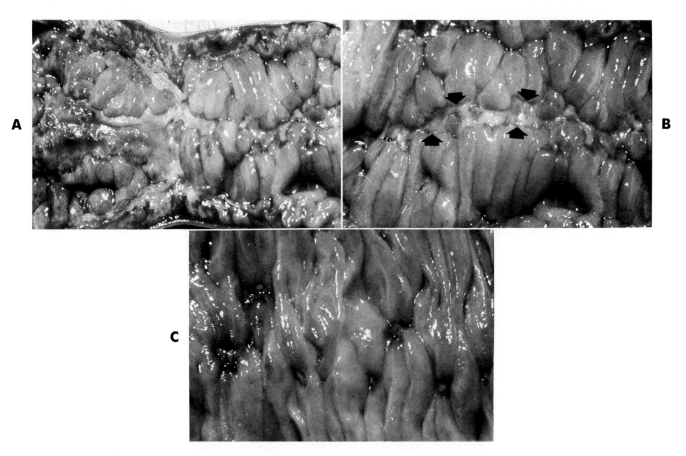

Fig. 7-29 Surgical specimen shows characteristic gradation in severity of lesion. **A,** Ulceronodular pattern. **B,** Longitudinal ulcer *(arrows)* along mesenteric border. **C,** Aphthoid ulcers and thickened edematous folds.

thickening, fistulas, sinuses, and abscesses (Figs. 7-30 to 7-32). In the distal segment, longitudinal fissures are distributed over the entire circumference of the intestinal loop and are intersected by transverse ulcers. This produces the *cobblestone pattern.* This pattern is occasionally caused by mucosa crisscrossed by epithelialized cracks. In the intermediary zone a longitudinal ulcer deeper than the others follows the mesenteric border of the affected intestine, extending proximally further than the other ulcers. The progressive shrinking from the antimesenteric border toward the mesenteric border, in which ulcers are located, is responsible for the formation of the asymmetric segments (Fig. 7-33). A more acute degree of shrinking produces short, eccentric stenoses and pseudodiverticula corresponding to zones unaffected by the shrinking. Free perforations seldom occur.

Imaging findings

CT findings in Crohn's disease include the following:

Mural changes: In Crohn's disease the most com-mon abnormality detected by cross-sectional imaging is the thickened small bowel wall. CT scans show symmetric wall thickening and a circular or tubular narrowing depending on the orientation of the diseased loop in a plane perpendicular or parallel to the plane of the transverse section. In Crohn's disease, an average mural thickness of 18 mm for the small bowel was found. The thickened bowel wall may show three different CT patterns. A homogeneous attenuation of soft tissue density of the thickened wall and contrast enhancement due to hypervascularity may be seen. The *double halo sign,* found on cross section through diseased segments, consists of two rings of different attenuation enclosing the intestinal lumen, an inner ring of water density surrounded by an outer ring of higher attenuation. On longitudinal section through the diseased bowel, the double halo sign consists of two linear zones of different attenuation levels, an inner submucosal zone of low attenuation and an outer zone of higher attenuation. The inner ring or line is thought to represent edematous inflamed mucosa, adherent mucus, and on occasion, submucosal edema; the outer ring or line is thought to represent the

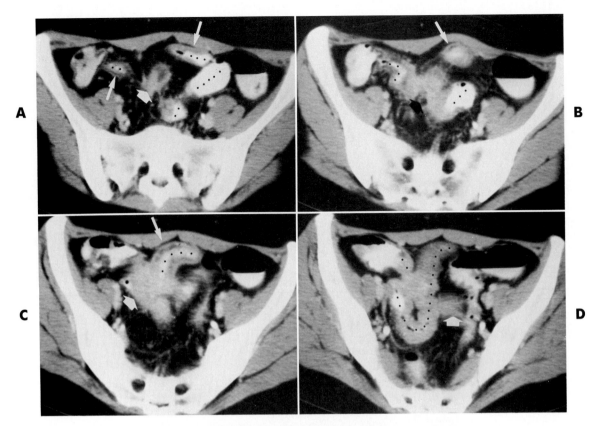

Fig. 7-30 For legend see opposite page.

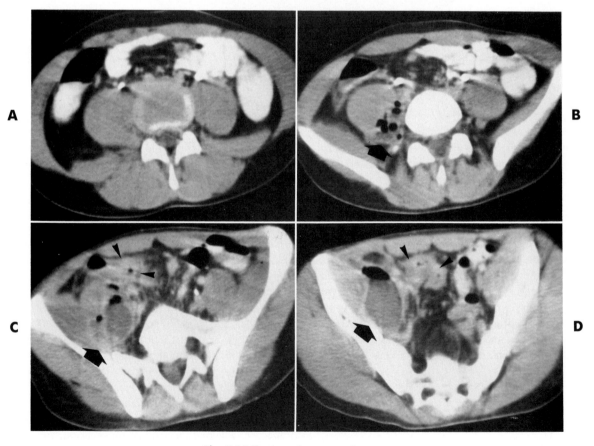

Fig. 7-31 For legend see opposite page.

Fig. 7-30 Nonhomogeneous mural thickening of diseased ileum *(dots);* low attenuation region *(arrows)* within thickened wall paralleling lumen is seen in longitudinal, **C** and **D,** and in transverse sections **A** and **B.** Note so-called target or double halo sign, **B.** Note also poorly defined interloop soft tissue density mass *(broad arrows).*

Fig. 7-31 Large abscess in sheath of right psoas muscle *(broad arrows),* **B, C,** and **D.** Abscess has enhancing rim, contains gas, and is contiguous to diseased small bowel *(arrowheads)* in right lower quadrant, **C.** Note swelling of psoas muscle above abscess in **A.**

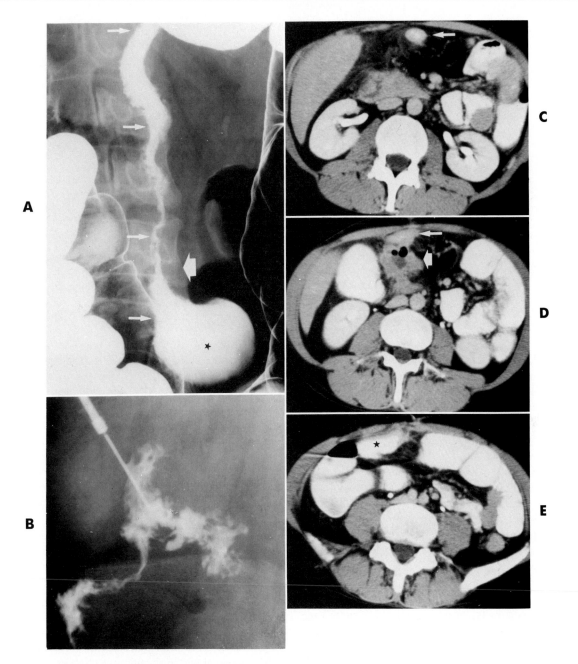

Fig. 7-32 Complicated recurrent Crohn's disease. **A,** Long stricture of preanastomotic small bowel *(arrows)* and impression *(broad arrow)* on bowel near point of dilatation *(star).* **B,** Noncommunicating abscess opacified through cutaneous fistula. **C,** CT scan shows thickened bowel wall *(arrow)* and fibrofatty changes. **D,** At level of bowel impression *(broad arrow)* is contiguous abscess. Thickened bowel *(narrow arrow)* is seen communicating with abscess. **E,** Normal wall thickness of proximal dilated bowel *(star).*

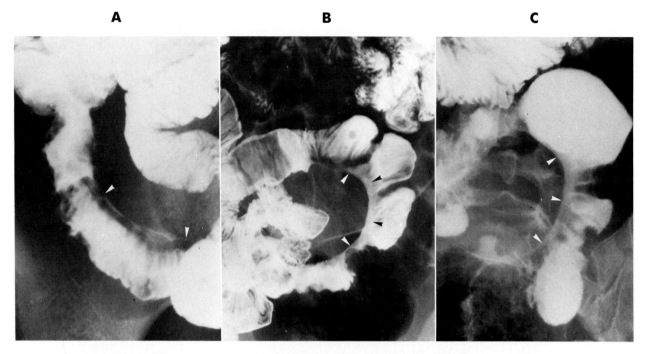

Fig. 7-33 Typical appearances of intermediary segment. **A** to **C,** Longitudinal ulcer *(arrows)* proximal to concentric lesions is located at concave mesenteric border of loop, the folds being arrested close to ulcer. Shrinking of antimesenteric border may be more, **C,** or less, **B,** marked. **D,** Sometimes longitudinal ulcer is not evident despite apparent convergence of mucosal folds.

remaining layers of the thickened bowel wall, reflecting the transmural characteristics of granulomatous disease.

In patients on long-term oral corticosteroid therapy and in whom the disease appears to be of low-grade activity on histologic examination, a zone of very low attenuation which is caused by submucosal accumulation of fat, exists. This zone, is from 1 to 5 mm in width with a CT density of 100 to 130 Hounsfield units (HU).

Mesenteric changes: Fibrofatty changes within the mesentery display an accentuated vascular pattern with several small nodules, probably lymph nodes. Lymph node enlargement of more than 1.5 cm in diameter or a conglomerate of enlarged nodes are found in only a minority of patients.

Fistulas and sinuses: CT is more sensitive than ultrasound for the demonstration of fistulas. Fistulas are seen as defined tracts, usually opacified by contrast material, which extend between adjacent thickened bowel loops from the bowel to the subcutaneous tissues and adjacent muscles or skeletal structures. CT should be regarded as the initial radiographic study in patients with suspected enterovesical fistula.

Interloop and extraintestinal abscesses: On sonograms, abscesses complicating Crohn's disease generally appear as rounded or oval fluid collections with fairly well defined irregular walls. The abscesses are attached to inflamed bowel loops or to the abdominal wall, or are located in the retroperitoneal space, particularly the psoas or iliopsoas muscles.

CT scans, however, appear more sensitive and more specific than ultrasound not only for the detection of abscesses, but also for the evaluation of their localization and extension in the extraintestinal spaces. Abscesses appear typically as low-density rounded masses with a thick wall that enhances after intravenous contrast, but they may also show a more crescentic or semilunar shape. The presence of gas or extraluminal contrast material indicates that the abscess is communicating with the intestinal lumen. In rare cases, the presence of gas results from gas-producing bacteria. MRI is useful only in depicting changes in the pelvis. Its value is in depicting the pericolonic disease, fistulas, sinuses, and abscesses. T_1 and T_2 weighted images are required. Imaging in all three orthogonal planes provides precise indentification and localization of changes.

Differential diagnosis

In our experience the radiographic findings that most simulate those of Crohn's disease are observed in certain cases of *segmental ischemia*. The ischemic lesion

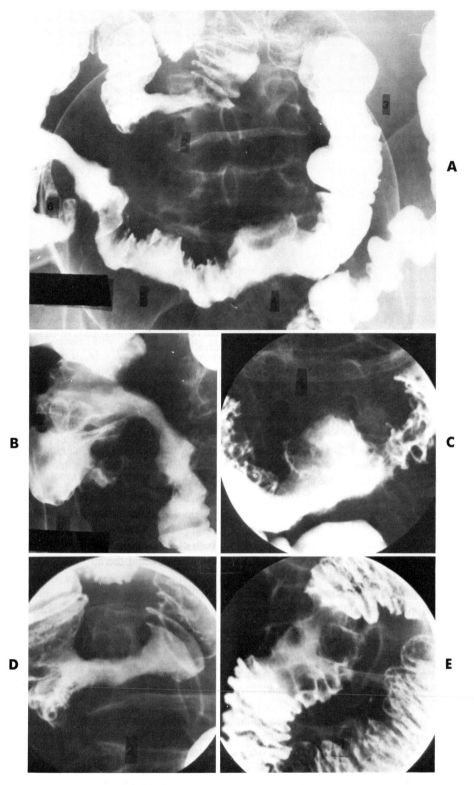

Fig. 7-34 A, Secondary ulcerative tuberculosis with multiple skip lesions in distal ileum. **B,** Detail of ileocecal lesions shows extensive ulcerative process of terminal ileum and ileocecal valve area. Cecal folds are thickened and converge toward ulcerated valve. **C,** Cavitating ulcer. **D,** Large circular stenotic ulcer. **E,** Irregular, shallow ulcer raised above normal mucosa.

darteritic lesions in the surrounding connective tissue. The lesions usually involve the ileal loops located within the pelvis and are often extensive and irregularly distributed throughout the ileum. In some cases they are segmental or even focal, particularly after intracavitary radiotherapy. Chronic radiation enteritis becomes progressively more severe and may be complicated by stenosis, perforation, or fistulization.

Plain films of the abdomen may show signs of an obstruction and/or increased density in the affected regions. Barium studies reveal the separation of intestinal loops with a greater or lesser degree of narrowing, as well as a straightening and thickening of the mucosal folds. Nodular filling defects and thumbprinting—the results of edema or fibrous nodule formations or both—are also observed within the submucosa. Because of the changes occurring within the mesentery, the bowel loops are fixed, angulated, and matted together and have serrated contours. The thickened mesentery gives the effect of an extrinsic mass. Contrast material outside the bowel lumen may indicate an ulceration but is more often the sign of a developing perforation or fistula.

The differential diagnosis is basically limited to differentiating x-ray lesions from a recurrence of a cancerous growth. Tumor spread is most common along the mesenteric border of the small intestine and should be suspected in cases of irregular nodular thickening at the mesenteric (concave) border of the loops. In postoperative adhesions there is no radiologic evidence of radiation damage, such as edematous thickening of valvulae conniventes and intestinal wall.

CT scanning in radiation ileitis demonstrates intestinal wall thickening that is distributed geographically, corresponding to the radiation field. The loops show mucosal folds with somewhat straightened contours. Thickened, crowded, and linear streaks of increased density in the mesenteric area are also seen.

DRUG-ASSOCIATED DISORDERS

Enteric-coated *potassium chloride tablets* (withdrawn from the market in the United States but still in use in other countries), *slow-release potassium chloride* (Slow-K), and *potassium gluconate* liquid have all been associated with small bowel strictures. Generally located in the midportion of the intestine, the stricture is usually single but may be multiple. It appears as a short, concentric, moderate to severe narrowing, with smooth borders and a conical transition to the efferent bowel loop, which is more or less dilated.

Clofazimine, a derivative of phendimetrazine tartrate, which is used in the treatment of leprosy, pyoderma grangrenosum, and chronic lupus erythematosus, causes segmental intestinal and mesenteric lesions that slowly regress after withdrawal of the drug. On radiographic examination, moderate segmental narrowing is revealed, along with a blunted and slightly nodular mucosal surface at the level of the affected segment.

Flucytosine, a systemic antifungal drug, is used for the treatment of cryptococcal meningitis and other fungal diseases. This treatment may produce extensive inflammatory infiltrates and edema, with multiple focal areas of mucosal necrosis in the small intestine and proximal colon, that can lead to bowel perforation. The radiologic pattern consists of severe luminal narrowing of the distal part of the small bowel, regular fold thickening, and marked separation of bowel loops. Discontinuation of the drug therapy results in total reversal of the radiologic abnormalities.

EOSINOPHILIC GASTROENTERITIS

Eosinophilic infiltration may extend to the small intestine alone or to both the small intestine and the ascending colon. In fact, eosinophilic infiltration may involve any part of the gastrointestinal tract from the esophagus to the colon. The obstructive form of eosinophilic enteritis or gastroenteritis has been reported to account for about half the cases, and surgery may be required for the relief of an obstruction or because of diagnostic uncertainty. Eosinophilic gastroenteritis is typically characterized by subacute, recurring episodes of abdominal cramps, diarrhea, and distention with nausea and vomiting, especially when the stomach is involved.

The typical radiographic pattern is a smooth, concentric narrowing of the distal gastric antrum and a focal or diffuse thickening of circular small bowel folds along with a moderately narrowed lumen and ill-defined transition to normal bowel. The narrowed small bowel may show a saw-toothed contour, or the infiltration may be sufficiently pronounced to completely blunt the valvulae. Separation and angulation of the intestinal loops are generally considered to result from thickening of the bowel wall and mesentery. In typical cases the diagnosis is presumed on the basis of clinical, radiologic, and hematologic abnormalities and is confirmed by a peroral intestinal biopsy. In doubtful cases the only means of determining the diagnosis is a laparotomy to obtain a full-thickness biopsy specimen.

PSEUDOMEMBRANOUS ENTERITIS OR ENTEROCOLITIS

In adults pseudomembranous enterocolitis usually involves only the colon. In the rare cases in which the small bowel is affected, plain films show gaseous distention and irregular thickening of the mucosal surface in the aerated bowel loops. Barium studies show a diffuse fold thickening and shaggy, irregular borders.

RECOMMENDED READING

1. Bodart P, Dive CH, Van Trappen G: Radiological differences between ileocaecal tuberculosis and Crohn's disease. II. Diagnosis of Crohn's disease, *Am J Dig Dis* 6:604, 1961.
2. Bray FJ: Filiform polyposis of the small bowel in Crohn's disease, *Gastrointest Radiol* 8:155, 1983.
3. Brombart M, Massion J: Radiological differences between ileocaecal tuberculosis and Crohn's disease. I. Diagnosis of ileocaecal tuberculosis, *Am J Dig Dis* 6:589, 1961.
4. Clemett AR, Chang J: The radiologic diagnosis of spontaneous mesenteric venous thrombosis, *Am J Gastroenterol* 63:209, 1975.
5. Crooks DJM, Brown WR: The distribution of intestinal nodular lymphoid hyperplasia in immunoglobulin deficiency, *Clin Radiol* 31:701, 1980.
6. Ekberg O, Lindstrom C: Superficial lesions in Crohn's disease of the small bowel, *Gastrointest Radiol* 4:389, 1979.
7. Federle MP et al: Computed tomographic findings in bowel infarction, *Am J Roentgenol* 142:91, 1984.
8. Goldberg JI et al: Computed tomography in the evaluation of Crohn disease, *Am J Roentgenol* 140:277, 1983.
9. Gore RM et al: The value of computed tomography in the detection of complication of Crohn's disease, *Dig Dis Sci* 30:701, 1985.
10. Hricak H, Bennadette C: *MRI of the pelvis,* Martin London, UK, 1991, Dunitz Ltd.
11. Jeffrey RB et al: Abdominal CT in acquired immunodeficiency syndrome, *Am J Roentgenol* 146:7, 1986.
12. Jones B et al: Granular small bowel mucosa: a reflection of villous abnormality, *Gastrointest Radiol* 12:219, 1987.
13. Koelbel G, Schniedl U, Majer MC et al: Diagnosis of fistulae and sinus tracts in patients with Crohn's disease: value of MR imaging, *Am J Roentgenol* 152(2):999, 1989.
14. Laufer I, Costopoulos LL: Early lesions of Crohn's disease, *Am J Roentgenol* 130:307, 1978.
15. Maizel H, Ruffin JM, Dobbins WO III: Whipple's disease: a review of 19 patients from one hospital and a review of the literature since 1950, *Medicine* 49:175, 1970.
16. Marshak RH, Lindner AE: *Radiology of the small intestine,* Philadelphia, 1970, WB Saunders.
17. Mathieu D et al: Periportal tuberculous adenitis: CT features, *Radiology* 161:713, 1986.
18. McLean AM, Simms DM, Homer MJ: Ileal ring ulcers in Behçet syndrome, *Am J Roentgenol* 140:947, 1983.
19. Morson BC: Pathology of Crohn's disease, *Clin Gastroenterol* 1:265, 1972.
20. Pringot J et al: Nonstenotic ulcers of the small bowel, *Radiographics* 4:357, 1984.
21. Rosen A et al: Mesenteric vein thrombosis: CT identification, *Am J Roentgenol* 143:83, 1984.
22. Teixidor HS et al: Cytomegalovirus infection of the alimentary canal: radiologic findings with pathologic correlation, *Radiology* 163:317, 1987.
23. Thoeni RF, Margulis AR: Gastrointestinal tuberculosis, *Semin Roentgenol* 14:283, 1979.
24. Wall SD et al: Multifocal abnormalities of the gastrointestinal tract in AIDS, *Am J Roentgenol* 146:1, 1986.
25. Weese WC, Smith IM: A study of 57 cases of actinomycosis over a 36 year period, *Arch Intern Med* 135:1562, 1975.

Neoplastic lesions

ROBERT KOEHLER

Neoplasms of the small bowel are rare, constituting only 2% to 3% of GI tumors. With the exception of metastatic disease, tumors tend to concentrate at the two ends of the bowel, the duodenum and proximal jejunum, and in the distal ileum.

BENIGN TUMORS

A variety of benign tumors occurs in the small bowel, but approximately 90% are adenomas, leiomyomas, lipomas, and hemangiomas. Of these, adenomatous polyps and leiomyomas are the most common and occur with roughly equal frequency.

When benign tumors of the small intestine are evident clinically, they usually present with abdominal pain, small bowel obstruction, bleeding, or a palpable mass. Obstruction is often caused by the intussusception of tumors that are intraluminal in location. Bleeding can occur when ulceration develops in an adenoma or in the mucosa covering a submucosal or intramural tumor.

Adenomas

Adenomas make up about 25% of benign small bowel tumors. They occur more frequently in the duodenum than in the jejunum, and more frequently in the jejunum than in the ileum. On radiographic examination, adenomas appear as intraluminal filling defects that are usually pedunculated and may have a lobulated surface. The stalk can be several centimeters long, leaving the polyp free to move back and forth in a segment of duodenum or jejunum.

Leiomyomas

Leiomyomas of the small intestine occur with slightly greater frequency in the jejunum than in the ileum. Leiomyomas that originate in the submucosa appear as smooth, oval, or rounded filling defects or as pedunculated intraluminal defects. Intussusception may occur. Some lesions are dumbbell-shaped, bilobed tumors that protrude both outside the bowel and into the lumen.

Gastrointestinal bleeding in a young to middle-aged adult is the most likely clinical presentation of intestinal leiomyomas. The bleeding often occurs in repeated episodes with the passage of melena or dark red blood through the rectum. Angiography is helpful in demonstrating small intestinal leiomyomas, even if performed at a time when the patient is not actively bleeding (Fig. 7-39). These tumors are hypervascular and show intense opacification during the capillary phase of the injection. Early opacification of mesenteric veins draining

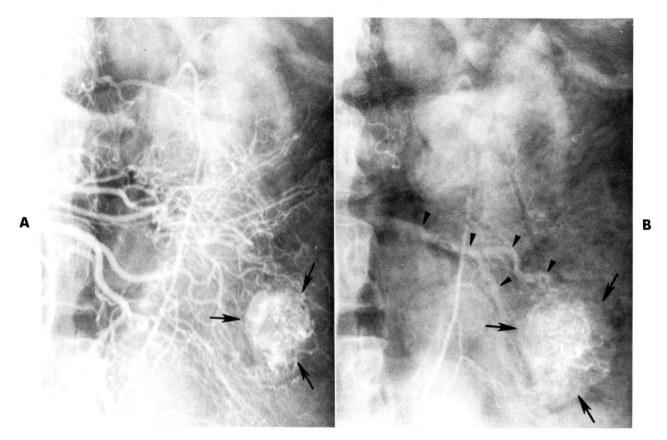

Fig. 7-39 Arteriographic demonstration of jejunal leiomyoma in 54-year-old woman with three major episodes of gastrointestinal bleeding in 2 years. Barium studies and endoscopic examinations were unrevealing. At surgery tumor was subserosal and did not protrude into lumen. **A,** Late arterial phase shows tumor stain *(arrows)* and irregular vessels within mass. **B,** Prominent veins *(arrowheads)* drain tumor *(arrows)*.

the tumor is also usually seen. *Leiomyoblastomas,* which resemble intestinal leiomyomas, may rarely occur in the small intestine.

Much has been learned recently about the CT appearance of small intestinal tumors of smooth muscle origin. Leiomyomas and leiomyoblastomas are typically spherical or ovoid and average 5 cm in diameter. Dense focal calcifications may be seen. The CT attenuation of these tumors is uniform, and contrast enhancement peaks about 10 seconds after bolus intravenous injection.

Lipomas

Lipomas occur somewhat less frequently in the small intestine than do adenomas or leiomyomas. Symptoms are not present in the majority of cases, but bleeding or intussusception may occur. Like leiomyomas, lipomas appear as smooth, round, or oval filling defects with an appearance suggesting an intramural location. Pressure on the abdomen may cause sufficient change in the

shape of a lipoma to indicate its soft, fatty nature (Fig. 7-40). As with lipomas elsewhere in the body, their appearance on a CT scan can be characteristic: a sharply demarcated round or ovoid mass with a low CT attenuation similar to that of normal fat. CT may also reveal signs of intussusception (Fig. 7-41) as can occur with many benign small bowel neoplasms.

Hemangiomas

Hemangiomas occur predominantly in the jejunum and, when clinically detectable, involve gastrointestinal bleeding or anemia. Calcified phleboliths are usually not seen. They occur more often in patients with Turner's syndrome, Sturge-Weber syndrome, tuberous sclerosis, and the blue rubber bleb nevus syndrome. Patients with hereditary hemorrhagic telangiectasia (Osler-Weber-Rendu disease) may have cavernous hemangiomas of the small bowel in addition to the more characteristic telangiectatic lesions.

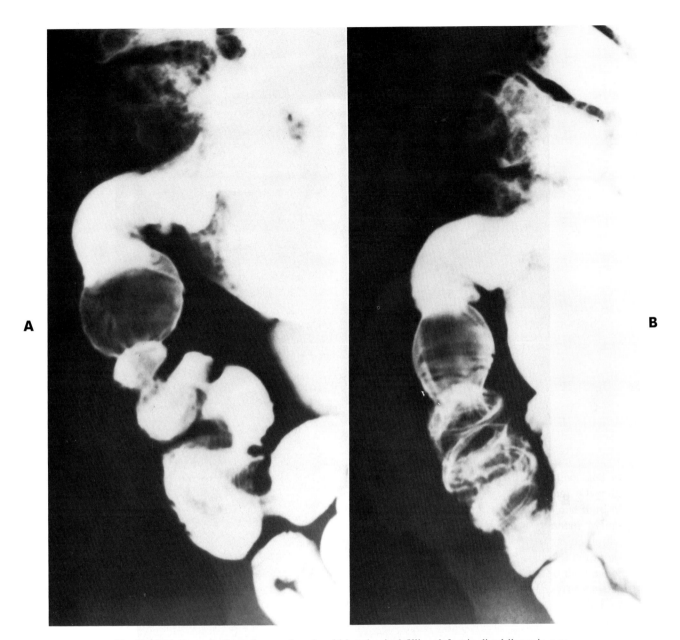

Fig. 7-40 Lipoma. **A,** Smooth, round, polypoid intraluminal filling defect in distal ileum in a patient with occult gastrointestinal blood loss. **B,** Soft nature of lesion is revealed in change from round to oval shape with peristaltic contraction of bowel.

Peutz-Jeghers syndrome

This autosomal dominant syndrome consists of polyps of the GI tract and characteristic brown pigmented lesions of the lips. The small bowel is affected in most cases and contains polyps ranging from tiny to 4 cm in size (Fig. 7-42). GI blood is common, and risk of GI malignancy is slightly increased.

Cronkhite-Canada syndrome

Cronkhite-Canada syndrome is a rare polyposis syndrome. The small bowel is involved in approximately half of the cases, whereas polyps occur in the stomach and colon in virtually all affected patients. The polyps are inflammatory and contain dilated interstitial glands that may become cystic. No true neoplastic tissue is

tumor is detected at this stage, it appears as a small, sharply defined submucosal lesion, typically in the distal ileum. Mechanical obstruction is not usually present at this stage unless the tumor is large enough to cause intussusception. As the carcinoid tumor grows outside the bowel lumen, it infiltrates the bowel wall, mesentery, and eventually the adjacent lymph nodes (Fig. 7-43). The bowel muscle may undergo hypertrophic thickening, presumably as a result of stimulation by serotonin or other hormones produced by the tumor. Even more striking is the fibroblastic proliferation induced in the adjacent mesentery. Together these effects cause kinking, angulation, and narrowing of the bowel lumen and sometimes the appearance of a mesenteric mass. Affected bowel loops become fixed and appear to be separated from each other. The desmoplastic response in the mesentery puts tension on the bowel wall at certain points, causing focal areas of spiculation and straightening of the mucosal fold pattern. Because radiographic findings can mimic those produced by a number of other conditions, the diagnosis of a small intestinal carcinoid tumor cannot usually be made with certainty on the basis of the barium examination unless the carcinoid syndrome is also present.

CT has proven to be very helpful in delineating the extent of spread in patients with carcinoid tumors. The primary tumor is rarely visible, but metastatic deposits in the liver and retroperitoneal adenopathy are detectable in many patients. Mesenteric involvement, reported to be visible on CT scans in 40% of cases, typically appears as an irregular mass in the lower right or middle abdomen. Linear strands extend out into the surrounding fat in a stellate pattern. Similar findings can be seen on MRI scans. Angiography is useful in demonstrating the presence of hepatic metastases that are almost uniformly hypervascular and therefore easy to demonstrate.

LYMPHOMAS
Clinical features

Malignant lymphomas make up about 20% of all malignant tumors that occur in the small bowel, being somewhat less common than adenocarcinomas in most series. A lymphoma may occur in the small intestine as a primary neoplasm or as part of a more widespread

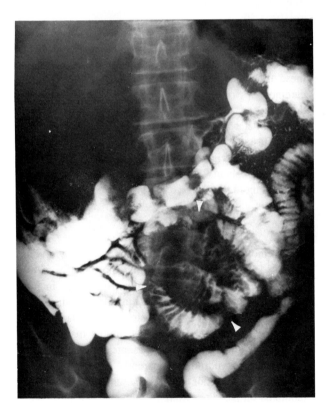

Fig. 7-43 Carcinoid tumor of ileum with mesenteric involvement *(arrowheads)*. Note straightened, spiculated appearance of small bowel folds and large liver, indicating hepatic metastasis.

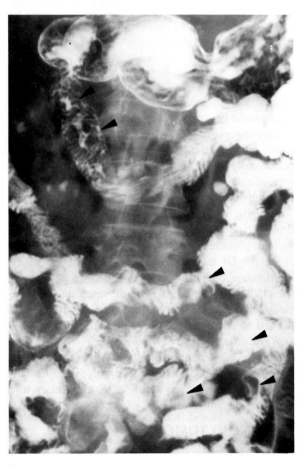

Fig. 7-44 Histiocytic lymphoma of small bowel. There are 1- to 2-cm mural nodules in duodenum, jejunum, and ileum *(arrowheads)*. Those in duodenum are ulcerated.

systemic process. Except for intestinal Hodgkin's lymphomas (which are of T-cell origin), gastrointestinal lymphomas are thought to be B-cell tumors. About 60% are of the diffuse histiocytic type. The next most common type is poorly differentiated lymphocytic lymphoma.

The majority of patients with malignant lymphoma involving the small bowel are symptomatic. Weight loss and diarrhea can occur, and perforation, which is quite unusual in patients with an adenocarcinoma of the small bowel, occurs in about 15% of patients with lymphoma. In 10% to 20% of patients, multiple small bowel lesions are found. As is the case with adenocarcinomas, lymphomas of the small bowel occur with an increased incidence in patients with celiac disease. Radiographic features of Crohn's disease and intestinal lymphoma are occasionally similar enough to prevent the distinction between the two by radiographic means.

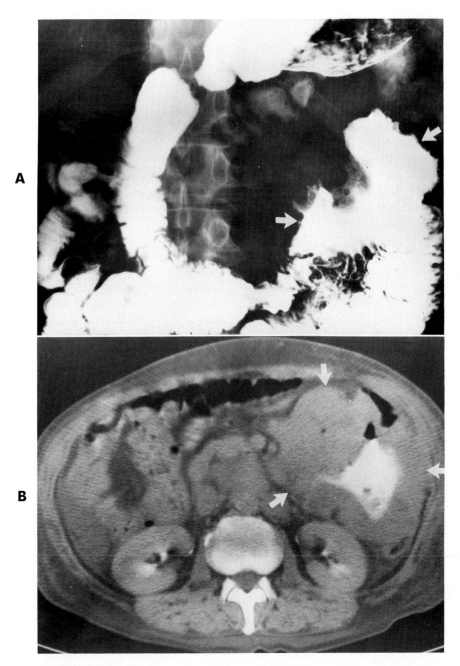

Fig. 7-45 Diffuse histiocytic lymphoma involving the jejunum. **A,** Barium study shows large irregular excavation *(arrows)* communicating with bowel lumen. **B,** Corresponding CT scan shows better the extent of tumor mass *(arrows).*

Radiographic features

Malignant lymphomas have a variety of different radiographic manifestations in the small bowel. These were classified by Marshak and co-workers into five different patterns: (1) multiple nodules, (2) an infiltrating tumor, (3) a polypoid mass, (4) an endoexoenteric form with excavation and fistula formation, and (5) mesenteric invasion with extraluminal masses or production of the sprue pattern.

When ulceration is present within the nodules, a central depression can sometimes be seen on radiographs (Fig. 7-44). When the terminal ileum is involved, multiple nodules are often seen in the adjacent cecum. In the infiltrating form, one or more areas of narrowing of the lumen are often present. The separation of adjacent loops of bowel may give further evidence of mural thickening. When lymphoma presents as a polypoid mass, it is often associated with a mechanical obstruction caused by intussusception. Such a mass may achieve a large size. In the endoexocenteric form of intestinal lymphoma, the tumor contains a large area of ulceration and sometimes multiple fistulas communicating with adjacent segments of bowel. On barium studies the ulcer or excavation appears to represent a large irregular collection that does not conform to the contour of a normal segment of bowel (Fig. 7-45). Sometimes, when such an excavation appears to represent a widened area of the lumen, the term *"aneurysmal dilatation"* is used. When the tumor is predominantly extraluminal, large areas of the mesentery and adjacent retroperitoneum may be filled with the tumor.

CT scans are useful in detecting, characterizing, and staging lymphoma of the small bowel. They are particularly adept at showing bowel wall thickening, which can be diffuse or quite focal. Enlargement of regional mesenteric lymph nodes and the finding of a large mass without mechanical bowel obstruction are features frequently seen on CT scans (Fig. 7-46). Ultrasonography can also be useful in demonstrating small intestinal lymphomas. Like lymphomas elsewhere in the body, those arising in the bowel tend to be relatively sonolucent. Intestinal lymphomas, however, typically have a central hyperechoic area representing mucosa and mucus or gas within the bowel lumen.

Lymphoma variants

Hodgkin's disease can produce some of the same radiographic findings as seen in patients with non-Hodgkin's lymphomas. In Hodgkin's disease, however, large excavations, fistulas, and aneurysmal dilatations are uncommon. Mesenteric fibrosis along with resultant angulation and narrowing of the bowel is occasionally seen because Hodgkin's disease sometimes stimulates a desmoplastic response in tissues surrounding the lymphoma.

Burkitt's lymphoma can also involve the small intestine. In younger patients jaw tumors are often seen, whereas in older patients abdominal and pelvic tumors are more typical. These B-cell tumors grow rapidly and are often large at the time of diagnosis. Involved loops of small bowel may show a narrowing and irregular thickening of folds.

The primary jejunal lymphoma of the type known as *Mediterranean lymphoma* appears to be a clinically distinct entity. It occurs predominantly among persons of Arabian and non-Ashkenazi Jewish descent, and is particularly prevalent in southern Iran. Mediterranean lymphomas affect younger persons and do not show a male predominance. The duodenum and jejunum are the areas primarily affected. Radiographic findings consist of

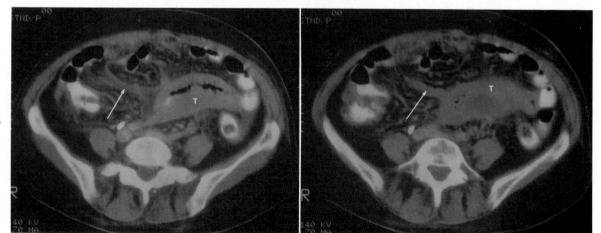

Fig. 7-46 A and **B,** Adjacent sections of a CT study showing a histiocytic lymphoma of proximal ileum *(T)*. The mass extends further into the mesenteric leaves *(arrows)*.

marked, uniform, diffuse thickening of mucosal folds due to massive infiltration of plasma cells. The portions of the small bowel that are uninvolved with lymphoma show a spruelike pattern, particularly in the ileum. In some patients there is a tendency to develop nodules superimposed on the thickened folds, and there may be separation of bowel loops by masses of enlarged lymph nodes in the mesentery.

ADENOCARCINOMAS

Adenocarcinomas constitute about one fourth of malignant tumors occurring in the small intestine. They are most common in the duodenum and proximal jejunum, and their likelihood of occurrence diminishes with increasing distance from the ligament of Treitz.

The radiographic appearance of an adenocarcinoma of the small intestine is similar to that of a carcinoma of the esophagus or colon. Infiltrating tumors are the most common and appear as short, well-demarcated segments of narrowing (Fig. 7-47) with an irregular lumen indicating replacement of the mucosa by the tumor (Fig. 7-48). These tumors tend to have overhanging edges. Not uncommonly there is ulceration within the mass. Infiltrating tumors of this type incite a local scirrhous reaction in the bowel wall, and there is usually mechanical obstruction of the jejunum by the tumor. Prestenotic dilatation can be quite marked. Small plaquelike polypoid adenocarcinomas involving one wall of the jejunum have been detected by enteroclysis.

Adenocarcinomas have also been found in the small intestine in the form of a pedunculated polyp, but this is a rare occurrence.

Small intestinal adenocarcinomas occur with a higher incidence in patients with adult celiac disease. A latent period of 20 years or more generally exists between the onset of malabsorption and the discovery of the tumor. Some evidence suggests a minor increase in the risk of small bowel adenocarcinoma developing in patients with regional enteritis.

SARCOMAS

Sarcomas of spindle cell origin are another type of primary malignant tumor likely to be found in the small bowel. The majority of these primary sarcomas arise from smooth muscle. Melena and abdominal pain are common symptoms that tend to occur when the tumor has reached considerable size and has undergone necrosis or ulceration. Mechanical obstruction is a relatively late manifestation. Many tumors are large enough to be palpable on abdominal examination at the time they are discovered.

On radiographic examination the tumor appears as an extrinsic mass with the displacement of overlying intestinal loops that may be adherent. A prominent transverse stretching of parallel mucosal folds can indicate the site of the tumor. When necrosis and ulceration occur, an irregular cavity develops within the tumor and may fill with barium. Barium also outlines fistulous

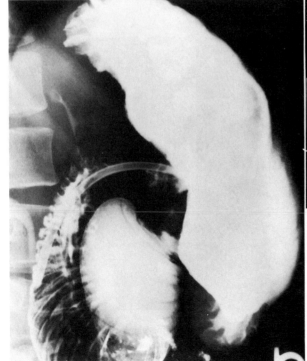

A

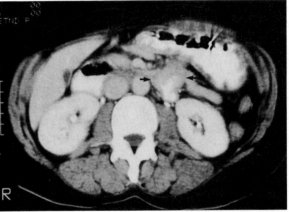

B

Fig. 7-47 Jejunal carcinoma in a middle-aged woman with abdominal pain and vomiting. **A,** Barium study shows high-grade obstruction by a tight annular mass at duodenal-jejunal junction. **B,** Soft-tissue mass of tumor itself *(arrows)* is better seen on CT.

nodules and subtle pleating of folds, which may be the first radiographic manifestations of metastatic small bowel disease (Fig. 7-49).

The signs and symptoms of secondary neoplasms of the small bowel are not specific. Gastrointestinal blood loss occurs in 20% to 30% of these patients and is most common in metastatic lesions that ulcerate or cavitate. Obstruction is most likely with tumors that stimulate a fibrotic reaction causing fixation, angulation, and narrowing of the bowel. Tumor cells can reach the small intestine through the blood (embolic) (Figs. 7-50, 7-51) through intraperitoneal spread (Fig. 7-52) through the lymphatic chain, or by direct extension from an adjacent tumor mass. Of these four routes, the first two are the most common modes of tumor spread to the small bowel.

Intraperitoneal seeding occurs most often from tumors of gastrointestinal origin in men and tumors of ovarian origin in women. The classic *Blumer's shelf* represents a tumor in the prerectal pouch of Douglas, a dependent recess of the peritoneal cavity in the pelvis. When a barium enema reveals the typical narrowing and irregularity of the rectum at the level of the upper sacrum, a careful search for evidence of intraperitoneal spread of tumor to the small intestine should be made.

The hematogenous spread of tumor to the small intestine occurs most commonly in patients with melanoma or carcinoma of the lung (see Fig. 7-50). The nodules are usually multiple and may be uniform or dissimilar in size (see Fig. 7-51). These nodules tend to occur on the antimesenteric border of the bowel and sometimes grow into large polypoid masses that may cavitate, particularly in patients with melanoma.

RECOMMENDED READING

1. Bessette JR et al: Primary malignant tumors in the small bowel: a comparison of the small bowel enema and conventional follow-through examination, *Am J Roentgenol* 153:741, 1989.
2. Brady LW, Asbell SO: Malignant lymphoma of the gastrointestinal tract, *Radiology* 137:291, 1980.
3. Cronkhite LW, Canada WJ: Generalized gastrointestinal polyposis: an unusual syndrome of polyposis, pigmentation, alopecia and onychotrophia, *N Engl J Med* 252:1011, 1955.
4. Dachman AH et al: Cronkhite-Canada syndrome: radiologic features, *Gastrointest Radiol* 14:285, 1989.
5. Dudiak KM et al: Primary tumors of the small intestine: CT evaluation, *Am J Roentgenol* 152:995, 1989.
6. Gourtsoyiannis NC, Nolan DJ: Lymphoma of the small intestine: radiological appearances, *Clin Radiol* 39:639, 1988.
7. Kerber GW, Frank PH: Carcinoma of the small intestine and colon as a complication of Crohn disease: radiologic manifestations, *Radiology* 150:639, 1984.
8. Modlin IM: Carcinoid syndrome, *J Clin Gastroenterol* 2:349, 1980.
9. Olmstead WW et al: Tumors of the small intestine with little or no malignant predisposition: a review of the literature and report of 56 cases, *Gastrointest Radiol* 12:231, 1987.
10. Picus D, Glazer HS, Levitt RG et al: Computed tomography of abdominal carcinoid tumors, *Am J Roentgenol* 143:581, 1984.
11. Ramos L et al: Radiological characteristics of primary intestinal lymphoma of the "Mediterranean" type: observations of 12 cases, *Radiology* 126:379, 1978.
12. Rubesin SE et al: non-Hodgkin lymphoma of the small intestine, *Radiographics* 10:985, 1990.
13. Traube J, Simpson S, Riddell RH et al: Crohn's disease and adenocarcinoma of the bowel, *Dig Dis Sci* 25:939, 1980.

Malabsorption and immune deficiencies

DANIEL MAKLANSKY
ARTHUR E LINDNER

DISEASES ASSOCIATED WITH MALABSORPTION
Sprue and sprue pattern

The name sprue is given to a group of three diseases of the small bowel that share a similar pathologic appearance: *celiac disease of children, nontropical sprue of adults,* and *tropical sprue.* Evidence now indicates that celiac disease and nontropical sprue are the same entity presenting at different times of life; the term *celiac sprue* is used to include both diseases. Tropical sprue is a distinct disease. Its cause has not been fully established, but it is related to small bowel infection.

The three diseases of the sprue group exhibit similar lesions on small bowel biopsy. There is flattening, broadening, and coalescence of the villi and sometimes even a complete loss of these structures. Since the crypts of Lieberkuhn become elongated, the overall thickness of the mucosa may not be much different from normal. The lamina propria is infiltrated with lymphocytes, plasma cells, and some eosinophils. The epithelial cells of the villi are flattened and cuboidal, and the nuclei of these cells, instead of maintaining a regular basal orientation, appear at irregular levels. All of these mucosal abnormalities associated with celiac sprue are more pronounced in the jejunum than in the ileum.

Celiac sprue has a particular relationship to diet, in that *gluten,* a water-soluble protein fraction, causes the symptoms. The cause of this toxicity, however, remains elusive. There is a high incidence of the histocompatibility antigen HLA-B8 in patients with celiac sprue, which suggests a genetic predisposition. Evidence has been presented that the intestinal damage induced by gluten may be mediated by local immune reactions. In adults, some improvement in the biopsy as a result of a gluten-free diet may be noted, but in most cases the lesions persist. When a patient on a gluten-free diet is in clinical remission, reintroduction of gluten into the diet increases fecal fat excretion to abnormal levels and causes a clinical exacerbation. Patients with celiac sprue have an increased risk of developing lymphoma or carcinoma.

Tropical sprue is distinct from celiac sprue and patients usually respond to folic acid or antibiotic therapy.

The radiographic findings described are those of celiac sprue, and they are present in virtually all patients in the clinically active phase of the disease. Because they are also found in patients suffering from other diseases associated with malabsorption, the term *sprue pattern* or *malabsorption pattern* is sometimes used. The radiographic findings of tropical sprue are the same as those of celiac sprue.

Inflammatory changes are rarely seen in patients with sprue. Almost all, however, exhibit some degree of dilatation and hypersecretion in the small bowel (Fig. 7-53). Segmentation and fragmentation of the barium column are seen in severe disease. The folds may appear thin or thickened. When there is dilatation but no associated hypoproteinemia, the folds are thin. In patients in remission, the radiographic findings may or may not return to normal.

Dilatation of the lumen of the small intestine is one of the important and common findings in sprue. It is usually best visualized in the middle and distal jejunum and is less often seen in the ileum. The dilated loops are flaccid and contract poorly, and they do not have the erectile configuration seen in mechanical obstruction.

Intussusceptions are frequently seen in sprue. They are nonobstructive, with a typical coiled-spring appearance. Usually they are transient (Fig. 7-54).

Hypersecretion, excessive fluid in the intestinal lumen, is a constant finding in most patients with sprue, and radiographs show marked segmentation of barium. *Segmentation* refers to masses of barium that are moderately large and definitely separated from adjacent clumps (Fig. 7-55). The phenomenon is a physical response to excessive fluid within the bowel lumen in patients with malabsorption. When micropulverized barium suspensions containing suspending agents are employed, segmentation is greatly reduced. Thus with modern barium preparations, segmentation is not a prominent finding in most cases of sprue.

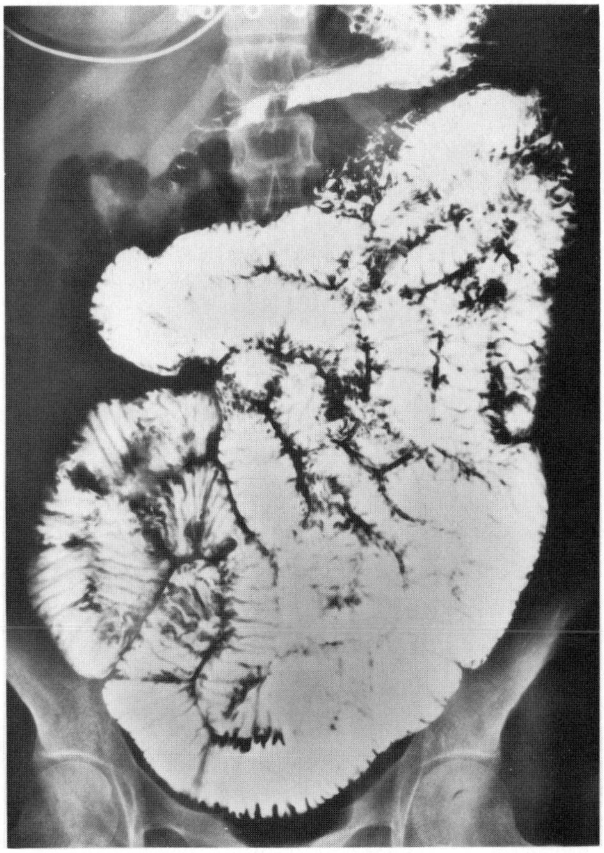

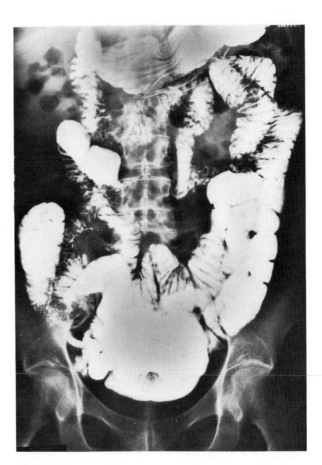

Fig. 7-53 Sprue. There is moderate dilatation of proximal jejunum. Intestinal loops are pliable and flaccid.

Fig. 7-54 Sprue. There is moderate dilatation of entire jejunum along with thinning of valvulae conniventes, minimal fragmentation, and increased secretions. Nonobstructive intussusception is noted in distal jejunum.

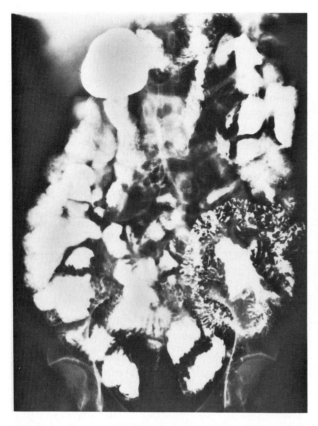

Fig. 7-55 Sprue. There is segmentation with stringlike strands of barium between the segmented loops. Dilatation and excessive secretions are also seen.

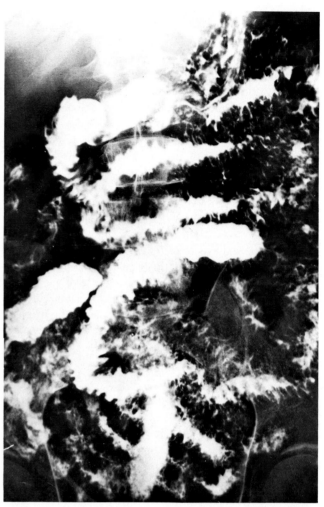

Fig. 7-56 Whipple's disease. Folds of jejunum and proximal ileum are blunted, redundant, thickened, and slightly nodular. Fragmentation and segmentation are minimal.

In the *moulage sign,* mucosal folds appear to be effaced, and the barium-filled lumen resembles a tube into which wax has been poured and allowed to harden. It is usually seen in association with marked segmentation and hypersecretion.

Whipple's disease

The clinical picture in Whipple's disease is one of weight loss, fever, diarrhea, steatorrhea, abdominal signs, and intermittent arthralgia or arthritis. Macrophages in the lamina propria have been found to contain a glycoprotein that reacts positively to periodic acid-Schiff (PAS) stain. Electron microscopy and histochemical studies show that the PAS-positive and gram-positive rods and granules seen under the light microscope are bacteria and bacterial substances.

The most prominent single radiographic finding in Whipple's disease is an alteration in the appearance of the mucosal fold pattern. The valvulae conniventes are thickened, even slightly nodular. At times the folds may appear to be wild and redundant (Fig. 7-56). *Intestinal lymphangiectasia* may simulate the radiographic findings in Whipple's disease, except for the distribu-

tion of the thickened folds. In Whipple's disease this finding is more prominent in the jejunum, whereas in intestinal lymphangiectasia it is usually diffuse. Other diseases that may mimic Whipple's disease on radiographs include amyloidosis, systemic mastocytosis, immune deficiencies, histoplasmosis, eosinophilic gastroenteritis, and lymphoma. On CT, enlarged mesenteric lymph nodes showing relative low attenuation are frequently present.

Scleroderma

Scleroderma is a systemic disease that may involve the small bowel and be associated with malabsorption syndrome. Involvement of the small intestine may occur at any time in the course of the disease but is usually preceded by skin changes, Raynaud's phenomenon, or arthropathy. When the small bowel is affected, pathologic examination shows atrophy of the muscular layers and replacement by collagen tissue. Both the mucosa and submucosa are atrophic, although the mucosa itself may be normal.

The vasculitis in scleroderma may contribute to a decrease in small bowel absorptive capacity. Replacement of the submucosal and muscular layers with fibrous tissue impairs motility, leading to bacterial overgrowth with alterations in the bile acids and consequent malabsorption. Long-term administration of broad-spectrum antibiotics improves absorption.

Delay in peristaltic activity in the stomach and duodenal bulb is usually minimal. The second portion of the duodenum demonstrates changes in its caliber, characterized by dilatation and delayed emptying (Fig. 7-57). Dilatation may be so marked that the changes suggest an obstruction at the ligament of Treitz from metastasis, an extension from carcinoma of the pancreas, or adhesions.

In the jejunum and ileum the most striking radiographic alteration is hypomotility with dilatation (Fig. 7-58). Segmentation, fragmentation, and increased secretions are usually absent. Sacculation with the formation of pseudodiverticula may occur, but this finding is more common in the colon in association with fecaliths. In scleroderma, dilatation is diffuse, rather than restricted to the jejunum as in sprue. The presence of sacculation suggests scleroderma.

Postoperative conditions

Radiographic examination may contribute to a diagnosis of malabsorption syndrome by demonstrating a surgical reconstruction of the gastrointestinal tract. Resection of the proximal small bowel reduces the area for absorption, and ileal resections promote loss of bile acids essential for digestion of fat, leading to malabsorption.

IMMUNE DEFICIENCIES

Intestinal infection with *Giardia lamblia* is now detected frequently in patients who have diseases associated with immunodeficiency (Fig. 7-59). The radio-

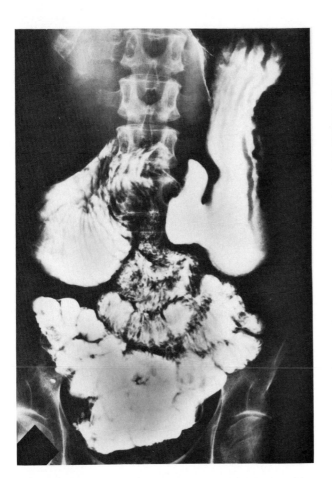

Fig. 7-57 Scleroderma. Marked dilatation of duodenum without organic obstruction at ligament of Treitz. There is moderate hypomotility of barium through small bowel.

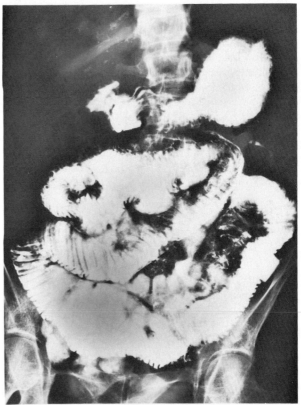

Fig. 7-58 Scleroderma. There is marked hypomotility with pseudosacculation, and dilatation is minimal. Pleating of valvulae conniventes is noted.

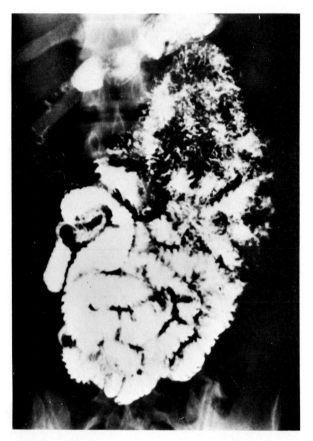

Fig. 7-59 Giardiasis. There is spasm and irritability of jejunum associated with increased secretions and thickening of valvulae conniventes. Findings are secondary to inflammatory process. Distal ileum is normal.

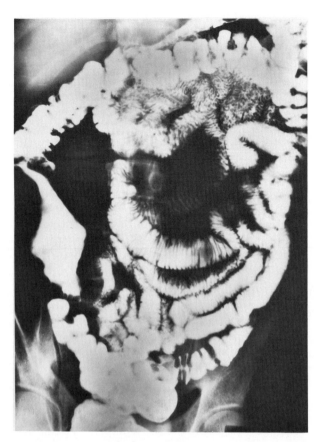

Fig. 7-60 Lymphoma. Aneurysmal dilatation of ileum surrounded by mass. Displacement of small bowel loops in central abdomen caused by retroperitoneal masses.

graphic manifestations of the enteropathic immunoglobulin deficiency syndromes have been organized into the following groups:

1. Sprue pattern, as seen in cases of hypogammaglobulinemic sprue and IgA-deficient sprue.
2. Multiple nodular defects.
3. Inflammatory changes secondary to infection.
4. Thickening of small intestinal folds as occurs in amyloidosis, lymphoma, macroglobulinemia, plasma cell dyscrasias, and intestinal lymphangiectasia (Fig. 7-60).
5. Tumor.

The radiographic alterations are not necessarily confined to one of these findings; a patient may exhibit more than one of these features either simultaneously or on successive examinations.

RECOMMENDED READING

1. Corner GM, Brandt LJ, Abissi CJ: Whipple's disease: a review, *Am J Gastrointest,* 78:107, 1983.
2. Ross IN: Primary immunodeficiency and the small intestine. In Marsh MN, editor: *Immunopathology of the small intestine,* New York, 1987, John Wiley & Sons.

8 *Colon*

GERALD D DODD
WYLIE J DODDS
PIERRE G MAHIEU
ALEXANDER R MARGULIS
PIERRE SCHNYDER
EDWARD STEWART
RUEDI F-L THOENI

RADIOLOGIC EXAMINATION OF THE COLON
Preliminary plain radiographs of the abdomen
Contrast examinations of the colon
Special examinations

DEFECOGRAPHY
Procedure for examination
Anatomic landmarks
Normal defecogram
Pathologic defecograms

DIVERTICULA
Technique of examination
Incidence
Pathogenesis
Diverticulitis
Complications
Diverticular disease with neoplasm
Classification

INFLAMMATORY DISEASE OF THE COLON
Indications for and techniques of barium enema
    examination
Ulcerative colitis
Granulomatous colitis
Differential diagnosis in inflammatory disease
Ultrasonography for inflammatory disease
Computed tomography for inflammatory disease
Magnetic resonance imaging for inflammatory bowel
    disease

POLYPS
Pathologic findings
Detection
Radiologic features
Specific polypoid lesions
Management of polypoid lesions
Polyposis syndromes

MALIGNANCIES
Etiology
Histologic tumor types and radiographic patterns
Metastases
Complications
Differential diagnosis
Neoplastic staging

Radiologic examination of the colon

RUEDI F-L THOENI
ALEXANDER R MARGULIS

The examination of the colon has undergone significant changes in the last decade, but barium enemas are still used for screening of the colon. Colonoscopy has become a complementary approach that contributes to the precision of the colonic examination and allows biopsies, as well as removal of small polypoid lesions. Ultrasonography has emerged as a method of identifying the location of large colonic masses, and it may offer a preliminary diagnosis of neoplastic masses and their staging. More recently, transrectal ultrasonography has been employed for staging rectal cancers, and the results for local invasion are very promising. Computed tomography (CT) has assumed an important role in demonstrating the extent of neoplasms, particularly in the rectum, and CT permits preoperative staging. In recent years magnetic resonance (MR) imaging has been increasingly used for evaluating colonic neoplasms.

Considerable information about the colon is obtainable from plain films of the abdomen, and both single- and double-contrast barium sulfate enema examinations are performed in radiology departments throughout the world to more clearly define colorectal pathology. In a multiinstitutional survey conducted in 1987, 40% of the surveyed institutions reported that during the last 5 years radiographic examinations of the colon have decreased by 20% to 30%, and 34% of the institutions reported decreases of 10% to 20%. These changes are largely due to the increased use of colonoscopy.

PRELIMINARY PLAIN RADIOGRAPHS OF THE ABDOMEN

The preliminary plain radiograph of the abdomen displays calcifications, unusual air or fat collections, and abnormalities of the intraperitoneal or retroperitoneal tissues and bone. Plain films also demonstrate changes in the size of organs, which is of great impor-

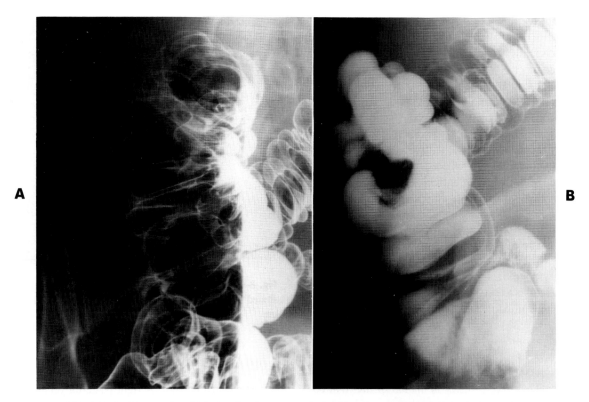

Fig. 8-5 A, Large polypoid lesion in distal ascending colon is seen with difficulty on double-contrast examination. **B,** It is seen very easily on single-contrast examination.

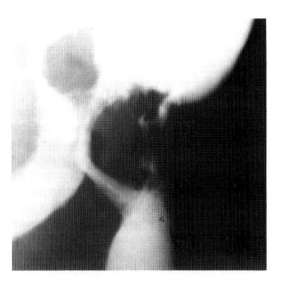

Fig. 8-6 Fistulas and sinuses are better demonstrated by single-contrast examination with careful fluoroscopic control. Spot film from barium enema of 24-year-old woman with colon-to-colon fistulas in left colon: Crohn's disease.

Contraindications to contrast examination

Because the double-contrast enema is the standard examination at many institutions, it is important to realize that certain contraindications exist. These include (1) obstruction of the colon, (2) debilitation or unconsciousness, (3) inability of the patient to be rotated on the table because too many devices are attached to him or to her or because movement is too painful, (4) the presence of severely acute or fulminating inflammatory colon disease, (5) severe diverticulitis (diverticulosis per se is not a contraindication), and (6) when fluoroscopic control of the examination is essential. During double-contrast examination, fluoroscopy is used to ensure technical adequacy of the examination and is only infrequently used to discover small lesions or fistulas. These are diagnosed during film interpretation.

The contraindications to single-contrast examination are (1) suspected acute fulminating ulcerative colitis, (2) suspected acute perforation, (3) immediately after deep biopsy, and (4) necessity to visualize mucosal detail and small lesions.

Examination through a colostomy

A double-contrast examination through a colostomy can be performed with ease in patients whose colon has been well cleansed and who have been on a clear liquid diet for 48 hours. The barium suspension is introduced through the stoma into the proximal transverse colon. The patient is rotated on the table as much as possible to obtain good coating. Air is introduced with the patient lying on the right side. Particular attention must be given to the most distal portion of the colon leading into the stoma, best seen in steep oblique spot films. When a double-barrel colostomy has been performed, the examination is again usually directed to the distal portion of the colon. Knowledge of the patient's history is very important.

The barium is introduced via soft catheter through a cone into the stoma. The patient holds the cone, pressing it into the stoma. Many other devices are also available; some have external suction cups and others have the appearance of large pacifiers with an enlarged hole in the rubber part. Packing towels or bandages around a soft rubber catheter can also be successful. Twenty percent of radiologists report using inflatable balloons inside the stoma. A catheter with an inflatable balloon inside the stoma should be inflated only under fluoroscopic guidance. The inflatable balloon catheter should be deeply inserted into the colon, and the balloon inflated only after the area of the stoma is visualized with barium. Perforation of the bowel with intraperitoneal or extraperitoneal spillage is often a fatal complication.

Ileostomy enema

A permanent ileostomy after total colectomy is most commonly performed in patients with chronic ulcerative colitis, granulomatous colitis, and familial multiple polyposis. With a normally functioning ileostomy, the distal prestomal ileum does not distend. Ileostomy dysfunction, resulting in copious uncontrolled discharge from the ileostomy, is a common complication. In administering the enema through the ileal stoma, the same precautions must be taken as for examination through a colostomy. A catheter with an inflated balloon can be inserted into the bowel and carefully distended as described for colostomies. The examiner may insert a soft catheter and surround the stoma with towels or use a stoma bag tightly closed around the end of the tubing used for administration of barium and air. The same devices used for colostomy enemas may be employed and can be held externally by the patient, with a soft catheter inside the stoma. Ileal pouches that are created as a reservoir after total colectomy can be examined by the rectum or ileostomy before definitive hookup after the initial surgery.

Retrograde examination of the small bowel

First described by Miller, retrograde barium sulfate examination of the small bowel was his preferred method for detecting and studying lesions obstructing the lower small bowel. The colon is filled with diluted barium sulfate, and the small bowel is filled until the lesion is encountered, studied, and recorded on spot films in various projections. The filling of the small bowel should not proceed beyond the proximal ileum. In most patients in whom difficulties are encountered because of pain, 1 mg of glucagon administered intravenously or intramuscularly may lead to an uneventful and satisfactory study. Also, the postevacuation film may be of great value, because barium present from retrograde flow in the small bowel may show the lesion to good advantage while the colon is collapsed.

Biphasic barium enema examination

The biphasic examination consists of a double-contrast barium enema followed by a single-contrast barium enema on the same day. The double-contrast examination of the colon under optimal conditions is the ideal examination for the demonstration of small lesions and mucosal detail. Nevertheless, very large lesions, whether polypoid or ulcerated, may sometimes escape detection (see Fig. 8-5). This is particularly true in patients in whom the ileocecal valve is widely patent so that haustral folds do not distend and often mask an annular lesion. Whenever the double-contrast barium examination shows a questionable or suspicious area on some of the views, it is advisable to follow it with a single-contrast examination (Fig. 8-7). The patient is sent to the bathroom for evacuation of some of the air and barium, and a single-contrast barium examination is performed. The combination of residual air and dilute low-density barium washes away some of the thick barium. The patient needs to be totally rotated on the table at least twice to mix the high-density and the dilute barium. Prone and supine views in an oblique projection and multiple spot films are then obtained.

Water-soluble contrast media for colon examination

Indications for the use of water-soluble contrast media include (1) suspected intestinal perforation with the need to demonstrate its exact location, (2) suspected vesicocolonic fistula, and (3) injection of a sinus tract from the skin and outlining of collections in the soft tissues. In the last situation the injection should always be done under fluoroscopic control through a soft rubber catheter placed in the sinus tract. Sterile technique is practiced by most radiologists to avoid introduction of additional infectious agents into the sinus tract. For the demonstration of fistulas and sinuses connecting to walled-off abscesses, however, barium sulfate remains the contrast medium of choice. Water-soluble iodinated contrast material can also be used for softening of

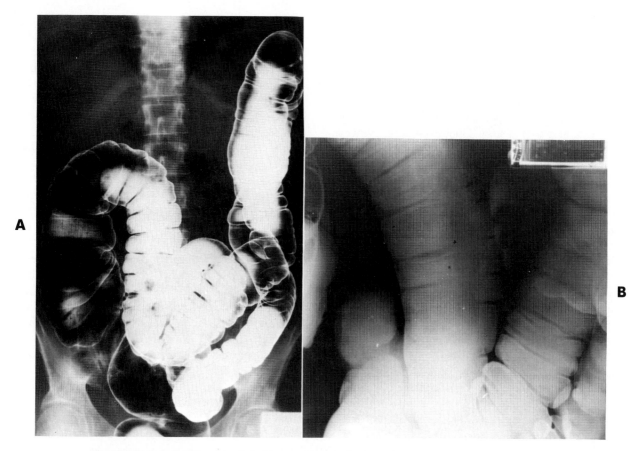

Fig. 8-7 Value of follow-up of double-contrast examination with single-contrast technique. **A,** Large defect is seen in proximal transverse colon. After patient evacuated barium and gas, barium was introduced into rectum, and spot films and prone and supine overhead films were obtained. No lesion was seen. **B,** Spot film of single-contrast enema after double-contrast examination.

meconium in newborns, to relieve fecal impaction in adults, and to outline the colon proximal to a complete obstruction.

SPECIAL EXAMINATIONS
Peroral double-contrast examination of the right colon and terminal ileum

Heitzman and Berne described the introduction of barium orally and air rectally during the same examination for visualization of lesions in the right colon, cecum, and ileocecal valve. The advantage of this type of examination is that the right colon can be visualized without interfering with the barium-filled loops of the sigmoid (Fig. 8-8). A further advantage is that in many diseases involving the ileocecal valve, a barium enema, particularly a double-contrast examination of the colon, is usually unsuccessful in demonstrating the terminal ileum.

The patient is prepared in the same manner as for a double-contrast enema examination of the colon. He or she receives a clear liquid diet, 13 ounces of magnesium citrate, and bisacodyl tablets and suppositories. The examination of the upper gastrointestinal tract and the small bowel proceeds in the usual way, with the patient receiving at least 10 to 12 ounces (300 to 350 ml) of barium sulfate. When the head of the barium column reaches the transverse colon and both the jejunum and proximal ileum are empty of barium, air is introduced into the rectum. Reflux into the terminal ileum is facilitated by injecting 1 mg of glucagon intravenously. Multiple spot films are then obtained. This examination is especially useful for visualizing lesions of the ileocecal valve, the cecum, and the last few inches of the terminal ileum.

Reduction of intussusception and volvulus

Intussusception should be reduced very carefully, observing the precautions outlined in Chapter 15. Reduction of volvulus should be done only after attempts at reduction with a sigmoidoscope, rectal tube, or both. A surgical procedure is often necessary, despite the transient reduction by barium enema.

Water-soluble contrast media for stool softening

Diatrizoate enemas have been administered to newborn infants with meconium ileus, resulting in prompt evacuation of the meconium. Water-soluble enemas can also be used in adults with fecal impaction.

Arteriography

Arteriography is widely employed to detect massive bleeding into the colon (Fig. 8-9). Bleeding rates as low as 0.5 ml/min can be detected with selective angiography, and although rates for detection of arterial bleed-

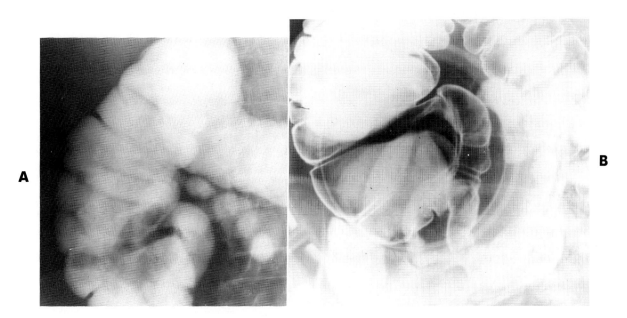

Fig. 8-8 Peroral pneumocolon in patient with large ileocecal valve. **A,** Valve is coated with fecal material and resembles large polypoid lesion. **B,** Peroral pneumocolon. Ileocecal valve appears normal.

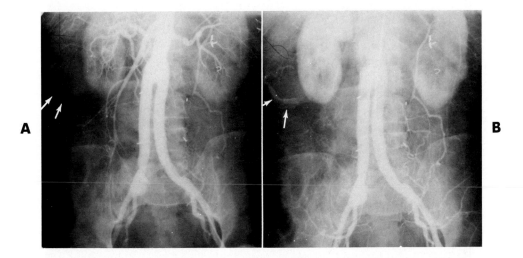

Fig. 8-9 Midstream aortogram injection in patient with massive rectal bleeding. **A,** Contrast material is leaking from ileocecal branch of superior mesenteric artery into cecum. Contrast medium has accumulated in lumen *(arrows).* **B,** Later aortogram shows massive accumulation of contrast medium in cecum *(arrows).* Patient was operated on minutes after aortographic study, and ischemic ulcer of cecum was found. Bleeding came from exposed artery.

ing into the bowel by digital angiography have not yet been determined, it is hoped that they will be in the same range. Nuclear medicine techniques using technetium-labeled red blood cells have been used recently to demonstrate active chronic bleeding. Bleeding rates lower than 0.5 ml/min can be detected by these radioisotope studies, and they have replaced selective arteriography unless direct infusion of vasoconstrictors is desired to stop the bleeding.

Computed tomography of the colon

CT has many advantages over barium sulfate luminal studies. It offers better density discrimination; allows visualization of the wall of the gut; permits demonstration of structures beyond the alimentary tube, allowing assessment of the extent of disease; provides reconstruction of images in any plane; and offers quantitative data from CT numbers, as well as bolus and perfusion approaches. CT is also an excellent method for guided control of needle biopsy of lesions of the alimentary tube.

CT, however, cannot approach the effectiveness of barium sulfate, particularly double-contrast studies, in providing excellence of mucosal detail, control of the distribution of contrast medium, and real-time fluoroscopic control of the movement of barium. Barium studies also can be better controlled, afford easy repeatability not possible with CT, and are less expensive than CT.

CT provides the first means of staging gastrointestinal neoplasms with an accuracy that approaches Duke's classification, which is based on histology. The Thoeni and Moss scheme for staging primary and secondary neoplasms of the colon and rectum by CT allows staging with a high degree of accuracy. This approach serves as a guide in determining the treatment of such neoplasms. In stage 1 the wall of the colon is normal, but an intraluminal polyp is present. In stage 2 the wall is locally thickened without extension outside of the bowel. In stage 3 extension is present beyond the bowel wall into neighboring organs and nodes. In substage 3A the extension does not involve the pelvic side walls, and in substage 3B the extension involves the pelvic side walls. In stage 4 distant metastases are present.

The technique that we use for examining the colon by CT consists of several steps. First, 300 to 400 ml of 1.5% to 2% solution of diatrizoate is administered per rectum. Also, oral contrast material is given to fill the distal small bowel loops (Fig. 8-10). The patient may drink 500 ml of water before the examination to distend the bladder. Cuts 1 cm thick with the patient supine and with the gantry at zero angulation are obtained from the anal verge to the dome of the liver. In most cases intravenous contrast material is administered. Optimal filling of the colon with contrast material avoids an erroneous diagnosis in a patient who has undergone colonic preparation.

CT has been extremely valuable in evaluating neo-

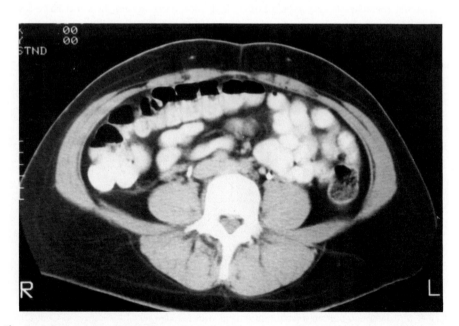

Fig. 8-10 CT of colon. Good filling of right and transverse colon with oral water-soluble contrast material and of rectum, sigmoid, and descending colon with rectal water-soluble contrast material is needed for adequate evaluation and for preclusion of mass lesions in colon. For optimal results, colonic cleansing is also necessary.

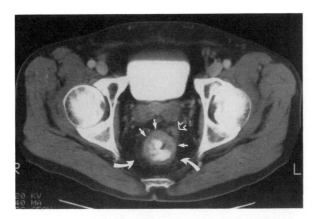

Fig. 8-11 In this patient with rectal carcinoma, CT demonstrates thickening of rectal wall *(straight arrows)*, perirectal stranding *(curved arrows)* and adenopathy *(open arrow)*. Whereas barium enema allows excellent assessment of mucosal changes, cross-sectional methods can provide information on depth of tumor involvement, as well as local and distant spread.

plasms (Figs. 8-11, 8-12), perirectal abscesses, and inflammatory masses, and in determining the presence and exact location of foreign bodies. At first, many rectosigmoid tumors were inaccurately staged because of microinvasion of surrounding perirectal fat and tumor foci in normal-sized nodes not seen on CT. The discrepancy between early and more recent reports is due to the larger number of advanced stages that were

included in the earlier reports. Advanced stages of rectosigmoid tumors with adrenal, liver, and distant nodal metastases are accurately diagnosed by CT. Therefore CT should not be used for routine preoperative staging of rectosigmoid tumors but should be reserved for diagnosing patients with suspected advanced disease who cannot undergo curative surgery, for selecting patients with inoperable tumor that could be radiated preoperatively to render the disease operable, and for detection of localized tumor in the rectal wall that could benefit from endocavitary radiation. In recurrent rectosigmoid cancer, high accuracy of CT in staging has been reported.

Transrectal ultrasonography of the rectum

With the development of transrectal ultrasonography, a new method became available to distinguish among the different layers of the rectal wall (Fig. 8-13). The first layer seen on transrectal sonograms represents the echogenic mucosa; the second layer is the echo-poor muscularis mucosae; the third layer is the echogenic submucosa; the fourth layer is the echo-poor muscularis propria; and the fifth layer is the echogenic serosa and perirectal fat. Preliminary studies indicate promise for the use of transrectal ultrasound in staging rectal tumors; accurate staging is important because the choice between anterior and abdominal perineal resection for tumors in the lower two thirds of the rectum depends on the stage of the colonic neoplasm.

With the transrectal approach, an ultrasonographic

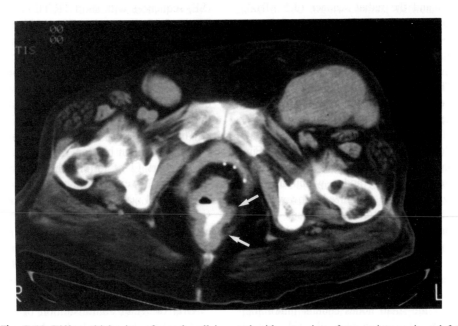

Fig. 8-12 Diffuse thickening of rectal wall is noted with extension of tumor into perirectal fat *(arrows)*. Very large nodes, particularly on left side, are noted in inguinal areas. Patient suffered from lymphoma of rectum with diffuse spread, stage 4.

of the puborectal sling (Fig. 8-17). The mean values of the ARA are 92 at rest and 137 on straining.

NORMAL DEFECOGRAM

During evacuation the pelvic floor descent should be less than 3.5 cm. The anorectal junction goes down and backwards, and in women the rectovaginal septum usually remains undeformed by straining. Before evacuation the patient is asked to squeeze; the impression of the puborectal sling becomes more evident, the anorectal junction moves up and forward, the ARA decreases (see Fig. 8-17), the pelvic floor rises, and the anal canal closes tightly.

PATHOLOGIC DEFECOGRAMS
Rectal intussusception and prolapse

Three stages of severity can be observed in rectal intussusception. At the first stage, a fold can be seen in the rectal wall, deepening gradually during rectal evac-uation to form an intussusception of the full thickness of the rectal wall in the rectal lumen. At the second stage the apex of the rectal intussusception passes into the anal canal and remains in it to form an intraanal rectal intussusception (Fig. 8-18). At the third stage, the intussusception passes through the anal canal to form an external rectal prolapse (Fig. 8-19).

There is usually no doubt regarding the clinical diagnosis of complete rectal prolapse. Lesser stages can, however, cause diagnostic difficulties. When the pouch of Douglas is deep, intestinal or sigmoidal loops may be enclosed in the anterior wall of a rectal prolapse to form an enterocele. Most intussusceptions originate from the anterior rectal wall or from an annular segment. The posterior wall is only rarely the origin of intussusception. Intussusception most often develops at the level of a Houston valve, 6 to 8 cm from the anal margin.

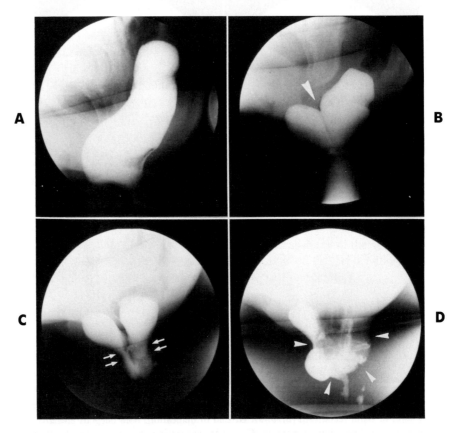

Fig. 8-19 Defecogram showing successive phases of external rectal prolapse. **A,** Beginning of defecation: puborectal muscle relaxes and anal canal opens. **B,** Infolding *(arrowhead)* appears in anterior wall of rectum and gives rise to the primary intussusception. **C,** Intussusception *(arrows)* invaginates into anal canal. **D,** Symmetric external rectal prolapse *(arrowheads)* is protruding.
(From Bartram DL, Mahieu PHG. In Henry M, Swash M, editors: *Coloproctology and the pelvic floor,* London, 1985, Butterworth.)

Rectocele

A rectocele is formed by an outpocketing of the anterior rectal wall, which becomes more pronounced during defecation. The compliance of the rectovaginal septum is abnormally increased, and part of the contrast material injected into the rectum is sequestered in this outpocketing. Fecal residue remains in a diverticulum, and evacuation cannot be achieved at the first attempt (see Fig. 8-18, *D*). Rectoceles may be associated with rectal intussusception, usually arising from the anterior wall.

Dyskinetic puborectal muscle

The puborectal sling normally relaxes when evacuation begins, and its impression on the posterior wall of the distal rectum is progressively obliterated. In some patients the impression increases in relation to paradoxic hypertonic muscular contractions, which can be intermittent or persistent, even though the anal canal remains open.

Descending perineum syndrome

Defecography reveals pelvic floor descent at rest expressed by a distance over 8.5 cm between the anorectal junction and the pubococcygeal line (Fig. 8-20). When a straining effort is made, the pelvic floor rapidly descends more than 3.5 cm, and the perineum bulges posteriorly between the coccyx and the anus.

Incontinence

Primary incontinence seems to be associated with an enlarged opacified anal canal (anal sphincter hypotony) and an abnormal increase of the ARA over 130 (hypotonic puborectal). In patients with prolapse, there is a significant difference in the ARA, depending on whether the patient is continent. The anal canal is displaced posteriorly and inferiorly, and the anopubic distance is increased.

RECOMMENDED READING

1. Mahieu PHG, Pringot J, Bodart P: Defecography. I. Description of a new procedure and results in normal patients, *Gastrointest Radiol* 9:247, 1984.
2. Mahieu PHG, Pringot J, Bodart P: Defecography. II. Constribution to the diagnosis of defecation disorders, *Gastrointest Radiol* 9:253, 1984.
3. Yang A, Mostwin JL, Rosenshein NB, Zerhouni EA: Pelvic floor descent in women: dynamic evaluation with fast MR imaging and cinematic display, *Radiology* 179:25, 1991.

Diverticula

PIERRE SCHNYDER

TECHNIQUE OF EXAMINATION

It is valuable to look at the plain films of the abdomen with great care, not so much for diverticulosis, but for diverticulitis. Sacs can occasionally be recognized as a row of appropriately sized gas-filled shadows run-

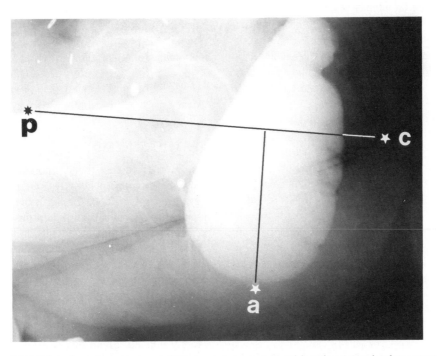

Fig. 8-20 Pelvic floor descent at rest. Distance between anorectal junction *(a)* and pubococcygeal line *(p* to *c)* is abnormally long. Posteriorly, pelvic floor bulges below coccyx.

ning parallel to the line of the colon, but a poorly contoured soft-tissue mass and obliteration of the peritoneal fat lines suggest inflammation. An irregular gas shadow may indicate an abscess. Although this is often not a reliable diagnostic picture, suspicion may influence the way in which further investigations are performed.

Demonstrating diverticular sacs and the distorted lumen of diverticular disease is easy, requiring no more than a well-performed enema on a well-prepared patient. The left posterior oblique view is a worthwhile component. Spasm of the sigmoid and lower descending colon is very common, and films taken at an early filling stage show a narrowed lumen, which at a later stage relaxes to the characteristic deformity. Careful spot films of any suspicious areas, taken with the colon in maximal distention, are essential. There is a good case for frequent use of smooth muscle relaxants, such as glucagon, 0.5 to 1.5 mg IV, which both abolishes spasm and allows full distention without causing pain or discomfort to the patient. Full distention reduces the number of overlapping lines in any picture, making the visual recognition of an abnormality easier. Inflammation is usually seen in the form of microperforations that rapidly seal, leading to small intramural or subserous abscesses. However, large abscesses and free perforation are well known.

Current thinking rejects the concept that the radiologist should delay the diagnostic enema as long as possible to allow a thick-walled barrier to form around any leak. Because free barium in the peritoneal cavity worsens the prognosis for an already severely ill patient, the enema should be achieved with any of the numerous available water-soluble contrast materials. During the acute phase, a gentle, low-pressure, water-soluble contrast enema should be performed. This study should be carefully controlled with fluoroscopy, and reconsidered at the first sign of a leak.

Isotope scanning and ultrasonography have proved their worth in the detection of abscesses in the abdomen (Fig. 8-21). CT performed in the acute phase of the disease may play an important role in assessing the site and the extent of an abscess and can predict the need for percutaneous drainage, surgery, or conservative therapy.

MR imaging shows promise as an alternative approach in studying the relationships of the abscess to the urinary bladder and colon. MR offers direct coronal and sagittal imaging, in addition to transverse imaging and a variety of other sequences giving information about soft tissue consistency (Fig. 8-22).

INCIDENCE

Diverticular disease was rare in western industrial nations during the 19th century, but it has become

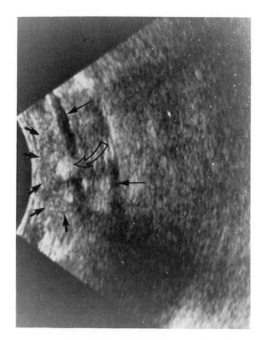

Fig. 8-21 Ultrasonographic examination demonstrating thickened wall of sigmoid colon *(long arrows)*, diverticulum filled with air *(open arrow)*, surrounded by an abscess *(small arrows)* infiltrating peritoneal fat and markedly modifying its echogenicity.

steadily more common during the last 80 years. Now at least 1 person in 2 can expect to acquire colon diverticula by 60 years of age. For all symptomatic patients, the age of onset was before 29 years in less than 1% of patients, before 40 years in only 11%, and between 50 and 70 years in 56%. The disease is virtually unknown in the native populations of Africa. The hospital admission rate for diverticulitis per 100,000 population is 80 times higher in Scotland than in Malaysia. The incidence is low in people who eat a large amount of roughage.

PATHOGENESIS

Diverticulitis has been reported at a very young age in patients with a number of rare syndromes. Marfan's syndrome, the Ehlers-Danlos syndrome, and intestinal ganglioneuromatosis come into this category.

Common colonic diverticula are acquired herniations of the mucosa and muscularis mucosae, and some at least are reducible hernias. Sacs seen easily on one enema study may never appear on a subsequent one. They vary in size from tiny spikes to 2 cm spheres, but most commonly they are 5 to 10 mm in diameter. In full distention they are spherical or ovoid in shape and are rarely bilobed. Small pieces of retained feces may give them an irregular outline.

Diverticula are found in all zones of the colon, al-

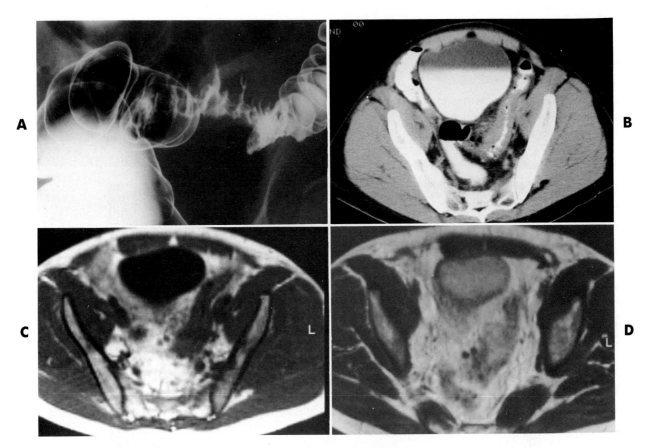

Fig. 8-22 Diverticulitis with abscess impinging on bladder in 66-year-old white male. **A,** Spot film from barium enema showing spasm and impression from abscess. **B,** Transverse CT section shows abscess impinging on urinary bladder. Small bubbles are seen within abscess. There is contrast material in colon and bladder. **C,** T_1-weighted MR image, and **D,** T_2-weighted image of abscess and its effect on surrounding organs is well seen. T_1- and T_2-weighting provides information equivalent to contrast-enhanced CT.

though by far the most common site is the sigmoid. The upper half of the rectum is rarely the site of sacs. In the left half of the colon the sacs emerge in four rows, one on each side of the mesenteric tenia and one on the mesenteric side of each antimesenteric tenia. The close relationship of these sites to the penetrating blood vessel has been known for half a century and confirmed by two investigations. According to this theory, an increase in the intraluminal pressure raises the pressure in the submucosa, which forces out the artery and the loose connective tissue around it, raising a small mound on the serosal surface. The emerging artery pulls the mucosa into the gap, and as the diverticulum moves outside the wall, it remains covered by a net-like collection of blood vessels that were originally lying in the submucosa. This theory does not explain all findings, however, since occasional sacs are found in the lateral wall and in the antimesenteric zone where there are no penetration vessels. Williams postulated that persistent

shortening of the bowel crumples the circular layer in the way that a coat sleeve wrinkles when it is pulled up the arm. This can crack the circular muscle in circumferential fashion and give rise to weak areas through which diverticula emerge. This is especially true of the short antimesenteric zone, where the cracking can lead to a ridge-shaped herniation.

DIVERTICULITIS

The term *diverticulitis* is used here to denote the presence of inflammation, not merely diverticular disease with symptoms. In some patients, clinical diagnosis of diverticulitis is simple—they present with a painful mass and local signs of peritoneal irritation, as well as fever and leukocytosis. Many in this group require surgery, which proves the diagnosis. In a larger number of patients, however, there is pain and tenderness, but no collateral evidence of inflammation. The radiologic diagnosis of diverticulitis has three signs: (1) deformed sacs (2) demonstration of an abscess, and (3) extravasation of water-soluble contrast material.

Deformed sacs

Diverticular sacs, which have a thin layer of longitudinal muscle over them, often look irregular or flattened when the colon is fully or partially contracted. It is possible that an irregularity could represent old fibrous scarring rather than an active abscess. Nevertheless, such minor deformities detected in a fully distended zone are a useful pointer to the common form of inflammation: *microperforations*.

Demonstration of abscess

Significant inflammation of the perforated diverticulum is very infrequent. This suggests that rupture

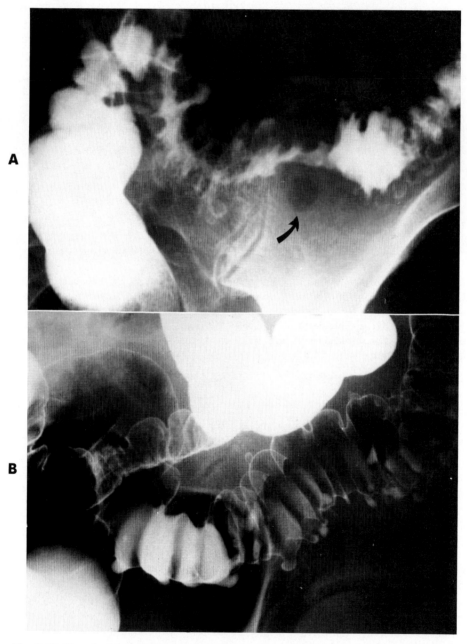

Fig. 8-23 Diverticulitis resembling carcinoma. This water-soluble enema shows partial obstruction, circumferential mass effect with shouldered ends resembling encircling carcinoma. Presence of gas collection *(arrow)* on antimesenteric side of colon was of value here to point to diagnosis of diverticular abscess. Single sac opens off middle of narrowed area.

caused by a transient surge of intraluminal pressure may more often be responsible. Concomitant or other etiologic factors include ischemia, stercoral ulcerations, and foreign bodies. A pericolic abscess can appear as a pressure defect of the filled colon (Fig. 8-23). Multiple spot films may be necessary to demonstrate an easily palpable abscess; even large abscesses may go undetected.

In the right clinical setting, other techniques can be used to demonstrate the abscess. Isotope scanning with gallium-67, as well as ultrasonography, have both proved useful (see Fig. 8-21). However, these are more and more being replaced by CT examinations, which can display subtle peridiverticular changes, such as discrete increase of the attenuation value of the mesenteric fat, thickening of the colonic wall, slight enlargement of the peritoneal fascia (Figs. 8-24, 8-25), or minute fluid collections in the paracolic spaces. Such abnormalities are displayed by 63% of CT scans obtained during an acute episode. CT is also the best and most reliable device to guide the drainage of large diverticular abscess and to demonstrate fistulas.

Extravasation of contrast material

The most reliable sign of diverticulitis, mimicked only by a perforated carcinoma, is the presence of contrast material outside the lumen (Fig. 8-26). A characteristic extravasation is seen as a track running parallel to the bowel wall in the region of the sigmoid and pelvic portions of the colon. This long abscess is located in the subserosal layer and communicates with several sacs (Fig. 8-27). This, with the original lumen, gives a *double-track sign* that can be up to 15 cm long and is also present when Crohn's disease is superimposed on diverticular disease.

COMPLICATIONS
Obstruction

Complete or almost complete clinical obstruction is seen in diverticulitis, but sigmoid carcinoma is a more common cause. Smooth muscle relaxants may help by widening the lumen to allow enough contrast material to pass and establish the exact diagnosis.

Bleeding

Elderly patients who have typical radiologic evidence of diverticulosis with numerous sacs, may experience a specific type of blood loss—unheralded, painless, and profuse enough to be exsanguinating. With arteriography and colonoscopy the bleeding area can be localized and limited resection performed. In almost half the cases, the source of the bleeding is not a diverticulum, but an angiomatous malformation in the submucosa. These may be multiple, and any remaining after surgery can be a source of recurrent bleeding. Identification of the actual bleeding diverticulum has shown that the damage to the blood vessel is not a consequence of inflammation. Instead, at the point where the

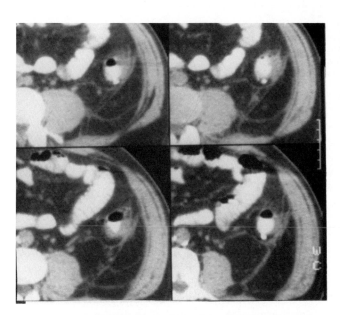

Fig. 8-24 4-mm CT sections obtained in area of small peridiverticular abscess. Small mass involves lateral aspect of distal descending colon, peritoneal fat, and fascia. Three scattered diverticula are also identified on posterior aspect of descending colon.

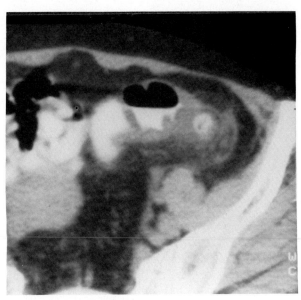

Fig. 8-25 4-mm sections obtained at junction of descending and sigmoid colon showing peridiverticular abscess, infiltrating mesenteric fat, thickening peritoneal fascia and lateral aspect of the colon. Abscess is centered by small amount of water-soluble contrast material located within lumen of perforated sac.

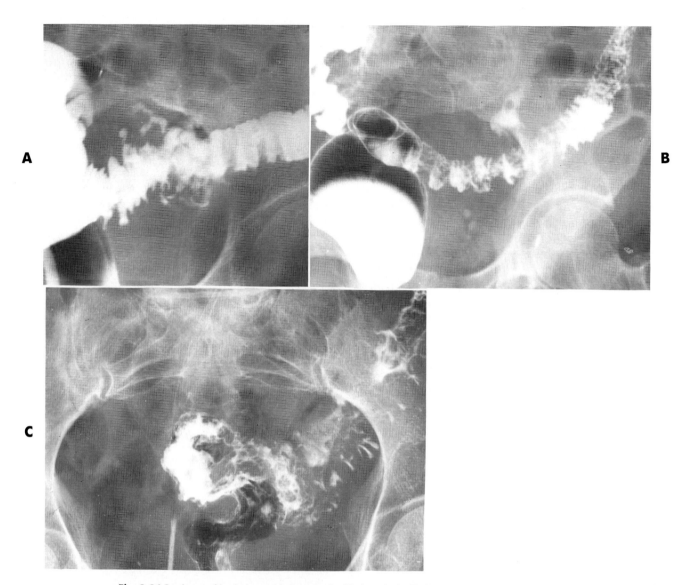

Fig. 8-26 Leakage of barium outside lumen. **A,** Obvious leak. **B,** Leak into circumscribed abscess cavity. **C,** Barium collection seen as triangular in *en face* view. This did not appear until post-evacuation film.

penetrating artery passes the neck of the sac, this small artery demonstrates a peculiar change, with intimal thickening, reduplication of the internal elastic lamina, and atrophy of the media. This histologic picture is not specific and may be found at other sites as the result of mechanical, thermal, or chemical trauma and in immunologic disease.

Spread of inflammation and fistula formation

Transperitoneal spread can result in fistulas to most organs in the lower half of the abdomen, including the bladder, vagina, fallopian tubes, other parts of the colon, the small intestine, and the ureter. More difficult to diagnose is the spread of pus in the retroperitoneal space. It may first be recognized in a perinephric site, tracking down the pararectal region to mimic Crohn's disease. The pus may also pass through the sacrosciatic notch to present as an abscess in the buttock or thigh. Ultrasonography, CT, and MR are currently the best modalities for an early diagnosis of peritoneal and extraperitoneal abscesses from diverticular origin (see Fig. 8-26).

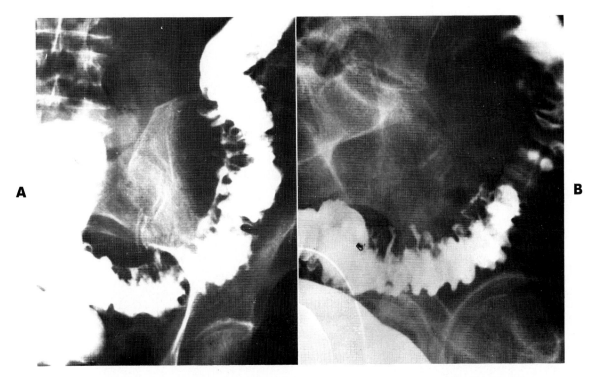

Fig. 8-27 Long-tracking subserous abscess. Long tract of barium runs beside sigmoid and pelvic colon, giving second channel beside main lumen. Note at proximal end localized low-filling defect caused by submucosal edema, which resembles flat carcinoma.

DIVERTICULAR DISEASE WITH NEOPLASM

The symptoms of diverticular disease and distal colon neoplasm can be very similar, and when they occur together radiologic interpretation is difficult. Obstruction, perforation, and fistulas are seen in both. Diverticular disease involves long lengths of colon, with varying patterns along the length. The problem is deciding whether one small part represents an added carcinoma (Fig. 8-28). Air contrast films in maximal distention, with spot films in various positions, are used to obtain a three-dimensional visual synthesis. With care, it is possible to eliminate spasms that can give an apple-core narrowing, but local submucosal or mucosal edema, especially in the double-track cases, can look like a flat neoplasm. Boulos and co-workers, in a study of 105 patients with symptomatic sigmoid diverticular disease, showed that colonoscopy revealed an associated carcinoma in 6.6% of patients and adenomas in 27.6%, with a peak incidence at 60 to 79 years and an equal sex distribution. Extensive diverticulosis was shown to represent an important factor limiting the sensitivity of barium enema studies for the evaluation of sigmoid masses. Indeed, only 3.1% of lesions are missed in patients with less than 15 diverticula, whereas in those with more than 15 diverticula, 20.4% of tumors remain undetected.

CLASSIFICATION

The classification that accomodates most clinical settings follows:

Scattered diverticula: A small number of sacs are visible in cases of scattered diverticula, but no muscular hypertrophy can be recognized.

Diverticulosis: There are many sacs, with shortening of the sigmoid and pelvic portions of the colon.

Diverticular disease without diverticula: There is usually a serrated edge to the colon and no sacs visible. This is the "prediverticular state" and in its pure form is rare. However, the pelvic colon may have this appearance despite obvious diverticulosis of the sigmoid.

Diverticular disease: This term includes diverticulosis with symptoms. At one end of the spectrum is the picture of gross zonal narrowing of the lumen with the pathologist finding a very thick muscle wall; this is *myochosis.*

Diverticulitis: Any of the patterns mentioned, with clear evidence of inflammation and diverticular perforation, represent diverticulitis.

RECOMMENDED READING

1. Baker SR, Alterman DD: False-negative barium enema in patients with sigmoid cancer and coexistent diverticula, *Gastrointest Radiol* 10:171, 1985.

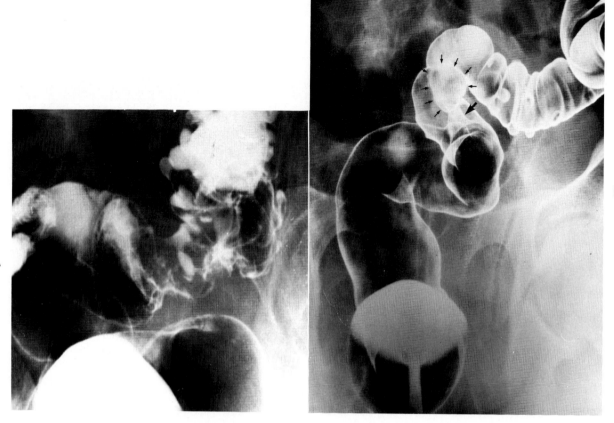

Fig. 8-28 Carcinoma with diverticular disease. Neoplastic filling defect encircling perhaps two thirds of lumen in area of diverticulosis.

2. Beighton PH, Mudoch JL, Votteler T: Gastrointestinal complications of the Ehlers Danlos syndrome, *Gut* 10:1004, 1969.

3. Fleischner FG, Ming SC: Revised concepts on diverticular disease of the colon. II. So-called diverticulitis: sigmoiditis and peridiverticulitis: diverticular abscess, fistula and frank peritonitis, *Radiology* 84:599, 1965.

4. Johnson CD et al: Diagnosis of acute colonic diverticulis: comparison of barium enema and CT, *Am J Roentgenol* 148:541, 1987.

5. Kyunghee CC et al: Sigmoid diverticulitis: diagnostic role of CT—comparison with barium enema studies, *Radiology* 176:111, 1990.

6. Miller WT et al: Bowler-hat sign: a simple principle for differentiating polyps from diverticula, *Radiology* 173:615, 1989.

7. Mueller PR, van Sonnenberg E, Ferrucci JT Jr: Percutaneous drainage of 250 abdominal abscesses and fluid collections. II. Current procedural concepts, *Radiology* 151:343, 1984.

8. Painter NS, Burkitt DP: Diverticular disease of the colon: a deficiency disease of western civilization, *Br Med J* 2:450, 1971.

9. Schnyder P et al: A double-blind study of radiological accuracy in diverticulitis, diverticulosis and carcinoma of the sigmoid colon, *J Clin Gastroenterol* 1:55, 1979.

10. van Sonnenberg E, Mueller PR, Ferrucci JT: Percutaneous drainage of 250 abdominal abscesses and fluid collections. I. Results, failures and complications, *Radiology* 151, 337, 1984.

11. Wada M, Kikuchi Y, Doy M: Uncomplicated acute diverticulitis of the cecum and ascending colon: sonographic findings in 18 patients, *Am J Roentgenol* 155:283, 1990.

12. Wilson SR, Toi A: The value of sonography in the diagnosis of acute diverticulitis of the colon, *Am J Roentgenol* 154:1199, 1990.

Inflammatory disease of the colon

RUEDI F-L THOENI
ALEXANDER R MARGULIS

INDICATIONS FOR AND TECHNIQUES OF BARIUM ENEMA EXAMINATION
Plain films of the abdomen

Plain films of the abdomen in patients with inflammatory bowel disease can provide useful information. In one study, colitis was diagnosed or strongly suggested in 45% of patients based on plain films. A combination of increased thickness of colonic wall, irregularity of the mucosal surface, and absence of stool in these areas can suggest colitis (Fig. 8-29). Ischemic

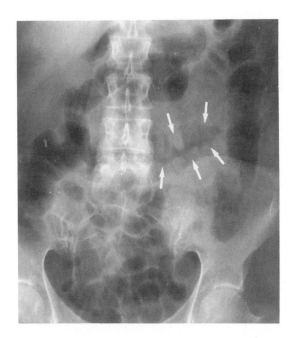

Fig. 8-29 Plain film shows thumbprinting *(arrows)* in transverse colon caused by pseudomembranous colitis. Colon is devoid of stool in absence of colonic cleansing.

changes may present in a similar fashion, but the extent of abnormal bowel segments follows the distribution of a major artery, which is different from inflammatory colitis. Feces do not accumulate next to inflamed mucosa, and increased peristalsis moves fecal material to distal segments of the colon.

In one study of 100 children with inflammatory bowel disease, plain film abnormalities were seen in 73% (76% with Crohn's disease and 72% with ulcerative colitis) and in 20% of 50 matched controls. No correlation between the barium enema and the plain film was obtained, because all patients had undergone a colonic preparation. An abnormal stool pattern was found in 47% and an abnormal gas pattern in 38% of these 100 children. Other findings—such as hepatosplenomegaly, bony abnormalities, or renal calculi— were noted in 9% of the children.

Barium examination

Before a barium enema examination is ordered for a patient whose condition is suggestive of inflammatory bowel disease, several factors must be considered: the patient's overall condition, the severity of the acute inflammatory disease, the information that can be gained from the radiographic procedure, and the relevance of this information to patient care and prognosis. Establishing the severity and extent of disease is important because patients with more severe or more extensive

disease have a more grave prognosis, and medical treatment in these patients is often unsuccessful.

The barium enema examination is indicated in patients with inflammatory bowel disease when it is necessary to establish the presence or extent of colitis, to determine the type of inflammatory disease, or to assess resulting complications (for example, carcinoma, stricture formation, and fistulas). This examination is contraindicated in patients with toxic megacolon (because of the risk of perforation and bacteremia), in patients with a suspected perforation, and immediately following endoscopy and deep biopsy. Delay of the examination is advisable in patients having a fulminant attack, evidenced by profuse diarrhea, high fever, and constant rectal bleeding, until the disease becomes less active.

A thorough evaluation of the single-contrast barium enema examination versus the double-contrast technique has not been accomplished in patients with inflammatory bowel disease. However, although severe disease can be detected accurately with both methods, the double-contrast method is superior for detecting superficial mucosal lesions and early changes. Therefore the extent of disease is more accurately assessed with the double-contrast method. Suspected fistulization, however, is better demonstrated by a single barium column.

For double-contrast examination patients are subjected to a 24- to 48-hour liquid diet, and water enemas are administered the evening of the day before the examination and in the morning immediately before the procedure. No additives should be used in the water enema. Some clinicians recommend mild laxatives, such as mineral oil or bisacodyl, although others prefer to use no laxatives at all.

A preliminary film of the abdomen should always be obtained to exclude the presence of toxic megacolon and to assess fecal residue. The number of overhead films can usually be limited to three or four (prone, upright, left lateral decubitus, and angled rectal) to minimize patient discomfort.

Glucagon should be used to relax spasms. A peroral pneumocolon examination may clarify involvement of the terminal ileum in examinations where there is a lack of reflux into the small bowel, or may be used to further evaluate the right colon. In cases of pancolitis, involvement of the terminal ileum can distinguish ulcerative colitis from granulomatous colitis.

The single-contrast method demonstrates severe and longstanding disease accurately and permits a determination of the presence of edema in the bowel wall on the basis of the postevacuation film. In general, the postevacuation film is not useful in the double-contrast technique. The single-contrast method may also be useful in patients with suspected fistulas or sinus tracts.

ULCERATIVE COLITIS
Clinical features

Radiographic assessment by itself is not a reliable indicator of the severity of ulcerative colitis. Diffuse disease may be seen in up to 20% of patients with mild colitis; however, diffuse disease with deep ulcerations points to a severe form of inflammatory bowel disease. Foreshortening and narrowing of the colon indicates chronicity rather than severity. Three arbitrary categories of severity have been established: a mild form, a moderate form, and a severe or fulminant form. The mild form is characterized by less than four bowel movements a day and the absence of systemic signs. Moderate disease, seen in about 25% of patients, is characterized by more intense symptoms and diarrhea is a major manifestations. Severe or fulminant disease is the rarest form, seen in about 15% of all patients with ulcerative colitis. Associated pathologic changes include musculoskeletal abnormalities sacroiliitis and spondylitis with an incidence of 1% to 26%) and peripheral arthritis (incidence of 10% to 12%). Spondylitis usually precedes the onset of bowel disease, whereas peripheral joint disease tends to present simultaneously with or subsequent to bowel disease.

Radiographic findings
Granularity

The early findings of ulcerative colitis are changes in the mucosa related to edema and granulation tissue. With sigmoidoscopy, submucosal inflammation and edema are evidenced by impaired translucency of the ramifying submucosal vessels and irregularity of the mucosa caused by subepithelial infiltration, edema, and crypt abscesses (Fig. 8-30), giving the mucosa a granular appearance.

The mucosa loses its even texture and reveals an amorphous or finely stippled appearance through the barium coating of the mucosa. This *granularity* of the mucosa may also be caused by microscopic colitis. On occasion these superficial changes cannot be seen, and the only sign of inflammation in the rectosigmoid colon is the blunting of the normally acute angles of the rectal valves (seen in 43% of cases of ulcerative colitis). With progressive disease, superficial erosions develop that give the mucosa a stippled appearance (Fig. 8-31). In the chronic stages, granulation tissue develops that creates a coarse granular mucosal appearance.

The single-contrast barium enema examination cannot demonstrate the early mucosal changes of ulcerative colitis but may demonstrate inflammatory disease by the failure of the colonic walls to collapse and by abnormal fold patterns on the postevacuation film. These signs are not very reliable. Innominate lines demonstrated by the single-contrast method may be confused with irregularities caused by inflammatory disease.

Ulceration

If an acute attack is superimposed on chronic disease, the mucosa shows multiple ill-defined collections of barium on a background of coarse granularity (Fig.

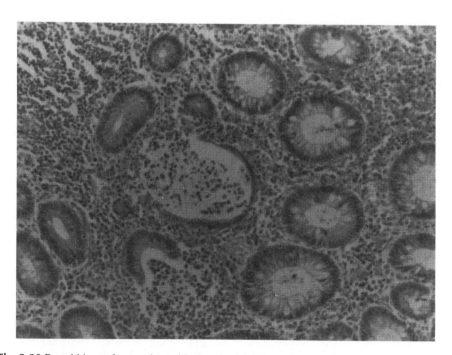

Fig. 8-30 Rectal biopsy from patient with chronic ulcerative colitis demonstrates mucosal atrophy, cellular infiltration, and crypt abscesses.

(Courtesy Dr. Caroline Montgomery.)

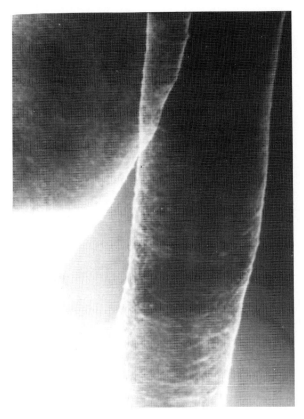

Fig. 8-31 Coarse granularity of colonic mucosa with multiple erosions in patient with chronic ulcerative colitis.

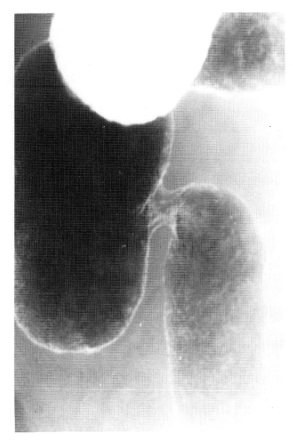

Fig. 8-32 Blotchy collections of barium represent ulcers superimposed on diffuse granularity.

8-32). These collections represent mucosal ulcerations. Ulcers are often seen best in profile because they are linear in relation to the tenial attachment and undermine the mucosa. They usually have a T-shaped, flask-shaped, or "collar button" appearance. The term *collar button ulcer* is most frequently used to describe ulcers in an acute exacerbation of a chronic stage of ulcerative colitis. These collections are not diagnostic of idiopathic inflammatory disease, however, because they can be seen in cases of tuberculous colitis, shigellosis, amebiasis, and ischemic colitis. In the chronic stages of disease, collar button ulcers may also be demonstrated by the single-contrast method because the ulcers are best demonstrated in profile.

Polypoid changes

Polypoid changes may be seen at any stage of ulcerative colitis. They may occur in the acute stage from ulcerations or in the healed and quiescent stage from mucosal tags.

Pseudopolyps, seen in acute severe attacks, are islands of inflamed edematous mucosa seen between denuded and ulcerated areas. They are called pseudopol-

yps because they represent the actual mucosa and not polypoid protuberances.

Inflammatory polyps are areas of inflamed mucosa resulting in polypoid elevations and are seen strung out on a background of granular mucosa in patients with low-grade activity of inflammatory bowel disease. These inflammatory polyps may be sessile or they may have a stalk.

Postinflammatory polyps are seen in the quiescent phase of ulcerative colitis. Seen in 10% to 20% of patients, they may be composed of normal or inflamed mucosa. They are thought to originate in elevations of the mucosa during severe undermining by deep ulcers. Epithelization prevents these mucosal lesions from fusing in a reparative phase, thus creating a multitude of polypoid changes such as *sessile nodules,* long finger-like outgrowths called *filiform polyps,* or mucosal bridges created by the fusion of two islands over an area of reepithelization (Fig. 8-33). These polyps may represent excessive repair. On occasion, however, these polyps are present in a normal-appearing colon and are the only indicators of previous inflammatory disease. Inflammatory polyps on a background of normal mu-

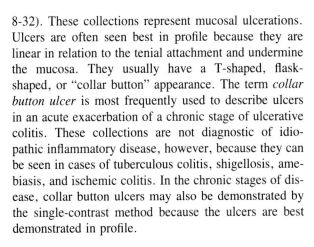

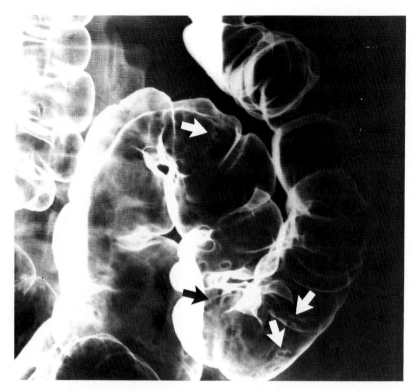

Fig. 8-33 Multiple filiform polyps *(arrows)*. Patient is in quiescent phase of chronic ulcerative colitis.

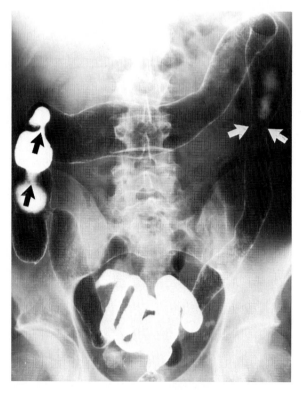

Fig. 8-34 Tubular colon with backwash ileitis and several strictures *(arrows)* as manifestations of chronic form of ulcerative colitis.

cosa may be confused with adenomas or even small carcinomas, and only endoscopy and biopsy can provide the correct diagnosis. In some cases, giant inflammatory polyps may develop.

Secondary changes

The main signs of chronic disease are foreshortening of the colon, lack of haustration, and tubular narrowing of the colon that gives the large bowel the appearance of a garden hose or stovepipe. Narrowing of the colon is often related to spasms and smooth muscle hypertrophy, which explain the reversion to normal of a colon that was severely affected by ulcerative colitis. Fibrosis and strictures may develop (Fig. 8-34).

Another secondary sign is increased presacral space. This sign is often used as an indicator of inflammatory disease that involves the rectum. A presacral space measuring 1 cm or less is considered normal. The width of the presacral space is usually inversely related to the width of the rectum.

Terminal ileum

In the great majority (74%) of patients with ulcerative colitis, the terminal ileum is normal. In as many as 39% of patients, the terminal ileum shows atonia, a

☐ **TABLE 8-2**
Radiographic features of ulcerative, granulomatous, and infectious colitis

Radiographic features	Ulcerative colitis	Granulomatous colitis	Infectious colitis
Granular mucosa	+	−	
Ulcerations			
Small, shallow	−	+	*Yersinia*, Behçet's, ischemia, tuberculosis, amebiasis, salmonellosis
Confluent, shallow	+	(+)	Amebiasis
Confluent, deep	−	+	Ischemia, amebiasis, tuberculosis, strongyloidiasis
Rectum			
Diffusely involved	+	−	Amebiasis, shigellosis
Patchy distribution	−	+	
Continuity	+	(+)	Shigellosis
Continuous			
Discontinuous	(+)	+	Lymphogranuloma venereum
Stricture			
Symmetric	+	−	Lymphogranuloma venereum (tuberculosis)
Asymmetric	−	+	Ischemia, tuberculosis
Fistulas	−	+	Lymphogranuloma venereum (tuberculosis, ischemia, Behçet's)
Terminal ileum	(+)	+	*Yersinia*, pseudomembranous colitis, tuberculosis
Inflammatory polyp	+	+	Schistosomiasis, colitis cystica profunda (ischemia), strongyloidiasis
Toxic megacolon	+	(+)	Ischemia, amebiasis (salmonellosis, pseudomembranous colitis)

(+), Occurs rarely.

widely gaping ileocecal valve, and occasionally, granularity of the mucosa. Ulcers in the terminal ileum are not features of so-called *backwash ileitis*. Whenever ulcers are seen in the terminal ileum, Crohn's disease, tuberculosis, or *Versinia* infection should be considered. The terminal ileum is usually abnormal in a patient with long-standing subacute disease. The most exact method of determining the presence or absence of inflammatory disease of the terminal ileum is a peroral pneumocolon examination.

Accuracy of radiographic examination

The differentiation of ulcerative colitis from granulomatous colitis can be made with high accuracy in the acute stage because the radiographic features of each disease are most distinct in this phase. Useful criteria for distinguishing between these two idiopathic diseases are summarized in Table 8-2. After multiple attacks, remission, and chronic disease, the typical mucosal patterns are distorted, and distinction becomes more difficult. In the acute stages, ulcerative colitis can be distinguished from granulomatous colitis in at least 95% of cases. However, an overlapping spectrum remains, which is estimated to amount to approximately 10% to 15% of cases.

Complications
Toxic megacolon

One of the most important complications of ulcerative colitis that radiography can detect is toxic megacolon. Its detection relies on the plain film. Because of the high risk of perforation during barium enema examination in a patient with a toxic megacolon, a preliminary film of the abdomen is mandatory before a barium enema examination is begun. Toxic megacolon is most frequently seen with ulcerative colitis, but it has been found in cases of Crohn's disease, Behçet's disease, amebiasis, ischemic disease, and salmonellosis.

Toxic megacolon is best defined as toxic dilatation associated with fulminant colitis. The radiographic diagnosis is based on colonic dilatation and, more important, abnormality of the colonic wall. In general a diameter of 5.5 to 6.5 cm is considered to be the upper limit of normal. Destruction of mucosa can often be seen on plain films and appears as thinned bowel wall, interrupted by segments of bowel wall thickened by subserosal edema and congested mucosa, and mucosal islands that often resemble polyps (Fig. 8-35). Some thumbprintlike impressions on the air column in the early stages of a toxic megacolon suggest a neuromuscular disorder, as well as edema in the bowel wall.

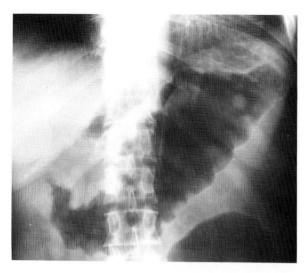

Fig. 8-35 Toxic megacolon in patient with chronic ulcerative colitis shows thickened edematous bowel wall and several polypoid masses.

Perforation

Spontaneous perforation does not occur frequently in ulcerative colitis except if a toxic megacolon develops.

Stricture

Strictures are seen more frequently in cases of ulcerative colitis (7% to 11%) than was previously thought. They may be benign or malignant, but the majority are benign. Many strictures are caused by muscular hypertrophy and are potentially reversible. Benign strictures occur only in longstanding and severe cases of colitis, and they may be multiple. Because of the risk of malignancy in ulcerative colitis, all strictures should be viewed with suspicion. Colonoscopy is indicated in these cases. If multiple strictures are present, ulcerative colitis may be difficult to differentiate from a cathartic colon, with abnormal contractions simulating the strictures found in chronic colitis.

Malignancy

Epithelial dysplasia is considered a precancerous lesion that occurs in longstanding cases of ulcerative colitis. It may be diagnosed radiographically on the basis of nodularity and irregularity of the mucosa with sharply angular edges. Its detection is an absolute indication for colonscopy with a biopsy.

Patients with ulcerative colitis are at increased risk of developing colorectal cancer. In one series, the observed-to-expected ratio of colorectal cancer was 8 in left-sided ulcerative colitis to 26 in pancolitis. It is therefore important to recognize that although patients with total colitis run a high risk of developing a cancerous lesion, cancer also may be seen in patients with left-sided ulcerative colitis. Cancerous lesions usually appear after a shorter duration in pancolitis than in left-sided disease. In patients with ulcerative colitis confined to the rectum, the risk of developing cancer is the same or minimally increased over that of the normal population. Colorectal cancer in patients with ulcerative colitis appears to be more often multiple (23% to 40%) and is reported to be more proximal in location than in the population without colitis.

The radiographic signs of carcinoma in ulcerative colitis include recognition of mucosal dysplasia based on small plaquelike or nodular, faceted filling defects. Irregularities or nodularity of the mucosa are changes typical of carcinoma of the colon in the general population. The carcinoma in ulcerative colitis is often flat, infiltrating, and difficult to detect because of its plaquelike appearance. Scirrhous carcinoma and annular carcinoma are seen frequently, but polypoid lesions are unusual (Fig. 8-36). Carcinoma associated with a stricture has been seen in 23% to 27% of cases of ulcerative colitis. Carcinomas that develop in ulcerative colitis tend to be high grade colloid or mucinous type.

The incidence of lymphomas and leukemia is also increased in patients with ulcerative colitis. The cause is unclear but is probably multifactorial, involving the immunologic deficiencies in inflammatory bowel disease as well as the immunosuppressive treatment used in these patients.

Surgical procedures for ulcerative colitis

For a long time, total colectomy with ileostomy was the procedure of choice for patients with severe, longstanding ulcerative colitis. However, because ileostomy was not a viable or acceptable surgical option for many young patients with active life-styles, other surgical procedures have been introduced. Another early procedure, the formation of a continent ileostomy following total colectomy, was successful in some cases, but is rarely performed today. The radiographic appearance of the continent ileostomy has been well described.

An ileal pouch and ileoanal anastomosis have more recently been used. This procedure consists of mucosal proctectomy and total colectomy with ileoanal anastomosis and an ileal pouch immediately above the anastomosis to maintain reservoir function. The reservoir is created from 15 to 20 cm of ileum, and may have a side-to-side configuration, a J shape, or an S shape. For this surgical procedure, patients usually undergo a total colectomy and a temporary ileostomy and creation of an ileal pouch with a mucocutaneous fistula. Before definitive hookup, most patients are examined radiographically either for a routine checkup or for suspected

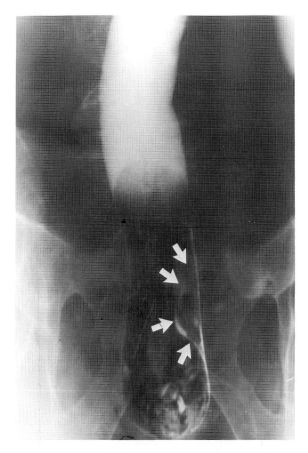

Fig. 8-36 Large plaquelike lesion *(arrows)* in left lateral rectal wall. Rectum and rectosigmoid colon appear to be narrowed. Patient had chronic ulcerative colitis for 20 years and now has cancer of the rectum.

complications. In these patients, a catheter with an inflatable balloon can be introduced, then a small amount of barium may be administered and the balloon carefully inflated.

GRANULOMATOUS COLITIS
Clinical features

The clinical picture of Crohn's disease may differ markedly from that of ulcerative colitis. Patients with granulomatous colitis often seek the help of a physician because of complications related to their disease, such as an anorectal fistula, perirectal sinuses and abscesses, intestinal obstruction, or symptoms of abdominal fistulas or abscesses. Often these patients have insidious symptoms (low-grade fever, mild or moderate diarrhea without blood, or mild weight loss and moderate anemia). A reduced concentration of conjugated bile salts and increased amounts of unabsorbed irritating bile salts cause steatorrhea and increased diarrhea. About 10% of patients with Crohn's disease have anal fissures, si-

nuses, or perirectal abscesses, and 20% to 30% have a palpable abdominal mass.

Behçet's syndrome involves the clinical triad of relapsing iritis and painful ulcers of the mouth and genitalia. The skin lesions tend to remit spontaneously and then recur. Other features such as arthralgia and thrombophlebitis have been described in this syndrome, and in some of these patients colitis similar to that found in Crohn's disease is seen. Behçet's syndrome therefore is not discussed separately in this chapter.

The incidence of musculoskeletal abnormalities in Crohn's disease reported in recent publications is higher (15% to 22%) than previously reported (2% to 4%). Peripheral joint disease is more common in Crohn's disease than in ulcerative colitis. Other extraintestinal manifestations in Crohn's disease include cholelithiasis and pericholangitis (60% of patients) and in rare cases sclerosing cholangitis, cirrhosis, and granulomatous hepatitis. Amyloidosis is uncommon, but occurs more frequently with Crohn's disease than with ulcerative colitis. Genitourinary complications, including urinary tract calculi, ureteral obstruction, and vesical fistulas, have been reported in 4% to 23% of patients.

Radiographic features

In contrast to ulcerative colitis, Crohn's disease is a transmural process, and in advanced cases it can be distinguished easily from ulcerative colitis. If the entire colon is involved, however, distinctions may be difficult. Some authors estimate that approximately 20% to 25% of all cases of Crohn's disease cannot be differentiated with certainty from those of ulcerative colitis. Discontinuity and asymmetry of disease are typical for Crohn's disease, which is remarkably different from ulcerative colitis. Unlike ulcerative colitis, Crohn's disease may involve any part of the small bowel, the stomach, the duodenum, and, on rare occasion, the esophagus. The most commonly involved areas are the cecum and the terminal ileum, and it is unusual to find Crohn's disease of the right colon that does not extend into the terminal ileum.

Early stages

On radiographs the earliest findings are tiny elevations or mammillations of 1 to 2 mm in diameter that probably represent exaggerated lymphoid follicles. Many of these lesions develop ulcerations in their centers and then become radiographically visible as *"target lesions"* or so-called *aphthous ulcers* (Fig. 8-37). Because these aphthous ulcers are shallow lesions, they are not seen in profile. They are usually multiple and are found on a background of normal mucosa, but detection of these ulcers is not diagnostic per se for Crohn's disease. Such ulcers have been seen in *Versinia*

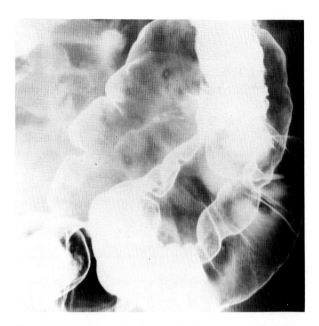

Fig. 8-37 Multiple collections of barium are surrounded by halo in patient with granulomatous colitis.

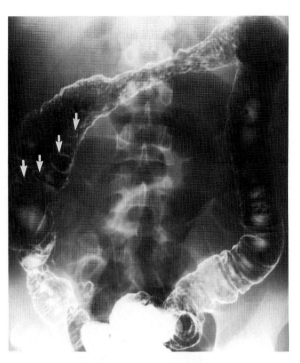

Fig. 8-38 Pseudosacculations *(arrows)*, skip lesions, and filiform polyposis are seen in patient with Crohn's disease of the colon.

enterocolitis, amebic colitis, and other specific inflammations. Aphthous ulcers can be demonstrated by single-contrast barium enema examination, but are best seen by the double-contrast technique. They are rapidly changing lesions, and they may regress or develop into the longitudinal and transverse folds commonly seen in advanced disease.

Advanced disease

The two most important features of advanced Crohn's disease are discontinuity of the disease and asymmetry. Even in the early stages, patches of aphthous ulcers on a background of normal mucosa are often separated by completely normal mucosa or located next to deep longitudinal and transverse ulcerations. Discontinuous disease is seen in 90% of patients.

Asymmetric involvement is another typical feature of Crohn's disease. In the early stages, one wall of bowel segment may be irregular and covered with aphthous ulcers and the opposite wall may be completely normal. In more advanced stages, fibrosis shrinks the involved bowel wall and creates pseudosacculations (Fig. 8-38) on the opposite normal wall, as seen in scleroderma and occasionally in ischemia.

Other findings in Crohn's disease of the colon are marked wall and mesenteric thickening. Deep longitudinal and transverse ulcers (Fig. 8-39) crisscrossing each other and the surrounding edematous mucosa create the well-known cobblestone pattern of advanced disease.

Giant inflammatory polyps occasionally develop, which may produce distinctive signs and symptoms.

Strictures are often found in Crohn's disease but need not be examined for malignancy (Fig. 8-40). Narrowing of the terminal ileum, often referred to as the *string sign,* originally was described as being related to spasms and not to actual stricture formation. Fistulas and abscesses, though uncommon in ulcerative colitis, are seen very frequently in Crohn's disease (Fig. 8-41). Fistulas, as mentioned previously, are best examined by the single-contrast technique. Intramural and paracolonic fistula tracts may be seen in patients with Crohn's disease, particularly in the presence of diverticula. They do not reliably indicate Crohn's disease because they may also be seen in patients with diverticulitis alone. As with ulcerative colitis, all three types of polypoid lesions (pseudopolyps, inflammatory polyps, and filiform polyps) can be seen in Crohn's disease.

Reversibility

Reversal, seen occasionally in Crohn's disease, is more common in the colon than in the small bowel. Aphthous ulcers may fluctuate or regress, but usually the disease progresses to more severe manifestations. Because of the transmural involvement in Crohn's disease, it is rare that the colon appears completely normal

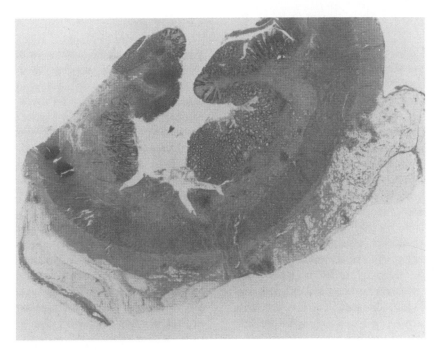

Fig. 8-39 Histologic section of colon from patient with granulomatous colitis shows deep fissure penetrating muscularis in center of figure.
(Courtesy Dr. Caroline Montgomery.)

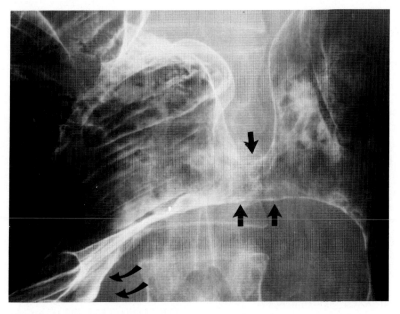

Fig. 8-40 Stricture *(arrows)* in patient with partial colonic resection and reanastomosis. Terminal ileum is on left side *(large curved arrows)*.

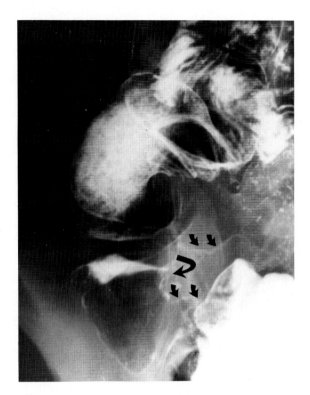

Fig. 8-41 Impressions on medial wall of cecum *(curved arrow)* and thin fistula tracts *(small arrows)* in patient with acute exacerbation of granulomatous colitis.

after regression of the acute manifestations of inflammation.

Terminal ileum

The terminal ileum is the most common site of involvement by Crohn's disease, and it can be examined by means of reflux from the cecum during a double-contrast barium enema examination. The terminal ileum can also be examined by a peroral pneumocolon examination that consists of a small bowel follow-through and air insufflation of the rectum to distend the cecum and terminal ileum. Reflux from the cecum into the terminal ileum often does not occur during barium enema examination because the ileocecal valve is edematous and spastic. During the early stages of Crohn's disease in the terminal ileum, nodularity of the folds, spasms, spiculation of the wall, and aphthous ulcers may be seen. In the more advanced stages, marked narrowing, deep ulcerations, cobblestoning, and fistulas are seen. Often an impression is noted on the medial cecal wall that is related to small bowel involvement and mesenteric thickening.

Recurrence

Postoperative recurrence of Crohn's disease is still a controversial subject. Some authors have reported post-

operative spread of disease to a previously normal colon. Recurrence in the new distal ileum, in addition to persistent granulomatous colitis, occurred in 11 of 12 patients. Disease also spread across the ileocecal anastomosis in 92 patients in an oral direction, but never in an aboral one. It appears therefore, that recurrence is largely related to exacerbation of disease in diseased colonic segments that were left behind.

Accuracy of radiographic examination

The extent of the disease is often underestimated by radiography even with the double-contrast technique.

Complications
Carcinoma

There is probably a slightly higher risk of carcinoma in patients with Crohn's disease than in the general population, but the incidence of colonic malignancies is certainly much lower than in patients with ulcerative colitis. Overall the risk of developing a carcinoma in Crohn's disease is similar to that in ulcerative colitis that involves the left side of the colon only. Malignancy is more likely to occur in patients who suffer from disease for several years. Malignancies may occur in the small bowel or colon but are more common in the colon. There is also a higher incidence of tumors in the area of the anal canal and in fistulas. Carcinomas in Crohn's disease frequently infiltrate through and along the bowel wall. Because of this type of spreading, the radiographic diagnosis of Crohn's carcinoma is often difficult. Any progressive change in the appearance of fistulas or strictures should be viewed with suspicion. CT can help in some of these cases, but biopsy is necessary for confirmation. For both ulcerative colitis and Crohn's disease, increased incidence of lymphomas and leukemias has been found.

Fistulas

Fistulas occur commonly in Crohn's disease and may extend from the cecum and ascending colon to the terminal ileum or to the sigmoid colon. Also, sinuses from the rectum or sigmoid to the perineum are highly suggestive of Crohn's disease. As previously mentioned, fistulas are best shown by a single-contrast barium enema examination.

Perforation

Spontaneous perforation of the colon related to Crohn's disease is rare but may occur.

DIFFERENTIAL DIAGNOSIS IN INFLAMMATORY DISEASE
Ischemic colitis

Today, many infectious types of colitis must be included in the differential diagnosis, but ischemic disease in particular has become a frequently recognized colonic disease that may mimic ulcerative colitis or Crohn's disease. Ischemia may cause a sudden onset of abdominal pain and tenderness over the involved colonic area. In severe ischemic disease, melena is seen. Ischemia of the colon may be related to vasculitis, arteriosclerosis, or administration of oral contraceptives.

Ischemia may be observed in three different stages: transient, gangrenous, and stricturing. In the early stages of ischemic colitis, spasm, thickening of the bowel wall, and spiculation may occur in the afflicted segments. If the disease is more severe, multiple defects are seen on the barium or barium-air column. These defects are referred to as *thumbprinting* and are caused by blood and edema accumulation in the bowel wall. Transverse ridging may be observed and is more common in patients with the stricturing type of colitis. If ischemic disease progresses ulcerations may be present, making it difficult to distinguish from Crohn's disease or ulcerative colitis. In many cases even a biopsy cannot distinguish between edema and inflammatory bowel disease.

The pattern of involvement in ischemic disease of the colon follows the distribution of a major artery, and the condition only rarely produces pancolitis. The splenic flexure is most commonly involved, and the rectum is usually spared. Even polypoid changes similar to those found in idiopathic inflammatory bowel disease may occur.

Inflammatory changes are occasionally seen in the bowel proximal to partially obstructing colonic malignancies. The ragged ulcerations in the large bowel found in these patients are difficult to distinguish from ulcerative colitis or Crohn's disease if the terminal ileum is involved. It is thought that these ulcers are related to bowel distention, stasis, ischemia, and bacterial infection.

Infectious colitis

Bacteria, viruses, fungi, and parasites are found as etiologic agents of the infectious types of colitis. Definite diagnosis is based on bacterial or viral cultures from stool specimens; stool analysis for blood, leukocytes, parasites, ova, and protozoa; and testing for serologic titers and specific toxins. In early stages of infectious colitis, the radiographic barium examination is often not useful in differential diagnosis but may be helpful in the patient's follow-up care.

Bacterial colitis
Actinomyces

Actinomyces israelii, a normal inhabitant of the gastrointestinal tract, causes pathologic changes once it has invaded the epithelium. Once the agent has invaded tissue, local growth causes multiple sinus tracts. Commonly the cecum and ascending colon are involved, with firm, fibrous masses that mimic neoplasms macroscopically and can be confused with amebiasis or Crohn's disease on radiographs.

Campylobacter

Campylobacter fetus probably invades directly and produces enterotoxins. On radiographic examination this entity mimics ulcerative colitis or Crohn's disease. Toxic megacolon, pseudomembranes, and lower gastrointestinal hemorrhage may be seen. *Campylobacter* infection should be considered in any case of acute colitis, and it can be excluded by bacteriologic and immunologic methods.

Chlamydia

Chlamydial infection may be quiescent and may become pathogenic in an immunocompromised host. Chronic proctitis is seen in men who practice anal receptive sex and in women.

Lymphogranuloma venereum can be diagnosed from radiographs based on a narrowing of the rectum and, on occasion, the descending and transverse colons. The sigmoid loop is often elevated and shortened by fibrosis. Sinuses commonly form in the pericolic, rectal, and vaginal areas. If these are untreated, rectovaginal and rectovesicular fistulas may develop.

Clostridium

Pseudomembranous colitis is caused by *Clostridium difficile,* a gram-negative bacillus with potent exotoxins. It produces foul-smelling greenish stools, usually has a fulminant course, and produces symptoms similar to those described for other types of colitis. Plain radiographs of the abdomen may show an adynamic ileus along with distention of the small and large bowel. The colon is frequently greatly dilated, and thumbprintlike indentations are often seen in the large bowel. Toxic megacolon has been reported in cases of pseudomembranous colitis. If a barium enema examination is performed, the barium column appears shaggy and irregular, and many thumbprintlike filling defects become evident. The irregularity of the colonic wall is related to pseudomembranes and superficial necrosis, and ulcers are shallow and partially covered by the membranes (Fig. 8-42).

Escherichia

E. coli causes acute *traveler's diarrhea* by adhering to the mucosa, altering fluid secretion in the small bowel, and producing toxins in the duodenum and upper ileum. On radiographs, this type of colitis resembles ulcerative colitis, but barium examinations are rarely used.

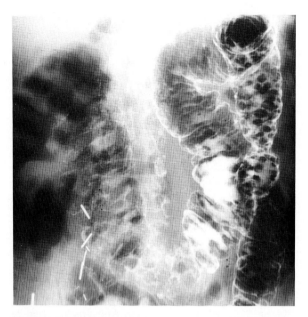

Fig. 8-42 Severe pseudomembranous colitis related to administration of penicillin. Multiple plaques are well shown, suggesting correct diagnosis.

Mycobacterium

Tuberculous colitis usually is not diagnosed before laparotomy, because it is difficult to demonstrate acid-fast mycobacteria in stool or in the colonic wall. Hoshino and co-workers have distinguished three types: type A, showing an extensive scarred area in the ileocecum and ascending colon; type B, showing annular stricture in the ascending colon and dilatation of its oral side; and type C, showing pouch formation (pseudodiverticulum) and deformity in the cecum. On radiographic examination, intestinal tuberculosis mimics Crohn's disease, and frequently the correct diagnosis is not made before surgery, particularly because many of the patients have a normal chest examination. Even fistula formation may occur. On rare occasions the more diffuse disease simulates ulcerative colitis.

Neisseria

Diagnosis of *Neisseria gonorrhoeae* (gonococcus) requires cultures of the organism. Rectal gonorrhea is characterized by rectal edema, friability and erythema, spasm, and small ulcers confined to the rectal ampulla. The small ulcerations in rectal gonorrhea are usually superimposed on a normal mucosa and can be distinguished from aphthous ulcers by their lack of halos. A fistula, ischiorectal abscess, or stricture may develop in rare cases.

Salmonella

Salmonella enteritidis is a common food infection. Patients who are suspected of suffering from salmonel-losis rarely undergo barium enema examinations because the symptoms are acute and suggest the underlying condition. If a barium enema is performed, the findings are nonspecific. Diffuse ulceration may be seen, and diffuse disease may produce a toxic megacolon.

Shigella

Shigella sonnei, S. dysenteriae, S. flexneri, and *S. boydii* are strictly pathogenic. *S. dysenteriae* is responsible for the typical *dysentery* of the Orient and Mexico. Radiographic findings for shigellosis are very similar to those for mild ulcerative colitis. Usually only the rectum and the rectosigmoid are involved, but the left side of the colon may be affected as well. Unusual manifestations include involvement of the entire colon or preferential involvement of the right side of the colon and the small bowel with small ulcers. Toxic megacolon may develop. In the chronic stages, stenosis may develop and rigidity of segments of the colon may be noted.

Yersinia

The diagnosis of *Yersinia enterocolitica* infection, a short-lived and spontaneously resolving disease, is based on stool cultures. In recent years there have been reports of patients with *Yersinia* enterocolitis showing a nodular pattern that is usually located in the terminal ileum and may extend into the colon. Ulcers similar to those found in Crohn's disease may be seen. They may be solitary or multiple. Fistulas or fibrosis are never seen.

Viral colitis

Viral infections of the colon can be caused by herpesviruses (herpes simplex types 1 and 2 or zoster-varicella) and by cytomegalovirus. Disseminated cytomegalovirus disease is fatal. The radiographic appearance of colonic herpes zoster depends on the stage of the disease. Small sharply marginated polygonal filling defects that resemble the skin manifestations are seen. Deep ulcerations, especially in the cecum, may be present with cytomegalovirus infection. Polyps can be distinguished from herpetic lesions by the segmental distribution and angular shape of the herpetic lesions.

Fungal colitis

Fungal disease of the gastrointestinal tract in humans is usually subacute or chronic. Invasive or noninvasive disease occurs in healthy individuals and invasive disease in immunocompromised hosts.

Blastomyces

Brazilian blastomycosis is caused by *Blastomyces* or *Paracoccidioides brasiliensis,* which is a yeastlike organism. It involves primarily the right side of the colon and is seen rarely in the United States.

Candida

Radiographically evident colonic changes caused by *Candida albicans* (moniliasis) are similar to those seen in pseudomembranous colitis.

Histoplasma

On radiographic examination, *Histoplasma capsulatum* infection (histoplasmosis) of the colon mimics ulcerative colitis or Crohn's disease. Extensive ulcers, nodules, polypoid masses, and annular strictures may involve the entire gastrointestinal tract, particularly the ileocecal area.

Parasitic colitis
Entamoeba

Infection with *Entamoeba histolytica* usually presents with diarrhea containing blood and mucus and may cause severe colicky abdominal pain. Typical radiologic findings of *amebiasis* are similar to those of Crohn's disease with two major differences. First, the terminal ileum is the site of the disease in less than 10% of patients, and then only a very short segment is involved. Second, defects similar to amebomas are seldom seen in any other disease. Amebomas appear as filling defects within the lumen of the colon or as a narrowing associated clinically with a mass. In the fulminating type of colitis, a toxic megacolon with or without perforation may occur, and a cavity may form that extends outside of the colonic lumen. In chronic disease, stenosis of the lumen may occur and is usually located in the transverse colon and in both colonic flexures. A cone-shaped cecum is occasionally seen. The most common form of amebiasis is *ulcerative rectal colitis* that manifests itself with collar button type ulcers. It usually involves the rectosigmoid, cecum, and ascending colon. Even skip lesions may be present, making the distinction from granulomatous colitis very difficult. Complete reversal to normal is usually seen after treatment.

Cryptosporidium

Cryptosporidium species are parasitic protozoans that infect only immunocompromised patients. The radiographic appearance is similar to that of ulcerative colitis—mucosal damage with edema, inflammatory cells, wall thickening, and ulcers.

Helminths

Strongyloides stercoralis colitis caused by mucosal and submucosal invasion may mimic ulcerative colitis. Manifestations are edema, ulcers, and subsequent stricture formation. In patients with *Schistosoma mansoni* infection (schistosomiasis, also called *bilharziasis*), hepatosplenomegaly and multiple small filling defects, stricture formation, and nodularity of the colon may be detected. These changes result from marked granulomatous reactions to eggs deposited in colonic venules, which compromise organ function. The rectum and sigmoid are most commonly involved, but the small bowel may be affected. If the granulomas become very large, they may obstruct the colonic lumen.

Noninfectious colitis
Anaphylactic changes

Chronic urticaria caused by an allergic reaction (to penicillin, for example) mimics herpetic colitis in every aspect of the colonic changes except that the lesions tend to be less segmental. In addition, no dermatomas are involved (Fig. 8-43).

Cathartic colon

Chronic irritation of the mucosa is caused by drugs such as senna, castor oil, bisacodyl, and podophyllum resin. The radiographic changes found in patients with chronic laxative abuse mimic those of ulcerative colitis. The mucosa is atrophic, with scattered shallow ulcers, submucosal chronic inflammation, and thickening of the muscularis mucosae. A narrowed colon with a complete lack of haustration is seen on radiographs. The cecum and ascending colon are usually and primarily involved

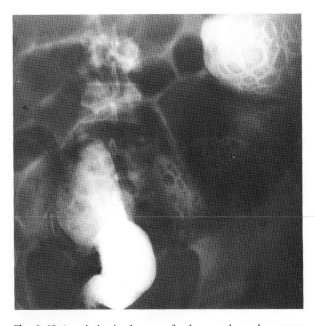

Fig. 8-43 Anaphylactic changes of colon are shown by means of polygonal angular filling defects. Colon is diffusely dilated.

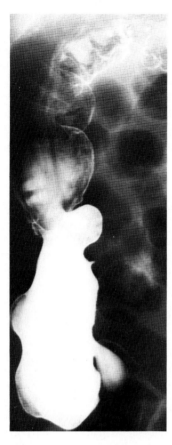

Fig. 8-44 Strictures, tubular narrowing, and pseudosacculations related to asymmetric fibrosis in patient with history of chronic senna abuse.

(Fig. 8-44); however, diffuse colonic involvement may occur. The terminal ileum may show superficial ileitis.

Radiation colitis

Radiation colitis may mimic ulcerative colitis or occasionally Crohn's, ischemic, and infectious colitis. On occasion, radiation strictures in the colon mimic a colonic adenocarcinoma or a stricture related to ischemia. Folds and spiculations in the acute phase are similar to those of ischemic colitis. Retractile mesenteritis may be difficult to distinguish from radiation or ischemic colitis, except for fatty infiltration of the mesentery.

Colitis cystica

Colitis cystica superficialis and *profunda* are both rare. The superficialis variety involves the colon diffusely with discrete gray blebs filled with mucus on the mucosal surface. It is usually of no significance and is found in pellagra and celiac disease. The profunda type, with submucosal cysts containing gelatinous material, however, is diagnostically important. Elevations mimicking polyps or indentations are seen in the rectum on radiograph. Colitis cystica profunda is usually confined to the rectum and occasionally may simulate the appearance of an adenocarcinoma.

ULTRASONOGRAPHY FOR INFLAMMATORY DISEASE

The use of ultrasonography for large bowel disease is limited because of artifacts from gas, but some applications have emerged. The most frequent indication for ultrasonography of the colon is assessing presence or absence of appendicitis.

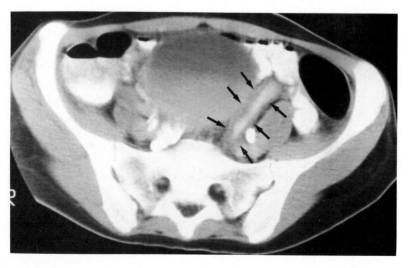

Fig. 8-45 CT of colon. Thickening of descending colon *(arrows)* is noted in patient with ulcerative colitis.

COMPUTED TOMOGRAPHY FOR INFLAMMATORY DISEASE
Idiopathic and infectious types of colitis

CT can be used to detect abnormalities of the colon produced by ulcerative colitis (Fig. 8-45) or granulomatous colitis (Fig. 8-46), infectious colitides including amebiasis or pseudomembranous colitis, (Fig. 8-47) ischemia, diverticulitis, and appendicitis (Fig. 8-48). Abdominal or pelvic abscesses and fistulas (with or without abscess formation) and colonic perforation can be detected and related to adjacent structures. In patients with Crohn's disease, CT can be used to assess the degree of thickening of the bowel and mesentery,

detect fistulous tracts around a stoma, and identify abscesses that cannot be demonstrated by conventional studies. In comparison with Crohn's disease, uncomplicated ulcerative colitis shows only minimal wall thickening and little change in the pericolonic fat. Wall thickening in inflammatory bowel disease is occasionally caused by submucosal fat deposition rather than inflammation. Such deposition may result from steroid therapy. Bowel wall thickening is nonspecific and may be caused by conditions other than inflammatory bowel disease. Such conditions include edema caused by cirrhosis, hypoproteinemia, ascites, ischemia, or a local inflammatory process (pancreatitis, for example).

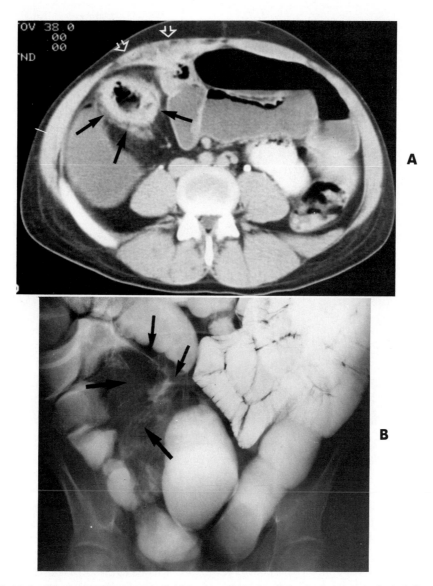

Fig. 8-46 A, CT of colon. Note marked thickening of cecal wall *(arrows)* and pericolonic inflammation. Anterior abdominal wall is also thickened *(open arrows)* in patient with Crohn's disease.
B, Multiple ileoileal and ileocolonic fistulas *(arrows)* and abnormal ileal segments are identified during entroclysis. Mesentery is thickened with displacement of loops of small bowel.

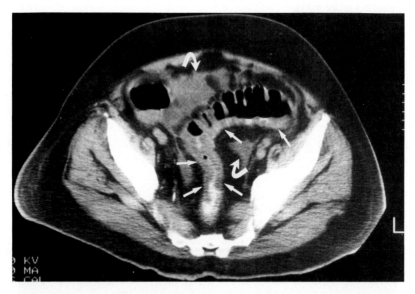

Fig. 8-47 CT of colon. Thickening of wall of rectosigmoid and sigmoid colon *(straight arrows)*. Some ascites *(curved arrows)* is also noted. Patient suffered from ischemic colitis.

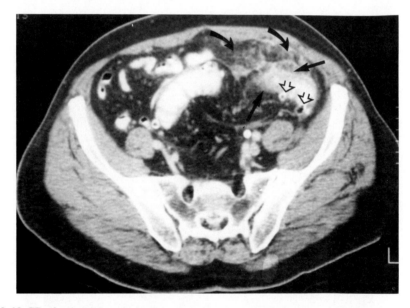

Fig. 8-48 CT of colon. Note thickening of sigmoid wall *(straight arrow)*, pericolonic stranding caused by inflammation *(curved arrows)*, and diverticula *(open arrows)*.

CT may be useful in patients with perirectal inflammatory disease and suspected perirectal abscesses. Such abscesses also can be seen after corrective surgery for Hirschsprung's disease or after total colectomy and ileoanal anastomosis with creation of a rectal pouch. In patients with perirectal inflammation, clinical examination without anesthesia may be difficult. CT provides a noninvasive means to assess the perirectal space reliably and can separate patients who need percutaneous drainage or surgery from those who can be managed conservatively. In particular, CT can be used to distinguish between supralevator and infralevator abscesses. It is important to differentiate between a simple perianal or ischiorectal abscess and an abscess that is a causal extension of a large supralevator abscess. Any failure to recognize such extension of a supralevator abscess leads to a recurrence of abscesses and inadequate surgical drainage.

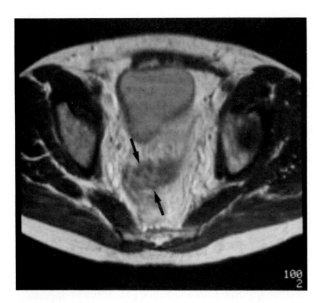

Fig. 8-49 MR examination of the colon, T_2-weighted image (TR, 2000 msec; MR, 60 msec), transverse image. Thickening and increased signal intensity of sigmoid wall in this patient with diverticulitis (arrows). Crohn's disease may appear in similar fashion.

MAGNETIC RESONANCE IMAGING FOR INFLAMMATORY BOWEL DISEASE

At present the use of oral and intravenous paramagnetic and diamagnetic substances for magnetic resonance imaging (MRI) is still in its research phase. To achieve the high resolution of the gastrointestinal tract seen with CT, many more trials need to be made with different scanning sequences and contrast media. Meticulous cleansing of the colon is needed to avoid confusion of feces with bowel wall thickening. No available data based on large series have addressed the use of MRI for diagnosing inflammatory changes in the large bowel (Fig. 8-49).

RECOMMENDED READING

1. Baba S et al: Intestinal Behçet's disease, *Dis Colon Rectum* 19:428, 1976.
2. Bablikian JP, Uthman SU, Khouri NF: Intestinal amebiasis a roentgen analysis of 19 cases including 2 case reports, *Am J Roentgenol* 122:245, 1974.
3. Balthazar EJ, Gordon R, Julnick D: Ileocecal tuberculosis: CT and radiologic evaluation, *Am J Roentgenol* 154:499, 1990.
4. Balthazar EJ, Megibow A, Schnella RA, Gordon R: Limitations in the CT diagnosis of acute diverticulitis: comparison of CT, contrast enema, and pathologic findings in 16 patients, *Am J Roentgenol* 154:281, 1990.
5. Bartram CI, Laufer I: Inflammatory bowel disease. In Laufer I, editor: *Double contrast gastrointestinal radiology with endoscopic correlation*, Philadelphia, 1979, WB Saunders.
6. Bartram CI, Walmsley K: A radiological and pathological correlation of the mucosal changes in ulcerative colitis, *Clin Radiol* 29:323, 1978.
7. de Dombal FT et al: Local complications of ulcerative colitis: stricture, pseudopolyps, and carcinoma of the colon and rectum, *Br Med J* 1:1442, 1966.
8. Dey C, Duvoisin B: CT findings in primary amyloidosis of the colon, *J Comput Assist Tomogr* 13:1094, 1989.
9. Dobbins WO: Dysplasia and malignancy in inflammatory bowel disease, *Ann Rev Med* 35:33, 1984.
10. Eade MN, Thompson H: Liver disease in Crohn's colitis, *Ann Intern Med* 74:518, 1971.
11. Epstein SE et al: Colitis cystica profunda, *Am J Clin Pathol* 45:186, 1966.
12. Federle MP et al: Computed tomographic findings in bowel infarction, *Am J Roentgenol* 142:91, 1984.
13. Gardiner GA: "Backwash ileitis" with pseudopolyposis, *Am J Roentgenol* 129:506, 1977.
14. Gelfand MD, Krone CL: Nonstaphylococcal pseudomembranous colitis, *Am J Dig Dis* 14:278, 1969.
15. Glick SN et al: Development of lymphoma in patients with Crohn's disease, *Radiology* 153:337, 1984.
16. Glick SN, Teplick SK, Amenta PS: Microscopic (collagenous) colitis, *Am J Roentgenol* 153:995, 1989.
17. Goodman PC, Federle MP: Pseudomembranous colitis, *J Comput Assist Tomogr* 4:403, 1980.
18. Greenstein AJ et al: A comparison of cancer risk in Crohn's disease and ulcerative colitis, *Cancer* 48:2742, 1981.
19. Greenstein AJ et al: Cancer in Crohn's disease after diversionary surgery: a report of seven carcinomas occurring in excluded bowel, *Am J Surg* 135:86, 1978.
20. Guillaumin E et al: Perirectal inflammatory disease: CT findings, *Radiology* 161:153, 1986.
21. Hammerman AM, Shatz BA, Sussman N: Radiographic characteristics of colonic "mucosal bridges": sequelae of inflammatory bowel disease, *Radiology* 127:611, 1978.
22. Harned RK et al: Barium enema examination following biopsy of the rectum or colon, *Radiology* 145:11, 1982.
23. Hoddick W, Jeffrey RB, Federle MP: CT differentiation of portal venous air from biliary air, *J Comput Assist Tomogr* 6:633, 1982.
24. Jones B, Abbruzzese AA: Obstructing giant pseudopolyps in granulomatous colitis, *Gastrointest Radiol* 3:437, 1978.
25. Kurchin A et al: Cholelithiasis in ileostomy patients, *Dis Colon Rectum* 27:585, 1984.
26. Larson JM et al: The validity and utility of sonography in the diagnosis of appendicitis in the community setting, *Am J Roentgenol* 153:687, 1989.
27. Laufer I, Costopoulos L: Early lesions of Crohn's disease, *Am J Roentgenol* 130:307, 1978.
28. Laufer I, Hamilton JD: The radiologic differentiation between ulcerative and granulomatous colitis by double contrast radiology, *Am J Gastroenterol* 66:259, 1976.
29. Levine SM et al: Ameboma: the forgotten granuloma, *JAMA* 215:1461, 1971.
30. Lockhart-Mummery HE, Morson BC: Crohn's disease (regional enteritis) of the large intestine, *Gut* 5:493, 1964.
31. Margulis AR et al: The overlapping spectrum of ulcerative and granulomatous colitis: a roentgenographic-pathologic study, *Am J Roentgenol* 113:325, 1971.
32. Medina JT et al: The roentgen appearance of schistomiasis mansoni involving the colon, *Radiology* 85:682, 1965.
33. Menuck LS et al: Colonic changes of herpes zoster, *Am J Roentgenol* 127:237, 1976.
34. Montagne JP et al: Radiologic evaluation of the continent (Koch) ileostomy, *Radiology* 127:325, 1978.
35. Munyer TP et al: Postinflammatory polypsis (PIP) of the colon: the radiologic-pathologic spectrum, *Radiology* 145:607, 1982.

36. Nelson JA et al: Ulcerative and granulomatous colitis: variation in observer interpretation and in roentgenographic appearance as related to time, *Am J Roentgenol* 119:369, 1973.

37. Schimmel DH et al: Bacteraemia and the barium enema, *Am J Roentgenol* 128:207, 1977.

38. Schofield PF, Mandal BK, Ironside AG: Toxic dilatation of the colon in salmonella colitis and inflammatory bowel disease, *Br J Surg* 66:5, 1979.

39. Stanley RJ, Nelson Gl, Tedesco FJ: The spectrum of radiographic findings in antibiotic-related pseudomembranous colitis, *Radiology* 111:519, 1974.

40. Tully TE, Feinberg SB: Those other types of enterocolitis, *Am J Roentgenol* 121:291, 1974.

41. Urso FP, Urso MI, Lee CM: The cathartic colon: pathological findings and radiological-pathological correlation, *Radiology* 116:557, 1975.

42. Vantrappen G et al: Yersinial enteritis and enterocolitis: gastroenterological aspects, *Gastroenterology* 72:220, 1977.

43. Zegel H, Laufer L: Filiform polyposis, *Radiology* 127:615, 1978.

Polyps

EDWARD STEWART
WYLIE J DODDS

Because colonic polyps may harbor a malignant tumor or lead to a malignancy, the detection of polypoid colonic lesions is an important diagnostic challenge (Table 8-3).

PATHOLOGIC FINDINGS
Histology

The histologic characteristics of colon polyps allow the pathologist to categorize most polypoid lesions of the colon with considerable accuracy. Hyperplastic polyps contain mucosal glands lined by a single layer of columnar epithelium with infoldings arranged in a coiled fashion. Hamartomas represent a malformation of cellular elements indigenous to the colonic mucosa. Juvenile polyps are classified as cystic hamartomas by some pathologists and as inflammatory retention cysts by others. The only polyps with significant malignant potential are neoplastic polyps. Therefore these polypoid lesions are the focus of attention. Neoplastic polyps are either benign or malignant. This distinction is essential. Benign neoplastic polyps are either simple tubular adenomas or have varying amounts of villous components. A tubular adenoma can therefore contain areas with villous architecture that may or may not dominate the histologic appearance of the polyp. When malignant degeneration occurs in a tubular adenoma, tubulovillous adenoma, or villous adenoma, the malignant process can either occupy a portion of the polyp or replace the entire polyp. Villous architecture appears to be more premalignant than is simple tubular epithelium.

Morphology

Polypoid colonic lesions show different morphologic characteristics. The three general morphologic forms are sessile plaques, sessile hemispheres, and pedunculated spheres.

Distribution

Although sporadic colonic polyps may occur as a solitary lesion, they are more commonly multiple. About half of the patients with an index lesion harbor one or more additional synchronous polyps. Many patients with a sporadic colonic adenoma or carcinoma subsequently develop one or more metachronous polypoid lesions. In some instances, however, polyps clas-

☐ **TABLE 8-3**
Summary of the features characterizing gastrointestinal polyposis syndromes

Syndrome	Usual age at symptom onset (yrs)	Hereditary transmission	Distribution (%)		
			Stomach	Small bowel	Colon
Multiple polyposis	15 to 30	Dominant	<5	<5	100
Gardner's syndrome	15 to 30	Dominant	~5	~5	100
Peutz-Jeghers syndrome	10 to 30	Dominant	25	95	30
Ruvalcaba-Myhre-Smith syndrome	Variable	Dominant	100	100	100
Turcot's syndrome	Teens	Recessive	—	—	100
Cronkhite-Canada syndrome	40 to 70	None	100	<50	100
Juvenile polyposis	<10	May be familial	>5	>5	100

See qualifying comments in text.

sified as metachronous lesions are undoubtedly polyps that were missed in the initial examination.

Cancer origin

The main function of the radiologic examination is to accurately identify polypoid colonic lesions. Once a polypoid lesion is demonstrated, histologic assessment is usually necessary to determine the presence of carcinoma.

DETECTION
Contrast enema

At present radiographic examinations and endoscopy are the two main methods for detecting polypoid lesions of the colon. The radiographic examination may be either a single-contrast barium enema or double-contrast pneumocolon examination. The pneumocolon examination appears to be more sensitive than the conventional barium enema, but either method may miss lesions. For example, it is common to find two or three polyps a centimeter or more in size and to overlook an additional polyp of similar size. The pneumocolon examination is 90% accurate in identifying index polyps in patients with one or more polyps at least 0.5 cm in size. It may be as high as 97% accurate in identifying index polyps in patients with one or more polyps at least 1 cm in size. At present, the pneumocolon is an accepted standard examination for patients with suspected colonic polyps or lower intestinal bleeding. With uncooperative, debilitated, or immobile patients and with patients with massive diverticulosis a single-contrast barium enema may be more appropriate. A good single-contrast barium enema examination is preferable to a poor pneumocolon examination. Interpreting the pneumocolon examination is more difficult than interpreting the single-contrast barium enema examination. On the second viewing of an air contrast study, it is not unusual to identify a polyp that was overlooked during the initial interpretation.

A relatively common occurrence is the demonstration of a rectal polyp with a pneumocolon examination that is not detected with proctoscopy. The polyps missed by proctoscopy are commonly hidden from view, because they are located on the proximal surface of rectal valves. To maximize the efficacy of the double-contrast examination of the rectum, it is desirable to avoid inflated rectal balloons that may obscure low-lying lesions, as well as cause injury.

Colonoscopy

During the past decade fiberoptic colonoscopy has substantially altered the diagnosis and management of polypoid colonic lesions. The colonoscopic method not only detects colonic polyps, but it also allows histologic diagnosis and therapeutic excision. Although colonoscopy is a more sensitive method than radiographic examination for detecting colonic polyps, radiographic examination accompanied by proctosigmoid endoscopy remains the major initial screening method in many centers. In particular, the double-contrast pneumocolon examination is especially well suited for detecting colonic polyps. Widespread use of the radiographic method continues to be recommended because (1) it nearly invariably examines the entire colon, whereas many colonoscopies fail to reach the right side of the colon; (2) the radiographic method requires less time and is much less expensive; (3) the radiographic examination is generally well tolerated by most patients; and

Histology	Additional features	Prognosis
Adenomas		Colon carcinoma
Adenomas	Soft tissue tumors, osteomatosis	Colon carcinoma
Cellular Hamartomas	Pigmented skin lesions	Occasional GI tract carcinoma
Hamartomas	Macrocephaly penile macules Mental retardation	Occasional GI tract pain
Adenomas	Central nervous system tumors	Central nervous system tumor
Inflammatory	Alopecia, onychia, hyperpigmentation, diarrhea, protein and electrolyte losses	Often die from cachexia
Glandular Dilatation		
Inflammatory	Diarrhea with protein loss may occur	GI tract carcinoma

(4) the capability for high-volume colonoscopy is not available in most areas. Colonoscopy is also likely to miss lesions on the inner margin of bowel curvatures.

Confidence level

Although radiographic images are often considered positive or negative, a considerable borderline area exists as well. As a consequence the radiologic report should convey a confidence level for any given study. Studies featuring a clean colon, good barium coating, and optimal anatomy elicit a high level of confidence. In contrast, studies with suboptimal colon cleansing, poor barium coating, and suboptimal display of redundant loops often result in a low confidence level in the identification of presence or absence of colonic polypoid lesions. A variety of maneuvers, such as the supplemental use of glucagon, compression techniques, additional films, and colon refilling, generally determine whether a filling defect is an artifact or a true lesion. In cases of equivocal polypoid lesions, additional studies are needed to resolve the issue.

The major error of experienced radiologists is overlooking polypoid colonic lesions rather than making false-positive diagnoses. Perceptive errors seem to account for the majority of mistakes. Even large lesions can be misinterpreted on double-contrast examinations because of perceptive errors. This occasional shortcoming has prompted the use of single-contrast examinations to supplement negative double-contrast examinations in very high-risk patients, especially those with significant blood loss. Perceptive errors for larger lesions may be reduced with the single-contrast technique. The possibility of a real lesion should not be dismissed on the basis of negative colonoscopic findings; rather an additional radiographic or colonoscopic examination should be performed to resolve the conflict.

RADIOLOGIC FEATURES
Differentiation from artifacts

Polypoid colonic lesions must be distinguished from intraluminal and extraluminal artifacts. Polyps may be simulated by intraluminal fecal material, gas bubbles, oil droplets, mucus, and foreign bodies. In general such intraluminal artifacts change location with shifts in the patient's position; however, fecal material may adhere to the mucosa. Adherent feces usually have an irregular shape, uneven barium coating, and fuzzy margins, but in some instances may simulate a sessile polyp (Fig. 8-50). Air bubbles less than 1 cm in size are generally perfectly round, whereas larger accumulations trapped within the dome of a bowel loop tend to be ovoid. Bubbles often occur in pairs or clusters. Wetting agents, such as simethicone, minimize trapped bubbles. The appearance of oil droplets from lubricating agents is similar to that of bubbles. Mucus may appear in strands or globs. The latter form may simulate a polypoid lesion, especially when anchored in a diverticulum and projecting into the bowel lumen. Ingested foreign bodies, such as seeds, occasionally simulate colonic polyps but often have a typical ovoid, elongated, or slightly triangular shape with very smooth margins.

Structures intrinsic to the bowel wall, such as diverticula, mucosal plications, and haustral folds, or knuckles at angulations may also simulate true polypoid lesions. On pneumocolon examination diverticula seen face on may simulate a sessile polyp. With multiple films, however, the diverticula may be seen to fill with barium, to have an air-fluid level, or to project clear of the bowel lumen. On face-on views, the ring projected by barium lining of an air-filled diverticulum tends to have a smooth outer margin and a hazy inner margin, whereas the reverse is the case for a barium-coated polyp (Fig. 8-51). This distinction, however, is not very reliable. Manual pressure over a diverticulum may change its size and shape or result in some filling with barium. Occasional stool-filled diverticula can project into the colon lumen, simulating a polyp. Mucosal plications or haustral folds seen end on may mimic a polyp. These filling defects tend to have a slightly teardrop shape, and their identity is generally evident on multiple views. Pseudotumors produced by angulations at flexures may also be confused with polyps. An inverted appendicial stump or plump ileocecal valve containing fat must also be differentiated from polypoid neoplasms.

Morphologic findings

On radiographs, polypoid colonic lesions appear either sessile or pedunculated. Sessile lesions have a broad base and are either moundlike protuberances or flattened plaques. Pedunculated polyps may have a long or short stalk. They may be attached at a point on a spherelike head. The specific radiologic findings differ somewhat between the barium enema and pneumocolon examinations and among *en face,* tangential, and oblique views (Fig. 8-52).

Polypoid lesions 0.5 cm or less in size are usually flat, occasionally rounded, and seldom pedunculated. On *en face* projections flat sessile polyps commonly escape detection in single-contrast examinations. Their shallow vertical height does not result in sufficient radiographic attenuation to project through the barium column. With the pneumocolon examination, however, such lesions are often identified face on as ringlike densities that are generally round or ovoid. When viewed tangentially, flat sessile lesions project into a barium or air column as a plaquelike filling defect. In cases of larger lesions, the margin of the colonic wall may lose

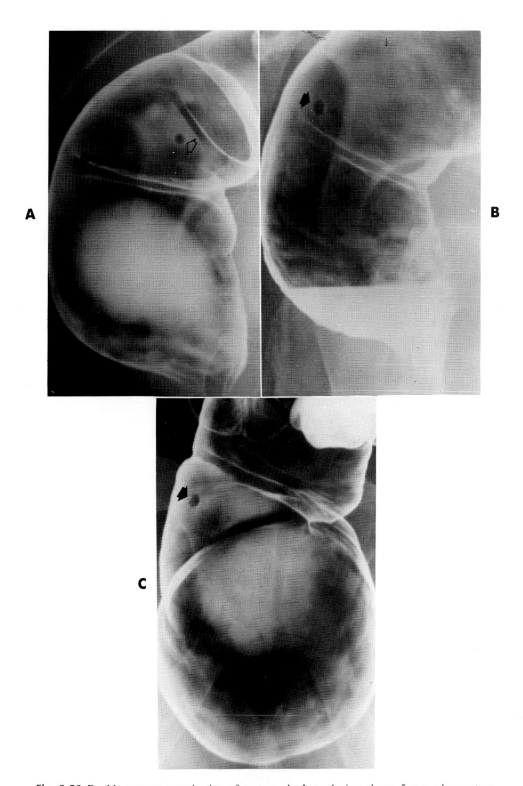

Fig. 8-50 Double-contrast examination of rectum. **A,** Lateral view shows 5 mm adenomatous polyp *(closed arrow)* and 4 mm air bubble *(open arrow)*. **B,** In upright lateral view taken subsequently air bubble has disappeared but small polypoid lesion *(arrow)* remains unchanged. This lesion, located immediately proximal to a rectal fold (Houston's valve), was not seen at initial proctoscopy. **C,** Posteroanterior projection confirms presence of small sessile polyp *(arrow)* that was located on posterolateral wall of proximal rectum.

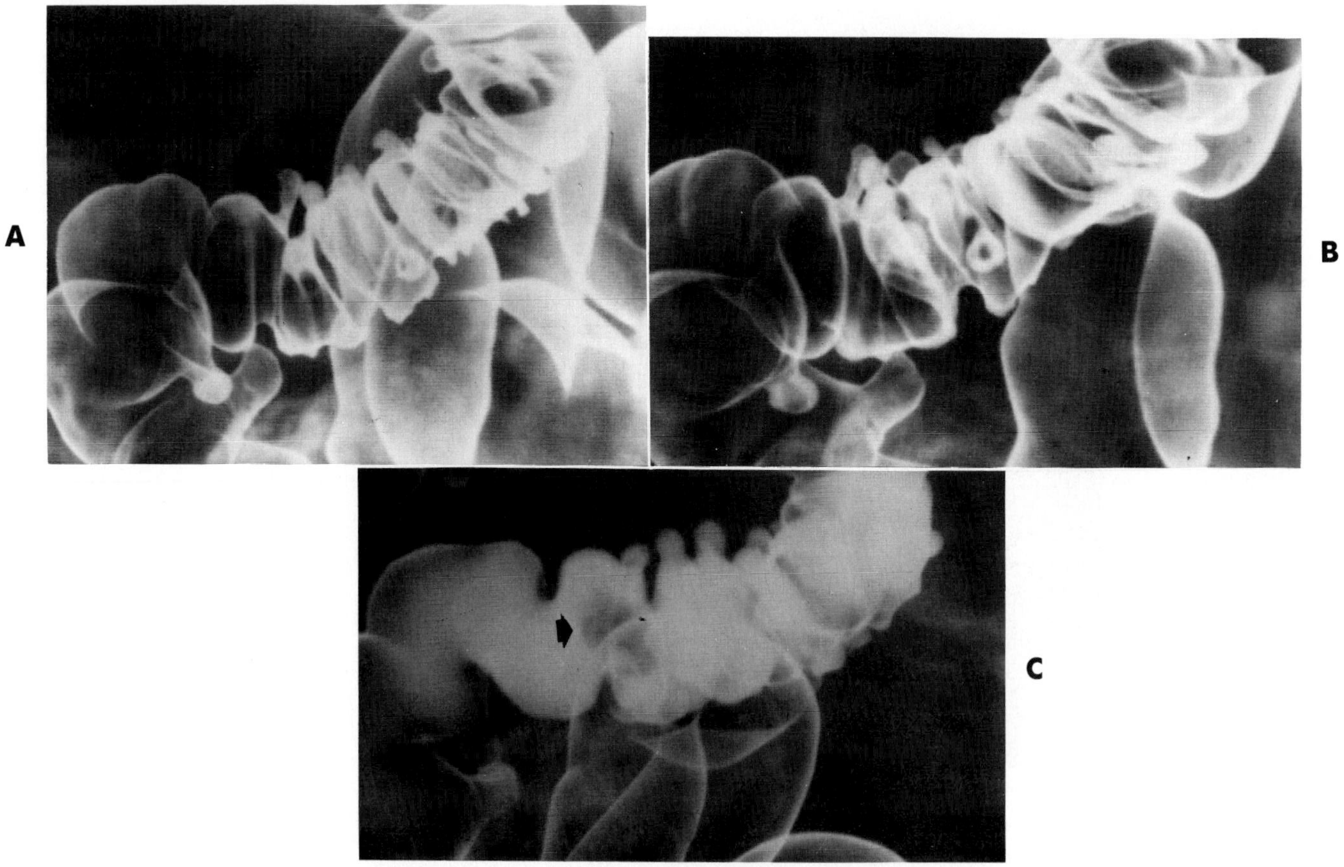

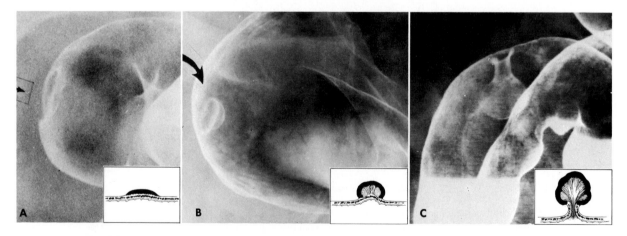

Fig. 8-51 On double-contrast images in pneumocolon examination, **A** and **B**, sessile sigmoid polyp is completely obscured by cluster of diverticula, despite films of excellent technical quality. Polyp *(arrow)* was visualized only on single-contrast image. **C**, when barium flooded loop.

Fig. 8-52 Morphologic forms of polypoid colonic lesions. **A**, Sessile plaque seen tangentially. **B**, Sessile hemispheric moundlike lesion seen obliquely. Slight undercutting at margins traps ring of barium that overlaps coated dome of polyp to create hat sign. **C**, Pedunculated sphere. Pedunculated polyp on short stalk is seen in profile.

(From Youker JE, Welin S: *Radiology* 84:610, 1965.)

its normal curved contour and appear as a flat, rigid area.

On single-contrast examinations protuberant sessile polyps have a vertical height that is 50% or more of their width. The base is broad with either flared or undercut margins. In the barium enema examination sessile lesions seen *en face* appear as a roundish or slightly oval filling defect. Thin barium (15% to 20% w/v) and high photon penetration (120 kV technique) are needed to image such lesions through the barium column. Manual palpation is useful for demonstrating the lesion and should be done routinely for the entire colon. In the tangential view protuberant sessile polyps project as a hemispheric defect into the contour of the barium column. In some instances undercutting at the margins can be appreciated.

On pneumocolon examinations protuberant sessile polyps are seen face on as a ringlike density that represents the side walls of the barium-coated lesion. Visualization requires a good coating with high-density barium (90% to 100% w/v). In addition to overhead and decubitus films, multiple spot films taken with the patient recumbent and erect will help detect such lesions. When undercutting is present, barium fills the crevice and may be seen as a crescent or oval ring if the lesion is viewed obliquely. In this circumstance the second barium ring from the undercut margin projected onto the barium outline of the moundlike contour of the polyp may produce the *hat sign*.

With pedunculated lesions the polyp head is always seen more or less *en face,* because the spherical head does not have a broad attachment with the colonic mucosa. On single-contrast barium enema examinations the head of a pedunculated polyp is usually identified by a roundish filling defect, whereas on the pneumocolon examination it appears as a coated sphere. In many instances the stalk is not clearly visualized, and thus the polyp may be judged to be a sessile lesion. In tangential views the polyp head often lies against the colonic wall, simulating a protuberant sessile lesion.

Pedunculated polyps generally shift in position during the radiographic examination. If the stalk is long (2 to 5 cm), the polyp head may move axially a distance of 4 to 10 cm along the bowel lumen. Polyps on short stalks move a shorter distance, and polyps attached to a point may be seen to jiggle back and forth. These phenomena are best seen with manual compression during the barium enema examination, but may also be appreciated during the fluoroscopic portion of the pneumocolon examination. In upright or decubitus views pedunculated polyps may hang suspended within the bowel lumen. When not stretched, the stalk is serpiginous and may mimic a lobulated broad-based lesion. On tangential views a polyp lying limp on a short stalk may simulate a flat sessile lesion.

Potential for malignancy

Estimates of the probability of malignancy can be made on the basis of radiologic findings.

Size

The single most important feature for estimating the probability of malignancy is the size of the polyp. Polyps less than 0.5 cm in diameter are rarely malignant. Polyps 1 cm or less in diameter have about a 1% to 2% incidence of malignancy; in polyps with a diameter greater than 1 cm the incidence of malignancy rises sharply. About 10% of polyps between 1 and 2 cm in diameter harbor malignancy, and 20% to 46% of polyps greater than 2 cm are cancerous.

Pedunculation

Polyps with a well-defined pedicle have a substantially lower incidence of malignancy than sessile lesions of comparable diameter. A smooth pedicle 2 cm or more in length almost always indicates a benign lesion. The adenoma is confined to the polyp head, and the stalk represents an elongation of normal mucosa, possibly caused by repeated tugging on the polyp by colonic contractions. Even when a focus of carcinoma exists in the head of a well-defined pedunculated polyp, metastases to regional nodes or distant sites are rare. In cases of frank polypoid cancers the pedicle is usually thick, short, and irregular.

Surface contour

In some instances the outline and surface contour of colonic polyps may provide clues to the underlying histologic condition, but radiographic findings in this category are usually unreliable. The presence of a reticular or filiform surface pattern suggests a villous tumor, but these findings are seldom present when villous tumors are less than 2 to 3 cm in size. A discrete surface ulceration is highly suggestive of a carcinoma. Another contour finding suggesting malignancy is an indentation of the polyp base when the lesion is seen in the tangential view. This suggests infiltration and invasion of the mucosa adjacent to the lesion.

With polyps greater than 1 cm in size an exquisitely sharp contour with smooth tapering margins seen on tangential views suggests a benign submucosal tumor or carcinoid tumor.

Location

Polyp location generally does not help in distinguishing benign from malignant lesions. In some instances, however, the location of a polypoid lesion may weight the diagnostic probabilities. For example, polypoid lesions at the cecal tip are likely to be related to the appendix—an inverted stump, prolapse, abscess, or mucocele. The ileocecal valve may simulate a polypoid neoplasm. Fatty infiltration of the valve may cause a pronounced filling defect. Even when prominent, however, the normal valve is smooth and symmetric. Any nodularity or asymmetry suggests malignancy.

Although sessile filling defects located low in the rectum may be caused by internal hemorrhoids, such rectal lesions suggest the possibility of a villous tumor, squamous carcinoma, or cloacogenic carcinoma.

Growth rate

Another useful factor in the evaluation for malignancy is the polyp's growth rate. An increase in the size of a colonic polyp should be considered an indication for removal.

SPECIFIC POLYPOID LESIONS
Adenomas

Most adenomatous polyps are sessile or pedunculated tubular adenomas. However, the remaining lesions are either tubulovillous adenomas or pure villous

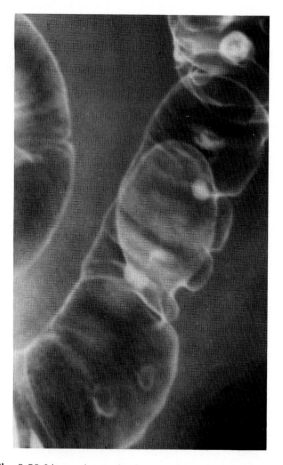

Fig. 8-53 Lipoma in proximal sigmoid. Smooth-walled, oval lesion has short broad pedicle. Exquisitely sharp margins of lesion are characteristic of lipoma. Scattered diverticula are present.

adenomas. About 10% of adenomatous polyps are probably completely villous in architecture, and these tend to be sessile lesions, which have a predilection for the rectum and the cecum. For a given size, the likelihood that a villous tumor harbors a carcinoma is 10 times greater than that for a tubular adenoma. In some instances, villous tumors greater than 1 cm can be identified on radiographs by a fine or coarse reticular pattern of barium on their surface that gives the lesion a wartlike appearance. The more proximal the lesion, the less likely it is to have a typical villous appearance. In some cases villous tumors appear as an annular plaque or spreading carpet lesion with surface irregularity or mamillation. Large rectal lesions are often seen as broad-based tumors that often have a soft consistency on the digital rectal examination. The extensive surface area of villous tumors may cause diarrhea with excessive loss of potassium or less commonly of albumen.

Lipomas

Among benign colonic tumors, lipomas are second in prevalence to adenomas. Patients with a colonic lipoma are commonly asymptomatic; when present, symptoms include abdominal pain, constipation, rectal bleeding, and diarrhea. Most colonic lipomas are submucosal, and about 10% are subserosal. About 40% are located in the right side of the colon and 20% in the sigmoid (Fig. 8-53). The usual radiographic appearance is one of a smooth, sharply outlined hemispheric mass. Because the tumors are soft, their contour is often altered by peristalsis or compression.

Juvenile polyps

Most juvenile polyps occur as an isolated colonic lesion in children less than 10 years old. The lesion is solitary in about 75% of cases. Rectal bleeding is the most common symptom. On the barium enema examination juvenile polyps are identified as roundish filling defects, often pedunculated, that are located most commonly in the rectum or sigmoid. Because the lesions are benign and have a tendency toward autoamputation or regression, their removal is not mandatory in the absence of significant bleeding or intussusception.

Carcinoid tumors

Approximately 15% of alimentary tract carcinoid tumors occur in the large bowel, and nearly all of these are in the rectum. Rectal carcinoid tumors constitute about 1% to 2% of rectal polyps greater than 0.5 cm in size. On contrast enema examinations rectal carcinoid tumors usually appear as sessile hemispheric lesions with sharp margins. They are occasionally bulky or annular.

Colonic carcinoid tumors should be considered to be

malignant lesions. About 15% of rectal carcinoids are accompanied by metastases. This figure soars to 75% to 90% for lesions 2 cm or more in size. Metastatic rectal carcinoid tumors rarely cause the carcinoid syndrome.

Endometriomas

After adenomas and lipomas, endometriomas are the third most common benign tumor of the rectum and colon. Intestinal implants of endometriosis are estimated to occur in about 4% of women, with rectosigmoid involvement in 85% of such cases. The symptoms often wax and wane in severity during the menstrual cycle (Fig. 8-54).

On barium enema examination endometrial implants of the large bowel are generally seen along the superior anterior rectal wall near the rectosigmoid junction (from seeding into the pouch of Douglas) or along the superior margin of the sigmoid (from implants at the attachment of the sigmoid mesentery). Involvement of the ap-

pendix and terminal ileum is an occasional finding. The implants generally appear as smooth, eccentric submucosal lesions that project for a variable distance into the bowel lumen. In some instances the implants evoke a hypertrophic response in the muscularis mucosae that causes pleating or transverse ridging of the overlying mucosa, giving the lesion a characteristic scalloped appearance. Most lesions are eccentric and cause only mild to modest luminal narrowing. On occasion, the lesions encircle the bowel and cause a significant obstruction. Endometriomas are well demonstrated by MRI as high signal masses.

Other tumors

In addition to the more common benign tumors described, a number of unusual or rare benign polypoid lesions of the colon may occur. These include leiomyoma, fibroma, neurogenic tumor, hemangioma, lymphangioma, endothelioma, granular cell myoblastoma, cysts, and duplication. In most cases, these tumors are

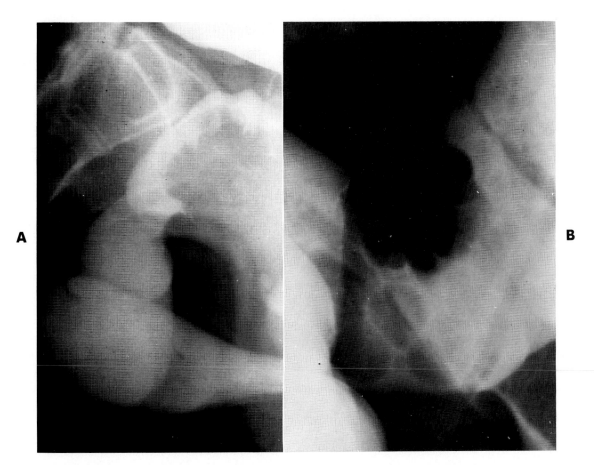

Fig. 8-54 Colonic endometriosis. In two patients endometrioma is seen, **A,** along anterior wall of rectosigmoid adjacent to pouch of Douglas and, **B,** along superior margin of sigmoid adjacent to its mesenteric junction. Both lesions are excentric and show scalloping or pleating of mucosa, findings typical of endometrioma.

located submucosally, the mucosa is intact, and their radiographic appearance suggests a benign lesion.

MANAGEMENT OF POLYPOID LESIONS

Current practice is to remove all polyps, whether sessile or pedunculated. Another important consideration is patient follow-up and surveillance. Patients who have had a colonic adenoma or carcinoma are at risk for the subsequent development of additional large bowel neoplasms. Such patients are generally considered to have a "tumor-prone" colon, and follow-up surveillance is indicated. At present a follow-up examination, usually endoscopic, should be performed 1 year after removal of a neoplastic polyp to detect any synchronous lesions missed initially or to search for new lesions.

POLYPOSIS SYNDROMES

The polyposis syndrome should be suspected when (1) a gastrointestinal polyp is identified in a young patient, (2) multiple polyps are demonstrated in any patient, and (3) a colon carcinoma is present in a patient less than 40 years old. Gastrointestinal polyposis syndromes that affect the colon may be classified as hereditary or nonhereditary. The three major hereditary syndromes—familial multiple polyposis, Gardner's syndrome, and Peutz-Jeghers syndrome—have autosomal dominant inheritance.

Familial multiple polyposis

Patients with multiple polyposis reveal an autosomal dominant mechanism of inheritance. The abnormal gene has high penetrance, estimated to be about 80%. About two thirds of afflicted individuals have a positive family history of colonic polyps or carcinoma, and about one third are sporadic cases. A high percentage of individuals with clinical symptoms have an existing colon carcinoma or develop a large bowel malignancy within 2 years.

The colonic polyps are numerous, ranging from pinhead lesions to those 1 cm or more in size, and may be sessile or pedunculated. The rectum and left side of the colon are more commonly involved than the right side of the colon, but often the entire colonic mucosa is carpeted with myriad polyps, such that normal mucosa is not seen. Recent reports, primarily from Japan, claim a high incidence of gastric, duodenal, and small bowel polyps in patients with familial multiple polyposis. Although Japanese patients with multiple familial polyposis might have a predilection to develop gastric and perhaps small bowel polyps, extracolonic polyps still appear to be uncommon in North American and European patients.

Colonic polyps in patients with familial multiple polyposis generally arise during the first or second decade

---

```
┌──────────────────────────────────────────┐
│   □   POLYPOSIS SYNDROMES INVOLVING   □   │
│                THE COLON                  │
│                                           │
│  1. Hereditary polyposis syndromes        │
│     a. Familial multiple polyposis        │
│     b. Gardner's syndrome                 │
│     c. Peutz-Jeghers syndrome             │
│     d. Ruvalcaba-Myhre-Smith syndrome     │
│     e. Turcot's syndrome                  │
│  2. Nonhereditary polyposis syndromes     │
│     a. Cronkhite-Canada syndrome          │
│     b. Juvenile polyposis (sometimes      │
│        hereditary)                        │
└──────────────────────────────────────────┘
```

of life, but are not usually evident until after puberty. As a rule, colon cancers develop in patients with familial polyposis between the ages of 20 to 40 years, and rarely occur before the age of 20 years. A colon carcinoma develops in nearly 100% of untreated patients. Radiographic examination should be performed in all susceptible patients to document the size, number, and distribution of the polyps and to search for a carcinoma (Fig. 8-55). Carcinomas may appear as polypoid filling defects, areas of symmetric segmental narrowing, or typical annular lesions with overhanging margins. Multiple carcinomas are common. The colon is a dispensable organ, not necessary for useful life, and a colon carcinoma is entirely preventable if afflicted patients are identified when they are young and a prophylactic total colectomy is performed. Colectomy with an ileorectal anastomosis is a suitable operation for reliable patients who will return for follow-up proctoscopy.

Gardner's syndrome

Gardner's syndrome is characterized by an autosomal dominant inheritance, multiple soft tissue tumors, osteomatosis, polyposis coli, and a potential for colon malignancy. About 20% of afflicted patients have the complete triad of soft tissue tumors, osteomatosis, and polyposis.

The cutaneous lesions consist of sebaceous or inclusion cysts that are most numerous on the scalp and back but may be present on the face or extremities. Benign mesenchymal tumors include fibromas, lipomas, lipofibromas, leiomyomas, and neurofibromas. Malignant sarcomas, such as fibrosarcomas and leiomyosarcomas, are unusual but do occur. The fibrous tissue in patients with Gardner's syndrome often has a pronounced tendency toward proliferation, thereby resulting in desmoid tumors, keloids, hypertrophied scars, mammary fibromatosis, peritoneal adhesions, mesenteric fibrosis, and retroperitoneal fibrosis. Fibrous tissue proliferation

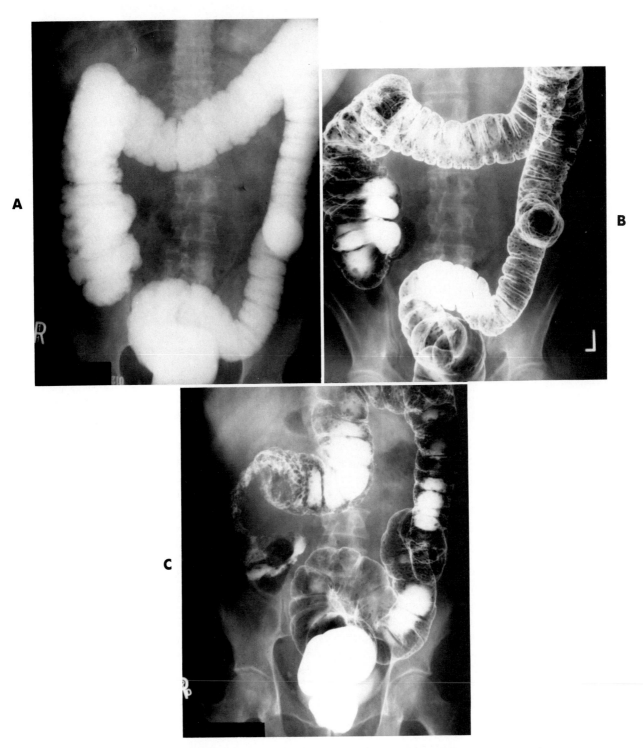

Fig. 8-55 Familial multiple polyposis. **A,** Single-contrast examination on this patient shows fine marginal contour irregularities caused by multiple polyposis. Myriad small polyps are not well seen on overhead film. **B,** Double-contrast examination nicely demonstrates voluminous number of small polyps of varying sizes, from several millimeters up to 1 cm. They involve entire colon. **C,** Patient refused colectomy and 4 years later returned with large fungating, infiltrating adenocarcinoma of right side of colon (cont'd).

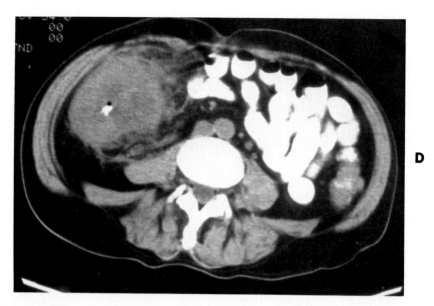

Fig. 8-55, cont'd D, CT scan done at this time demonstrates large, bulky tumor that encompasses entire circumference of right side of colon with extension into mesentery. Patient had numerous liver metastases by this time as well.

may arise either spontaneously or in response to injury or surgery.

Localized areas of dense bone *(osteomas),* appearing as exostoses or enostoses, are commonly present in the maxilla, mandible, or skull. The long bones, particularly the femur and tibia, are often abnormal and demonstrate localized cortical thickening, wavy cortical thickening, or exostoses. The long bones may also be slightly shortened and bowed. Dental abnormalities frequently include odontomas, unerupted supernumerary teeth, hypercementosis, and a tendency toward numerous caries. The bone and soft tissue lesions often appear before or during puberty and may precede the development of polyps.

The polyps in Gardner's syndrome tend to be limited to the colon, although some recent reports suggest that a higher than normal incidence also exists for polyps in the stomach, duodenum, and small bowel. Patients have a predilection for a duodenal carcinoma. In gross and histologic examinations, the polyps do not differ from the adenomatous polyps present in patients with familial multiple polyposis. Further, virtually all patients with Gardner's syndrome eventually develop a colon carcinoma if the colon is not removed. In patients with a colon carcinoma the average age at death is 41 years, which is essentially identical to that of patients with familial multiple polyposis dying from large bowel cancer.

Peutz-Jeghers syndrome

Peutz-Jeghers syndrome is worldwide in its distribution and has no racial predilection. About 50% of re-

ported cases have a positive family history, whereas the remaining 50% are sporadic. The characteristic mucocutaneous pigmented lesions usually develop during infancy or early childhood and are present in nearly all patients. These mucocutaneous lesions appear as brown or black, oval or slightly irregular macules 1 to 5 mm in diameter (Fig. 8-56). They are most common on the lips, particularly the mucosal surface of the lower lip, and the buccal mucosa. Pigmentation occurs less commonly on the face or volar aspect of the hands and feet.

The clinical symptomatology is usually related to gastrointestinal polyposis. The most common clinical symptom is cramping abdominal pain, caused by small bowel intussusception. Most of the intussusceptions are transient, but some persist and cause a significant small bowel obstruction. Rectal bleeding, or melena, occurs in about 30% of cases, but massive gastrointestinal bleeding is rare. Chronic anemia caused by low-grade intestinal blood loss is commonly present. In some instances colonic intussusception or prolapse of a rectal polyp brings the patient to clinical attention.

The polyps in cases of Peutz-Jeghers syndrome occur predominantly in the alimentary tract but are occasionally located in the urinary or respiratory tracts. The small bowel is involved in more than 95% of patients, the colon and rectum in about 30%, and the stomach in about 25%. Jejunal or ileal polyps are usually identified during a carefully performed small bowel examination using compression and spot films. Colonic polyps, when present, number from two to a dozen or more. The polyps are most commonly multiple and range in size from 0.1 to 3 cm. Numerous 1 to 2 mm nodules may be present in the small bowel, but carpeting has not been observed in the stomach or colon. The small bowel and gastric polyps, once considered precancerous adenomas, are currently regarded as benign hamartomatous malformations without malignant potential. Most colonic polyps in Peutz-Jeghers syndrome are proliferative mucosal lesions that are indistinguishable from adenomatous polyps. The overall incidence of alimentary tract carcinomas in these patients is estimated to be about 2% to 3%. Most of the gastrointestinal carcinomas occur in the stomach, duodenum, and colon. Carcinomas are rare in the jejunum and ileum. Sessile lesions greater than 1 to 1.5 cm in diameter, lesions demonstrating rapid growth, and annular lesions should be regarded as suggestive of carcinoma.

Ruvalcaba-Myhre-Smith syndrome

Ruvalcaba-Myhre-Smith syndrome is characterized by macrocephaly, pigmented genital lesions in males, and intestinal polyposis; it appears to be transmitted by autosomal dominant inheritance. Other possible features include mental retardation, lipid storage myopathy, and subcutaneous lipomas.

The genital skin lesions consist of hyperpigmented macules that are present on the glans and shaft of the penis. Pigmented macules are absent on the scrotum or on the genitalia of female patients. The intestinal lesions involve the bowel, with reports of multiple scattered polyps involving the gastric antrum, duodenum, small bowel, and colon. Available biopsy material from colonic polyps indicates that the lesions are hamartomas. There has been no evidence of malignant potential.

Turcot's syndrome

An association between polyposis coli and central nervous tumors was suggested by Turcot and co-workers in 1959. To date, about 15 patients (10 from 4 families) with the syndrome have been identified. The fact that neither brain tumors nor colonic polyps appeared in the parents of affected individuals suggests an autosomal recessive mode of inheritance. Most of the patients died as a result of their central nervous system malignancy. The polyps are multiple, range in diameter from 0.1 to 3 cm, and are limited to the rectum and colon. They appear to be benign adenomas, but the histologic description has often been incomplete. A colon carcinoma was present in four of the reported patients.

Cronkhite-Canada syndrome

The Cronkhite-Canada syndrome develops during middle or old age (from 42 to 75 years of age, with an average age of 60 years) and shows no sexual, familial, racial, or geographic predilection. The most common initial symptom is diarrhea of several months duration

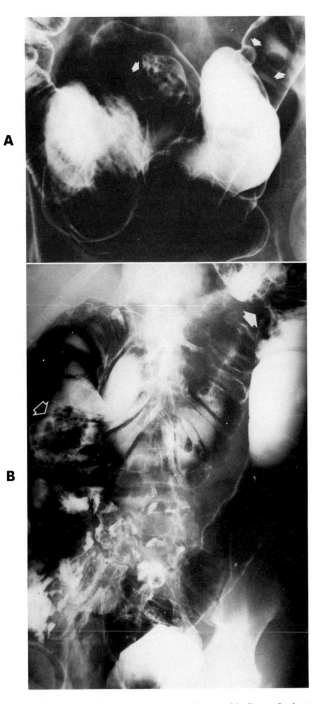

Fig. 8-56 Colon lesions in two patients with Peutz-Jeghers syndrome. **A,** Three benign sigmoid polyps *(arrows)* but no other colon lesions are present. **B,** Constricting carcinoma *(arrow)* is seen in splenic flexure; resected colon also demonstrated about 1 dozen benign polyps scattered throughout large bowel. Sessile hamartoma *(open arrow)* is present in cecum.

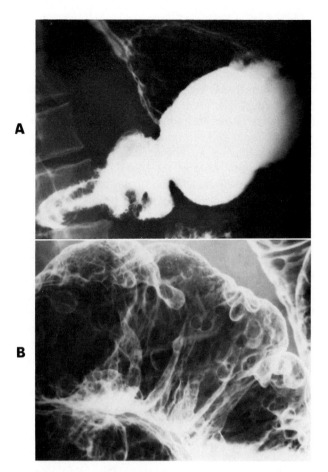

Fig. 8-57 Cronkhite-Canada syndrome. **A,** Hundreds of polypoid lesions, pinhead in size, mammillate distal half of stomach. Several larger polypoid lesions are also present in antrum. **B,** Numerous polypoid lesions are well shown on spot film of splenic flexure.

or more. The stools are watery and often contain blood, mucus, or both (Fig. 8-57). The diarrhea is usually accompanied by anorexia, vomiting, abdominal pain, and severe weight loss. Marked weakness results from electrolyte loss, and hypocalcemia often causes tetany. Protein is also lost in the stool, and most patients develop peripheral edema from hypoalbuminemia. The ectodermal abnormalities invariably present include alopecia, brownish hyperpigmentation, and atrophy of the fingernails and toenails.

Radiographic examinations demonstrate multiple gastric and colonic polyps. More than half the patients have evidence of small bowel polyps that may be accompanied by thickened mucosal folds and increased intraluminal fluid. Esophageal polyps have been described in two patients.

On histologic examination the polyps, once regarded as adenomas, reveal inflammatory changes of the juve-

nile type. The lesions do not appear to be associated with any potential for gastrointestinal malignancy.

In women the disease generally has an inexorable downhill course resulting in death from inanition and cachexia within 6 to 18 months after the onset of diarrhea. In men there is a tendency for remission.

Juvenile polyposis

Juvenile polyps, although occasionally present in adults, are so named because they generally develop during childhood. These polyps, also called *retention polyps* or *inflammatory polyps,* have typical gross and histologic features that distinguish them from adenomatous polyps and cellular hamartomas. The juvenile polyp usually has a smooth, round contour, whereas adenomatous polyps often have a fissured, lobulated appearance. The lesions are nonneoplastic and have no potential for malignancy.

Most juvenile polyps occur in children as isolated colonic lesions that are either solitary or few in number. Colonic juvenile polyps are less likely to develop as multiple lesions referred to as *juvenile polyposis coli.* Multiple juvenile colonic polyps may (1) exist without extracolonic lesions in cases of juvenile polyposis coli, (2) involve the stomach and small bowel in cases of generalized juvenile polyposis, (3) occur as numerous lesions carpeting the colon in infants, (4) coexist with adenomatous polyps (see Table 8-2) in some patients with familial multiple polyposis or Gardner's syndrome, and (5) develop in the colon in patients with the Cronkhite-Canada syndrome.

Numerous juvenile polyps occasionally develop in the colon and in some instances also in the stomach or small bowel or both. These forms of intestinal juvenile polyposis may be encountered in teenagers and adults, as well as in children. A positive family history is commonly present. In hereditary forms, an autosomal dominant pattern appears to be present. Some patients with juvenile polyposis coli, however, come from families with a history of colon carcinoma. Colonic juvenile polyps and a carcinoma may coexist in rare cases.

A rare, nonfamilial juvenile polyposis syndrome has been described in infants. Most of the affected children have died before 17 months of age.

Differential diagnosis

The differentiation of polyposis coli syndromes from other conditions that may cause multiple filling defects in the colon is summarized in Table 8-1.

RECOMMENDED READING

1. Arminski TC, McLean DW: Incidence and distribution of adenomatous polyps of the colon and rectum based on 1,000 autopsy examinations, *Dis Colon Rectum* 7:249, 1964.

2. Cronkhite LW Jr, Canada WJ: Generalized gastrointestinal polyposis: an unusual syndrome of pigmentation, alopecia, and onychotrophia, *N Engl J Med* 252:1001, 1955.

3. Dodds WJ et al: Peutz-Jeghers syndrome and gastrointestinal malignancy, *Am J Roentgenol* 115:374, 1972.

4. Ecker JA, Doane WA, Dickson DR: Endometriosis of the gastrointestinal tract, *Am J Gastroenterol* 41:405, 1964.

5. Foster MA, Kilcoyne RF: Ruvalcaba-Myhre-Smith syndrome: a new consideration in the differential diagnosis of intestinal polyposis, *Gastrointest Radiol* 11:349, 1986.

6. Itai Y et al: Radiographic features of gastric polyps in familial adenomatosis coli, *Am J Roentgenol* 127:73, 1977.

7. Olmstead WW et al: The solitary colonic polyp: radiologic-histologic differentiation and significance, *Radiology* 160:9, 1986.

8. Orloff MJ: Carcinoid tumors of the rectum, *Cancer* 27:175, 1971.

9. Sachatello CR, Pickren JW, Grace JT: Generalized juvenile gastrointestinal polypsis: a hereditary syndrome, *Gastroenterology* 58:699, 1970.

10. Smith TR: Pedunculated malignant colonic polyps with superficial invasion of the stalks, *Radiology* 115:593, 1975.

11. Ushio K et al: Lesions associated with familial polypsis coli: studies of lesions of the stomach, duodenum, bones and teeth, *Gastrointest Radiol* 1:67, 1976.

Malignancies

GERALD D DODD

In males, colorectal carcinoma is second only to carcinoma of the lung as a cause of cancer death. In females, it is third after carcinoma of the lung and breast cancer. The overall incidence is approximately equal in men and women, with carcinoma of the colon occurring 2.5 times more frequently than carcinoma of the rectum. About 5% of all cases occur in individuals under 30 years of age.

ETIOLOGY

The role of environment in the etiology of colorectal cancer is underscored by epidemiologic studies of migrant populations. The risk of developing carcinoma of the colon is four times greater in native-born citizens of the United States than in Japanese nationals. However, in Japanese who migrate to Hawaii or the continental United States, the incidence of carcinoma of the colon rises to a level equal to that of native-born inhabitants. A high intake of fat and a deficiency in dietary fiber are strongly associated with large bowel carcinogenesis.

It is well established that malignant epithelial tumors are more common in patients with ulcerative colitis than in the general population. Malignancies tend to occur at an early age, primarily in patients with extensive involvement of the colon over many years.

In addition, adenocarcinoma of the colon is a well-documented complication of Crohn's disease. However, no direct link appears to exist between adenocarcinoma and diverticular disease. Patients who have received pelvic radiation are at increased risk, as are those who have had uretero-sigmoidostomy. There is also an increased incidence in women with carcinoma of the breast and/or uterine fundus. A very high incidence of carcinoma of the colon occurs in patients with familial polyposis and with Gardner and Turcot syndromes. A moderate decrease of incidence has been noted in Peutz-Jeghers syndrome. Recently the gene for familial polyposis has been localized on chromosome 5.

Solomon and Voss and co-workers have suggested that loss of an allele on chromosome 5 may also be a critical step in the development of sporadic carcinoma of the colon.

A rare inherited disorder, retinitis pigmentosa, has also been reported to be associated with colon cancer.

Sporadic adenomatous polyps are a definite predisposing factor; malignant changes are found in 5% of tubular adenomas and 40% of villous adenomas. Not all tumors can be shown to arise from preexisting adenomas, and presumably a carcinoma may arise de novo from the colonic mucosa.

Approximately 4% to 5% of patients with colorectal

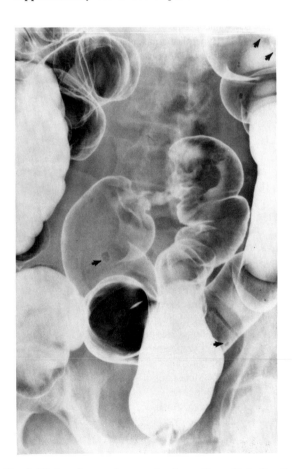

Fig. 8-58 Annular carcinoma of colon with multiple "sentinel" polyps. Of patients with primary colorectal carcinoma, 6.5% will have multiple tumors, including polyps *(arrows)*.

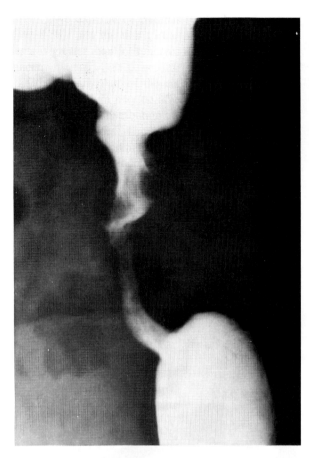

Fig. 8-61 Scirrhous carcinoma of descending colon. Margins of tumor show tapered appearance usually associated with inflammatory disease. Nodular component is seen proximally, but distal lumen is smooth. These tumors tend to infiltrate submucosally, and mucous membrane may be intact. Pathologic appearance is similar to linitis plastica type of carcinoma of stomach.

Tumors developing in patients with chronic ulcerative colitis, presumably because of longstanding mucosal disease and attendant scarring, tend to spread submucosally through the lymphatics and resemble strictures (Fig. 8-62). Because about 11% of patients with ulcerative colitis will develop strictures, all abnormal narrowings of the lumen should be considered potential malignancies and must be evaluated accordingly.

Ulcerative pattern

The least common radiographic appearance of colonic carcinoma is the primary ulcerative type. Ulceration may occur early and produce a deep, excavating lesion. The margins of the ulcers are usually elevated and sometimes have a nodular appearance. When seen in profile, the ulcer is meniscoid and surrounded by a collar of tumor tissue (Fig. 8-63).

Squamous cell carcinoma

Squamous cell carcinomas are rare except in the anal area. The radiographic characteristics do not differ significantly from those of adenocarcinoma. In a few reported cases, tumors of this type have shown a tendency toward annular constriction. Differentiation from other tumors is made only at biopsy.

Cloacogenic carcinomas

Cloacogenic carcinomas, which arise from the transitional cloacogenic remnants of the anorectal junction, present definite pathologic and radiographic appearances. These carcinomas are from the anal ducts and vary in their histologic structures. Three different types have been described: (1) transitional cell carcinomas, (2) squamous cell carcinomas, and (3) mucoid adenocarcinomas. Cloacogenic carcinomas spread predominantly by direct invasion of adjacent structures. Lymphatic involvement with spread to the regional nodes is also common. On radiographic examination the lesions appear plaquelike and have a smooth or finely irregular surface. In profile, the borders form a tapered, obtuse angle with the bowel wall, in contrast to the acute angle associated with sessile and polypoid masses. Ulceration is usually present, and fistulas may occur. Because the lesions lie in the distal rectal area, the enema tip may completely obscure the tumor (Fig. 8-64).

Villous adenoma

In villous adenomas the stroma is characterized by delicate fronds of connective tissue. Its surface is covered with columnar epithelial cells, which are often multilayered and active in mucous production. The lesions are usually sessile and bulky, and occur more often in the rectum. The mass of the tumor rarely obstructs the bowel, but it can produce intussusception and secondary bowel obstruction. On radiograph the tumors are recognized by linear streaks produced by barium lodged between the frond ends (Fig. 8-65). It is not possible to distinguish between the benign and malignant varieties on radiographic examination. Size is not a good criterion of benignity or malignancy.

Argentaffin carcinomas

Argentaffin carcinomas or *carcinoid tumors* rarely occur in the large bowel; they are found most often in the rectum. They usually present as a submucosal tumor, and a rounded, well-circumscribed mass is the most common radiographic appearance. After invasion of the bowel wall, the intense proliferation of fibrous tissue caused by the tumor may produce contraction and kinking of the large bowel.

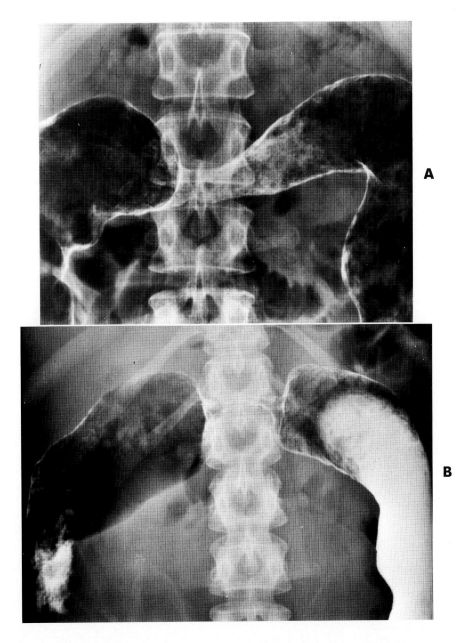

Fig. 8-62 Carcinoma of colon in case of chronic ulcerative colitis. **A,** Transverse colon shows narrowed segment with tapered margins. There is nothing to suggest mass, but characteristic changes of ulcerative colitis are seen elsewhere in bowel.

Mesodermal sarcomas

Mesodermal sarcomas of the large bowel are uncommon. The most frequent are those of smooth-muscle origin, and they have a predilection for the rectal region. The lesions are frequently rounded and lobulated but may sometimes be pedunculated. The tumors may grow extramurally, and when the overlying mucosa ulcerates, necrosis and cystic cavitation may develop (Fig. 8-66).

Kaposi's sarcoma can involve any portion of the

gastrointestinal tract and presents as a typical extramucosal mass or masses. Formerly a rare entity, this sarcoma is now seen with increasing frequency in patients with acquired immunodeficiency syndrome.

Lymphomas of the colon

Colonic lymphoma, whether primary or a manifestation of systemic disease, is rare. Primary lymphoma affects the cecum and rectum more often than other parts

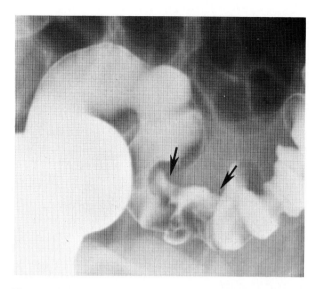

Fig. 8-63 Ulcerative carcinoma of sigmoid colon. All features of Carman-Kirklin complex are present. Extensively ulcerated tumor is surrounded by nodular collar of tumor tissue *(arrows)*.

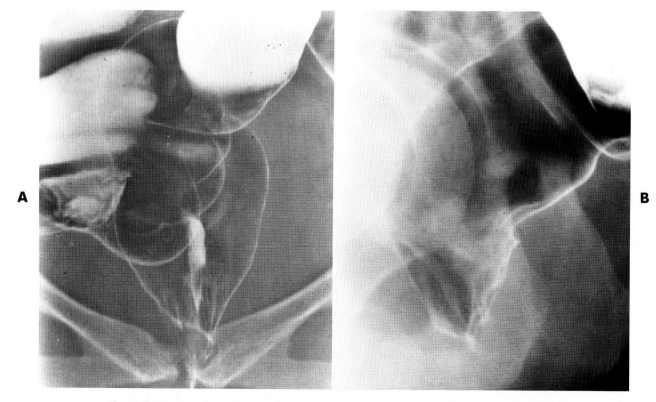

Fig. 8-64 Cloacogenic carcinoma. **A,** Linear ulcer in lower rectum extends to point just above internal sphincter. There is also infolding of mucous membrane on either side of inferior aspect of ulcer. **B,** Plaquelike defect is seen on posterior rectal wall. This is covered by mucous membrane but shows central irregularity that corresponds to ulceration. Location of tumor and submucosal component are typical of cloacogenic carcinoma.

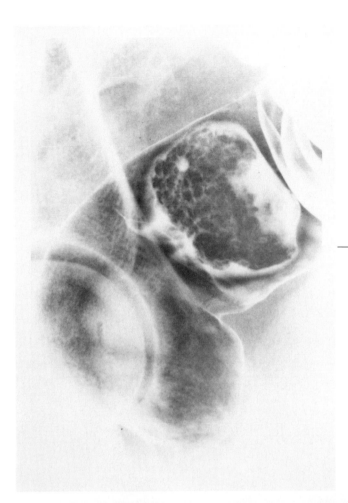

Fig. 8-65 Villous adenoma of rectum. Pedicle is broad, and tumor fills majority of lumen. Fine lacelike pattern results from seepage of barium into interstices between individual tumor fronds. Size is not necessarily indicative of malignancy with villous adenomas, but all have malignant potential.

Fig. 8-66 Ulcerating leiomyosarcoma of rectum. **A,** In anteroposterior view there is smoothly marginated mass with submucosal characteristics. Large ulcer is present in center of tumor. **B,** In lateral projection irregular nature of ulcer is easily appreciated. Combination of extramucosal mass and central excavation should suggest tumor of mesenchymal origin.

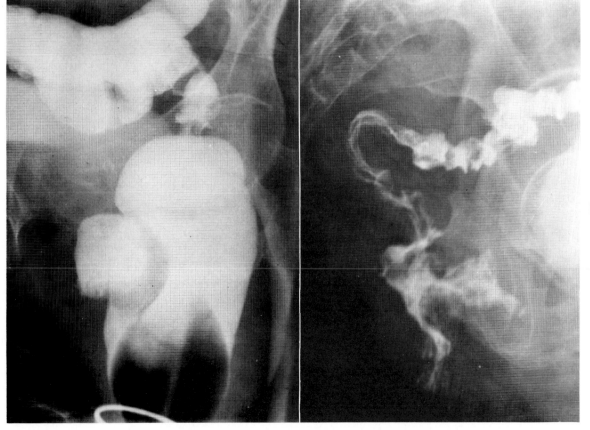

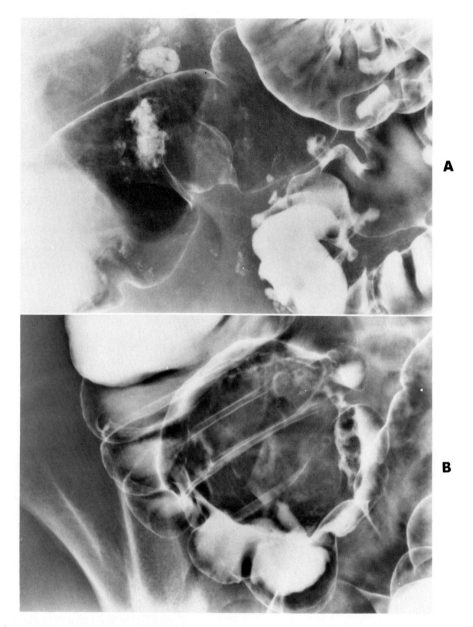

Fig. 8-67 Localized polypoid lymphoma of colon. **A,** Rectosigmoid. **B,** Cecum. Masses exhibit extramucosal characteristics.

of the colon. Secondary involvement is usually widely distributed and often multicentric. There are two main radiographic patterns. In the localized form the lesion is either a polypoid mass that protrudes into the colonic lumen (Fig. 8-67) or a constricting lesion that simulates an annular carcinoma. In the diffuse form, multiple small nodular lesions, varying in diameter from 0.5 to 2.0 cm, are usually seen. The defects are characteristically submucosal in origin, with the overlying mucous membrane intact. When lymphoma involves the mesentery, large masses may compress the colon.

METASTASES

Tumors that most commonly metastasize to the colon include stomach, breast, pancreas, and gynecologic pelvic malignancies. Secondary involvement of the colon can occur by direct invasion from contiguous neoplasms or by spread along mesenteric fascial planes and/or lymphatic channels. It can also occur by intraperitoneal seeding of tumor along pathways or intraperitoneal fluid movement or by embolic hematogenous spread. The classic radiographic appearance includes indentations, spiculation, angulation, narrowing, displacement, fixation, and serosal plaques (Fig. 8-68). When the metastases are produced by hematogenous spread, as in melanoma, the lesions present as smoothly marginated, submucosal masses, sometimes with ulceration. Lymphogenous spread of tumors to the colon is characterized by the involvement of long segments, variable areas of narrowing, loss of haustral markings, and a granular mucosal pattern with or without superficial ulceration. Associated primary tumors usually arise in the breast or stomach. Radiologic differentiation from primary scirrhous tumors of the colon may not be possible.

COMPLICATIONS

Obstruction produced by a carcinoma that surrounds and narrows the lumen occurs most frequently in the descending and sigmoid segments of the bowel. The narrowing is often augmented by inflammation, fibrosis, and impacted fecal material. With single- or double-contrast studies, the distal margins of the lesion stand out in abrupt relief against the normal adjacent mucosa. On occasion, some of the contrast material will enter the narrowed segment, but overdistension of the distal segment of bowel will frequently compromise the residual lumen and produce complete obstruction to the retrograde flow of the opaque material.

Perforating carcinoma of the colon is also a relatively common complication if all types are included. Free perforation, localized perforation with pericolic abscess, and perforation with fistula formation into adjacent organs may occur.

Carcinomas involving the transverse portion of the colon tend to be constrictive; however, they also tend toward intramural growth and direct extramural extension to contiguous organs such as the stomach. Gastrocolic fistulas are occasionally encountered, mainly in advanced cases. Perforating carcinomas involving the splenic flexure may produce a left subphrenic abscess. Rectal carcinomas involving the anterior wall may grow into the rectovaginal septum and lead to a rectovaginal fistula. Invasion of the urinary bladder may result in a rectovesical fistula.

Intussusception of the large bowel is rare in adults. The usual cause is a polypoid neoplasm of the cecum or ascending colon (Fig. 8-69). If barium enters the lumen of the intussuscipiens, the picture of narrow parallel folds surrounded by a coillike pattern (intussusceptum) is pathognomonic. The CT appearance of intussusception is also distinctive. Both the intussusceptum and intussuscipiens are readily identified (Fig. 8-70). The tumor itself is usually not identifiable by either method of examination until the intussusception is reduced.

In longstanding colonic obstruction, ischemic colitis may develop proximal to the point of obstruction. The

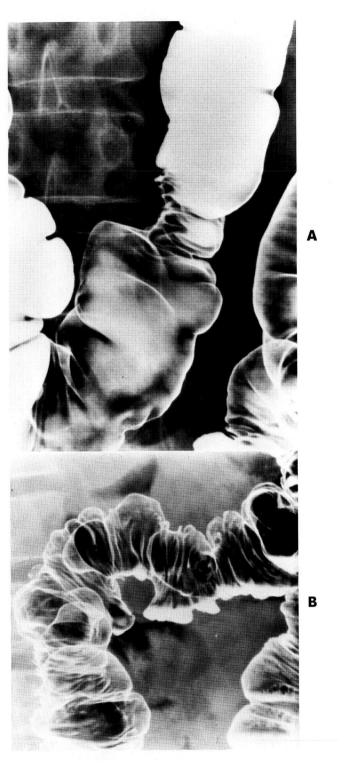

Fig. 8-68 Metastatic carcinoma of breast to colon. **A,** There is solitary deposit in mesocolon adjacent to bowel wall. Lumen is reduced in caliber, and incisurae are apparent on opposing side. Mucous membrane overlying defect shows typical pleating or tacking appearance. Residuum of trauma or inflammatory disease may produce similar changes. **B,** Pseudodiverticula formation as result of irregular infiltration of opposing bowel margin. Bizarre configuration of mucosal folds is most apparent in proximal transverse colon.

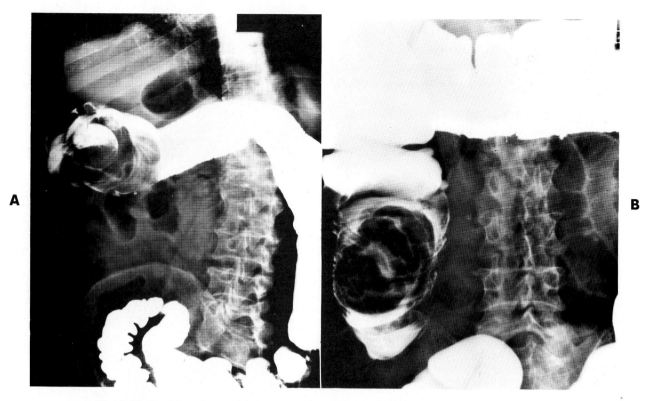

Fig. 8-69 Cecal lymphoma with intussusception. Patient complained of crampy abdominal pain and bleeding through rectum. **A,** Typical appearance of intussuscepting mass in transverse colon. **B,** Cecal mass is apparent following reduction of intussusception by hydrostatic pressure.

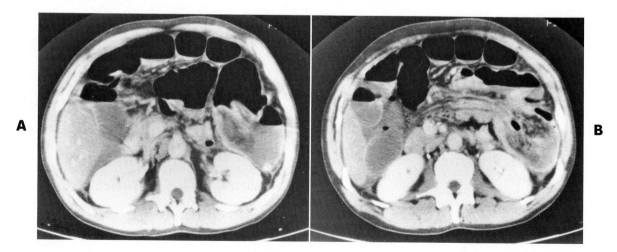

Fig. 8-70 Intussuscepting villous adenoma of cecum. **A,** Abdominal CT demonstrates intussusceptum and intussuscipiens with invaginated bowel pushed eccentrically by radiolucent mesenteric fat. The small bowel is obstructed. **B,** At lower level small bowel is included in intussusception. (Courtesy Dr. Rajani Surapaneni.)

mucosa becomes ulcerated, resembling ulcerative colitis. Air can leak through the ulcers and dissect the colonic wall, producing an acute form of extraluminal pneumatosis.

DIFFERENTIAL DIAGNOSIS

Benign strictures caused by peridiverticulitis are the most common differential problem. Destruction of the mucous membrane is the most reliable radiographic criterion for differentiating carcinoma from a peridiverticular abscess (Fig. 8-71). Inflammatory lesions simulating carcinoma, such as tuberculosis and amebic colitis, are rare. The transverse colon is a common site of involvement following cholecystitis, pancreatitis, and gastric or pancreatic carcinoma. Radiation strictures of the large bowel are common sequelae of therapy for carcinoma of the cervix, bladder, or uterus. The most common sites of stricture formation are the rectosig-

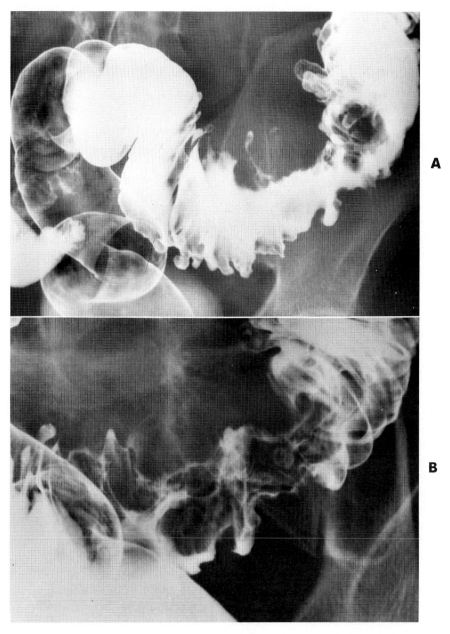

Fig. 8-71 Carcinoma of colon simulating peridiverticular abscess. **A,** Presence of diverticula and indistinct tumor margins suggests possibility of inflammatory origin. **B,** Double contrast technique shows destruction of mucous membrane, central ulceration, and typical shelving margins of primary tumor. There is adenomatous polyp at proximal end of carcinoma.

☐ **DIFFERENTIAL DIAGNOSIS OF MULTIPLE COLONIC FILLING DEFECTS** ☐

1. Foreign material
   a. Fecal material
   b. Gas bubbles
   c. Ingested foreign bodies
2. Inflammatory pseudopolyps
   a. Ulcerative colitis
   b. Granulomatous colitis
   c. Amebiasis
   d. Schistosomiasis
   e. Antibiotic colitis
   f. Ischemic colitis
   g. Radiation
3. Pneumatosis
4. Lymphoid tissue
   a. Benign lymphoid hyperplasia
   b. Lymphonodular hyperplasia
   c. Lymphgiectasis

5. Nonneoplastic processes
   a. Cystic fibrosis
   b. Tuberous sclerosis
   c. Amyloidosis
   d. Urticaria
   e. Herpes zoster
   f. Ischemic thumbprints
   g. Cowden's disease
   h. Giant hyperplastic polyposis
6. Benign neoplasms
   a. Lipomatosis
   b. Hemangiomatosis
   c. Lymphangiomatosis
   d. Neurofibromatosis
   e. Ganglioneuromatosis

7. Malignant tumors
   a. Lymphoma
   b. Leukemia
   c. Kaposi's sarcoma
   d. Metastases
8. Polyposis syndromes
   a. Familial multiple polyposis
   b. Gardner's syndrome
   c. Peutz-Jeghers syndrome
   d. Turcot's syndrome
   e. Cowden's disease
   f. Cronkhite-Canada syndrome
   g. Juvenile polyposis

---

moid and sigmoid regions. Abscess formation secondary to perforation of the colon following radiation therapy is indistinguishable from tumor or peridiverticulitis. Strictures resulting from endometriosis may cause symptoms of partial bowel obstruction. The most common areas of involvement are the rectum and the sigmoid colon. Extrinsic masses, including endometriomas, may cause a narrowing of the colonic diameter, but when they are visualized in profile, the extracolonic origin is usually apparent. Filling defects caused by benign tumors and fecal material must also be distinguished from polypoid carcinomas.

NEOPLASTIC STAGING

Modern radiography plays two roles in the evaluation of colonic tumors. In the first instance, radiography is used primarily for diagnostic purposes. Second, radiography is employed to assess the extent of colonic and extracolonic involvement (staging) or to determine the response to therapy or the presence of recurrent tumor in the posttreatment state.

The prognosis of carcinoma of the colon depends on the degree of intramural and extramural extension and on whether lymph nodes or other structures are involved. Survival rates decrease as the extent of disease increases. Limited or moderate degrees of submucosal extension or lymphatic involvement are usually not detected by conventional barium studies. Extracolonic spread may be assumed only when there is obvious invasion of an adjacent organ or perforation into adjacent organs or cavities. Experience has also shown that CT is not a reliable routine preoperative staging procedure for colorectal carcinomas. Small areas of periluminal infiltration may not be visualized, and involvement of nodes less than 1.5 cm in size is infrequently detected (Fig. 8-72). In general, CT should be reserved for patients in whom extensive disease is suspected. CT is helpful in evaluation of the liver and, on occasion, may be of value in patients whose conditions suggest complications such as intussusception or perforation (Fig. 8-73; see Fig. 8-70).

The accuracy of CT in the evaluation of suspected recurrences is significantly better than for preoperative staging. CT examination has proved accurate in detecting local recurrences, as well as lymph node metastases (Fig. 8-74), but difficulties are encountered in distinguishing recurrence from postoperative changes such as hematomas, abscesses, fibrosis, and displaced pelvic structures. In patients with equivocal changes, a final determination can frequently be made by means of a CT-guided aspiration biopsy.

In a series of advanced cases, Butch and co-workers found CT and MR imaging to be equally effective in staging rectal cancer (Figs. 8-75 to 8-77). Both techniques identified the primary tumor and invasion into the perirectal fat and regional organs. Neither was able to assess the degree of bowel wall infiltration or the presence or absence of tumor within normal-sized lymph nodes.

In posttreatment states, despite early hopes, MRI imaging probably cannot distinguish between recurrent tumor, fibrosis, and inflammation.

Transrectal sonography shows great promise in the staging of rectal cancers. It can distinguish the normal

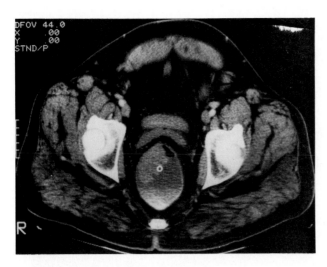

Fig. 8-72 Villous adenoma of rectum. Intraluminal mass is obvious, but presence or absence of serosal or small lymph node involvement cannot be determined.

layers of the bowel wall and demonstrate disruption of one or more of these by tumor. The detection of regional lymph node metastases is less satisfactory, with a sensitivity of 50% to 57%.

Monoclonal body imaging and positron emission tomography have shown considerable promise as staging procedures, but general use depends on further equipment development and availability of appropriate radionuclides.

Pulmonary metastases may be diagnosed by conventional chest radiography. Hepatic imaging by any of several methods may be used in cases of suspected liver metastases. Bone metastases occur in the later stages of the disease, and are usually blastic; they most often involve the axial skeleton.

RECOMMENDED READINGS

1. Adalsteinsson B, Pahlman A, Glimelius B et al: Computed tomography in early diagnosis of local recurrence of rectal carcinoma, *Acta Radiol* 28:41, 1987.
2. Baker HL, Good CA: Smooth-muscle tumors of the alimentary tract; their roentgen manifestations. *Am J Roentgenol* 74:246, 1955.
3. Balthazar EJ, Rosenberg HD, Davidian MM: Primary and metastatic scirrous carcinoma of the rectum, *Am J Roentgenol* 132:711, 1979.
4. Balthazar EJ, Megibow AJ, Hulnick D et al: Carcinoma of the colon, detection and preoperative staging by CT, *Am J Roentgenol* 150:301, 1988.
5. Bodmer WF et al: Localization of the gene for familial adenomatosis polyposis on chromosome 5, *Nature* 328:Aug 13, 1987.
6. Burkitt DP: Large-bowel cancer: an epidemiologic jigsaw puzzle, *J Natl Cancer Inst* 54:3, 1975.
7. Dodd GD: Genetics and cancer of the gastrointestinal system, *Radiology* 123:263, 1977.

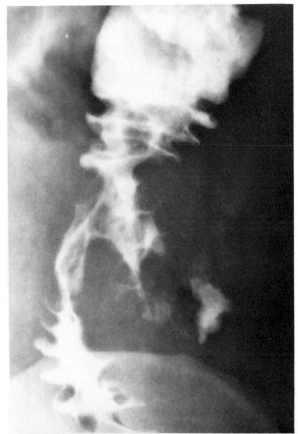

A

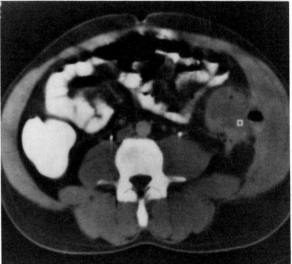

B

Fig. 8-73 Perforated carcinoma of colon. **A,** Single-contrast enema. No diverticuli are seen, but mucosal detail is lacking. Differentiation is not possible. **B,** CT confirms perforation, but necrotic mass could be of inflammatory origin.

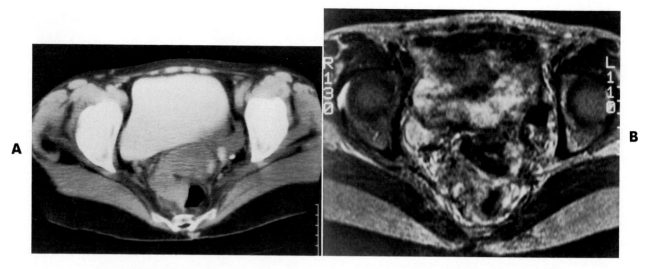

Fig. 8-74 Squamous cell carcinoma of rectum with invasion of uterosacral ligament. **A,** CT scan showing rectal deformity with extraluminal mass and involvement of the uterosacral ligament and posterior uterine surface on right. **B,** MR T_2-weighted image. Extent of involvement is the same.

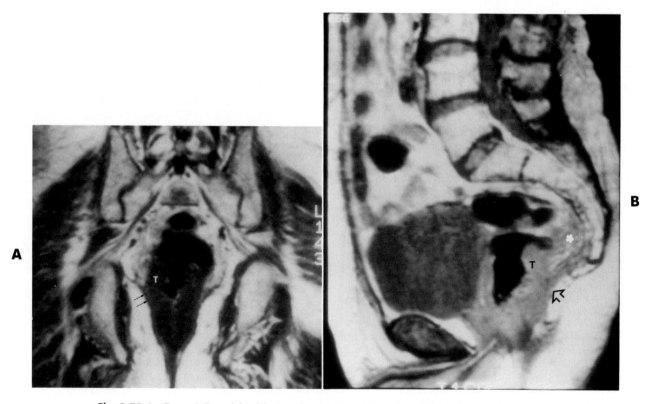

Fig. 8-75 A, Coronal T_1-weighted image showing large circumferential carcinoma of rectum extending into anal canal. Note extension well below levator ani insertion *(arrow)*. This extension totally changes surgical approach and makes anterior resection impossible. In such cases, colostomy with abdominoperineal resection is needed. **B,** Proton density sagittal image shows extension of carcinoma *(c)* below insertion of pubococcygeal muscle *(open arrow)* almost to anal verge. Tumor extends into fat posteriorly.

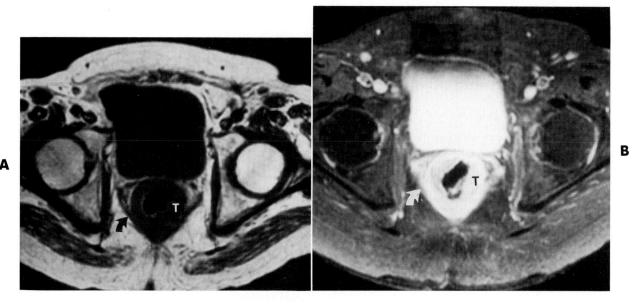

Fig. 8-76 A, T_1-weighted axial image showing carcinoma of rectum *(T)* at level of puborectalis sling. **B,** Same level; T_1-weighted fat-saturated image following intravenous gadolinium DTPA injection. Note tumor extent throughout wall of rectum enhanced by signal, and invasion of the puborectalis muscle *(curved arrow)*.

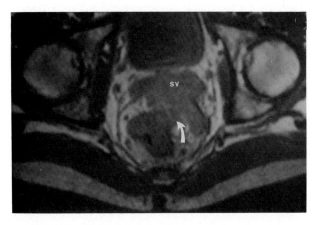

Fig. 8-77 Proton density axial image of carcinoma of prostate invading left seminal vesicle *(sv)* and rectum *(arrow)*.

8. Ebner F, Kressel HY, Mintz MC et al: Tumor recurrence versus fibrosis in the female pelvis, differentiation with MR imaging at 1.5T, *Radiology* 166:333, 1988.

9. Freeny PC et al: Colorectal carcinoma evaluation with CT; preoperative staging and detection of postoperative recurrence, *Radiology* 158:397, 1986.

10. Glotzer DJ, Roth SI Welch CE: Colonic ulceration proximal to obstructing carcinoma, *Surgery* 56:950, 1964.

11. Hildebrandt U, Feifel G: Preoperative staging of rectal by intrarectal ultrasound, *Dis Colon Rectum,* 28:42, 1985.

12. Holdsworth PJ, Johnston D, Chalmers, AG et al: Endoluminal ultrasound and computed tomography in staging of rectal cancer, *Br J Surg* 75:1019, 1988.

13. Kelly WE et al: Penetrating, obstructing and perforating carcinomas of the colon and rectum, *Arch Surg* 116:381, 1981.

14. Kyaw MM, Gallagher T, Haines JO: Cloacogenic carcinoma of anorectal junction: roentgenographic diagnosis, *Am J Roentgenol* 115:384, 1972.

15. MacDougall IPM: The cancer risk in ulcerative colitis, *Lancet* 2:655, 1964.

16. O'Connell DJ, Thompson AJ: Lymphoma of the colon: the spectrum of radiologic changes, *Gastrointest Radiol* 2:377, 1978.

17. Rafto SE, Amendola MA, Gefter WB: MR imaging of recurrent colorectal carcinoma versus fibrosis, *J Comput Assist Tomogr* 12(3):521-523, 1988.

18. Rifkin MD, Erlich SM, Marks G: Staging of rectal carcinoma: prospective comparison of endorectal US and CT, *Radiology* 170:319, 1989.

19. Skucas J, Spataro R et al: The radiographic features of small colon cancers, *Radiology* 143:355, 1982.

20. Thompson WM, Halvorsen RA Jr: Computed tomographic staging of gastrointestinal malignancies. II. The small bowel, colon and rectum, *Invest Radiol* 22:96, 1987.

21. Thoeni RF: Colorectal cancer: cross-sectional imaging for staging of primary tumor and detection of local recurrence, *Am J Roentgenol* 156:909, 1991.

22. Winzelberg GG, Greenstein R, Ferrucci JT: Retinitis pigmentosa and colon cancer: a previously unreported association, *Cancer* 45:28976, 1980.

23. Zornoza J, Dodd GD: Lymphoma of the gastrointestinal tract, *Semin Roentgenol* 15:272, 1980.

9 *Pancreas*

PATRICK C FREENY
BRIAN C LENTLE
GEORGE R LEOPOLD
DAVID KB LI
CHARLES A ROHRMANN JR
DAVID H STEPHENS

ANATOMY

DIAGNOSTIC EXAMINATION
  Computed tomography
  Ultrasonography
  Magnetic resonance imaging
  Radionuclide examination
  Endoscopic retrograde cholangiopancreatography
  Percutaneous transhepatic cholangiography
  Angiography
  Transhepatic pancreatic venography
  Fine-needle aspiration biopsy
  Fine-needle fluid aspiration and percutaneous
    pancreatography

NONNEOPLASTIC LESIONS OF THE PANCREAS
  Pancreatitis
  Congenital abnormalities

NEOPLASTIC LESIONS OF THE PANCREAS
  Adenocarcinoma (ductal carcinoma)
  Unusual carcinomas of the exocrine pancreas
  Cystic neoplasms
  Islet cell neoplasms (apudomas)
  Nonepithelial neoplasms
  Metastic neoplasms

Anatomy

Normal anatomy

The pancreatic features assessable by imaging include gland size and parenchymal texture pattern, pancreatic duct caliber, wall thickness and regularity, the presence of intraductal filling defects (calculi or neoplasms), peripancreatic blood vessels, and intrapancreatic and extrapancreatic bile duct anatomy. The pancreatic duct usually measures only 2 to 3 mm. High-resolution transducers typically display the celiac, superior, mesenteric, hepatic, splenic, superior mesenteric, and portal veins.

Regional anatomy

The splenic vein serves as a marker for the body and tail of the pancreas. Identification of the inferior vena cava helps to localize the pancreatic head, which abuts the anterior (ventral) surface of the inferior vena cava, and is usually apparent on both transverse and sagittal scans. The position of the head relative to the portal vein varies considerably. If sagittal scanning is carried out slightly medial to the pancreatic head, the superior mesenteric vein is seen ventral and parallel to the inferior vena cava or abdominal aorta. The uncinate process may be seen just posterior to the vein.

Transverse scans of the pancreatic head provide information about the intrapancreatic portion of the common bile duct. In most individuals the duct appears as an echogenic line in the center of the gland. A width of more than 4 mm is abnormal.

Diagnostic examination

Pancreatic disease produces a variety of morphologic changes that can be detected by different imaging mo-

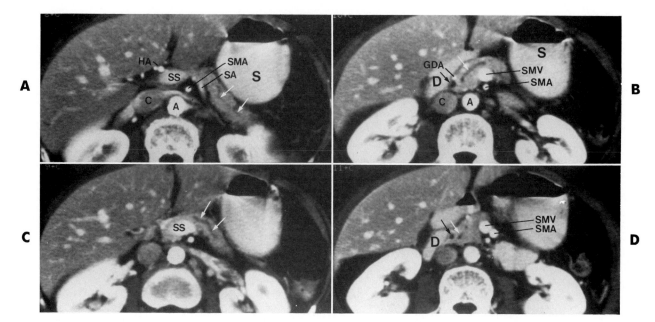

Fig. 9-1 Pancreatic CT. **A** and **B,** Contiguous 10 mm bolus-dynamic scans show normal pancreatic duct *(white arrows)* in body and tail of gland. **C** and **D,** Scans at level of head show pancreatic duct *(white arrows)* and common bile duct *(black arrows)* on cross section. Contrast opacifies stomach *(S)* and duodenum *(D)*. *HA,* hepatic artery; *GDA,* gastroduodenal artery; *SA,* splenic artery; *SMA,* superior mesenteric artery; *SMV,* superior mesenteric vein; *A,* aorta; *C,* inferior vena cava; *SS,* junction of splenic vein and superior mesenteric vein.

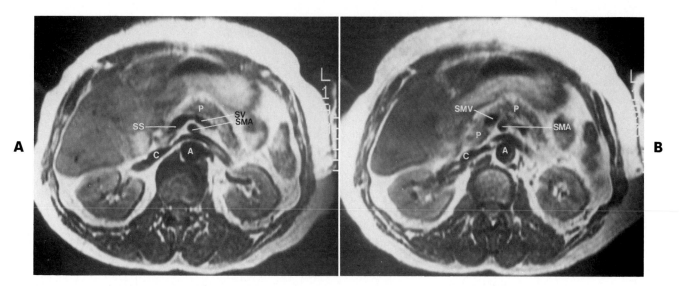

Fig. 9-2 Pancreatic MRI. **A** and **B,** Normal pancreas MRI (1.5 T; SE, TR 2000/TE 25) shows gland parenchyma *(P)* as area of low signal intensity. Gland is surrounded by peripancreatic fat of high signal intensity. Peripancreatic vessels have no signal (flow void), indicating vessel patency. *A,* aorta; *C,* inferior vena cava; *SMA,* superior mesenteric artery; *SMV,* superior mesenteric vein; *SV,* splenic vein; *SS,* junction of superior mesenteric and splenic veins.

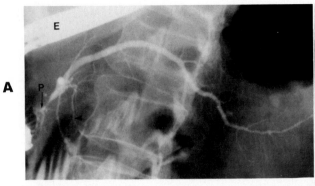

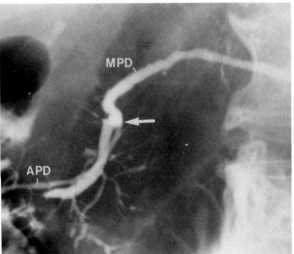

Fig. 9-3 Normal ERCP. **A,** Main pancreatic duct shows smooth, tapering walls from papilla *(P)* to tail. Lateral side branches are evenly spaced. Larger branches from uncinate are seen *(arrowheads)*. *E,* endoscope. **B,** Close-up of normal ERCP of head of pancreas shows junction *(arrow)* of accessory (APD) and main (MPD) pancreatic ducts.

dalities. Although plain radiographs depict changes in the chest or abdomen that result from pancreatic disease, they do not image the gland directly, with the exception of showing pancreatic ductal calcifications or a soft tissue mass in the region of the pancreas. The cross-sectional imaging modalities of ultrasonography (US), computed tomography (CT) (Fig. 9-1), and magnetic resonance imaging (MRI) (Fig. 9-2) visualize the pancreatic parenchyma, main pancreatic duct and biliary tract, major peripancreatic blood vessels, and the organs and structures surrounding the pancreas. Endoscopic retrograde cholangiopancreatography (ERCP) (Fig. 9-3) images only the pancreatic or biliary ducts. Percutaneous needle aspiration is employed to obtain blood or tissue samples for laboratory evaluation.

The initial diagnostic procedure and subsequent sequence of examination for evaluation of patients with suspected pancreatic disease depends on the specific disease and the structures of the gland (for example, parenchyma, blood vessels, ducts) most likely to be involved by the pathologic process.

The techniques of ERCP and percutaneous transhepatic cholangiography (PTC) have been extended to encompass *interventional procedures*. Endoscopic placement of biliary and pancreatic duct stents and endoscopic papillotomy can be used for treatment of ductal obstruction caused by both neoplastic and inflammatory diseases. Biliary duct obstruction also can be relieved by percutaneous transhepatic catheter or endoprosthesis placement.

COMPUTED TOMOGRAPHY

CT is currently the most important imaging technique for the pancreas. It has a high diagnostic accuracy rate for both neoplastic and inflammatory disease, and most clinicians and radiologists now agree that if symptoms are clearly related to the pancreas, CT is the test of choice. Possible exceptions are children and pregnant patients. The best anatomic detail is obtained using 5 or 10 mm collimation and contiguous scans. Intravenous contrast material is administered as a bolus (see Fig. 9-1).

ULTRASONOGRAPHY

Now the preferred test for evaluating the gallbladder, ultrasonography often uncovers unsuspected pancreatic disease. The lower cost and the ability to bring the imaging equipment to the bedside of a critically ill patient are major advantages. Radiologists interested in gastrointestinal disease now wield real-time ultrasound machines with the same aplomb once accorded the fluoroscope. Yet, as before, instrumentation is far less important than the examiner's understanding of anatomy and pathology (Fig. 9-4).

Techniques
Real-time sonography

Current real-time scanners usually employ transducers that operate at a frequency of 3 to 7.5 MHz. The transducers can be oriented in virtually any plane. Because intestinal gas interferes with sonographic imaging, the liver, spleen, and kidneys often are used as acoustic windows. As an alternative, the stomach and duodenum can be filled with orally ingested fluid, yielding a temporary window. The examiner quickly observes the orientation of the major upper abdominal viscera, such as the liver and gallbladder. An assessment of the left hepatic lobe is important, because a large or

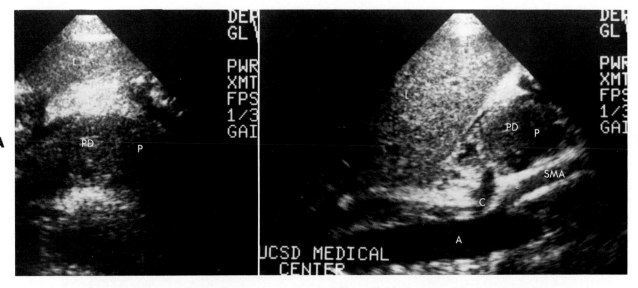

Fig. 9-4 A, Transverse US scan showing markedly enlarged, sonolucent pancreas *(P)* as compared to the more echogenic left lobe of liver *(L); PD,* pancreatic duct. **B,** Sagittal scan of same patient demonstrates relationships of the enlarged pancreas to the celiac *(C)* and superior mesenteric arteries *(SMA). A,* Aorta.

prominent left lobe usually facilitates pancreatic scanning.

Endoscopic sonography

The combination of ultrasonography with endoscopy has several compelling advantages. In addition to elim-

inating bowel gas problems, it permits use of high-frequency transducers (7.5 MHz), which have much improved resolution. Early reports indicate considerable success with endoscopic sonography in pancreatic diagnosis.

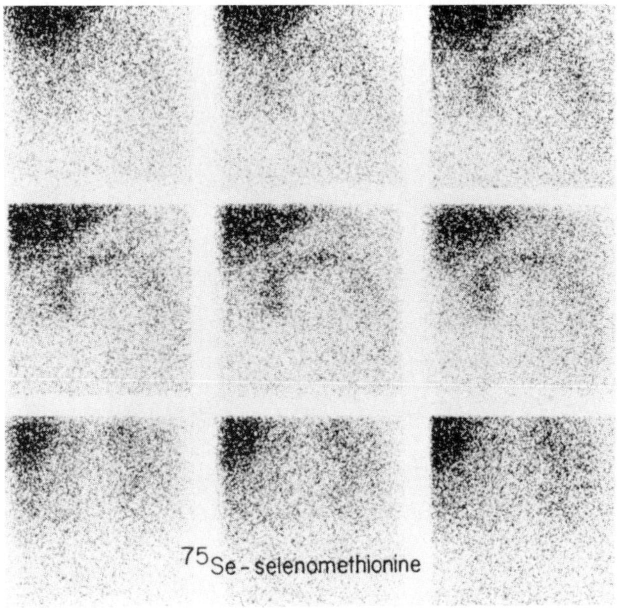

MAGNETIC RESONANCE IMAGING

MRI is the newest imaging technique to be applied to the pancreas. Though it has not yet significantly improved diagnosis of pancreatic disease, MRI holds much promise for the future. MRI displays the normal pancreatic parenchyma, peripancreatic blood vessels, and upper abdominal solid organs, but it does not reliably show the pancreatic duct or surrounding hollow organs as well as does CT.

RADIONUCLIDE EXAMINATION

It is something of a paradox that the pancreas is metabolically active but that its examination by radionuclide methods has virtually ceased to have any role in day-to-day clinical practice (Fig. 9-5).

ENDOSCOPIC RETROGRADE CHOLANGIOPANCREATOGRAPHY

The pancreatic ducts can be altered by both inflammatory and neoplastic disease. Thus ERCP is highly sensitive for diagnosis of ductal carcinoma and pancreatitis. Interventional ERCP techniques applicable to the pancreas include *endoscopic papillotomy* and *endoscopic placement of biliary and pancreatic duct stents*

Fig. 9-5 Coronal sectional images of a normal pancreas made with ^{75}Se-selenomethionine. Note uptake of tracer in liver.

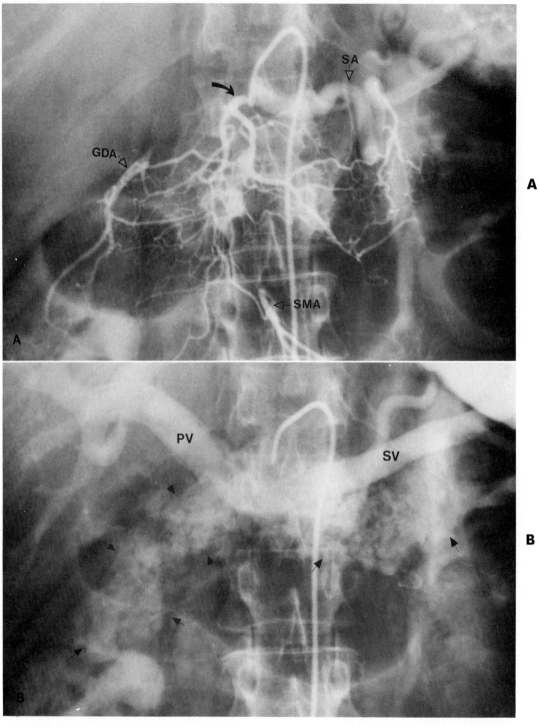

Fig. 9-6 Pancreatic angiogram. **A** and **B,** High-volume selective dorsal pancreatic artery *(curved arrow)* injection. **A,** (Arterial phase) shows filling of intrapancreatic vessels and retrograde filling of splenic *(SA)*, gastroduodenal (GDA), and superior mesenteric (SMA) arteries *(arrows)*. Parenchymal phase, **B,** shows normal lobular pattern of pancreatic parenchyma *(arrows)* and filling of splenic vein *(SV)* and portal vein *(PV)*.

for treatment of benign and malignant ductal obstruction.

PERCUTANEOUS TRANSHEPATIC CHOLANGIOGRAPHY

The intrapancreatic segment of the common bile duct is often altered by carcinoma or pancreatitis, and PTC can be used for diagnostic evaluation of the biliary ducts if obstructive jaundice is present. The technique may also be extended for percutaneous placement of transhepatic or endoprosthetic biliary drainage catheters.

ANGIOGRAPHY

CT and ERCP have replaced angiography for diagnosis of most pancreatic diseases. However, angiography continues to play an important role in evaluating patients with equivocal CT or ERCP findings, in assessing vascular anatomy before pancreatic surgery (Fig. 9-6), and in diagnosing and controlling pancreatic hemorrhage, which is usually caused by severe pancreatic inflammatory disease.

TRANSHEPATIC PANCREATIC VENOGRAPHY

In some patients with functioning islet cell tumors, the primary tumor cannot be localized preoperatively by CT, MRI, US, or angiography. In these patients, transhepatic pancreatic venography (TPV) with selective venous sampling is a useful method for tumor localization.

FINE-NEEDLE ASPIRATION BIOPSY

Pancreatic masses often have a nonspecific appearance and may be caused by inflammatory disease or by different types of neoplasm. Though ductal adenocarcinoma is usually incurable, other neoplasms, such as islet cell carcinoma and lymphoma, may respond to chemotherapy or radiation therapy, or may be curable by surgical resection. Thus a specific pathologic diagnosis must be made to ensure proper patient management. This can be accomplished safely and effectively with radiologically-guided fine-needle aspiration biopsy (FNAB) (Fig. 9-7).

Most pancreatic biopsies are performed with a 22- or 23-gauge needle. Precise guidance that permits visualization of the needle tip results in a positive biopsy in about 80% to 85% of cases. Examples of guidance techniques are fluoroscopic guidance with ERCP, angiography, PTC, bile duct drainage catheter, or endoprosthesis for targeting; CT; or sonography with transducer biopsy guide. Recent reports indicate improved results with similar safety using an 18-gauge cutting biopsy needle operated with a spring-driven biopsy gun.

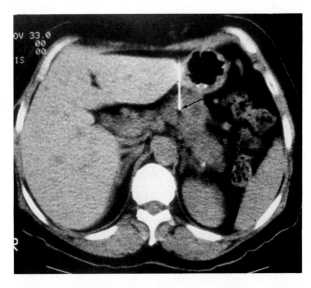

Fig. 9-7 FNAB. CT-guided FNAB shows 23-gauge needle *(arrow)* in focal mass (adenocarcinoma) in pancreatic body.

FINE-NEEDLE FLUID ASPIRATION AND PERCUTANEOUS PANCREATOGRAPHY

Using the same techniques as described for aspiration biopsy, 22- and 23-gauge needles can be placed in pancreatic fluid collections in patients with pancreatitis to determine the presence of infection. The pancreatic duct can also be punctured percutaneously under imaging guidance and contrast material may be injected to delineate the ductal anatomy.

Nonneoplastic lesions of the pancreas

PANCREATITIS
Radiologic diagnosis
Acute pancreatitis
PATRICK C FREENY
CHARLES A ROHRMANN JR

The diagnosis of acute pancreatitis is based on clinical and laboratory findings. Included in the differential diagnosis are gastric or duodenal ulcers, primary biliary tract disease, mesenteric vascular insufficiency or infarction, abdominal aortic aneurysm, gynecologic or renal disease, and some rare hematologic dyscrasias.

Conventional radiographs of the chest and abdomen are often abnormal during acute pancreatitis, but they rarely yield a specific diagnosis. The most common findings include pleural effusion, basilar atelectasis, and a focal or generalized ileus. Two findings that are quite suggestive of primary pancreatic disease include a focal *duodenal ileus* and the *colon cutoff sign* (Fig. 9-8). The most characteristic findings of acute pancreatitis are found in the duodenum. These include widening of the

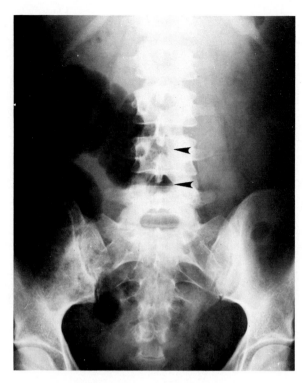

Fig. 9-8 Acute pancreatitis (colon cutoff sign). Conventional radiograph of abdomen shows dilatation of proximal transverse colon and abrupt termination of gas shadow *(arrowheads)*.

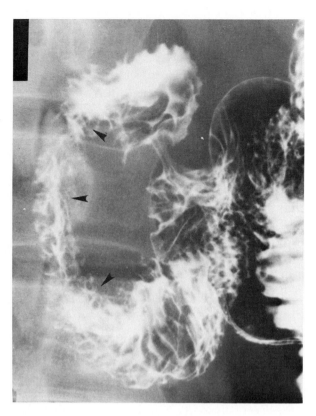

Fig. 9-9 Acute pancreatitis. Double-contrast examination of duodenum shows persistent spasm, effacement of medial wall, and spiculation of folds *(arrowheads)*.

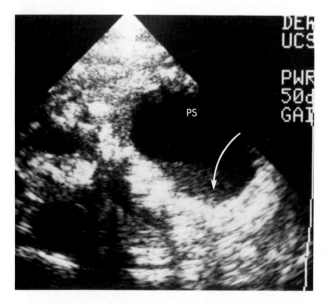

Fig. 9-10 Transverse scan of patient with pancreatic pseudocyst *(PS)*. Note debris *(arrow)* in dependent portion of cyst.

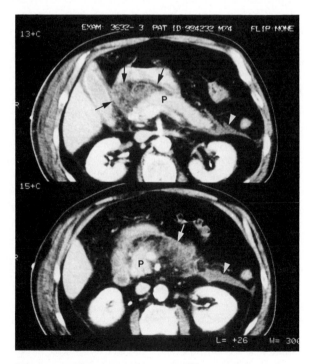

Fig. 9-11 Acute pancreatitis. **A** and **B,** Bolus-enhanced CT scan of pancreas shows peripancreatic fluid collection *(arrows)* and fluid ventral to anterior pararenal fascia *(arrowheads)*. Pancreatic parenchyma *(P)* shows normal, homogeneous contrast enhancement.

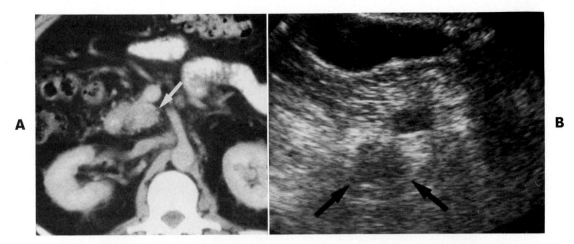

Fig. 9-12 Carcinoma of uncinate process; complementary use of ultrasound. **A,** CT scan showing subtle enlargement and rounding of uncinate process *(arrow)* as only positive CT finding in man with otherwise unexplained abdominal pain. **B,** Sonogram of pancreatic head, which shows uncinate process to contain small hypoechoic mass *(arrows). st,* Water-filled stomach. Workup also revealed pulmonary metastases. Carcinoma of pancreas was confirmed by CT-guided biopsy, and pulmonary metastases were confirmed by transthoracic needle aspiration.

C-loop caused by enlargement of the head of the pancreas, mucosal edema, and spiculation of the fold (Fig. 9-9).

A radiologic diagnosis of acute pancreatitis can be made by identifying fluid collections or pseudocyst formation. CT is the preferred method for initial evaluation of patients with acute pancreatitis.

Ultrasonographic findings in acute pancreatitis are characterized by gland enlargement and decreased parenchymal echogenicity. Complications of acute pancreatitis, such as intrapancreatic or peripancreatic fluid collections, pseudocysts (Fig. 9-10), phlegmons, and abscesses, often can be recognized by carefully performed ultrasound.

With *computed tomography,* the morphologic changes of acute edematous pancreatitis include enlargement and indistinctness of the gland margins, parenchymal inhomogeneity, thickening of the anterior pararenal fascia, and—on occasion—small fluid collections within or adjacent to the pancreas (Fig. 9-11). Acute hemorrhagic pancreatitis usually results in more marked gland enlargement. Parenchymal hemorrhage can be seen as an area of increased attenuation, and parenchymal necrosis can be identified as an area of non–contrast-enhancing parenchyma during bolus-dynamic contrast-enhanced CT (Fig. 9-12).

As with US, the CT diagnosis of acute pancreatitis is aided by the identification of complications of the inflammatory process, such as intrapancreatic and peripancreatic fluid collections, pancreatic ascites, pseudocyst, phlegmon, and abscess.

Chronic pancreatitis

Radiologic evaluation often plays a crucial role in the initial diagnosis of chronic pancreatitis. Conventional radiographs of the abdomen show pancreatic calcifications in 27% to 65% of patients (Fig. 9-13). The great majority of pancreatic calcifications seen radiolog-

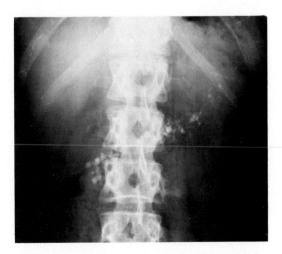

Fig. 9-13 Chronic pancreatitis. Conventional radiograph of abdomen shows small calcifications distributed throughout pancreas.

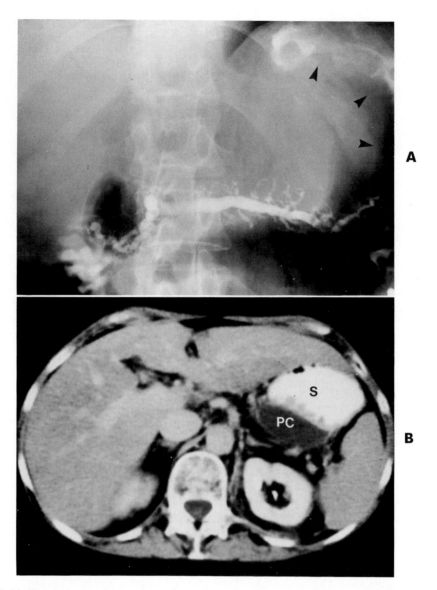

Fig. 9-14 Chronic pancreatitis: marked changes. **A,** ERCP shows marked main pancreatic duct dilatation, ectasia of lateral side branches, and small calculi. Note evidence of displacement of stomach *(arrowheads);* contrast is from duodenal gastric reflux during ERCP. **B,** Bolus-dynamic CT scan shows pseudocyst *(PC)* displacing stomach *(S)*.

(From Freeny PC: Acute and chronic pancreatitis: current concepts of diagnosis. In Margulis AR, Gooding CA, editors: *Diagnostic radiology 1987.* San Francisco, 1987, University of California in San Francisco.)

ically are caused by chronic alcoholic pancreatitis. They are intraductal in location. Calcifications may also occur in patients with cystic fibrosis, kwashiorkor, hyperparathyroidism, pancreatic carcinoma, and cystic pancreatic neoplasms.

CT findings in chronic pancreatitis include alterations in gland size (focal or diffuse enlargement or gland atrophy), irregular margins, pancreatic duct dilatation, and intraductal calculi. Secondary findings include intrapancreatic or peripancreatic cysts or fluid col-

lections, thickening of peripancreatic fascia, and evidence of vascular involvement (arterial pseudoaneurysm formation or venous occlusion and varices) (Fig. 9-14).

ERCP is the most sensitive modality for detection of chronic pancreatitis. The ERCP findings include clubbing and dilatation of the lateral side branches, narrowing ("nipping") of the origins of the side branches from the main duct, main duct marginal irregularities, strictures, focal or diffuse dilatation, or multifocal strictures and intervening areas of dilatation *("chain of lakes")*

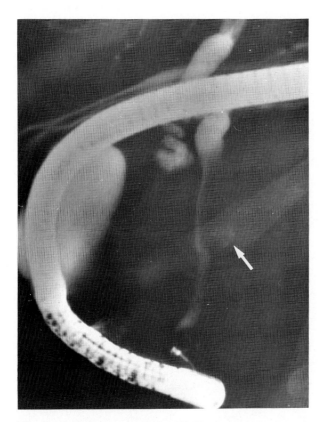

Fig. 9-15 Chronic pancreatitis. ERCP shows long, smooth narrowing of common bile duct. Pancreatic calcification *(arrow)* is seen adjacent to duct.

and intraductal protein plugs or calculi. These findings may be diffuse or focal. Communicating cysts may be small or large and can be filled during contrast injection. The intrapancreatic segment of the common bile duct also may be narrowed (Fig. 9-15). In rare cases the main pancreatic duct is completely obstructed by an intraductal calculus or ductal fibrosis. In the latter case, differentiation from a pancreatic neoplasm may be difficult, necessitating angiography (Fig. 9-16).

ERCP is more sensitive than CT for detecting the changes of chronic pancreatitis because mild to moderate changes, limited to the main duct and side branches, are very difficult to detect with CT.

Clinical and radiologic staging of pancreatitis
Parenchymal necrosis

Parenchymal necrosis is the most important prognostic CT finding, short of frank pancreatic abscess. Necrosis is identified by CT as areas of non–contrast-enhancing pancreatic parenchyma. The approximate percentage of gland necrosis correlates with patient mortality. The only reliable method of diagnosing the presence of bacterial contamination, short of surgery, is guided percutaneous fine-needle aspiration.

Fluid collections

Fluid collections have a spontaneous resolution rate of about 40% to 50% within the first 6 weeks.

Pancreatic ascites

Pancreatic ascites is caused by disruption of the pancreatic duct with leakage of pancreatic juice into the peritoneal cavity. The presence of free fluid within the peritoneal cavity can be detected with US or CT; the diagnosis of pancreatic ascites is then confirmed by percutaneous aspiration of the fluid and amylase determination, and the site of the duct rupture is documented by ERCP.

Pancreatic abscess

Pancreatic abscess is a focal collection of liquid pus. Diagnosis of infection can be suspected if gas is present within the collection, but percutaneous aspiration is the only reliable method for confirming the diagnosis.

Etiology of pancreatitis

Radiology plays a crucial role in identifying correctable causes of pancreatitis.

Biliary tract disease

Biliary tract disease is the most common cause of acute pancreatitis in the United States. In most patients calculi are found within the gallbladder or common bile duct. A diagnosis of cholelithiasis or choledocholithiasis and associated acute edematous pancreatitis can be made in many patients by US and ERCP soon after hospital admission.

The current use of ^{99m}Tc-HIDA has been shown to be efficacious in differentiating acute pancreatitis from acute cholecystitis.

A variety of inflammatory, neoplastic, and congenital abnormalities of the common bile duct have been associated with pancreatitis. These include choledochal cysts, parasitic infestations, sclerosing cholangitis, stenosis of Oddi's sphincter, and bile duct tumors.

Stomach and duodenum

Primary abnormalities of the stomach and duodenum have also been associated with pancreatitis. These may be diagnosed by barium studies and include penetrating ulcers and tumors of the stomach and duodenum, intraluminal and conventional duodenal diverticula, afferent loop obstruction, and regional enteritis involving the stomach and duodenum.

Pancreas divisum

Pancreas divisum is the failure of the dorsal and ventral ducts of Wirsung and Santorini to fuse. Its incidence is about 9%. If minor papillary stenosis occurs in

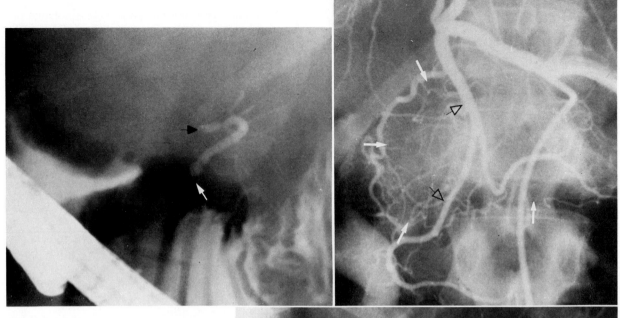

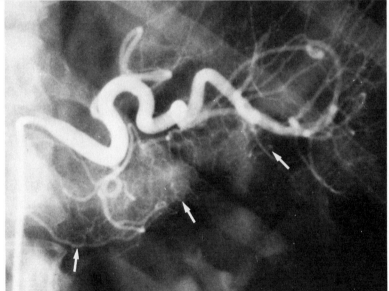

Fig. 9-16 Pancreatitis or carcinoma? **A,** ERCP shows nonspecific obstruction of main pancreatic duct *(arrow).* Papilla is in transverse duodenum *(white arrow).* Selective hepatic, **B,** and splenic, **C,** arteriograms show typical changes of pancreatitis: gland is moderately enlarged and hypervascular, and small intrapancreatic vessels *(white arrows)* are minimally deformed and tortuous. Gastroduodenal artery *(open arrows)* is displaced anteromedially. Venous phases (not shown) were normal. Inflammatory ductal stricture and chronic pancreatitis were found at surgery.

a patient with pancreas divisum, recurrent attacks of pancreatitis, caused by obstruction, are likely to result (Fig. 9-17). Minor duct papillotomy produces good results in most patients.

Traumatic pancreatitis

Traumatic pancreatitis follows blunt or penetrating abdominal trauma in about 3% to 12% of cases. The injury may vary from a simple contusion to complete transection of the gland, resulting in either acute or chronic pancreatitis.

Complications of pancreatitis

One of the most important roles of radiology is the diagnosis and evaluation of complications of acute and chronic pancreatitis. These complications are responsible for a significant proportion of the morbidity and mortality of inflammatory disease of the pancreas. However, if detected early, they often can be treated appropriately without sequelae.

Pancreatic and extrapancreatic fluid collections

An intrapancreatic or extrapancreatic fluid collection is a potential complication of either acute or chronic pancreatitis and occurs in up to 50% of patients. These fluid collections are composed of blood, pancreatic enzymes, fluid, and debris. Although the term *pseudocyst* implies the presence of a wall or containing structure, the fluid collections are often uncontained and poorly circumscribed. They are most frequently found in the

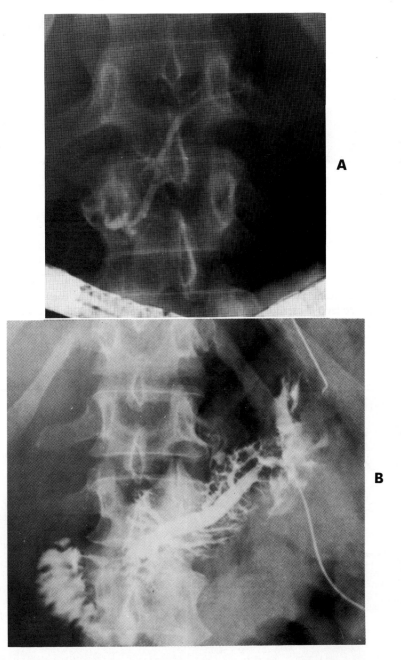

Fig. 9-17 Pancreas divisum. **A,** ERCP shows large ventral pancreas with changes of chronic pancreatitis. **B,** Operative pancreatogram shows more severe inflammatory changes in dorsal duct system.

lesser sac and anterior pararenal space, and about 20% are multiple. Less common sites include perihepatic and perisplenic spaces, the mediastinum, the mesentery, and the pelvis. Continuity with the pancreatic ductal system is common and can be demonstrated by pancreatography in 50% to 80% of cases.

On *conventional chest radiographs,* pancreatic or extrapancreatic fluid collections may produce findings that include elevation of the left diaphragm, pleural ef-

fusion, atelectasis or consolidation, and rarely, a mediastinal mass. *Abdominal films* may show displacement of the gastric air bubble or bowel gas shadows, a soft tissue mass, or pancreatic calcifications, possibly of a curvilinear type in a cyst wall.

On *barium studies* pancreatic fluid collections displace some part of the upper gastrointestinal tract in 75% of cases. If the fluid collection ruptures into the adjacent stomach or bowel, it may fill with gas or inter-

Since the pancreas does not have an effective capsular covering, carcinomas arising from the organ have a tendency to involve *adjacent organs* by direct extension. On CT scans, involvement of the stomach or intestine is best appreciated when the lumen of the involved viscus is distended with contrast material. Other organs sometimes affected by direct extension are the spleen and either the adrenal gland or kidney.

Metastases are very common CT findings in patients with pancreatic carcinoma. Liver metastases—hypovascular lesions, best displayed on contrast-enhanced scans—are found by CT most often.

Ultrasonography

Primary US signs of pancreatic carcinoma are similar to those demonstrated by CT. Most bulky pancreatic tumors are readily demonstrated as masses. A more important contribution of ultrasound is the demonstration of altered parenchymal texture. Most pancreatic adenocarcinomas are hypoechoic relative to normal parenchyma.

Real-time ultrasonography is especially well suited to demonstrate the *secondary signs* of pancreatic and biliary ductal dilatation.

Complementary roles of CT and US

It is perhaps not well recognized that US can complement CT studies. Ultrasonography is especially worthwhile in differentiating between a subtle pancreatic mass and a normal variation in pancreatic configuration. Differentiation is accomplished by demonstrating whether the region of concern has a normal echo pattern relative to the adjacent pancreatic tissue. Directed real-time ultrasonographic examination is only rarely unsuccessful in solving such a problem. In that case a more invasive procedure, such as endoscopic pancreatography, may be required.

Magnetic resonance imaging

Significant improvements have been made in MRI of the pancreas. On T_1- or T_2-weighted images the signal intensities of tumor range from hyperintense to isointense with those of normal pancreatic tissue. Advantages of MRI include delineation of vessels without the need for contrast material and the production of images that are free of artifactual degradation caused by metal clips in postoperative patients.

Differential diagnosis

Occasional variations in the size or shape of the normal pancreas can resemble a pancreatic mass, as can extrapancreatic structures, especially neighboring parts of the GI tract. Mass tumors originating from neighboring structures may also simulate primary pancreatic tu-

mors, but often an interface can be identified between the mass and the pancreas.

Pancreatic neoplasms other than ductal adenocarcinomas often have radiologic and clinical characteristics that indicate they are something other than the ductal type of pancreatic cancer.

The diagnosis of *pancreatic carcinoma versus pancreatitis* can be difficult, since the two have many gross pathologic features in common. Pancreatic enlargement, ductal obstruction and dilatation, cyst formation, infiltration of adjacent tissues, and ascites can occur with both conditions. To further complicate the diagnosis, cancer of the pancreas may be accompanied by inflammation, and a pancreas already involved with chronic inflammation may develop a carcinoma.

Despite their similarities, carcinoma and pancreatitis can usually be distinguished from each other, especially when clinical and laboratory information is correlated with radiologic findings. Although phlegmonous swelling of the pancreas might sometimes resemble a neoplasm, the clinical picture in that condition is one of acute or recently acute pancreatitis. Extrapancreatic spread of acute inflammation usually occurs in the form of an effusion that extends into the anterior pararenal space or lesser sac, whereas neoplastic extension tends to be perivascular and retropancreatic.

Chronic pancreatitis is more difficult to distinguish from carcinoma. It is particularly difficult to determine the nature of a focal enlargement, although additional findings may be influential. The presence of hepatic or nodal metastases, for example, indicates malignancy, whereas intraductal pancreatic calcification indicates chronic pancreatitis.

The most difficult diagnostic problem is presented by a focal solid mass with no ancillary features to indicate whether it is inflammatory or neoplastic. Since a sample biopsy that is negative for carcinoma does not exclude the possibility of malignancy, it may be more prudent to follow the appearance of the mass with serial noninvasive imaging.

Direct ductography: pancreatic and biliary
Endoscopic retrograde cholangiopancreatography

In current practice ERCP may be used to clarify ambiguous information from CT or US. Because it affords an endoscopic view of the duodenum, ERCP has advantages in differentiating duodenal or ampullary carcinomas from periampullary cancers of the pancreatic head. Endoscopy is also used for placement of endoprostheses to relieve biliary obstruction. With cancer of the pancreas the most frequent positive findings involving the main pancreatic duct are stenosis and complete obstruction (Fig. 9-31).

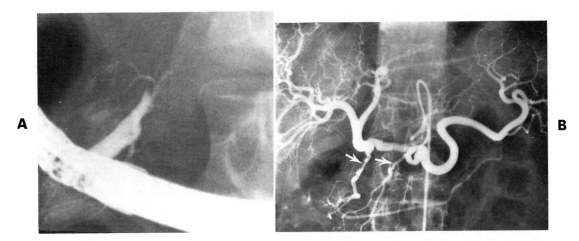

Fig. 9-31 Carcinoma of pancreatic head. **A,** ERCP showing abrupt obstruction of main pancreatic duct in head of pancreas. **B,** Celiac arteriogram showing irregular narrowing of gastroduodenal and dorsal pancreatic arteries *(arrows)* as result of neoplastic encasement.

Percutaneous transhepatic cholangiography

The information provided by transhepatic cholangiography is limited to a depiction of the biliary system. The ductal dilatation often ends in an abruptly tapered deformity with a nipple-like terminal extension or an asymmetric rattail configuration.

Angiography

At present, angiography is most often used to search for evidence of unresectability or as an attempt to define vascular anatomy before surgical intervention. Most authorities employ selective catheterization of the celiac and superior mesenteric arteries. The sign generally regarded to be most characteristic of pancreatic cancer is *arterial encasement.*

Gastrointestinal examinations

Barium examinations are no longer among the principal diagnostic procedures to search for evidence of pancreatic cancer. Masses that arise from the head of the pancreas tend to involve the inner curvature of the duodenal loop (Fig. 9-32). In advanced cases upper gastrointestinal examination may be useful to indicate the degree of duodenal or gastric obstruction.

Percutaneous biopsy

Biopsy of pancreatic tumors by percutaneous needle aspiration has become a standard radiologic procedure. The safety and efficacy of percutaneous fine-needle biopsy of pancreatic tumors is established. Complications are extremely rare, although at least one case of seeding of tumor cells along the needle path has been reported.

Clinical benefits of radiologic advances

The potential for earlier diagnosis of pancreatic carcinoma in symptomatic patients has not had a noticeably favorable effect on the extremely poor survival rates associated with this disease. Among the patients who benefit most from modern pancreatic imaging are those whose conditions are suggestive of pancreatic

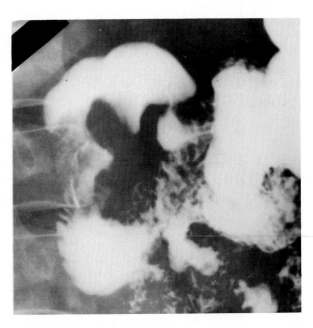

Fig. 9-32 Carcinoma of head of pancreas. Barium upper GI tract examination showing compression and invasion of second portion of duodenum with ulceration on inner wall. This configuration has been called reverse-3 sign of Frostberg.

cancer but are not. In these patients the demonstration of a pancreas that appears entirely normal in form and substance is an important finding that allows attention to be directed toward other possible explanations for the symptoms. The decline in the use of exploratory laparotomy to search for the cause of vague abdominal symptoms is a fairly accurate measure of the effectiveness of contemporary abdominal imaging to accomplish the same goal.

UNUSUAL CARCINOMAS OF THE EXOCRINE PANCREAS
Pleomorphic carcinoma

Pleomorphic, or *sarcomatoid,* carcinoma of the pancreas is a rare form of pancreatic cancer characterized histologically by anaplastic mononuclear cells, multinucleated giant cells, and spindle cells. The striking feature on abdominal imaging, in addition to the pancreatic mass, is massive lymphadenopathy, which is so extensive that the disease is likely to be mistaken for lymphoma.

Acinar cell carcinoma

Another uncommon cancer of the exocrine pancreas is acinar cell carcinoma. A peculiar proclivity of this type of pancreatic carcinoma is the production of a clinical syndrome resulting from focal necrosis of subcutaneous and intraosseous fat. Awareness of the association between the syndrome of metastatic fat necrosis and an otherwise occult pancreatic neoplasm should lead to an imaging examination of the pancreas in patients afflicted with the syndrome.

Mucin-hypersecreting tumor of the pancreatic duct

Yet another rare carcinoma of the pancreas is this relatively well-differentiated papillary tumor that arises from and is confined to the mucosal lining of the main pancreatic duct. The tumor produces mucin in such quantity that it causes pronounced dilatation of the main pancreatic duct with consequent thinning of the pancreatic parenchyma. The markedly dilated duct, which is filled with radiolucent mucin, and the thinned parenchyma constitute the main findings on CT.

Solid and papillary epithelial neoplasm

Solid and papillary epithelial neoplasm begins as a solid tumor but undergoes varying degrees of cystic degeneration caused by necrosis and hemorrhage. Examined by sectional imaging, these lesions consistently appear as large, rounded, well-defined pancreatic masses. The interior of the tumor may be either solid or cystic or, as occurs in most cases, of mixed solid and cystic composition. These tumors can resemble serous or mucinous cystic neoplasms or islet cell carcinomas.

CYSTIC NEOPLASMS

Cystic neoplasms have traditionally been classified as either cystadenoma or cystadenocarcinoma. Two

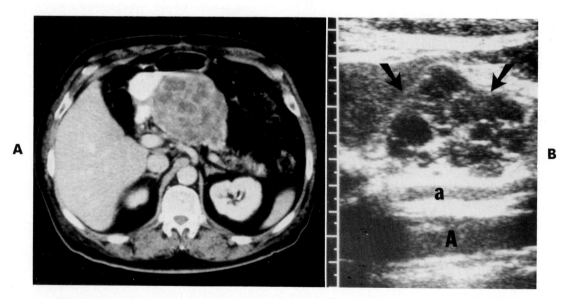

Fig. 9-33 Microcystic adenoma (serous cystadenoma). **A,** Contrast-enhanced CT showing large pancreatic mass composed of numerous small cysts with enhancing walls. **B,** Sagittal sonogram showing the multicystic appearance of another microcystic adenoma *(arrows).* Note enhanced through-transmission of sound, which clearly defines aorta *(A)* and superior mesenteric artery *(a)* behind mass.

types are recognized: microcystic adenoma, also called serous or glycogen-rich cystadenoma; and mucinous cystic, or macrocystic, neoplasms.

Microcystic adenoma (serous cystadenoma)

Sectional imaging accurately depicts the morphology and internal architecture of most microcystic adenomas (Fig. 9-33). Ultrasound is especially suited to display the cystic structure of these tumors, even in masses that do not appear conspicuously cystic on CT. Experience to date indicates that some microcystic adenomas have appearances characteristic enough to permit a confident diagnosis of this benign tumor.

Mucinous cystic neoplasms (macrocystic cystadenoma and cystadenocarcinoma)

The cysts that occur in mucinous cystic neoplasms are usually larger than those in microcystic adenomas (Fig. 9-34). In mucinous cystic tumors the cysts may be solitary or multiple, unilocular or multilocular. Calcifications tend to be peripherally located. All mucinous cystic tumors should be removed if possible.

Sometimes it is difficult to distinguish one of these tumors from a microcystic adenoma having larger than usual cysts, from a ductal adenocarcinoma that has undergone cavitary necrosis, or from a large islet cell tumor with cystic degeneration. The CT appearance of *cystic lymphangioma*, a rare benign tumor, may be identical to that of mucinous cystic neoplasms.

ISLET CELL NEOPLASMS (APUDOMAS)

Since the diagnosis of functioning islet cell tumors is usually established or suspected on the basis of clinical and laboratory information, the primary role of radiology is to provide preoperative assessment of the location and number of tumors.

Insulinoma

About 85% of insulinomas are benign adenomas. Angiography, ultrasonography (Fig. 9-35), and venous sampling have all been shown to be effective in their preoperative localization. Angiography has been reported to localize insulinomas in up to 90% of cases. Success rates as high as 97% have been reported with pancreatic venous sampling, but this invasive, technically difficult, and time-consuming procedure has not met with widespread acceptance. Intraoperative ultrasonography has recently been shown to be the most sensitive. Combined with surgical palpation, almost all solitary insulinomas can be detected. In addition, intraoperative ultrasound is useful for determining the proximity of the insulinoma to the pancreatic and biliary ducts.

Gastrinoma

A sizable proportion of gastrinomas can be detected with dynamic contrast-enhanced CT scans. If the tumor is sufficiently vascular, it becomes hyperdense with dynamic enhancement, and if it is sufficiently large or superficial, it may be obvious as a mass.

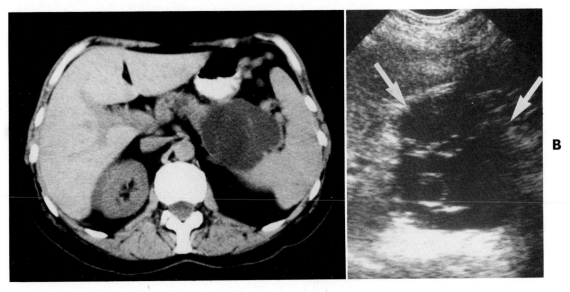

Fig. 9-34 Mucinous cystic (macrocystic) neoplasm. **A,** CT scan showing large cystic mass arising from pancreatic tail. Mass has internal septations, but individual cystic compartments are considerably larger than those of microcystic adenoma in Fig. 9-33. **B,** Sonogram of same tumor *(arrows)*. At pathologic examination no malignant tissue was found.

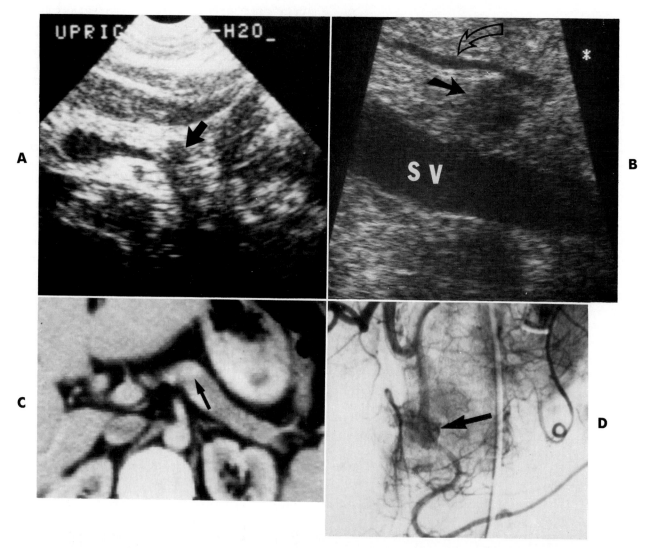

Fig. 9-35 Solitary insulinomas *(black arrows)*, each about 1 cm in diameter. Each tumor is depicted by different modality. **A,** Preoperative sonogram showing hypoechoic lesion in pancreatic body. **B,** Intraoperative sonogram showing discrete hypoechoic lesion in substance of pancreas, between main pancreatic duct *(open arrow)* and splenic vein *(sv)*. **C,** CT scan showing enhancing tumor in body of pancreas (same tumor as in **A**). **D,** Subtraction angiogram showing hypervascular tumor in pancreatic head.

(**A** and **B** from Gorman B et al: Benign pancreatic insulinoma: preoperative and intraoperative sonographic localization, *Am J Roentgenol* 147:929-934, © by American Roentgen Ray Society, 1986.)

Nonfunctioning islet cell carcinoma

Nonfunctioning islet cell carcinomas are sometimes radiographically indistinguishable from ductal carcinoma. As a general rule, islet cell carcinomas tend to be larger than ductal carcinomas at the time of discovery. Approximately 25% of islet cell carcinomas contain calcification (Fig. 9-36), whereas calcification is rare in ordinary pancreatic carcinoma. One feature notably lacking in islet cell carcinomas is the type of ret-

ropancreatic periarterial extension that is a common CT feature of ductal carcinoma.

NONEPITHELIAL NEOPLASMS
Lymphoma

Pancreatic lymphoma is usually of a non-Hodgkin's variety and is often associated with generalized disease. In cases of widespread disease there is seldom any difficulty distinguishing lymphoma from a primary pancre-

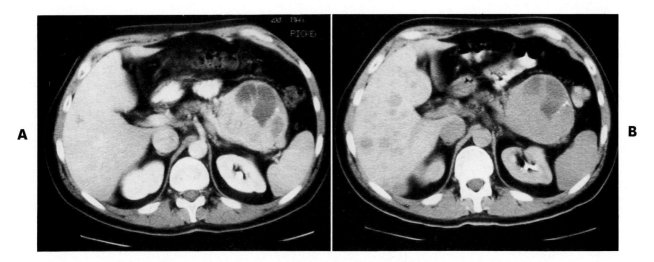

Fig. 9-36 Nonfunctioning islet cell carcinoma with hypervascular hepatic metastases. Advantage of delayed scanning. **A,** Contrast-enhanced CT scan showing large pancreatic tumor containing small calcification. Tumor has both solid enhancing tissue and necrotic unenhancing components. **B,** Delayed scan, taken about 4 hours after administration of intravenous contrast material, shows multiple hepatic metastases, most of which were invisible on earlier scan **(A).**

atic carcinoma, but one type of pancreatic carcinoma that can resemble extensive lymphoma is pleomorphic carcinoma, which typically produces massive metastatic lymphadenopathy. Often a precise classification of lymphoma requires more tissue than can be obtained by needle aspiration.

Connective tissue tumors

Primary pancreatic neoplasms of connective tissue origin are rare. They occur in benign, as well as malignant, forms. Radiologic experience with these rare tumors is limited.

METASTATIC NEOPLASMS

Metastatic involvement of the pancreas is possible from almost any type of primary malignancy. Common primary sites include breast, lung, kidney, skin (melanoma), and GI tract.

RECOMMENDED READING

1. Balthazar EJ et al: Solid and papillary epithelial neoplasm of the pancreas: radiographic, CT, sonographic, and angiographic features, *Radiology* 150:39, 1984.
2. Balthazar EJ et al: Acute pancreatitis: Value of CT in establishing prognosis, *Radiology* 174:331, 1990.
3. Bilbao MK, Katon RM: Neoplasms of the pancreas. In Stewart ET et al, editors: *Atlas of endoscopic retrograde cholangiopancreatography,* St Louis, 1977, Mosby–Year Book.
4. Block S et al: Sensitivity of imaging procedures and clinical staging for necrotizing pancreatitis, *Digestion* 30:102, 1984.
5. Classen M, Phillip J: Endoscopic retrograde cholangiopancre-

atography (ERCP) and endoscopic therapy in pancreatic disease, *Clin Gastroenterol* 13:819, 1984.
6. Cotton PB et al: Gray-scale ultrasonography and endoscopic pancreatography in pancreatic diagnosis, *Radiology* 134:453, 1980.
7. Doppman JL et al: The role of pancreatic venous sampling in the localization of insulinomas, *Radiology* 138:557, 1981.
8. Freeny PC: Computed tomography of the pancreas, *Clin Gastroenterol* 13:791, 1984.
9. Freeny PC, editor: *Radiology of the pancreas,* Radiologic Clinics of North America, vol 27, Philadelphia, 1989, WB Saunders.
10. Freeny PC, Lawson TL: *Radiology of the pancreas,* New York, 1982, Springer-Verlag.
11. Froelich JW, Swanson D: Imaging of inflammatory processes with labeled cells, *Semin Med* 14:128, 1984.
12. Galiber AK et al: Localization of pancreatic insulinoma: comparison of pre- and intraoperative US and CT and angiography, *Radiology* 166:405, 1988.
13. Gerzof SG et al: Percutaneous drainage of infected pancreatic pseudocysts, *Arch Surg* 119:888, 1984.
14. Hall-Craggs MA, Lees WR: Fine-needle aspiration biopsy: pancreatic and biliary tumors, *Am J Roentgenol* 147:399, 1986.
15. Jeffrey RB Jr et al: Extrapancreatic spread of acute pancreatitis: new observations with real-time US, *Radiology* 159:707, 1986.
16. Jenkins JPR et al: Quantitative tissue characterization in pancreatic disease using magnetic resonance imaging, *Br J Radiol* 60:333, 1987.
17. Kim SY et al: Papillary carcinoma of the pancreas: findings of US and CT, *Radiology* 154:338, 1985.
18. Kuligowska E, Olsen W: Pancreatic pseudocysts drained through a percutaneous transgastric approach, *Radiology* 154:79, 1985.
19. Lammer J, Neumayer K: Biliary drainage endoprostheses: experience with 201 placements, *Radiology* 159:625, 1986.
20. Lees WR: Pancreatic ultrasonography, *Clin Gastroenterol* 13:763, 1984.
21. Maier W: Computed tomography in chronic pancreatitis. In Mal-

fertheiner P, Ditschuneit H, editors: *Diagnostic procedures in pancreatic disease,* Berlin, 1986, Springer-Verlag.

22. May GR et al: Diagnosis and treatment of jaundice, *RadioGraphics* 6:847, 1986.
23. Megibow AJ et al: Thickening of the celiac axis and/or superior mesenteric artery: a sign of pancreatic carcinoma on computed tomography. *Radiology* 141:449, 1981.
24. Rösch W: Report on a symposium, "10 years of ERCP": diagnostic and therapeutic aspects, European Society of Gastrointestinal Endoscopy, Newsletter 15:7, 1981.
25. Smith R et al: Gallbladder perforation: diagnostic utility of cholescintigraphy in suggested subacute or chronic cases, *Radiology* 158:63, 1986.
26. Steiner E et al: *MR imaging of pancreatic carcinoma: comparison with CT,* Paper presented at the 73rd Scientific Assembly and Annual Meeting of the Radiological Society of North America, Chicago, Nov 29–Dec 4, 1987.

27. Stewart ET et al: *Atlas of endoscopic retrograde cholangiopancreatography,* St Louis, 1977, Mosby–Year Book.
28. Tscholakoff D et al: MR imaging in the diagnosis of pancreatic disease, *Am J Roentgenol* 148:703, 1987.
29. vanSonnenberg E et al: Percutaneous drainage of infected and noninfected pancreatic pseudocysts: experience in 101 cases, *Radiology* 170:757, 1989.
30. Ward EM et al: Computed tomographic characteristics of pancreatic carcinoma: an analysis of 100 cases, *RadioGraphics* 3:547, 1983.
31. Weinstein D, Weinstein B: Ultrasonic demonstration of the pancreatic duct: an analysis of 41 cases, *Radiology* 130:729, 1979.
32. Wolfman N et al: Cystic neoplasms of the pancreas: CT and sonography, *Am J Roentgenol* 138:37, 1982.
33. Welch TJ et al: CT guided biopsy: prospective analysis of 1000 procedures, *Radiology* 171:493, 1989.

10 *Liver and Biliary Tract*

ROBERT N BERK
H JOACHIM BURHENNE
ARTHUR R CLEMETT
ROY A FILLY
GRETCHEN AW GOODING
FAYE C LAING
DIETER J MEYERHOFF
LEONARD ROSENTHALL
PREMYSL SLEZAK
DAVID D STARK
MICHAEL W WEINER
RALPH WEISSLEDER
JACK WITTENBERG

JAUNDICE

TRAUMA

LOCALIZED IMAGING DEFECTS

NEWLY DEVELOPING FIELDS
Liver transplants
Duplex scanning
Magnetic resonance imaging

GALLBLADDER

LIVER AND BILIARY TRACT
Congenital lesions
Diffuse liver diseases
Vascular diseases
Increased density of the liver
Liver calcifications
Inflammatory lesions
Liver cysts
Benign liver tumors
Malignant liver tumors
Bile duct carcinoma
Benign bile duct tumors
Sarcoma botryoides

IMAGING TECHNIQUES
Magnetic resonance imaging of the liver
Ultrasonography
Nuclear medicine
Endoscopy
Magnetic resonance spectroscopy

Radiology of the liver and biliary tract has advanced significantly. The addition of ultrasound (US) and computed tomography (CT) has changed the diagnostic approach to almost all pathologic conditions in the liver and biliary tract. These new biliary imaging modalities have resulted in decreased use of some of the more conventional radiographic techniques such as oral cholecystography, and have almost completely eliminated the use of intravenous cholangiography.

Jaundice

Extrahepatic ductal dilatation is the earliest change that occurrs with biliary obstruction. Dilatation precedes elevation of the serum bilirubin level. Thus the radiologic diagnosis of extrahepatic bile duct distention can be obtained before the clinical onset of jaundice. The early diagnosis of bile duct obstruction is clearly in the domain of the radiologist (Fig. 10-1).

An early differentiation between hepatocellular and obstructive jaundice greatly influences good patient care. The prompt surgical relief of bile duct obstruction prevents further hepatocellular damage and lowers the operative risk of complications such as superimposed cholangitis. Ultrasonographic evaluation is best performed on jaundiced patients at or before hospital admission.

The next best diagnostic procedure in the evaluation of jaundice is direct cholangiography. The choice be-

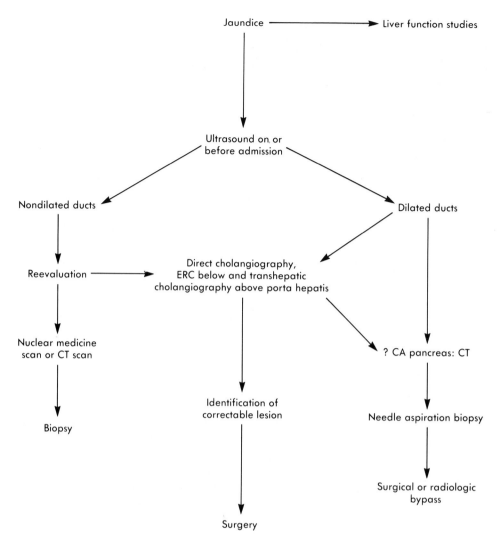

Fig. 10-1 Algorithm for jaundice.

tween transhepatic cholangiography and endoscopic retrograde cholangiography (ERC) depends on the expertise available. Most examiners use transhepatic cholangiography for intrahepatic lesions and lesions at the portal fissure (porta hepatis). Transhepatic cholangiography is also added if ERC is inconclusive or demonstrates only the distal extent of the lesions.

Trauma

Liver injury is less common than splenic laceration, but it carries a higher mortality. Plain film radiography should not be neglected because about one half of affected patients have associated rib fractures. CT and arteriography are the methods of choice for detecting subcapsular hematomas. Serial abdominal CT studies have become an integral part of conservative treatment of

blunt hepatic injuries and are useful in monitoring resorption of hemoperitoneum and the pattern of healing of intrahepatic hematomas, lacerations, and fractures.

Localized imaging defects

New and improved imaging modalities are changing the approach to screening for focal hepatic lesions (Fig. 10-2). Because of the rapid development of new and improved CT techniques—including incremental bolus dynamic scanning, CT arteriography, and delayed iodine scanning—radionuclide scans are no longer considered the initial imaging modality. A recent report on hepatic metastasis detection, however, indicates that magnetic resonance (MR) imaging may be more accurate in identifying focal hepatic lesions than is contrast-enhanced CT.

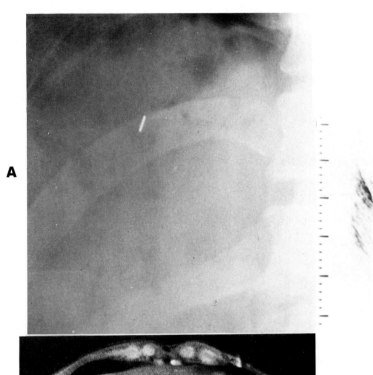

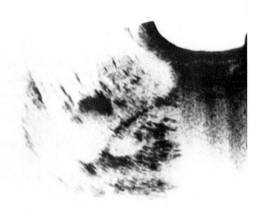

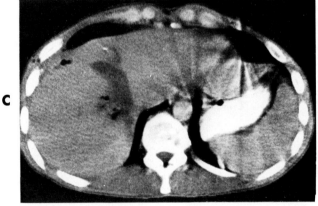

Fig. 10-2 A, Postoperative plain radiograph of right upper quadrant after surgery shows presence of air in liver. **B,** Ultrasonography demonstrates fluid collection with air-fluid level. **C,** CT again shows air and also pyogenic postoperative liver abscess.

Patients whose condition suggests primary or metastatic hepatic neoplasms must be imaged before surgery. Patients often undergo a sequence of imaging procedures including US, nuclear medicine studies, CT, angiography, and MR imaging (Fig. 10-3). Further studies with state-of-the-art technology are needed to compare ultrasound, CT, and MRI.

Another significant advance has been fine-needle aspiration biopsy, which is now well established as a method for diagnosing malignant disease. The sensitivity of the technique has been reported to be 78% for pancreatic tumors and 60% for biliary malignancy.

Newly developing fields

LIVER TRANSPLANTS

Radiographic assessment of the biliary tract is often essential in patients who have undergone liver trans-

plantation. Complications diagnosed by cholangiography include obstruction, bile leaks, and tube drainage problems that sometimes require transhepatic biliary drainage or balloon catheter dilatation of strictures to restore drainage tube patency.

DUPLEX SCANNING

Duplex Doppler techniques have been used for the qualitative assessment of splanchnic venous hemodynamics in patients with portal hypertension. The direction of blood flow in splenic, superior mesenteric, portal and intrahepatic portal, and portasystemic collaterals can be assessed. Duplex sonography is also a valuable portable technique for evaluating patients before and after liver transplants.

MAGNETIC RESONANCE IMAGING

Although MR imaging of the liver and biliary tract is in its early stages, this new modality already shows

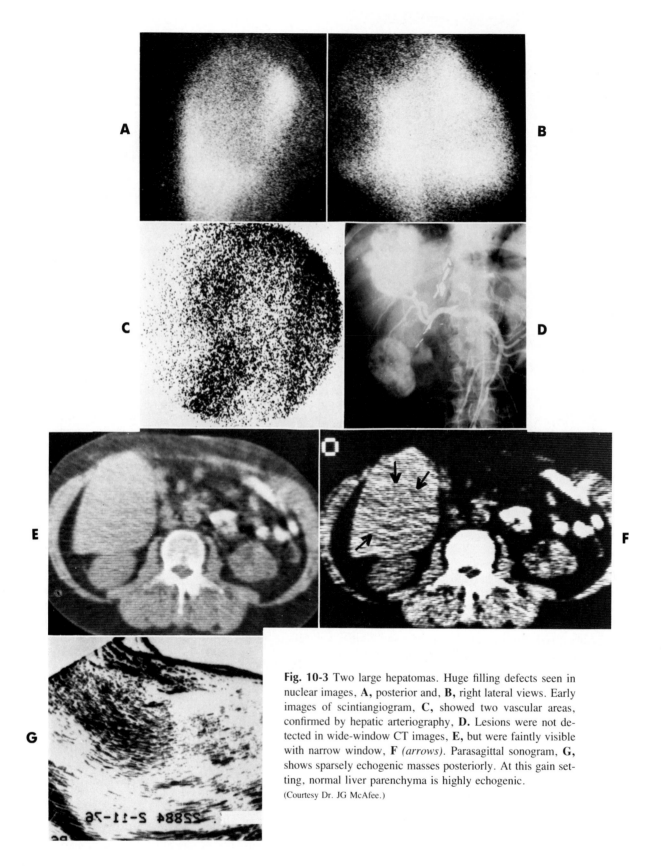

Fig. 10-3 Two large hepatomas. Huge filling defects seen in nuclear images, **A,** posterior and, **B,** right lateral views. Early images of scintiangiogram, **C,** showed two vascular areas, confirmed by hepatic arteriography, **D.** Lesions were not detected in wide-window CT images, **E,** but were faintly visible with narrow window, **F** *(arrows)*. Parasagittal sonogram, **G,** shows sparsely echogenic masses posteriorly. At this gain setting, normal liver parenchyma is highly echogenic.
(Courtesy Dr. JG McAfee.)

great promise for the detection of hepatic metastases and focal lesions.

Despite excellent soft-tissue contrast, the introduction of MR contrast agents has proved that the diagnostic performance of MR can be dramatically improved. A large variety of MR liver contrast agents have been synthesized, characterized, and studied in animal models. Several of these contrast agents are already in clinical use. Extracellular, extravascular *gadolinium (Gd) chelates* show pharmacokinetic and contrast-enhancement patterns similar to those of iodinated contrast agents used in CT imaging. *Intravascular contrast agents* such as Gd-DTPA- (gadolinium diethylene-triamine-pentaacetic acid)-labeled albumin are retained within the vascular system because of their larger size. The vascular agents selectively enhance tissues in proportion to their fractional blood volume. A series of *paramagnetic hepatobiliary agents* have been investigated in clinical trials. Gd-EOB-DTPA (gadolinium ethoxbenzyl-diethylene-triamine-pentaacetic acid) is a lipophilic agent with hepatobiliary excretion. Mn-DPDP (manganese dipyridoxal diphosphate) is recognized by the hepatocyte membrane transport system of the coenzyme pyridoxal-5'phosphate. Targeting of *Kupffer cells* has been achieved by administration of colloidal polycrystalline and monocrystalline iron oxide preparations.

GALLBLADDER
ROBERT N BERK
H JOACHIM BURHENNE

Plain abdominal radiography
Cholelithiasis

Estimates are that in the United States 10% of men and 20% of women between the ages of 55 and 65 have *gallstones*. Some gallstones contain calcium, but in only 10% to 15% of patients is the concentration of calcium sufficient to make the calculi radiopaque on plain abdominal radiographs. Gas-containing fissures are sometimes seen within gallstones, a finding referred to as the *Mercedes-Benz sign*. Eighty percent of gallstones identified by ultrasonography or at surgery can be detected with CT.

Not all round or oval calcifications in the right upper quadrant are caused by gallstones. Careful consideration must be given to calcification of the kidney, which may be caused by a wide variety of renal diseases. A calculus in the appendix or calcifications in the liver, adrenal gland, costal cartilages, lymph nodes, arteries, and veins may also have the appearance of gallstones.

Acute cholecystitis

Acute cholecystitis nearly always results from obstruction of the cystic duct by a gallstone. The findings on abdominal radiographs depend on the stage and severity of disease. With mild disease the radiographs may be normal or may reveal only the gallstones. With extension of the inflammatory process to adjacent peritoneal surfaces, however, there is reflex inhibition of motility in segments of the intestine *(sentinel ileus)*. If the colon is not affected by the paralytic ileus, the radiographic findings may simulate a mechanical small bowel obstruction. If empyema of the gallbladder develops, a mass adjacent to the liver may be apparent. Radiographs made at least 24 to 48 hours after the onset of cholecystitis show gas in the lumen of the gallbladder, in the gallbladder wall, and, on occasion, in the tissues adjacent to the gallbladder, indicating a pericholecystic abscess.

Emphysematous cholecystitis is an uncommon variant of acute cholecystitis in which gas is present in the gallbladder wall and in the lumen (Fig. 10-4). Twenty percent of patients with emphysematous cholecystitis have diabetes.

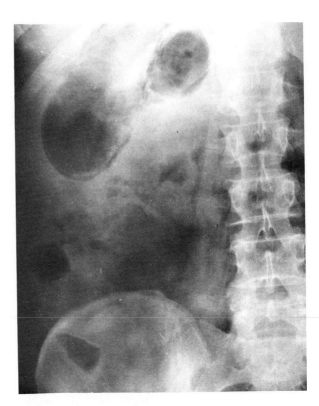

Fig. 10-4 Plain abdominal radiograph showing emphysematous cholecystitis. Intraluminal and intramural air are visible in body and neck of gallbladder.

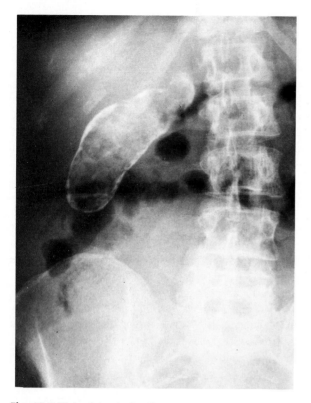

Fig. 10-5 Plain abdominal radiograph showing porcelain gallbladder. Large lower abdominal mass caused by uterine fibroid is also apparent.

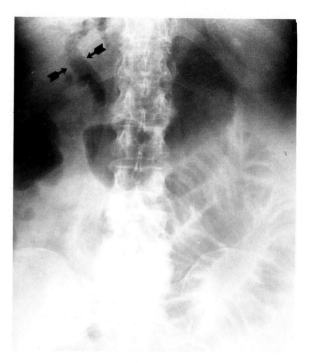

Fig. 10-6 Plain abdominal radiograph showing gallstone ileus. Loops of dilated small intestine and air in biliary tree *(arrows)* are evident.

Porcelain gallbladder

The condition in which extensive calcification is found in the wall of the gallbladder has been named *porcelain gallbladder* (Fig. 10-5). Plain abdominal radiographs show a characteristic ring of calcification that conforms to the shape and location of the gallbladder. Porcelain gallbladder must be distinguished from a single, large, calcified gallstone. Most authors agree that the incidence of carcinoma in cases of porcelain gallbladder is sufficient to warrant prophylactic cholecystectomy.

Milk of calcium bile

Milk of calcium bile, or the *limy bile syndrome,* is characterized by the presence of sufficient radiopaque material in the gallbladder to produce opacification on plain abdominal radiographs. The cystic duct is obstructed by a gallstone, and the gallbladder is chronically inflamed.

Spontaneous biliary-enteric fistula

Ninety percent of cases of spontaneous communication between the biliary tract and intestine result from erosion of a gallstone. If the gallstone is larger than 2.5 cm, it may cause an obturation type of intestinal obstruction *(gallstone ileus)*. The radiologist is in a unique position to establish the diagnosis of gallstone ileus because of the classic features of the disease on the plain abdominal radiographs. The cardinal plain film findings are (1) hoop-shaped, dilated loops of small bowel, (2) air in the biliary tree, and (3) a gallstone in an ectopic location in the abdomen (Fig. 10-6). Gas in the gallbladder or biliary tree, visible in nearly two thirds of patients with gallstone ileus, may also result from previous surgery, including a choledochoduodenostomy, cholecystojejunostomy, or sphincterotomy. In rare cases, gas may be caused by ascending cholangitis, a gas-forming organism, or—in older patients—by the reflux of air through a patulous Oddi's sphincter. Gas in the portal venous system usually collects toward the periphery of the liver, whereas gas in the bile duct is more prominent in the region of the porta hepatis.

Oral cholecystography

Where available, cholecystosonography has largely replaced oral cholecystography as the first technique

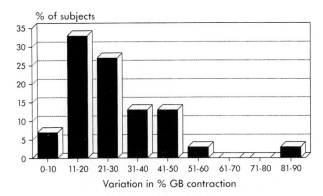

% of subjects

Fig. 10-7 Thirty healthy volunteers studied on three separate occasions for the degree of gallbladder contraction after a fatty meal demonstrated wide variations of normal. Variations of percentage gallbladder contraction greater than 5%, 10%, 20%, and 40% occurred in 100%, 93%, 60%, and 20% of the subjects respectively.

used to evaluate the patient with suspected gallbladder disease. The accuracy of the two techniques for the diagnosis of cholecystolithiasis is comparable, with sensitivity and specificity greater than 95%, but cholecystosonography with real-time high-resolution sector scanners is less time consuming.

Before undergoing oral cholecystography, patients should be evaluated for a history of previous allergic reaction to any of the radiographic contrast materials. A preliminary plain abdominal radiograph (to detect radiopaque gallstones that might be obscured by contrast material in the gallbladder and to recognize milk of calcium bile) should be obtained before the administration of contrast material.

Care must be taken to make the radiographs of the gallbladder at the appropriate time following the administration of contrast material. Poor gallbladder opacification occurs if the radiographs are taken prematurely or if they are delayed. On average, opacification of the gallbladder occurs between 14 and 19 hours after ingestion of Telepaque contrast material.

The routine use of a fatty meal for oral cholecystography has sometimes been recommended. In view of the considerable inconvenience, expense, and additional radiation exposure involved, however, there is little objective data to justify routine use. Also, gallbladder contraction varies greatly from one day to another in the same individual (Fig. 10-7).

Failure to visualize the gallbladder after the administration of two consecutive doses of cholecystographic contrast material is reliable evidence of gallbladder disease if other causes of nonvisualization can be excluded.

□ EXTRABILIARY CAUSES OF □ NONVISUALIZATION OF THE GALLBLADDER ON ORAL CHOLECYSTOGRAPHY

1. Fasting
2. Failure to ingest contrast material
3. Vomiting
4. Nasogastric suction
5. Esophageal disease
   a. Zenker's diverticulum
   b. Epiphrenic diverticulum
   c. Esophageal obstruction
   d. Hiatus hernia
6. Gastric retention
7. Gastrocolic fistula
8. Acute pancreatitis
9. Acute peritonitis
10. Severe trauma
11. Postoperative ileus
12. Liver disease
13. Dubin-Johnson syndrome
14. Previous cholecystectomy
15. Cholestyramine
16. Infants under 6 months of age
17. Crohn's disease
18. Pregnancy
19. Pernicious anemia

Hyperplastic cholecystoses

Hyperplastic cholecystoses is a general term for a group of abnormalities of the gallbladder that appear to be separate from inflammatory diseases. Hyperplasia implies a benign proliferation of normal tissue elements, whereas cholecystosis indicates a pathologic process that is distinct from inflammation. The two main categories of hyperplastic cholecystoses are *cholesterolosis* and *adenomyomatosis*.

CHOLESTEROLOSIS

Cholesterolosis, or *strawberry gallbladder,* is characterized by abnormal deposits of cholesterol esters. When the cholesterol deposits are of sufficient size, the cholecystogram shows fixed radiolucencies, either localized or generalized, in the opacified gallbladder (Fig. 10-8). Indirect radiographic findings include hyperconcentration and hyperexcretion, which are general features of all the hyperplastic cholecystoses. Cholesterolosis can be differentiated from cholelithiasis by determining that the radiolucent defects are fixed in position.

ADENOMYOMATOSIS

Adenomyomatosis consists of proliferation of mucosa, increased thickness of the muscle coat, and the

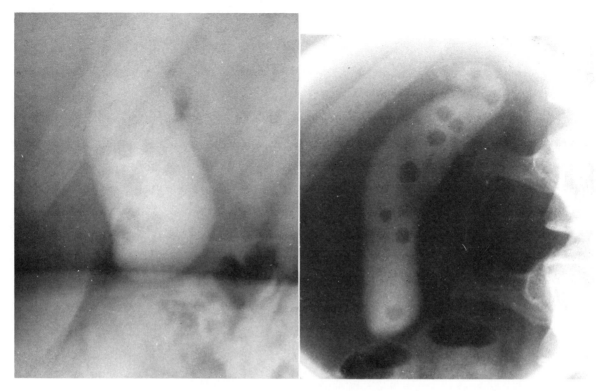

Fig. 10-8 Oral cholecystograms showing cholesterolosis of gallbladder in two patients. Numerous filling defects are visible in gallbladder. Defects maintained same location in gallbladder despite changes in patient's position, indicating that they are fixed to wall.

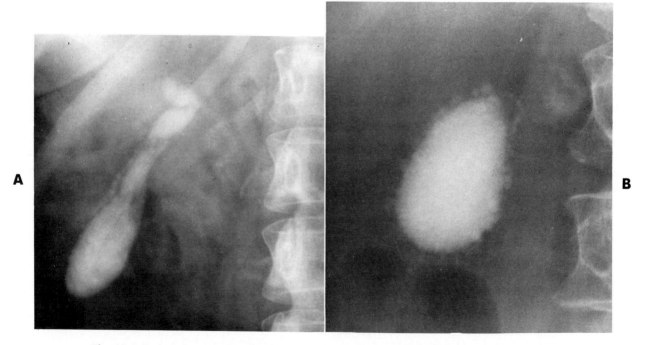

Fig. 10-9 Oral cholecystogram showing adenomyomatosis of gallbladder in two patients. Small outpouchings of gallbladder wall filled with contrast material are visible. **A,** Localized. **B,** Generalized.

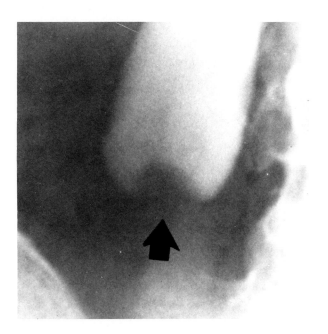

Fig. 10-10 Oral cholecystogram showing fundal adenomyoma of gallbladder *(arrow).*

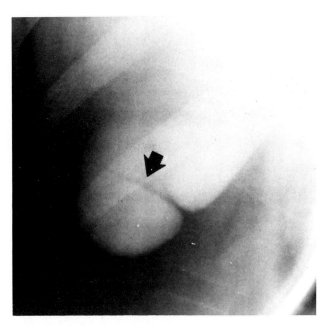

Fig. 10-11 Oral cholecystogram showing phrygian cap of gallbladder *(arrow).*

formation of outpouchings of mucosa into or through the muscularis (Figs. 10-9, 10-10). These diverticula, termed *Rokitansky-Aschoff sinuses,* may be segmental or diffuse throughout the gallbladder.

Normal variations

The size, shape, and position of the gallbladder as seen on cholecystography vary considerably in normal patients, depending on the body habitus of the patient.

A *phrygian cap* is a normal variation in the shape of the gallbladder in which the fundus appears to be folded on the body (Fig. 10-11).

Layering of contrast material is another normal variation. With the patient erect, layers of bile in the gallbladder increase in specific gravity from the neck to the fundus. Visual demonstration of this layering phenomenon occurs during cholecystography.

Congenital anomalies

Several congenital disorders of the gallbladder can be identified with oral cholecystography.

ANOMALIES OF POSITION

An abnormal position of the gallbladder occurs in association with situs inversus. When the gallbladder lies completely within the parenchyma of the liver, a liver scan, ultrasound studies, and hepatic angiography suggest the presence of a hepatic abscess. The gallbladder may also be located behind the liver (retrohepatic) or

may even be retroperitoneal or interposed between the liver and the diaphragm (suprahepatic).

If the gallbladder is on a long mesentery, it may be unusually mobile. In such cases, herniation into the foramen of Winslow is possible. The key radiologic finding is displacement of the gallbladder medial to the duodenal bulb.

DUPLICATION

The diagnosis of a double gallbladder on cholecystography is established if two separate gallbladder lumina and two distinct cystic ducts are demonstrated.

AGENESIS

Agenesis of the gallbladder is virtually impossible to distinguish from acute cholecystitis with obstruction of the cystic duct. However, two thirds of these patients have other malformations, such as congenital heart lesions, imperforate anus, or rectovaginal fistulas.

Cholelithiasis

An estimated 15 million Americans have gallstones, 85% of which are composed primarily of cholesterol. Cholecystography may demonstrate gallstones as large as 4 or 5 cm, as well as some that are no larger than 1 or 2 mm. The stones usually fall (by gravity) to the dependent portion of the gallbladder. They sometimes form a layer in the bile, depending on their specific gravity in relation to that of bile (Fig. 10-12).

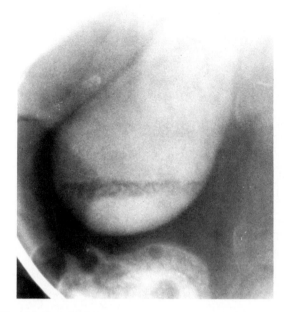

Fig. 10-12 Oral cholecystogram (upright projection) showing gallstones floating in gallbladder.

☐ **CAUSES OF FIXED FILLING DEFECT(S)** ☐
IN OPACIFIED GALLBLADDER

1. Cholesterolosis
2. Adenomyomatosis
3. Adherent gallstone
4. Adenoma
5. Papilloma
6. Carcinoid tumor
7. Carcinoma
8. Metastasis
9. Mucosal hyperplasia
10. Inflammatory polyp
11. Epithelial cyst
12. Mucous retention cyst
13. Spurious defect of infundibulum
14. Heterotopic pancreatic or gastric tissue
15. Parasitic granuloma
16. Varices
17. Arterial tortuosity and aneurysm

Neoplasms

True benign tumors of the gallbladder are exceedingly rare. Adenomas, the most common type, usually occur as flat elevations located in the body of the gallbladder. When a benign tumor is present, the cholecystogram discloses one or more small, round or oval radiolucent defects. Other causes of fixed filling defects in the opacified gallbladder are summarized in the following box.

Primary carcinoma of the gallbladder is nearly always a rapidly progressive disease, with a mortality approaching 100%. When bloodborne metastases to the gallbladder occur, they are often caused by melanoma.

Liver and biliary tract
ARTHUR R CLEMETT

Recent advances in imaging techniques for the liver and biliary tract have resulted in significant improvements in the ability of the radiologist to make precise diagnoses of diseases of the liver. Direct cholangiography remains the most efficient and efficacious modality for biliary tract imaging. In centers where requisite endoscopy skills are available, endoscopic retrograde cholangiopancreatography (ERCP), is the primary method of direct cholangiography. In some institutions percutaneous cholangiography is the primary study for patients with suspected lesions in the liver or at the porta hepatis, whereas ERCP is the preferred technique for direct cholangiography of lesions below the hilum; in the ex-

trahepatic ducts; and at the junction of the common duct, pancreatic duct, and duodenum. Additional studies, such as angiography (Fig. 10-13), US, CT, MR imaging, and nuclear medicine scans, are performed as indicated on a case-by-case basis.

The liver is a complex organ noted for the diversity of its function, the mixture of its cell types, and its dual vascular supply. The parenchymal cells of the liver form plasma proteins and clotting factors, and they participate in lipid and carbohydrate metabolism. Two additional functions of parenchymal cells are the secretion of specific bile salts to aid in digestion and the excretion of molecules harmful to the organism. The liver is abundantly supplied by both the portal vein, drawing blood from the intestinal tract, and by the hepatic artery, which supplies as much as 20% of the total blood flow to the liver.

Knowledge of the internal architecture of the liver is important and sometimes essential for the proper interpretation of liver angiograms, particularly cholangiograms. The hepatic arteries, portal vein branches (Fig. 10-14), and bile ducts (Fig. 10-15) follow the internal segmental anatomy of the liver, but the hepatic veins have an arrangement unrelated to the segmental distribution.

CONGENITAL LESIONS
Bile duct variations

A number of variations may occur in the junctional arrangement of the segmental or divisional ducts (Fig. 10-16).

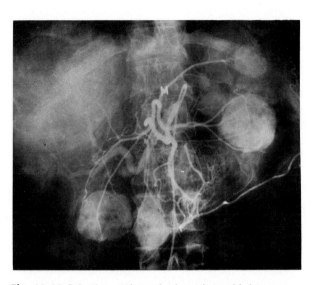

Fig. 10-13 Selective angiography in patient with known carcinoid tumor demonstrates four metastases in periphery of left lobe of liver.

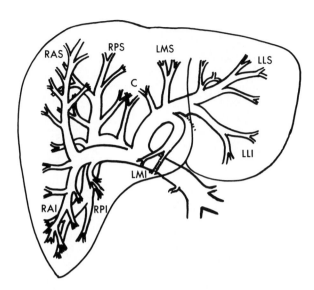

Fig. 10-14 Diagram of segmental anatomy of intrahepatic portal veins. Right and left lobes are divided by plane extending from gallbladder fossa to inferior vena cava. *RAS*, Right anterior superior; *RAI*, right anterior inferior; *RPS*, right posterior superior; *RPI*, right posterior inferior; *LMS*, left medial superior; *LMI*, left medial inferior (quadrate lobe in classical anatomy); *LLS*, left lateral superior; *LLI*, left lateral inferior; *C*, caudate lobe.

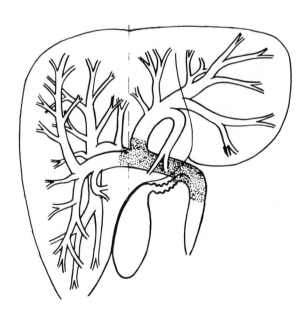

Fig. 10-15 Segmental anatomy of bile ducts. Shaded portion indicates area in which numerous variations in junctional arrangement occur.

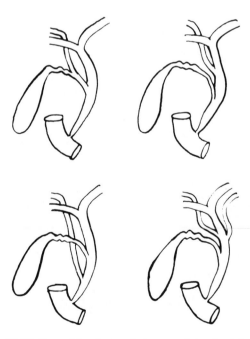

Fig. 10-16 Some bile duct variations as determined in 400 consecutive biliary operations.

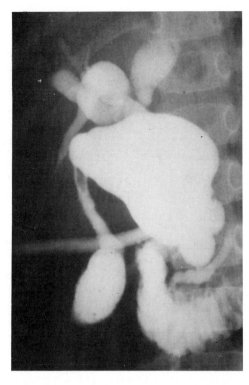

Fig. 10-17 Choledochal cyst in 7-year-old child. Operative cholangiogram. Note that distal common duct enters lateral aspect of main pancreatic duct about 2 cm proximal to duodenal papilla.

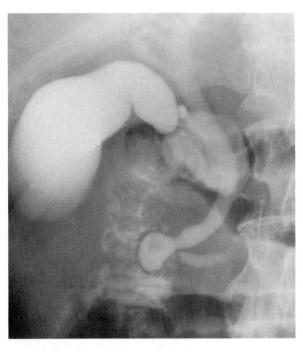

Fig. 10-18 Direct cholangiogram shows clublike configuration of distal common duct caused by choledochocele. Also note stone within.

Choledochal cyst

A choledochal cyst is a segmental dilatation of the extrahepatic bile duct that at times also involves the adjacent cystic duct or contiguous intrahepatic bile ducts. These lesions may be demonstrated by CT scanning, ultrasound, or cholescintigraphy. Direct cholangiography, however, best defines the anatomic extent of the choledochal cyst (Fig. 10-17).

Choledochocele

A choledochocele is a benign cystlike dilatation of the intramural segment of the distal common bile duct protruding into the duodenal lumen (Fig. 10-18). The diagnosis is difficult and has been missed even at cholecystectomy.

Caroli's disease

Caroli's disease (Fig. 10-19), or communicating cavernous ectasia, is characterized by segmental saccular dilatations of intrahepatic bile ducts, a predisposition to biliary calculus formation and cholangitis, and absence

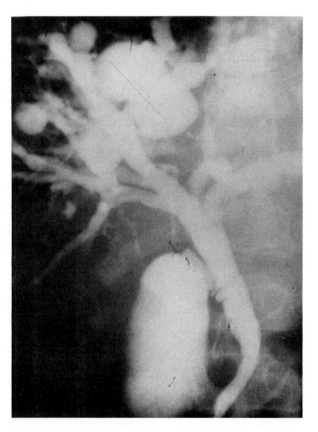

Fig. 10-19 Percutaneous cholangiogram demonstrating Caroli's disease in 10-year-old child with recurrent fever and right upper quadrant pain.

(Courtesy Plinio, R; from Berk RN, Clemett AR: *Radiology of the gallbladder and bile ducts,* Philadelphia, 1977, WB Saunders.)

of cirrhosis or portal hypertension. The disease is familial. Although the diagnosis can be made or suggested by CT scanning, ultrasound, or hepatic scintigraphy, direct cholangiography should be performed in all cases to confirm the diagnosis and to evaluate the possible formation of stasis calculi.

DIFFUSE LIVER DISEASES
Hepatomegaly

Gross hepatomegaly is readily recognized on plain films supplemented by cross-sectional imaging. It may be caused by a large number of diffuse diseases, by a single lesion, or by multiple focal lesions, such as abscesses, cysts, or tumors.

Cirrhosis

Radiologic findings in cirrhosis vary with the stage of the disease. The liver may be large, with features of diffuse hepatomegaly. When collapse, contraction, and scarring become prominent, the hepatic artery branches of the affected area become tortuous, or corkscrewlike in appearance (Fig. 10-20). Regenerating nodules cause stretching of hepatic artery branches. Contraction of the right lobe with extensive regeneration of the left is a common pattern in cirrhosis, but a dominant regenerating nodule may be found in any location. In biliary cirrhosis diffuse narrowing and diminished branching of intrahepatic bile ducts are frequent.

VASCULAR DISEASES
Portal hypertension

Cirrhosis is the major cause of portal hypertension in North America. Several other entities must be considered in any given case, especially when liver function is

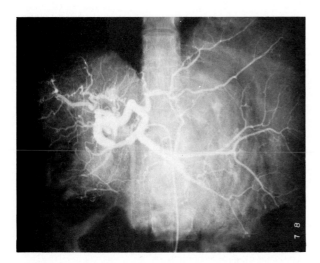

Fig. 10-20 Cirrhosis. Arteries in right lobe are tortuous and distorted because of contraction, whereas those on left are elongated and narrowed because of regenerating nodules.

relatively normal. These include schistosomiasis, portal vein thrombosis, splenic vein thrombosis, hepatic vein obstruction, sarcoidosis, hepatoportal sclerosis, congenital hepatic fibrosis, partial nodular transformation of the liver, hepatic artery–portal vein shunts, cystic fibrosis, and portal vein aneurysm.

INCREASED DENSITY OF THE LIVER

When sufficient concentrations of elements of high atomic number are deposited in the liver, radiographic density increases and the liver is visualized. An excessive burden of body iron, the most frequent cause of this phenomenon, usually comes from one of three sources: (1) increased absorption in hemochromatosis, (2) multiple transfusions in patients with refractory anemia, and (3) increased dietary iron.

Thallium intoxication has also been reported to cause increased radiographic density of the liver. Thorium is the other principal element causing diffuse liver opacification (Fig. 10-21). Following intravascular injection of colloidal thorium dioxide, about 70% is found in the liver, 30% in the spleen, and the remainder in other tissues, principally bone marrow and abdominal lymph nodes. Thorium dioxide is notorious for causing liver tumors, which develop after a mean latent period of 15 years.

LIVER CALCIFICATIONS

Conditions causing calcification of the liver are listed in the box on p. 332. Those in which calcifications occur with any real frequency include tuberculosis, granulomatous disease of childhood, echinococcal infestation, portal venous thrombosis, metastatic adenocarcinoma, giant hemangioma, hepatoblastoma, and mixed malignant tumor.

INFLAMMATORY LESIONS
Pyogenic, amebic, and fungal liver abscesses

In almost all cases diagnosis of liver abscess is possible with present radiologic techniques. An analysis of several large series reveals that abscesses are multiple in about half of the cases. Most are pyogenic, about 10% are amebic, and 1% to 2% are fungal. Plain film findings include hepatomegaly, loss of the hepatic angle, gallbladder distention, elevation of the right diaphragm, pleural effusion, and right lower lobe atelectasis or infiltration. Identification of gas in the abscess is a rare event usually associated with *Klebsiella* infections (Fig. 10-22).

Primary and secondary sclerosing cholangitis

Primary sclerosing cholangitis is a rare lesion, which nevertheless is an important cause of right upper quadrant pain and jaundice. Criteria for diagnosis include

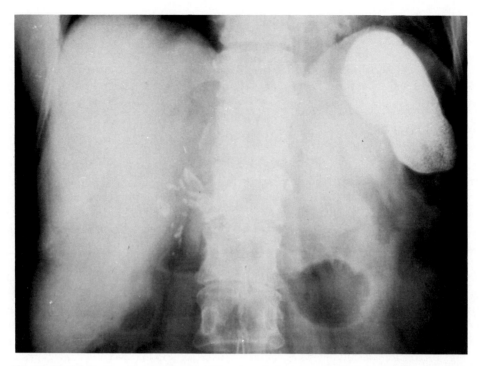

Fig. 10-21 Old thorium dioxide injection. There is reticular pattern in liver and stippled pattern in spleen and regional lymph nodes. Small dense spleen and opacified lymph nodes indicate that injection occurred several years earlier.

☐ **HEPATIC CALCIFICATIONS** ☐

INFECTION

Tuberculosis

Histoplasmosis

Gumma

Brucellosis

Pyogenic abscess (especially in granulomatous disease of childhood)

Amebic abscess

Echinococcus granulosus

Echinococcus multilocularis

Intrauterine infection by toxoplasmosis and herpes simplex

Schistosomiasis japonica

Fasciola gigantica

VASCULAR

Hepatic artery aneurysm

Portal venous thrombosis

PRIMARY TUMOR

Cavernous hemangioma

Giant hemangioma

Infantile hemangioendothelioma

Hepatocellular carcinoma

Hepatoblastoma

Mixed malignant tumor

Hamartoma

METASTATIC TUMOR

Adenocarcinoma (colon, stomach, breast, ovary)

Melanoma

Mesothelioma

Osteosarcoma

Leiomyosarcoma

Carcinoid

Adrenal rest tumor

Myeloma

Hodgkin's disease

Neuroblastoma

MISCELLANEOUS

Hematoma

Intrahepatic calculi

Posteclampsia

Regenerating nodule in cirrhosis

Congenital cyst

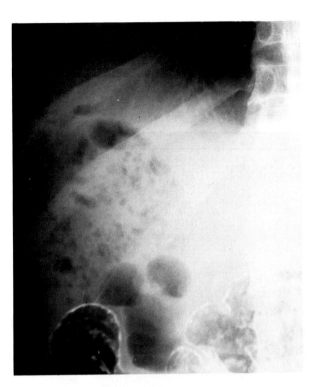

Fig. 10-22 Gas-containing abscess of liver.

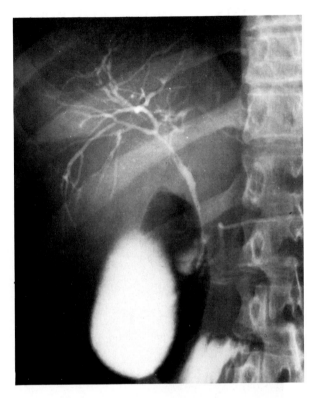

Fig. 10-23 Primary sclerosing cholangitis. ERCP demonstrates diffuse narrowing and irregularity of intrahepatic and extrahepatic ducts.

generalized thickening and stenosis of extrahepatic and intrahepatic ducts; absence of calculi; and exclusion of previous biliary surgery, primary biliary cirrhosis, and malignancy. Many cases occur in patients with chronic ulcerative colitis, and an association with pancreatitis has also been identified.

The cause of primary sclerosing cholangitis is unknown; theories include bacterial infection in the portal system and an autoimmune reaction. The autoimmune mechanism is supported by associated diseases, including regional enteritis, retroperitoneal fibrosis, Riedel's struma, follicular lymph node hyperplasia, and orbital pseudotumor.

In primary sclerosing cholangitis direct cholangiography reveals either diffuse narrowing of the extrahepatic and intrahepatic ducts or multiple strictures of varying lengths, most often without much proximal dilatation. The success rate for diagnosis is high with ERCP, which is clearly the procedure of choice (Fig. 10-23).

Echinococcal cyst

Humans are accidental intermediate hosts of the dog tapeworm, *Taenia echinococcus*. The patient's geo-graphic and ethnic origins are important clues to the diagnosis. Radiologic evaluation is essential for the preoperative diagnosis of echinococcal disease.

Ascariasis

Invasion of the biliary tract by *Ascaris lumbricoides* does occur. Adult ascarids may be demonstrated on direct cholangiography. This infestation is fairly prevalent in the Orient and South America.

Liver flukes

Infestation with the Chinese liver fluke *Clonorchis sinensis* is endemic in southern China and Indochina. *Clonorchis* infestation is associated with an increased incidence of intrahepatic bile duct carcinoma and has been implicated as the cause of hepatolithiasis. Only 30% to 40% of *Clonorchis sinensis* infestations are associated with ductal cholelithiasis in the Orient. Cases seen in the United States usually occur in Oriental immigrants. The flukes are flat and about 10 to 15 mm long.

Fasciola hepatica is similar in form and structure to *Clonorchis sinensis*. *F. hepatica* is associated with a high incidence of choledocholithiasis.

small focal liver masses. In comparison with CT, sonography is superior for determining the internal morphology of cystic hepatic lesions.

Gallbladder

During the past decade *cholecystosonography* has replaced oral cholecystography as the modality of choice for imaging the gallbladder. Advantages of ultrasound include the following:

1. Lack of ionizing radiation
2. Possible detection of more calculi than with oral cholecystography
3. No need for contrast material
4. Ability to use with acutely ill patients
5. Independence from gastrointestinal, hepatic, and biliary function
6. Ability to image multiple other organs in the upper abdomen

Normal gallbladder

A normal gallbladder, physiologically distended following an 8 to 12 hour fast, can be visualized in virtually all cases. In rare cases, massive obesity or overlying distended loops of bowel may preclude visualization. For most patients a 3.5 MHz transducer is required. The gallbladder should be examined during suspended respiration, usually following a deep inspiratory effort.

The examination is usually performed with the patient lying supine or in a left posterior oblique position. A special effort should be made to examine the region of the gallbladder neck, which, because of its dependent position, is where most calculi are found.

Calculus disease

Ultrasound has been reported to have sensitivities, specificities, and accuracies greater than 95% for detecting gallstones. The most reliable features for stone detection include (1) the presence of a high-amplitude, intraluminal reflection that casts an acoustic shadow and (2) gravity-dependent movement. It is easier to detect the high-amplitude reflection caused by the stone than to demonstrate the accompanying acoustic shadow (Fig. 10-46).

As the gallbladder progressively contracts about multiple intraluminal stones or as the lumen progressively fills with stones, the sonographic appearance of the gallbladder changes dramatically. Instead of a well-defined gallbladder outline, a high-amplitude echo with prominent acoustic shadowing is seen in the region of the gallbladder fossa. The echo-shadow complex is caused by reflections and absorption of sound from the most superficial layer of stones. One artifact that can be particularly troublesome results from shadowing that appears to arise from the neck region of the gallbladder. Because refraction can cause shadowing in this anatomic location, it is mandatory to visualize the stone and not merely an acoustic shadow before diagnosing cholelithiasis. In addition, shadows posterior to the gallbladder that emanate from bowel should not be misconstrued as features suggestive of primary gallbladder pathologic condition.

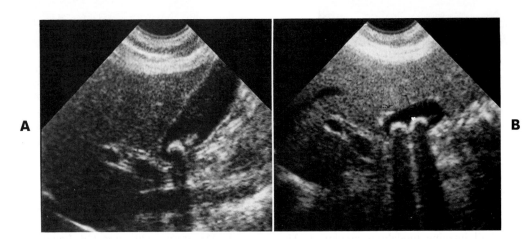

Fig. 10-46 A, Two echogenic foci are visible near gallbladder neck. Acoustic shadowing is visible behind one of these foci, consistent with calculus. Etiology for second mass is indeterminate on this scan. **B,** Repeat scan now shows acoustic shadowing behind both foci, consistent with two gallstones. It is important for gallstones to be contained within central portion of ultrasound beam in order to crease acoustic shadow.

(From Laing FC: Ultrasonography of the biliary tree. In Sarti DA, editor: *Diagnostic ultrasound: text and cases,* ed 2, Chicago, 1987, Mosby–Year Book.)

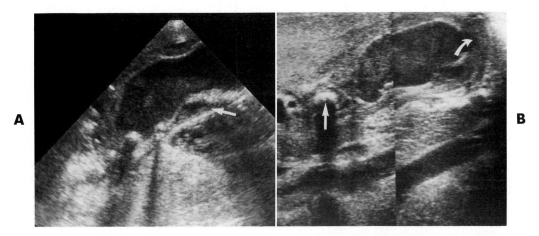

Fig. 10-47 Two longitudinal scans obtained from different patients, each of whom were proved surgically to have acute gangrenous cholecystitis. **A,** In addition to multiple gallstones, intraluminal sludge and irregular thickening *(arrow)* of the gallbladder wall are present. **B,** In addition to intraluminal stones and sludge, stone is impacted in cystic duct *(straight arrow)*, and focal wall irregularity appears in fundus of gallbladder *(curved arrow)* because of impending perforation. *H,* Head.

(From Laing FC: Ultrasonography of the gallbladder and biliary tree. In Sarti DA, editor: *Diagnostic ultrasound: text and cases,* ed 2, Chicago, 1987, Mosby–Year Book.)

Acute cholecystitis

Many different pathologic entities must be considered in patients with acute right upper quadrant pain. Because ultrasound allows rapid survey of the entire abdomen and diagnosis of acute cholecystitis, as well as many other conditions that may mimic acute gallbladder disease, sonography should be the imaging modality of choice for initial evaluation of these patients. The ultrasonographic diagnosis of acute cholecystitis can be made if a patient has focal tenderness over the gallbladder fossa in association with calculi. The presence of sludge and a thickened gallbladder wall lend further support to the diagnosis (Fig. 10-47).

Gallbladder wall

On sonograms the gallbladder wall is normally perceived as a thin (3 mm or less) echogenic line. When the gallbladder wall thickens, it usually does so in a diffuse and symmetric fashion. *Diffuse gallbladder wall thickening* is neither sensitive nor specific for primary gallbladder inflammation. Only 50% to 75% of patients with acute cholecystitis have thickened gallbladder walls, which may be seen with hepatic dysfunction (associated with alcoholism, hypoalbuminemia, ascites, and hepatitis), congestive heart failure, renal disease, neoplasm, and sepsis.

A more specific observation for primary gallbladder disease is *focal gallbladder wall thickening.* This condition can occur with various pathologic processes, including primary gallbladder carcinoma (Fig. 10-48),

polyps, cholesterolosis, papillary adenomas, metastases, adenomyomatosis, and—on occasion—tumefactive sludge.

Pericholecystic fluid

Localized pericholecystic fluid most often results from acute cholecystitis with associated gallbladder perforation and abscess formation.

Sludge

Intraluminal sludge *(echogenic bile)* is usually caused by crystalline particles and can be seen in several unrelated clinical conditions (Fig. 10-49). In most cases these nonshadowing echoes are situated dependently within the gallbladder. Because echo-free bile usually layers on the sludge, a fluid-fluid level is generally visible. The most frequent predisposing factors leading to true sludge are bile stasis, a prolonged fast, or hyperalimentation.

Bile ducts

Ultrasonography is particularly well suited for tracking and identifying tubular, fluid-filled structures such as blood vessels and bile ducts. Because with ultrasound it is possible to detect early changes associated with intrahepatic and extrahepatic duct dilatation, many consider this modality the procedure of choice in the initial evaluation of a patient with jaundice (Fig. 10-50).

Intrahepatic bile ducts

When intrahepatic bile ducts dilate, they cross a threshold of visibility and can be seen lying parallel to the normally visible branches of the intrahepatic portal veins (Fig. 10-51).

Intrahepatic pneumobilia can also be recognized on ultrasound and should be distinguished from the appearance of intrahepatic calculi or parenchymal gas collec-

tions. The characteristic sonographic appearance of pneumobilia consists of long or short echogenic foci, with associated reverberative comet-tail artifacts that are located in the distribution of the bile ducts. Because the left duct is anatomically superior and anterior to the right duct, gas tends to localize preferentially to the left duct.

On occasion, intrahepatic dilatation may be difficult to detect if the bile ducts are filled with echogenic material that is isoechoic with hepatic parenchymal tissue or if the ducts are obscured by associated shadowing. Most often, recurrent pyogenic cholangiohepatitis is responsible for this appearance.

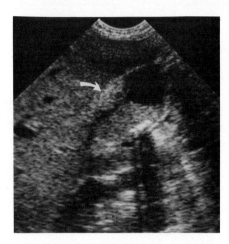

Fig. 10-48 Localized thickening is visible along anterior gallbladder wall *(arrow)* and is caused by primary gallbladder carcinoma. In addition, sludge and multiple gallstones are present in dependent portion of gallbladder.

(From Laing FC: Ultrasonography of the gallbladder and biliary tree. In Sarti DA, editor: *Diagnostic ultrasound: text and cases,* ed 2, Chicago, 1987, Mosby–Year Book.)

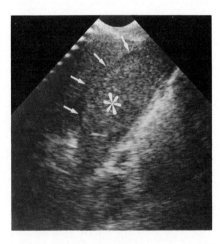

Fig. 10-49 Occasionally gallbladder may be filled with echogenic sludge *(asterisk)* such that its echo texture is similar to hepatic parenchymal tissue. Careful scanning usually can identify gallbladder wall *(arrows),* which aids in identification of gallbladder. *H,* Head.

(From Laing FC: Ultrasonography of the gallbladder and biliary tree. In Sarti DA, editor: *Diagnostic ultrasound: text and cases,* ed 2, Chicago, 1987, Mosby–Year Book.)

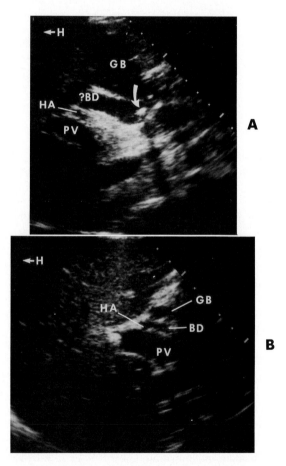

Fig. 10-50 A, Calculus with acoustic shadowing *(arrow)* is visible in what might be misconstrued as dilated bile duct *(BD).* Gallbladder *(GB)* is situated anteriorly, whereas portal vein *(PV)* and hepatic artery *(HA)* are situated posterior to this structure. This stone actually was within redundant gallbladder neck, not in dilated bile duct. *H,* Head. **B,** Longitudinal scan obtained in slightly more medial direction reveals normal-sized bile duct *(BD)* just behind gallbladder neck *(GB).* Also visible are more posteriorly located portal vein *(PV)* and hepatic artery *(HA). H,* Head.

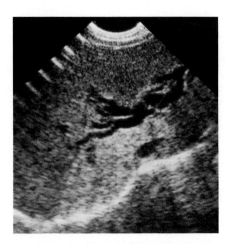

Fig. 10-51 Within substance of right lobe of liver are irregular, tortuous tubular structures that appear to converge centrally. In addition to stellate and tortuous configuration of bile ducts, enhanced sound transmission is present. These features are diagnostic for dilated intrahepatic bile ducts.

(From Laing FC: Ultrasonography of the gallbladder and biliary tree. In Sarti DA, editor: *Diagnostic ultrasound: text and cases,* ed 2, Chicago, 1987, Mosby–Year Book.)

Extrahepatic bile ducts

The most easily visualized portion of the extrahepatic ductal system is the *common hepatic duct*. This structure, which is visible in virtually all patients regardless of their size or body habitus, is located within the portal fissure (porta hepatis) (Fig. 10-52).

As the *common bile duct (CBD)* descends within the hepatoduodenal ligament toward the second duodenum, it is accompanied by two other tubular structures: the main portal vein and the proper hepatic artery. The distal CBD should be examined initially by placing the patient in a semierect, right posterior oblique position and obtaining transverse (as opposed to parasagittal) scans. This procedure minimizes antral and duodenal bowel gas because gas tends to rise to the fundus of the stomach. In addition, retained gastric fluid enters the antrum and duodenum.

It is generally accepted that the size of the extrahepatic bile duct is the most sensitive indicator for distinguishing *obstructive* from *nonobstructive jaundice*. Normally the diameter of the common hepatic duct or CBD is 5 mm or less. Measurements of 6 to 7 mm are considered equivocal, and measurements of 8 mm or greater are considered dilated. The size of the common hepatic duct or CBD may be somewhat larger in patients who have previously undergone biliary surgery.

A patient with obstructive jaundice may fail to exhibit dilatation of either the intrahepatic or extrahepatic biliary ducts. Sclerosing or AIDS-related cholangitis,

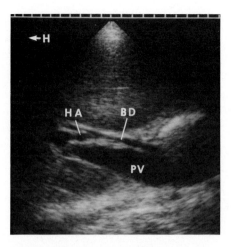

Fig. 10-52 Parasagittal oblique scan obtained over portal fissure (porta hepatis) demonstrates normal anatomic structures in this region, which consist of posterior portal vein *(PV)*, anterior bile duct *(BD)*, and interposed right hepatic artery *(HA)*. *H,* Head.

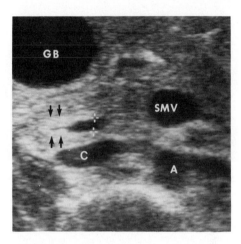

Fig. 10-53 Transverse magnified scan reveals stricture of distal common bile duct *(arrows)*. In this patient AIDS cholangitis accounted for this finding. *A,* Aorta; *C,* inferior vena cava; *SMV,* superior mesenteric vein; *GB,* gallbladder.

(From Dolmatch BL et al: AIDS-related cholangitis: radiographic findings in nine patients, *Radiology* 163:314, 1987.)

partial obstruction, or intermittent obstruction from choledocholithiasis is usually responsible in these cases.

Strictures, an uncommon cause of distal obstruction, are difficult to detect by sonography, but on occasion can be seen in thin patients (Fig. 10-53).

NUCLEAR MEDICINE
LEONARD ROSENTHALL

The normal liver is variable in configuration, but the guiding lines are smooth borders and a uniform distribution of radiocolloid. Liver size is generally assessed

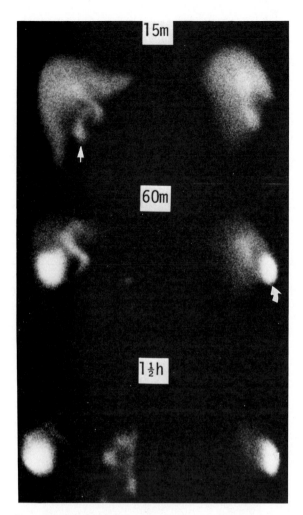

Fig. 10-54 Anterior and right lateral views of normal gallbladder study with ^{99m}Tc-diisopropyl-IDA (DISIDA). At 15 minutes common duct and duodenum *(arrow)* are seen. At 60 minutes gallbladder contains high concentration of ^{99m}Tc-IDA. Note its anterior position in right lateral projection *(arrow)*. By 90 minutes liver is virtually washed out.

subjectively; the simplest measurement is the maximum cephalocaudal dimension, which is reported to be approximately 17 cm in normal adults. Single-photon emission computerized tomography (SPECT) permits programmed determinations of liver volume by integrating liver slices of known thickness. The peak uptake of ^{99m}Tc-iminodiacetic acid (^{99m}Tc-IDA) in the liver usually occurs about 10 to 12 minutes after intravenous injection (Fig. 10-54). The times for biliary tract, gallbladder, and duodenal visualization are variable, but normally all three should be identified within 1 hour. The liver should be visually washed out by 2 hours.

Liver

Abnormalities of the liver present as single or multiple focal functional defects or as diffuse involvement.

Diffuse disease

Diffuse disease of the liver is appreciated only when the liver becomes enlarged or when the process decreases blood flow or interferes with Kupffer cell function to the point that radiocolloid shifts to the spleen and bone marrow. In *cirrhosis* associated with alcohol abuse, enlargement of the liver in the early phases of the disease is caused by fatty infiltration. As cirrhosis advances, the liver shrinks in size and becomes less fatty and more fibrotic. This may be followed by atrophy of the right lobe with compensatory hypertrophy of the left lobe and the production of ascites.

Focal disease

Since the resolution of a focal lesion by the gamma camera decreases as the distance from the face of the collimator increases, cold lesions 1.5 to 2 cm in diameter on the surface of the liver may be disclosed, whereas lesions 3 cm in diameter located in the depths of the right lobe may be missed. SPECT imaging improves the resolution.

Metastatic disease

Some controversy exists regarding the use of liver scans for screening patients with known primary carcinomas for purposes of staging and subsequent management. In patients without hepatomegaly and with normal liver function tests, no true positive liver scans occurred in a series of 109 patients with bronchogenic carcinoma. When at least one clinical finding suggested liver disease, however, 23 of 154 (15%) had true positive radiocolloid liver scans. Results of this kind prompted some investigators to conclude that it is not financially efficacious to perform preoperative liver scans routinely if there is no clinical or biochemical reason to suspect liver disease, and that high-risk patients should be screened with biochemical tests such as alkaline phosphatase, SGOT, LDH, and serum bilirubin. Others argue that baseline liver scans could disclose nonneoplastic lesions or variations in anatomic configuration, which might confuse the diagnosis when biochemical abnormalities develop later.

Primary malignant neoplasms

There are no distinguishing radiocolloid features of hepatomas or cholangiocarcinomas, and in a cirrhotic context they may resemble pseudotumors. Pseudotumors are areas of absent radiocolloid uptake caused by scarring, regenerating nodules, necrosis, and arteriovenous shunting in a cirrhotic liver.

Benign tumors

In cavernous hemangioma (Fig. 10-55), ^{99m}TC-labeled erythrocyte imaging shows a characteristic hypo-

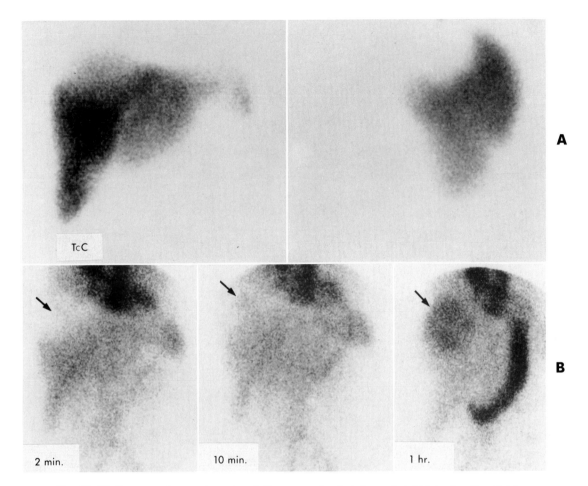

TcC

2 min.   10 min.   1 hr.

Fig. 10-55 Cavernous hemangioma in adult woman. **A,** Anterior and right lateral radiocolloid (TcC, technetium colloid) liver images demonstrate large solitary lesion in upper posterior part of right lobe. **B,** ^{99m}Tc-labeled red blood cell blood pool images taken at various times after administration, showing progressive accumulation within lesion. Hemangioma is not seen at 2 minutes, but early entry is observed at 10 minutes, and lesion has higher concentration than adjacent normal liver at 1 hour *(arrows)*.

perfusion and decreased initial blood pool activity, followed by progressive accumulation of labeled erythrocytes over the next hour or two. The sensitivity of detection approaches 90%. SPECT imaging with ^{99m}Tc-labeled erythrocytes has been shown to detect small hemangiomas that escaped planar imaging.

Abscesses

Pyogenic liver infection can be imaged with radiocolloids.^{67}Ga concentrates in abscesses, but it also has a tropism for tumors, particularly hepatoma, and therefore lacks the desired specificity.

Amebic liver abscesses produce a photon-deficient lesion on radiocolloid scans.^{67}Ga images have been reported to show a central photon deficiency surrounded by a rind of increased uptake.

Biliary tract
Cholecystitis

Obstruction of the cystic duct is the initiating cause of acute cholecystitis in about 95% of patients. Visualization of the gallbladder with^{99m}Tc-IDA therefore virtually excludes acute disease. Acute acalculous cholecystitis, an infrequently occurring entity, may be associated with gallbladder filling, but in that case the administration of cholecystokinin (CCK) fails to induce a normal contraction. In most of these cases, however, the gallbladder is not visualized, presumably a result of cystic duct occlusion by edema. Failure to visualize the gallbladder within 4 hours, or complete liver washout in the presence of normal or mildly impaired liver function, should not be considered pathognomonic of acute disease. The disease could be either acute or chronic,

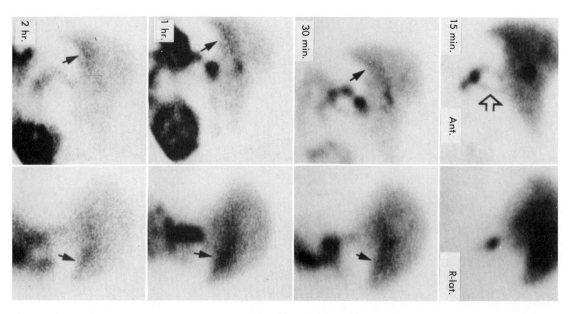

Fig. 10-56 Rim sign or pericholecystic accumulation of ^{99m}Tc-IDA in acute cholecystitis—anterior and right lateral views. At 15 minutes common duct is identified; it is deviated and bowed medially *(open arrow)*, reflecting enlarged nonvisualized gallbladder. As liver washes out, rim of relatively higher concentration develops *(solid arrows)*, but gallbladder does not visualize with time. *Ant,* Anterior; *R-Lat,* Right lateral.

Fig. 10-57 Various causes of jaundice shown with ^{99m}Tc-IDA. *1,* Hepatitis in patient with serum bilirubin of 4.7 mg/dl. Poor liver concentration is noted, but gallbladder and duodenum are visualized. *2,* Incomplete obstruction due to carcinoma of pancreas in patient with serum bilirubin of 3.2 mg/dl. At 90 minutes there is no entry into gut, but gallbladder is visualized, and there is stasis in dilated common and intrahepatic bile ducts. *3,* Complete obstruction showing retention in liver and no bowel radioactivity at 24 hours, but kidneys are seen because they are alternate channel of excretion. *4,* End-stage liver failure in patient with serum bilirubin of 35 mg/dl. No liver uptake was seen at 8 hours, and excretion via horseshoe kidneys was demonstrated.

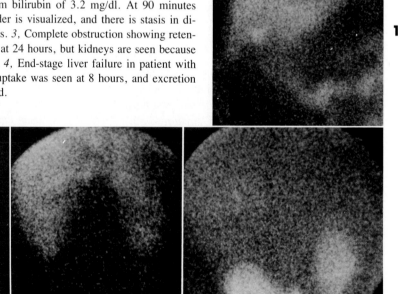

and the finding must be interpreted within the clinical context.

The *rim sign* (Fig. 10-56), when it appears, is a diagnostic aid in the presence of nonvisualization. It consists of a faintly increased concentration of ^{99m}Tc-IDA in the liver tissue bordering the gallbladder fossa, and has been observed in acute cholecystitis, gangrenous cholecystitis, gallbladder perforation, and—in rare cases—in chronic cholecystitis when the gallbladder did not visualize.

The true positive frequency (that is, the sensitivity) of ^{99m}Tc-IDA nucleography for acute cholecystitis is high, varying from 95% to 100%. Although some reports have stated that delayed filling indicates chronic disease, not all chronically diseased gallbladders demonstrate delayed filling, and some normal gallbladders do. For example, normal gallbladders in patients receiving total parenteral nutrition, as well as chronic alcoholics with liver disease, are reported to have showed delayed visualization or no visualization at all when followed for 24 hours.

Acalculous biliary pain

Biliary dyskinesia, chronic acalculous cholecystitis, and *cystic duct syndrome* are terms applied to abnormal gallbladder contractions associated with right upper quadrant pain in the absence of gallstone detection by radiographic cholecystography and ultrasonography.

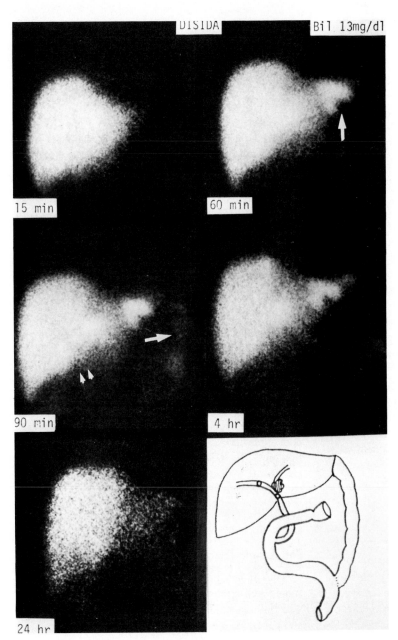

Fig. 10-58 Cholangiocarcinoma at common hepatic duct. A stent was inserted in right and common hepatic ducts to sustain biliary drainage. In addition, partial left lobe hepatectomy and anastomosis of left hepatic duct to a Roux-en-Y segment of jejunum were effected (Longmire's procedure). The ^{99m}Tc-diisopropyl-IDA (DISIDA, Disofenin) study performed 5 days postoperatively showed drainage through this bypass *(arrow)* but no biliary flow through common duct *(twin arrows)*. Latter pathway was obstructed. Note differential drainage between right and left lobes at 24 hours as compared with 15 minutes. Serum bilirubin was 13 mg/dl at time of study.

Cholestasis

Hepatobiliary scintigraphy is capable of distinguishing an extrahepatic cause of jaundice from an intrahepatic or prehepatic cause. Complete *extrahepatic obstruction* is characterized by an absence of liver-to-bowel transit over a 24-hour period of monitoring (Fig. 10-57). A secondary feature is nonvisualization of the biliary ducts and gallbladder. Hepatocyte concentration is usually good when the obstruction is of recent onset. *Intrahepatic jaundice* includes hepatocellular failure and intrahepatic cholestasis, which give rise to unconjugated and conjugated hyperbilirubinemia, respectively. The ^{99m}Tc-IDA portrayal is inconstant. Liver uptake is variably reduced, and liver-to-bowel transit may be normal, delayed, or—with extreme impairment—absent. Although no biliary tract pooling exists to suggest dilatation, the gallbladder may be seen sometime within 24 hours of administration. *Prehepatic jaundice* (for instance hemolytic anemia) generally shows a normal time course of liver concentration and washout. Progressive accumulation of ^{99m}Tc-IDA within the biliary tract plus gut entry beyond 1 hour is the hallmark of *incomplete mechanical choledochal obstruction*. With these criteria the reported sensitivity rates for medical jaundice, complete obstruction, and incomplete obstruction are 77% to 90%, 98% to 100%, and 74% to 78%, respectively.

Overall, the limitations encountered with ^{99m}Tc-IDA in the differential diagnosis of jaundice weigh against its use as a primary screening procedure. Ultrasonography is preferred over CT in terms of economy. ^{99m}Tc-IDA imaging plays an adjuvant role in patients with jaundice who have had no previous cholangioenteric reconstructive procedures, when ultrasonography is indeterminate, when the results of ultrasonography do not correspond to the clinical and biochemical parameters, or when there is a need to gain some insight into the bile flow dynamics.

Postcholecystectomy syndrome occurs in approximately 10% to 50% of patients following gallbladder resection. Causes include retained stones, biliary dyskinesia, common bile duct stricture or tumor, papillary stenosis, common bile duct obstruction secondary to pancreatitis, and cystic duct remnant. Many of these complications can be disclosed by ^{99m}Tc-IDA imaging.

Surgically altered biliary and gastrointestinal anatomy

The technique of monitoring the bile pathway with ^{99m}Tc-IDA analogs offers an innocuous, dynamic, and clinically useful procedure for clarification of postsurgical complications associated with cholecystointestinal and choledochointestinal anastomoses and gastroenteric bypasses (Fig. 10-58).

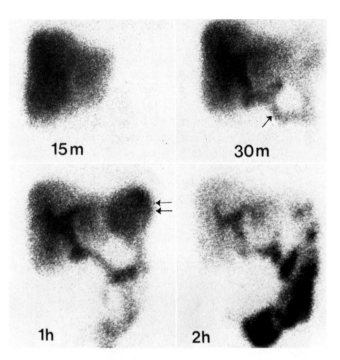

Fig. 10-59 Unobstructed dilated biliary tract and gastric reflux in patient with cholecystojejunostomy and Billroth II gastroenterostomy. Whipple's procedure for carcinoma of pancreas had been previously performed, and there was no jaundice at time of ^{99m}Tc-IDA study. Serial images demonstrate dilated hepatic and common ducts, but there was no obstruction because gut entry occurred within ½ hour of administration *(arrow)* and liver parenchyma showed normal washout. Gastric reflux is clearly seen at 1 hour *(twin arrows)*, and it progressively disappears with time. Afferent and efferent loop transit is normal, and there is no evidence of afferent loop stasis.

Normally functioning *cholangiointestinal conduits* exhibit bowel radioactivity within 1 hour. Extrahepatic obstruction is manifested as delayed gut entry with dilatation and stasis within the proximal biliary tract. In patients with normally functioning *gastroenterostomies* the afferent and efferent loops are seen within 1 hour, and afferent loop washout is usually achieved by 2 hours. Obstruction appears as a progressive accumulation of ^{99m}Tc-IDA in the segment proximal to the stenosis and as a delay or absence of antegrade movement (Figs. 10-56 to 10-60).

ENDOSCOPY
PREMYSL SLEZAK

Endoscopic retrograde cholangiopancreatography

The diagnostic and therapeutic potential of endoscopic retrograde cholangiopancreatography (ERCP), which includes the esophagus, stomach, duodenum, and pancreas, is much broader than that of percutaneous

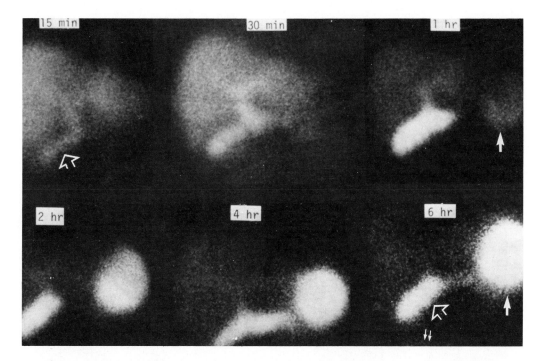

Fig. 10-60 Inlet-outlet obstruction in patient who had Whipple's procedure for papillary carcinoma of ampulla of Vater. It included partial gastrectomy, choledochojejunostomy, end-to-end pancreaticojejunostomy, and retrocolic gastrojejunostomy. Chief complaint was copious bile vomiting. ^{99m}Tc-IDA images depict efferent loop entry at 15 minutes *(open arrow)*, gastric reflux at 1 hour *(solid arrow)*, and persistent stasis in afferent loop and stomach remnant as late as 6 hours. Efferent loop entry is recorded only after 2 hours. Findings are consistent with partial inlet-outlet obstruction.

transhepatic cholangiography (PTC). ERCP, usually performed in a sophisticated radiology unit, can be undertaken as either a cooperative venture between the radiologist and a skilled endoscopist or as an individual effort for a radiologist who is also a skilled endoscopist. ERCP is impossible to perform in patients with obstruction in the gastrointestinal tract above the papilla, is difficult in patients with Billroth II partial gastrectomy, and may be impossible when the duct is blocked at the papilla. The most important indication for ERCP is obstructive jaundice.

Technique and anatomy

ERCP is performed with the patient sedated and preferably in the left lateral decubitus position. A side-viewing duodenoscope is passed to the papilla for cannulation under direct vision. Experts favor a straight endoscope for cannulation, which is achieved by hooking the tip of the instrument in the second part of the duodenum and bringing the lens up the medial wall of the duodenum to the longitudinal fold and papilla. The papilla minor is classically 2 to 3 cm above Vater's papilla and has no longitudinal fold. In 55% of cases the main pancreatic duct (PD) and the CBD form a common duct a few millimeters long. In 42% of patients, the CBD and the PD open separately into the papillary orifice, demanding a separate cannulation of each of the ducts.

Diagnostic accuracy and success rate

Reports of the diagnostic accuracy of ERCP vary from 67% to 100%. The overall accuracy rate has been reported to be 90%, 80% to 95%, and greater than 95%. The range of success rates is reported to be from 50% to 98%.

Complications

ERCP is currently the least invasive technique for obtaining detailed images of the pancreatic and biliary ductal system. ERCP performed by an expert is now accepted as a safe procedure. It is considered a safe technique even in patients with a previous history of allergic reactions to iodized contrast media, despite the fact that the contrast media is absorbed primarily from the PD, as seen by the pyelography in ERCP, in as many as 35% of cases. Nonetheless, ERCP may be followed by

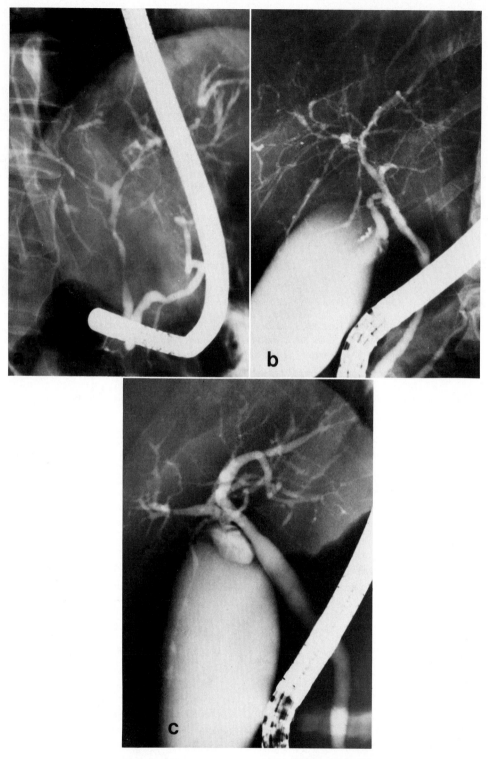

Fig. 10-61 Primary sclerosing cholangitis. Three cases associated with ulcerative colitis. **A,** Severe changes in intrahepatic bile ducts (pruning and beading), as well as in extrahepatic bile duct. **B,** Severe changes in intrahepatic and extrahepatic biliary ducts. **C,** Moderate changes mainly in intrahepatic biliary tree. Only slight narrowing of common hepatic duct close to hilum of liver can be seen.

serious complications and even death. The overall rate of complications after ERCP ranges from 0.38% to 12%. The overall incidence may be regarded as 2% to 5%. Overall mortality ranges from 0% to 2.9%.

Injection pancreatitis, one of the more common and important complications, varies in severity from slight hyperamylasemia, appearing in as many as 75% of patients undergoing ERCP, to a fatal necrotizing pancreatitis. The cause of injection pancreatitis is poorly understood. Fluoroscopic control during PD injection is recommended to prevent overfilling. The contrast injection should be stopped as soon as a large branch filling is recognized on the fluoroscopic screen.

Although less frequent, *cholangitis, cholangitic sepsis,* and *pancreatic sepsis* are not entirely uncommon after ERCP and can be very serious. The pathogenesis is bacterial and occurs most commonly in obstruction of the CBD.

Radiologic diagnosis and differential diagnosis

The most important radiologic findings are stenosis, dilatation, contrast defects in the biliary duct and leakage of contrast medium outside the biliary duct, and functional signs.

Stenosis
INTRAHEPATIC STENOSIS AND COMBINED INTRAHEPATIC AND EXTRAHEPATIC STENOSIS

Although stenoses are easily visualized on ERCP, its sensitivity (its ability to reveal an intrahepatic lesion that can cause stenosis) is low. The differential diagnosis can be difficult. With *cirrhosis,* generalized crowding of the intrahepatic ducts and zigzagging and corkscrewing of the fine radicles occur. *Infiltrative parenchymatous processes* show straightening and elongation of intrahepatic ducts that are spread apart. *Hepatic tumors* are characterized by mass lesions that cause displacement of the intrahepatic ducts, and may show signs of invasion such as enveloping, compressing, and stenosing to complete block of intrahepatic ducts. *Iatrogenic lesions* following biliary surgery are more common in the extrahepatic part of the biliary tract. *Recurrent pyogenic cholangitis* and *hepatolithiasis* involve strictures and stones in both the intrahepatic and extrahepatic bile ducts. *Primary sclerosing cholangitis (PSC)* is an uncommon disease of unknown cause characterized by inflammation and fibrosis of the biliary tree with diffuse stricture formation (Figs. 10-61, 10-62). *Cholangiocarcinoma (diffuse sclerosing carcinoma)* of

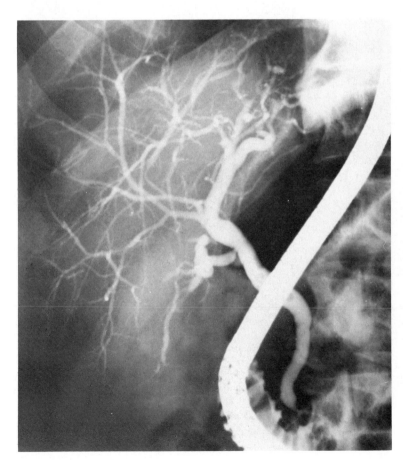

Fig. 10-62 Primary biliary cirrhosis. Moderate changes—corkscrewing and zigzagging of radicles—in left liver lobe and very discrete diffuse changes in ducts of right liver lobe. Extrahepatic biliary ducts are normal in PBC, unlike in most cases of PSC.

the bile ducts may mimic PSC. Since decompression plus drainage seem to be the proper treatment for both PSC and cholangiocarcinoma, it is not essential to make the exact differential diagnosis. In *cholangitis associated with acquired immunodeficiency syndrome* (AIDS), ERCP often reveals all the classic signs of PSC in the intrahepatic and extrahepatic bile ducts. *Lymphoma* (Hodgkin's and non-Hodgkin's) may cause encasement of the intrahepatic and extrahepatic bile ducts.

EXTRAHEPATIC STENOSIS

There are similar difficulties with the differential diagnosis in stenosis of the extrahepatic bile ducts. *Cholangiocarcinoma* (Fig. 10-63) may arise at any point, but more than half the lesions appear in the upper third of the CBD, classically at the hepatic hilum. All members of the congenital fibropolycystic family, including congenital hepatic fibrosis, Caroli's disease, choledochal cysts, polycystic liver, and von Meyenburg complexes such as microhamartoma, as well as liver

fluke infestations, may be complicated by cholangiocarcinoma. Most of the tumors are annular scirrhous infiltrating lesions with a tendency to infiltrate extensively in the submucosal plane. *Strictures in the middle duct must be presumed to be malignant if no prior biliary surgery or trauma has occurred.* Those caused by cholangiocarcinoma generally have an abrupt cutoff or rattail appearance (Fig. 10-64). A normal pancreatogram does not exclude a pancreatic malignancy as a cause of CBD involvement. *Pancreatic carcinoma* classically involves the lower part of the CBD and leaves none or almost none of the lumen patent at the time of ERCP (Figs. 10-65, 10-66). A combination of papillary stenosis and intrahepatic ductal strictures appears unique to AIDS-related cholangitis. Ninety percent of benign strictures result from surgery (Fig. 10-67). One in 400 to 500 cholecystectomies result in bile duct injury.

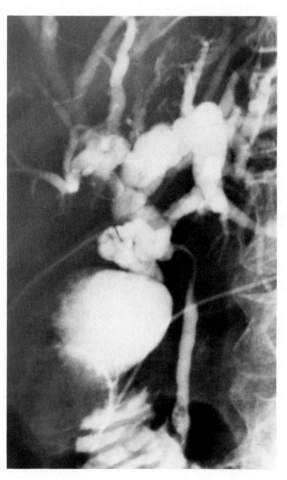

Fig. 10-63 Cholangiocarcinoma causing severe circular stenosis of middle duct—usual localization of CBD tumors.

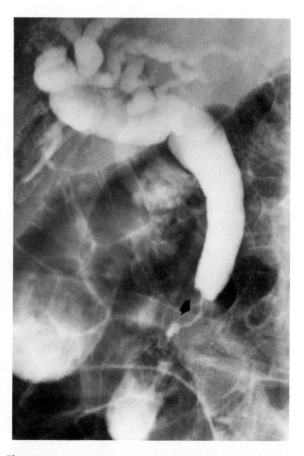

Fig. 10-64 Intraampullary carcinoma. Duodenoscopy did not reveal any abnormality of Vater's papilla. Intraampullary carcinoma causes severe stricture of intramural part of CBD *(arrow)*. Narrowing of such long segment of CBD, as well as irregular outline of stenotic segment, is abnormal finding. Prestenotic dilatation of CBD.

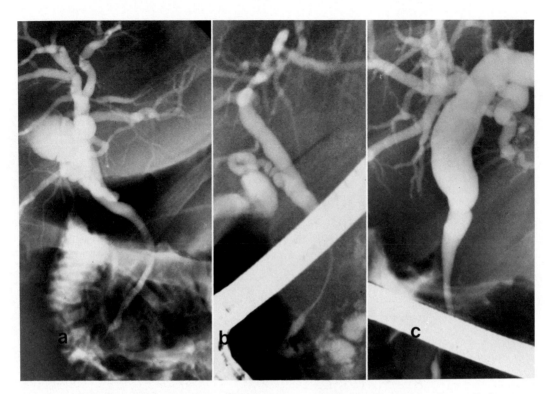

Fig. 10-65 Three cases of severe stenosis of lower part of CBD. **A,** Cholangiocarcinoma. **B,** Pancreatitis (calcifications in head of pancreas). **C,** Pancreatic cyst. Radiologic distinction between benign and malignant stenosis is often impossible.

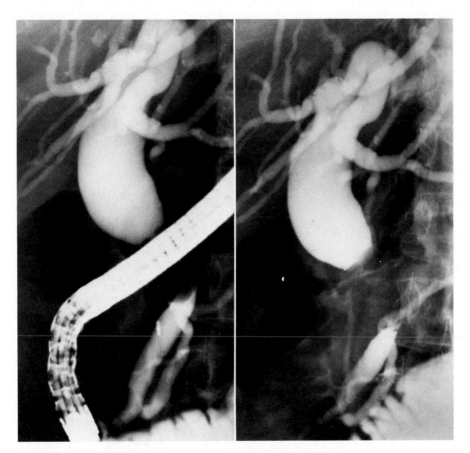

Fig. 10-66 Case of malignant stenosis in middle part of CBD caused by carcinoma of head of pancreas. Pancreatogram was normal.

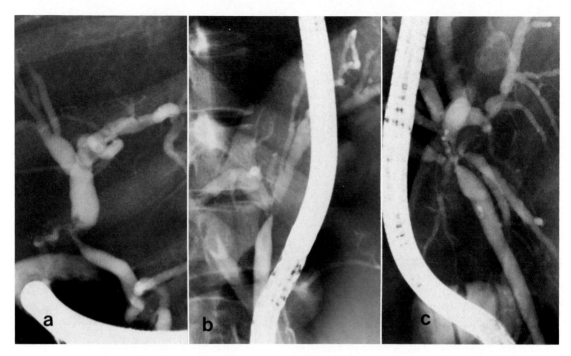

Fig. 10-67 Three cases of biliary duct stenoses. **A,** Classic localization of postsurgical stenosis in CBD at level of cystic duct. **B,** Severe iatrogenic stenosis of common hepatic duct at hilum. ERCP was performed 6 months after cholecystectomy. **C,** Severe stricture of common hepatic duct at hilum without previous history of biliary surgery. This stenosis was due to cholangiocarcinoma. Differential diagnosis between benign and malignant stenosis may be very difficult.

Dilatation

For the purpose of cholangiography, *choledochal cysts* are the most important dilatations of the bile ducts. Todani's classification divides the cysts into five types. Type I, the most common (80% to 90%), is subdivided into (a) choledochal cyst, (b) segmental choledochus dilatation, and (c) diffuse cylindrical dilatation. Type II, which is rare (2%), is a diverticulum anywhere in the extrahepatic ducts. Type III, also rare (1% to 5%), is a choledochocele. Type IV is not common (19%) and is subdivided into (a) multiple cysts of the intrahepatic and extrahepatic ducts and (b) multiple cysts in the extrahepatic ducts only. Type V is an intrahepatic bile duct cyst (single or multiple), also known as Caroli's disease.

The *choledochal cyst* is a dilatation of the CBD (Fig. 10-68). The gallbladder, cystic duct, and hepatic ducts above the cyst are normal. The cyst may obstruct the portal vein, leading to portal hypertension. There is an increased incidence of carcinoma associated with choledochal cyst, estimated at 2% to 5% (the incidence in a normal population is 0.012% to 0.4%).

Caroli's disease is a hereditary autosomal recessive disease often associated with nephrospongiosis. The intrahepatic bile ducts are ectatic and form rounded or oval dilatations 2 to 10 cm in size. The surrounding parenchyma is normal. The incidence of a biliary carcinoma in patients with Caroli's disease is 20 times that in the normal population.

Contrast medium defects

Stones are in general the most common cause of filling defects in the biliary ducts. Stones must be differentiated from air bubbles in the CBD, and apart from noting changes in size, number, and shape of air bubbles during the examination, the traditional maneuver for differentiation is to put the patient in an upright position so that stones move down in the biliary duct and air moves up. This maneuver is, however, not reliable. Stones less than 7 mm in size are able to pass without causing any significant symptoms.

Hepatolithiasis is a specific subtype of biliary lithiasis. This disease is very rare in Western countries but has been reported to have an incidence of 51% in East Asia. In this disorder, soft brown calcium-bicarbonate stones are found in the dilated intrahepatic duct proximal to a stricture. Stricture of the left hepatic duct at the hilum is common, and the left liver lobe is more often

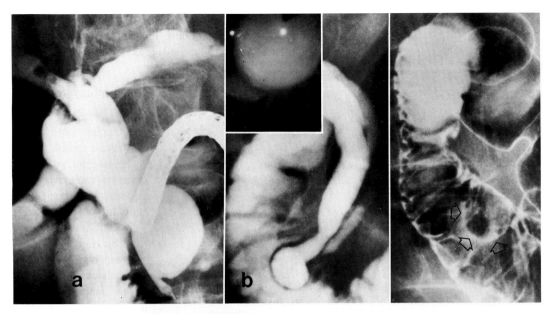

Fig. 10-68 A, Case of choledochal cyst classified as either type Ia or IVa according to Todani. **B,** Case of choledochocele. Duodenoscopy revealed enlarged papilla covered by normal mucosa. *(insert).* Radiograph is characteristic, showing clubbing of terminal end of CBD, producing contrast defect in descending part of duodenum *(open arrows).*

involved. Bile stasis and infection are the main factors responsible for the clinical signs, which are pain in the right upper quadrant, fever, and jaundice. Large stones may lead to the *Mirizzi syndrome,* characterized by large stone impaction in the gallbladder neck, erosion into and obstruction of the common hepatic duct, and proximal biliary tree dilatation. In Mirizzi syndrome the CBD is undilated.

Intrahepatic biliary papillomatosis, which is both uncommon and histologically benign, produces multiple filling defects in the biliary tree. This tumor discharges large quantities of mucus.

Hepatocellular carcinomas may sometimes produce lobulated, irregular filling defects in the major bile ducts.

Hemobilia is hemorrhage arising from pathologic changes in the intrahepatic biliary tract. Its main causes include iatrogenic (Fig. 10-69) and noniatrogenic trauma, cholangitis, tumors, and coagulopathies. Hemobilia occurs in 4% to 13% of cases after diagnostic and therapeutic interventions such as PTC, percutaneous transhepatic biliary drainage, and endoscopic papillotomy.

Parasites in the biliary tract may cause filling defects of various shapes and sizes. The organisms most commonly involved are trematodes or flukes, including

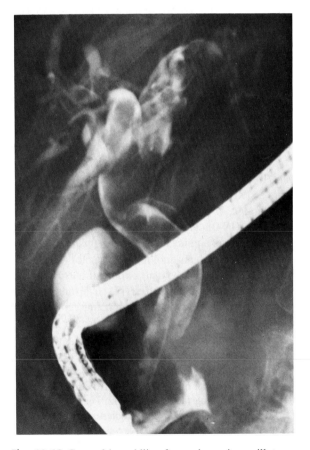

Fig. 10-69 Case of hemobilia after endoscopic papillotomy. ERCP performed 5 days later shows large contrast defects with typical appearance of casts in lumen of intrahepatic and extrahepatic biliary tree.

4. Berk RN et al: Hyperplastic cholecystoses: cholesterolosis and adenomyomatosis, *Radiology* 146:593, 1983.

5. Bernardino ME et al: Delayed hepatic CT scanning: increased confidence and improved detection of hepatic metastases, *Radiology* 159:71, 1986.

6. Burhenne HJ et al: Single-visit oral cholecystography for inpatients, *Radiology* 140:505, 1981.

7. Callen PW et al: Ultrasonography and computed tomography in the evaluation of hepatic microabscesses in the immunosuppressed patient, *Radiology* 136:433, 1980.

8. Choi TK, Wong J: Endoscopic retrograde cholangiopancreatography and endoscopic papillotomy in recurrent pyogenic cholangitis, *Clin Gastroenterol* 15:393, 1986.

9. Cooperberg PL, Burhenne HJ: Real-time ultrasound: diagnostic technique of choice in calculus gallbladder disease, *N Engl J Med* 302:1277, 1980.

10. Ehman RL et al: Relative intensity of abdominal organs in MR images, *J Comput Assist Tomogr* 9:315, 1985.

11. Federle MP et al: Cystic hepatic neoplasms: complementary roles of CT and sonography, *Am J Roentgenol* 136:345, 1981.

12. Ferrucci JT: MR imaging of the liver, *Am J Roentgenol* 147:1103, 1986.

13. Freeny PC, Marks WM: Computed tomographic arteriography of the liver, *Radiology* 148:193, 1983.

14. Freeny PC, Marks WM: Patterns of contrast enhancement of benign and malignant hepatic neoplasms during bolus dynamic and delayed CT, *Radiology* 160:613, 1986.

15. Frietas JE et al: Suspected acute cholecystitis: comparison of hepatobiliary imaging versus ultrasonography, *Clin Nucl Med* 7:364, 1982.

16. Gelfand DW: The liver: plain film diagnosis, *Semin Roentgenol* 10:177, 1975.

17. Goldberg HI et al: Hepatic cirrhosis: magnetic resonance imaging, *Radiology* 153:737, 1984.

18. Johnson CD, Rice RP: Acute abdomen: plain radiographic evaluation, *RadioGraphics* 5:259, 1985.

19. Laing FC et al: Biliary dilatation: defining the level and cause by real-time US, *Radiology* 160:39, 1986.

20. Liguory C, Canard JM: Tumors of the biliary system, *Clin Gastroenterol* 12:269, 1983.

21. Mauro MA et al: Hepatobiliary scanning with ^{99m}Tc-PIPIDA in acute cholecystitis, *Radiology* 142:193, 1982.

22. Meyers MA: *Dynamic radiology of the abdomen,* New York, 1976, Springer-Verlag.

23. Moss AA et al: Hepatic tumors: magnetic resonance and CT appearance, *Radiology* 150:141, 1984.

24. Nelson RC et al: Focal hepatic lesions: detection by dynamic and delayed computed tomography versus short TE/TR spin echo and fast field echo magnetic resonance imaging, *Gastrointest Radiol* 13:115, 1988.

25. Okada K et al: Diagnostic evaluation of CT and ERCP based on a retrospective analysis of hepato-biliary and pancreatic diseases, *Jap J Surg* 11:277, 1981.

26. Ott DJ, Gelfand DW: Complications of gastrointestinal radiologic procedures. II. Complications related to biliary tract studies, *Gastrointest Radiol* 6:47, 1981.

27. Pereiras R: Special radiologic procedures in liver disease. In Schiff L, Schiff ER, editors: *Diseases of the liver,* ed 5, Philadelphia, 1982, JB Lippincott.

28. Pickleman J et al: The role of sincalide cholescintigraphy in the evaluation of patients with acalculous gallbladder disease, *Arch Surg* 120:693, 1985.

29. Rosenthall L: Cholescintigraphy in the presence of jaundice utilizing Tc-IDA, *Semin Nucl Med* 12:53, 1982.

30. Shuman WP et al: PIPIDA scintigraphy for cholecystitis: false positives in alcoholism and total parenteral nutrition, *Am J Roentgenol* 138:5, 1982.

31. Stark DD et al: Hepatic metastases: randomized, controlled comparison of detection with MR imaging and CT, *Radiology* 165:399, 1987.

32. Stark DD et al: Magnetic resonance imaging of cavernous hemangioma of the liver: tissue specific characterization, *Am J Roentgenol* 145:213, 1985.

33. Wegener M et al: Gallbladder wall thickening: a frequent finding in various nonbiliary disorders—a prospective ultrasonographic study, *J Clin Ultrasound* 15:307, 1987.

34. Wittenberg J et al: Differentiation of hepatic metastases from hemangioma and cysts by MR, *Am J Roentgenol* 151:79, 1988.

35. Zeeman RK, Burrell MI: *Gallbladder and bile duct imaging,* New York, 1987, Churchill-Livingstone.

36. Ziessman HA et al: Atlas of hepatic arterial perfusion scintigraphy, *Clin Nucl Med* 10:675, 1985.

11 *Spleen*

ROY A FILLY
GRETCHEN AW GOODING
PETER F HAHN
FAYE C LAING
DAVID C PRICE
DAVID STARK
RALPH WEISSLEDER
WERNER WENZ

IMAGING OF THE SPLEEN

NORMAL SPLEEN

SPLENIC ABNORMALITIES
  Absence of spleen (asplenia syndrome, Ivemark's syndrome)
  Polysplenia
  Ectopic spleen
  Splenomegaly
  Abscesses
  Cysts
  Tumors
  Perisplenic masses
  Vascular diseases
  Trauma

INTERVENTIONAL RADIOLOGY

ULTRASONOGRAPHY
  Technique for ultrasound examination of the spleen
  Size of the spleen
  Contour of the spleen
  Consistency of the spleen
  Pitfalls in interpretation of splenic sonograms

MAGNETIC RESONANCE IMAGING
  Techniques for MR examination of the spleen
  MR examination in benign disease of the spleen
  Splenic tumors
  Future developments in MR imaging of the spleen

NUCLEAR MEDICINE
  Radiopharmaceuticals
  Clinical indications for spleen scintigraphy
  Scintigraphic examination of benign lesions
  Accessory spleens
  Functional asplenia
  Born-again spleen
  Nonimaging radionuclide studies

The spleen is one of the largest units of the reticuloendothelial system in the human body. About the size of a fist, it has an abundant blood supply, which allows it to serve as a major filtration site for blood, removing erythrocyte inclusions and culling dammed and effete erythrocytes. The spleen is also an immunologically competent organ, with both T cells and B cells present in the white pulp. Many systemic human diseases are associated with splenic enlargement, including systemic inflammatory diseases, generalized hematopoietic disorders, and a variety of metabolic disturbances (some genetic in origin).

The splenic parenchyma, or pulp, is largely composed of vascular sinuses, which are large channels of lymphatic tissue carrying venous blood. The organ is enclosed in a thin membranous capsule of elastic tissue. Fibrous cords called trabeculae run from the capsule to the depth of the pulp to give the organ a firm structural framework.

The methods of choice for examining the normal and diseased spleen are ultrasound (US) and computed tomography (CT). Earlier roentgenographic techniques, such as plain film radiography, visualization of the adjacent organs by barium meal or barium enema, or selective or superselective angiography, have lost relevance. Newer modalities, such as US, CT, magnetic resonance (MR) imaging, and in some cases radionuclear scintigraphy, provide optimal information about the spleen and surrounding organs.

Imaging of the spleen
WERNER WENZ

Abdominal *ultrasonographic screening* is presently the method of choice for investigation of upper abdominal disorders. Therefore many splenic lesions are readily detected by ultrasound in clinically asymptomatic patients (Fig. 11-1). *Plain film radiography* is primarily helpful in detection of splenic calcifications, which are summarized in Table 11-1. Thorotrast, which is no longer used because it is an α-particle emitter, is picked up by the reticuloendothelial cells and opacifies the spleen (Fig. 11-2). *Color Doppler sonography* is useful for studying arterial perfusion and evaluating portal blood flow in liver disease. Splenorenal shunts can be more obvious sonographically with color-coded Doppler. Other uses of vascular sonography of the spleen include the evaluation of splenic artery and vein patency, splenomegaly, collateral venous varices, and aneurysms. *MR imaging* can demonstrate arteries and veins in the various planes without the need for injection of contrast media. Until the introduction of these new imaging techniques, *angiography,* by way of the splenic artery, had been the diagnostic method of choice for many years. Vascular mapping by contrast injections into the celiac trunk or the splenic artery is still indicated in primary vascular lesions such as aneurysm, arterioportal fistula, hemangioma, and splenic vein thrombosis, as well as in preoperative demonstration of the vascular system after trauma. Splenic arteriography is also a prerequisite for interventional procedures, such as those involving visceral transcatheter emboliztaion. A more detailed discussion of the various imaging techniques follows.

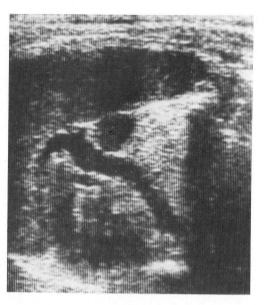

Fig. 11-1 Abdominal ultrasound image of accessory spleen close to hilum.

Normal spleen

Ultrasonography can rapidly and reliably help to determine the size of the spleen. In 95% of patients, the length of the spleen is less than 11 cm, and the weight, as determined by the rotation ellipsoid formula, is less than 190 g. The spleen diminishes in size with age and is slightly smaller in women than in men. The organ moves 2 to 3 cm with normal breathing and as much as 7 cm with deep inspiration. The dimensions of the normal spleen are summarized in Table 11-2.

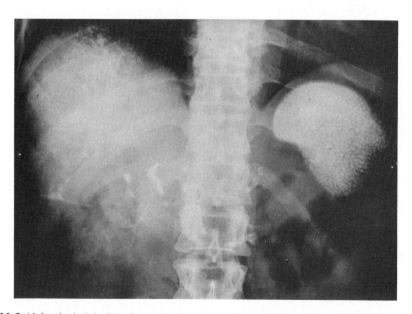

Fig. 11-2 Abdominal plain film shows thorotrastosis of spleen, liver, and periportal lymph nodes.

☐ **TABLE 11-1**
Splenic calcifications

	Common	Uncommon
Solitary calcifications	Splenic artery aneurysm Splenic artery atherosclerosis	Abscess Ascites Cysts Granuloma Hematoma Hemangioma (phleboliths) Previous infarction
Multiple calcifications	Hemangiomatosis Histoplasmosis (healed) Tuberculosis	Brucellosis Hamartoma Hemosiderosis Infarction Parasites Sickle cell anemia

☐ **TABLE 11-2**
Dimensions of the normal spleen

Method of determination	Size
Clinical	7 cm (by percussion)
Anatomic	12 × 8 × 3 cm
Scintigraphic	8 × 12 cm
Sonographic	10 × 6 × 14 cm

Splenic abnormalities

ABSENCE OF SPLEEN (ASPLENIA SYNDROME, IVEMARK'S SYNDROME)

Splenic agenesis is often associated with cardiac anomalies, disturbances of pulmonary circulation, trilobed left lung (dextroisomerism) with horseshoe kidney, malrotation of the gastrointestinal tract, and liver anomalies. The juxtaposition of the abdominal aorta and inferior vena cava can be easily identified on sonograph. Two additional abnormalities, absent splenic vein and midline portal vein, can also be demonstrated. The method of choice for outlining the features of Ivemark's syndrome, however, is isotopic scan.

POLYSPLENIA

Polysplenia is a syndrome characterized by multiple individual splenules, cardiac anomalies, atypical confluence of the pulmonary veins, and the presence of biliary, urogenital, and bronchial disorders. Chest radiographs and abdominal CT demonstrate multiple masses consistent with splenules in association with partial visceral heterotaxia and concomitant levoisomerism (bilateral left-sidedness).

ECTOPIC SPLEEN

Pedicle torsion of a *"wandering" spleen* is a rare phenomenon that can cause lower abdominal symptoms similar to those caused by a twisted hemorrhagic ovarian cyst. Chronic splenic pedicle torsion may result in subcapsular hematoma or ileus of unknown origin. A wandering spleen should always be considered when examination of the left upper quadrant indicates absence of the spleen.

SPLENOMEGALY

The following guidelines are helpful to establish an approximate diagnosis based on the size of the spleen only:
1. Slight splenomegaly suggests infarction.
2. Moderate splenomegaly may be related to portal hypertension.
3. Marked splenomegaly suggests hematologic disease (possibly leukemia).

Table 11-3 provides a complete differential diagnosis of splenomegaly, as provided by Felson and Reeder.

ABSCESSES

Splenic abscess occurs infrequently. Abdominal ultrasound allows precise diagnosis by showing sonolucent areas within an enlarged spleen. On CT, low-density areas with air bubbles and absent contrast enhancement are typical findings. In immunosuppressed patients, CT and ultrasound examinations suggestive of splenic cyst or hematoma must be followed by needle aspiration to rule out abscess.

CYSTS

Primary *splenic cysts* are rare. Almost all are the result of previous splenic trauma and evolve from a subcapsular hematoma that has not ruptured. On ultrasound, parasitic and nonparasitic cysts can be easily identified as sonolucent masses with distal echo enhancement. In some cases plain film studies reveal calcification of the cystic wall. CT and MR imaging are more precise and clearly outline the fluid collection.

TUMORS

Primary neoplasms of the spleen are rare; exceptions are malignant lymphoma and plasmacytoma. Other tumors, listed in decreasing order of frequency, include hemangioma, lymphangioma, hamartoma, fibroma, myxoma, chondroma, osteoma, hemangiosarcoma, and fibrosarcoma. Metastases to the spleen are seen only in terminal stages. Tumors that often metastasize to the spleen are those of the lung, breast, ovary, colon, prostate, and skin (melanoma).

☐   **TABLE 11-3**
Differential diagnosis of splenomegaly

Cause	Disease
Blood dyscrasias	Anemia
	Dysgammaglobulinemia
	Extramedullary hematopoiesis
	Hemochromatosis
	Myelofibrosis (hypersplenism)
	Osteoporosis
	Polycytopenic purpura
Infection	Bacterial
	Fungal
	Parasitic disease
	Viral
Neoplasm	Cyst
	Hemangioma, lymphangioma
	Lymphoma
	Metastases
	Neoplasm (benign)
	Sarcoma (especially angiosarcoma)
Portal hypertension	Congestive splenomegaly
	Nutritional or alcoholic cirrhosis
	Schistosomiasis
	Splenic or portal vein obstruction
Storage diseases	Gaucher's disease
	Glycogen storage disease
	Histiocytosis X
	Mucopolysaccharidosis
	Niemann-Pick disease
	Wilson's disease
Trauma	Hematoma
	Hemorrhagic pseudocyst
Other	Antitrypsinase deficiency

Splenic tumors do not necessarily cause splenomegaly and are clearly shown on sulfur colloid scintigraphy. Ultrasound, however, is the best screening method for this purpose and demonstrates whether the lesion is cystic or solid.

Despite numerous publications about the CT appearances of lymphatic disorders of the spleen, especially in Hodgkin's disease and non-Hodgkin's lymphoma, no specific imaging criteria exist except for the presence of low attenuation areas, circumscript or generalized enlargement of the organ, and possible infiltration into adjacent organs. Even in a case of primary angiosarcoma, CT showed no contrast enhancement.

Angiography reveals a characteristic hypervascular network in hemangioma and hamartoma. Vascular lakes and malignant tumor vessels can be seen in hemangiosarcomas. In hemangiomatosis of the liver and spleen, a rare condition, selective arteriography of the celiac trunk provides excellent information (Fig 11-3).

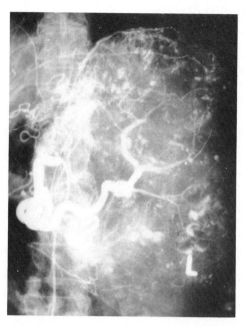

Fig. 11-3 Selective splenic arteriography shows hemangiomatosis of spleen with multiple contrast pools and massive splenic enlargement.

Almost all modern imaging techniques provide accurate localization of benign or malignant splenic tumors but indicate little about their nature. Ultrasound- or CT-guided needle biopsies are indispensable for definitive diagnosis in most cases.

PERISPLENIC MASSES

The distance from the spleen to the diaphragm is normally variable. On occasion, omentum extending to the left upper quadrant may mimic tumors in the splenic hilum. Pseudocysts of the pancreatic tail penetrating the spleen may mimic splenic cysts. When the left liver lobe is seen draped around the spleen, CT or ultrasound differentiation of the two organs may be impossible; angiography may be indicated in such cases (traumatized spleen, splenic tumor, etc).

VASCULAR DISEASES

Plain film studies of the abdomen in older patients frequently reveal atherosclerotic changes in the splenic artery. The tortuous, calcified vessel sometimes even shows aneurysmal dilatation. Celiac or superselective splenic angiography is indicated when occlusive disease is suspected. Stenosis of the splenic artery causes collaterals to develop through the tail of the pancreas, through the gastroepiploic arteries, and over the left and short gastric arteries.

Occlusion of one of the segmental arterial branches leads to splenic infarction. The diagnosis is easily made by demonstration of occluded branches and a wedge-shaped parenchymal defect.

Chronic pancreatitis causing repeated exposure of the splenic artery to pancreatic enzymes during acute attacks may cause aneurysm formation. Noncalcified aneurysms may rupture spontaneously, especially in pregnant women.

Arterioportal shunts, causing portal hypertension, can be congenital in origin or may be acquired traumatically. Arteriography demonstrates rapid contrast filling of the splenic vein and poor parenchymal opacification.

Splenic vein occlusion by thrombosis or compression leads to marked splenomegaly. The diagnosis can be made by ultrasound, angiography and CT, or arteriography. Larger than usual amounts of contrast material are necessary to visualize the patent portions of the splenic vein.

Direct measurement of portal pressure is possible after splenic puncture for splenoportography. The examination is justified only in very rare cases that require preoperative clarification of the venous anatomy.

TRAUMA

The spleen is the organ most frequently injured in blunt abdominal trauma. Clinical examination and plain film findings of lower rib fractures, elevation of the left hemidiaphragm, and splenic enlargement are insufficient criteria to indicate surgical exploration. CT is the basic imaging method in blunt abdominal trauma, since it may demonstrate free intraperitoneal fluid, as well as a splenic lesion, in addition to other traumatic lesions of perisplenic organs. Amounts as small as 50 to 100 ml of free blood can be recognized. Ultrasound examina-

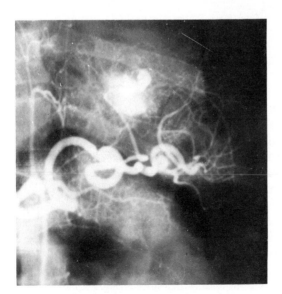

Fig. 11-4 Selective splenic arteriography demonstrates intrasplenic hematoma after traffic accident.

tions also can give information about the traumatized spleen indirectly: size of the organ, subcapsular or pericapsular hematoma, parenchymal contusion, or rupture with concomitant bleeding.

The rapid evaluation of splenic trauma includes thoracic and abdominal plain films, CT, and angiography (Fig. 11-4).

Interventional radiology

Transcatheter embolization of splenic artery branches or the main splenic artery can be lifesaving. Using Gianturco coils, detachable balloons, Gelfoam, or other occlusive agents, acute posttraumatic bleeding can be stopped. However, the intrasplenic branches are end arteries that do not anastomose. Therefore, complete embolization leaves no opportunity for development of an anastomotic blood supply. Splenic infarction or abscess formation may develop after complete or partial therapeutic embolization; therefore embolization should be undertaken only in extreme cases and should be used judiciously.

Abscess formation within the spleen or under the diaphragm can be treated by percutaneous ultrasound- or CT-guided needle puncture and drainage.

Ultrasonography
FAYE C LAING
ROY A FILLY
GRETCHEN AW GOODING

Ultrasonography offers useful information in the diagnosis of a variety of splenic disorders (Fig. 11-5). Although exact volume measurements may be difficult to obtain, ultrasound permits ready visualization of splenomegaly and can be used to easily determine changes in the spleen's size with serial examinations.

TECHNIQUE FOR ULTRASOUND EXAMINATION OF THE SPLEEN

The ultrasonographic examination of the spleen varies depending on size of the organ and, to some degree, on the body habitus of the patient. The easiest way to visualize a normal-sized spleen is to place the patient in a right lateral decubitus position and to scan obliquely along the axis of the spleen, that is, between the tenth and eleventh ribs. In all cases the sonograms should be obtained with suspended, deep inspiration (Fig. 11-6).

Longitudinal scans of the spleen are usually coronal and are obtained with the patient lying in a right lateral decubitus position. The transducer is normally placed either intercostally or subcostally (Fig. 11-7).

As splenomegaly becomes increasingly pronounced,

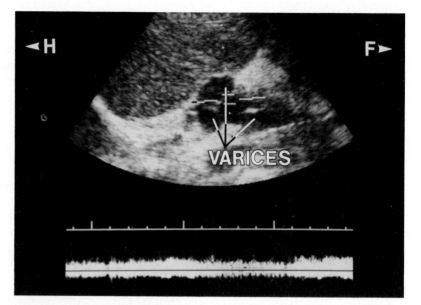

Fig. 11-5 Splenic varices are evident in region of splenic hilus in this patient with portal hypertension. Doppler signal confirms patency of vessels and displays typical venous flow pattern. *H*, Head; *F*, feet.

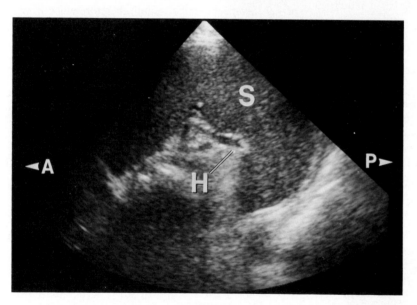

Fig. 11-6 Normal transverse scan over spleen shows homogeneous low-level echoes throughout splenic parenchyma *(S)*. Hilus of spleen *(H)* normally contains stronger echoes than remainder of spleen because of entry of vascular pedicle into this region. Patient is lying in right lateral decubitus position. *A*, Anterior; *P*, posterior.

the spleen becomes progressively easier to visualize on ultrasonograph. The enlarged spleen descends beneath the left costal margin and displaces the gas-filled stomach medially. When this occurs, the spleen may be satisfactorily visualized on sonograph even with the patient in a supine position. Longitudinal and transverse scans are performed through the spleen in a manner identical to that used in hepatic ultrasonographic examination.

SIZE OF THE SPLEEN
Normal spleen

Because of its posterior and superior location in the left upper quadrant, and because of the interposition of

the ribs, the normal spleen is sometimes difficult to examine with either palpation or ultrasonography. CT and MR imaging, on the other hand, are not limited by the overlying ribs or aerated lung, and thus do not suffer several of the technical difficulties encountered when imaging small spleens with ultrasound.

When seen, the normal-sized spleen does not usually extend more than 2 cm anterior to an imaginary line drawn tangentially to the anterior border of the aorta and parallel to the back. This is generally a reliable index for determining whether splenomegaly exists. Although the size of the spleen varies somewhat depending on the amount of blood it contains, the average adult spleen measures approximately 12.5 cm in length,

7.5 cm in transverse diameter, and 3.5 cm in thickness. Its normal weight is about 150 g, with a range of about 50 to 250 g.

Splenomegaly

Often the sonographic appearance of splenomegaly is nonspecific. However, with ultrasound, it is usually possible to determine whether a clinically palpable mass in the left upper quadrant represents an enlarged spleen or a mass arising from a neighboring organ. On occasion, focal pathologic processes affect the spleen, in which case ultrasound can be extremely useful in assessing the consistency of the lesion and suggesting the cause.

Because of its noninvasive nature, ultrasound can be used sequentially in the evaluation of patients with primary or secondary diseases involving the spleen. When the spleen enlarges, it frequently causes displacement of adjacent organs, particularly the left kidney. Ultrasound can easily assess whether the renal displacement is secondary to an enlarged spleen, an intrinsic renal pathologic process, or a mass arising in another contiguous organ.

CONTOUR OF THE SPLEEN

The spleen is normally well defined and smooth along its superior and lateral borders, both of which have a convex margin. The undersurface and medial aspect of the spleen are more lobulated because of focal impressions made on the surface by surrounding viscera. On occasion, a medial lobulation arising from the spleen can be observed projecting between the tail of the pancreas and the left kidney. This variant is seen in approximately 10% of patients with splenomegaly and should not be confused with lesions arising in the tail of the pancreas or adrenal gland.

The hilar region is normally umbilicated or lobulated because of the entry of the vascular pedicle at this point. A highly reflective group of echoes is frequently seen within the spleen in this region, in part secondary to perihilar fat, as well as air in the stomach. High amplitude echoes in this area should not be misinterpreted as representing a pathologic condition.

In approximately 10% of individuals a single *accessory spleen* is present (Fig. 11-8). Ultrasonographic identification is based on (1) its appearance, which is usually round or oval with an echo texture identical to that of the main spleen; (2) its location at or near the splenic hilum, or in relation to the gastrosplenic and splenocolic ligaments; and (3) demonstration of its vascular supply from the splenic artery or vein.

CONSISTENCY OF THE SPLEEN

The internal consistency of the spleen normally causes a very homogeneous echo pattern to be displayed. Normal splenic tissue has higher amplitude echogenicity than does hepatic tissue. Attempts to classify splenic pathologic conditions according to echo texture have led to considerable confusion in the ultrasound literature. Normal splenic parenchyma displays a remarkably uniform pattern. Lymphomatous nodules within the spleen are usually hypoechoic (Fig. 11-9). In general, splenic congestion and enlargement in cases of hepatocellular disease cause a hyperechoic pattern with the splenic parenchyma. Unlike that of the liver, the internal vasculature of the spleen cannot ordinarily be identified.

Although ultrasound is sensitive for detecting *focal*

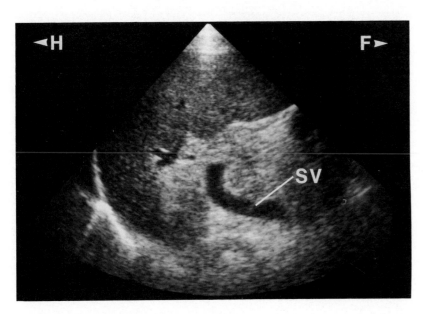

Fig. 11-7 Longitudinal subcostal sonogram shows normal contour of spleen with entry of splenic vein *(SV)* at splenic hilus. *H,* Head; *F,* feet.

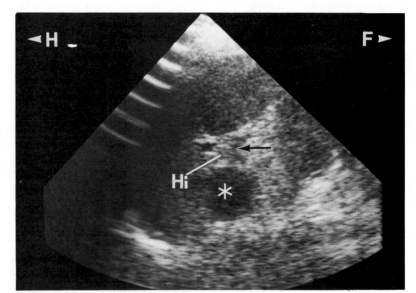

Fig. 11-8 Longitudinal scan showing accessory spleen *(asterisk)* near splenic hilus *(Hi)*. Branch of splenic artery *(arrow)* is seen entering accessory spleen. *H,* Head; *F,* feet.

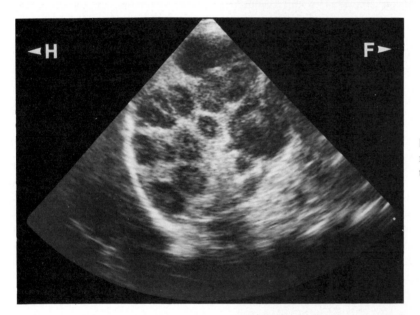

Fig. 11-9 Longitudinal sonogram reveals multiple hypoechoic splenic masses in patient with lymphoma. *H,* Head; *F,* feet.

Fig. 11-10 Using ultrasound guidance it is possible to pass needle between parallel lines to obtain tissue or fluid for diagnostic purposes. In this patient sonolucent mass *(arrow)* proved to be splenic abscess. *H,* Head; *F,* feet.

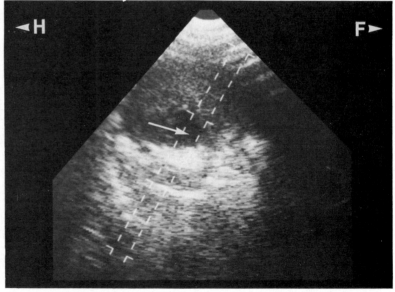

splenic lesions, it is limited, as are other noninvasive imaging modalities, in providing information sufficient to make a specific diagnosis. Inflammatory, neoplastic, and even posttraumatic processes can appear remarkably similar. Furthermore, the ultrasonographic appearances of a particular pathologic process can vary greatly. Even lymphomatous nodules, which are characteristically sonolucent, may contain large focal echogenic deposits. Splenic metastases, which are most often caused by melanoma, are also typically hypoechoic (but of higher echo amplitude than lymphoma); on occasion, however, these lesions may be predominantly echogenic. Other less common tumors that metastasize to the spleen include carcinoma of the lung, breast, stomach, ovary, and choriocarcinoma. To obtain a precise tissue diagnosis, ultrasound can be used as a guide for fine-needle aspiration biopsy (Fig. 11-10).

Predominantly fluid-filled splenic masses are usually caused by *splenic cysts.* These lesions are classified as true cysts when they are lined by a specific secreting membrane, or as false cysts when they contain serous, hemorrhagic, or inflammatory fluid or are caused by a degenerating infarct.

Acute *splenic infarction* typically appears as a well-demarcated wedge-shaped hypoechoic area with its apex directed toward the splenic hilus and its base directed toward the periphery of the spleen. During the acute phases of splenic infarction, when edema, inflammation, and necrosis predominate, the ultrasonographic appearance is primarily hypoechoic. As the infarct becomes more chronic and is associated with fibrosis and shrinkage, the ultrasonographic pattern gradually changes toward increased echogenicity and reduction in the size of the lesion. A healed infarct is characteristically seen as a dense, hyperechoic focus.

Similar to abscesses elsewhere in the body, the ultrasonographic appearance of a *splenic abscess* varies greatly with respect to number, size, echo texture, wall definition, and sound penetration. The most expeditious way to diagnose a splenic abscess is to direct a needle into the questionable lesions.

Although CT is the modality of choice for detecting and diagnosing intrasplenic and perisplenic *traumatic processes,* on occasion a history of trauma may be withheld or may be remote, in which case ultrasound may be performed because of vague left upper quadrant symptoms. The ultrasound findings are based on the age of the hematoma, its size, and its location (intrasplenic, perisplenic, or both). The ultrasonographic appearances for clotted blood have been shown to vary greatly and depend primarily on the age of the hematoma. An acute hematoma is a highly echogenic lesion that may be well or poorly defined.

Because it is becoming increasingly common to adopt a nonsurgical approach to patients with injured spleens, ultrasound has gained acceptance as an ideal modality for monitoring those individuals and observing the natural progression of splenic morphology as the hematoma evolves.

PITFALLS IN INTERPRETATION OF SPLENIC SONOGRAMS

On occasion it is difficult to discern whether a cystic mass in the left upper quadrant is splenic in origin. For example, fluid in the stomach may sometimes be mistaken for a splenic lesion; the reverse may also occur. Pseudocysts in the tail of the pancreas and left subphrenic fluid collections are two situations that may be difficult to differentiate from splenic fluid collections. The normal splenic hilus may also be confused with an

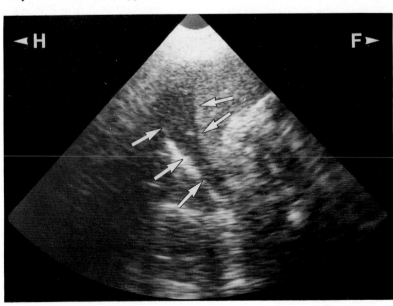

Fig. 11-11 This longitudinal sonogram demonstrates relatively sonolucent crescentic region *(arrows)* superior to spleen. Although this appearance can mimic subcapsular hematoma, it was subsequently shown to be left lobe of liver that extended superior to spleen. *H,* Head; *F,* feet.

echogenic intrasplenic abnormality. This confusion occurs in patients with splenomegaly in whom normal hilar echoes become more easily visualized. Another normal anatomic structure that can cause confusion is the left lobe of the liver, which in some individuals extends between the spleen and left hemidiaphragm and can resemble a perisplenic (subcapsular) fluid collection (Fig. 11-11). This confusion can be avoided by carefully observing that during real-time examination the "perisplenic abnormality" appears to move independently of the spleen during shallow respiration. Last, a subcapsular pseudohematoma can be distinguished from a true hematoma by the fact that the pseudolesion is predominantly situated superior to the spleen, whereas a true subcapsular hematoma is localized primarily lateral to the spleen.

Magnetic resonance imaging
RALPH WEISSLEDER
PETER F HAHN
DAVID STARK

MR imaging of the spleen has been fraught with difficulties for many reasons. Most important, motion artifacts can severely decrease image quality in the abdomen and commonly result in nondiagnostic MR studies. New techniques to suppress motion artifacts are under clinical investigation and have been shown to improve image quality. Second, splenic neoplasms have been difficult to detect with MR imaging because of the small difference in tumor-spleen relaxation times and proton densities. Administration of particulate MR contrast agents such as iron oxide has proved to increase tumor-organ contrast greatly, thus improving tumor detectability. Although the spleen has not been studied as extensively as have other abdominal organs, these recent advances are likely to increase the utility of MR in detecting splenic disease.

TECHNIQUES FOR MR EXAMINATION OF THE SPLEEN
Pulse sequences

A routine MR examination of the spleen includes acquisition of images with different contrast dependencies. Spin echo (SE) pulse sequences with T_1-dependent contrast (T_1-weighting; TR < 500 msec and TE > 30 msec) are routinely acquired in abdominal imaging because of excellent anatomic resolution (high signal-to-noise ratio [SNR]). Reduction of TR to less than the tissue T_1 relaxation time increases SNR per unit time and allows extensive signal averaging to reduce motion artifacts. Tissue composition and relaxation times are presented in Table 11-4.

Spin echo pulse sequences with T_2-dependent image

□ **TABLE 11-4**
Tissue composition and relaxation times

Parameter	Spleen		Liver	
Water (%)	77%	(72%-79%)	71%	(64%-74%)
Lipid (%)	1.6%	(1%-3%)	7.9%	(1%-11%)
Protein (%)	19%	(18%-20%)	18%	(16%-22%)
Blood content (ml)	60-120		250	
Iron (mg/g wet tissue)	0.049	(0.02-0.12)	0.32	(0.13-0.58)
T_1 (msec, 20 MHz)	805 ± 263		499 ± 140	
T_2 (msec, 20 MHz)	70 ± 20		48 ± 11	
N(H)	481 ± 143		583 ± 151	

contrast (T_2-weighting; TR = 2000 to 3000 msec and TE > 60 msec) techniques are usually acquired to detect splenic lesions with a long T_2 time (such as necrosis) and to characterize lesions with different T_2 times (for example, cysts versus solid tumors).

The spleen is readily displayed on routine abdominal MR scans. The transverse plane of section demonstrates the upper third of spleen posterior to small bowel loops, and the inferior third lateral to the left kidney (Fig. 11-12).

MR EXAMINATION IN BENIGN DISEASE OF THE SPLEEN

Splenic hemorrhage occurs most frequently after trauma and in patients with coagulopathy. Trauma commonly leads to subcapsular bleeding, and if the splenic capsule remains intact, blood accumulates under pressure, changing the normally convex splenic contour. Coagulopathy-induced splenic hemorrhages most commonly cause intraparenchymal bleeding (Fig. 11-13). Acute hematomas (less than 24 hours) consist predominantly of oxyhemoglobin and deoxyhemoglobin and are still isointense with spleen parenchyma on T_1- and T_2-weighted images. Chronic hematomas contain methemoglobin and, because of its T_1 shortening effect, are markedly hyperintense on both T_1- and T_2-weighted pulse sequences. T_2 shortening of hemosiderin produces a peripheral hypointense ring.

Iron overload leads to massive iron deposition (hemosiderin and ferritin) in both the liver and spleen. Regardless of the underlying pathologic process, iron overload shortens T_2 and reduces signal intensity.

In patients with *sickle cell anemia* (hemolysis of rigid and deformed erythrocytes), the spleen demon-

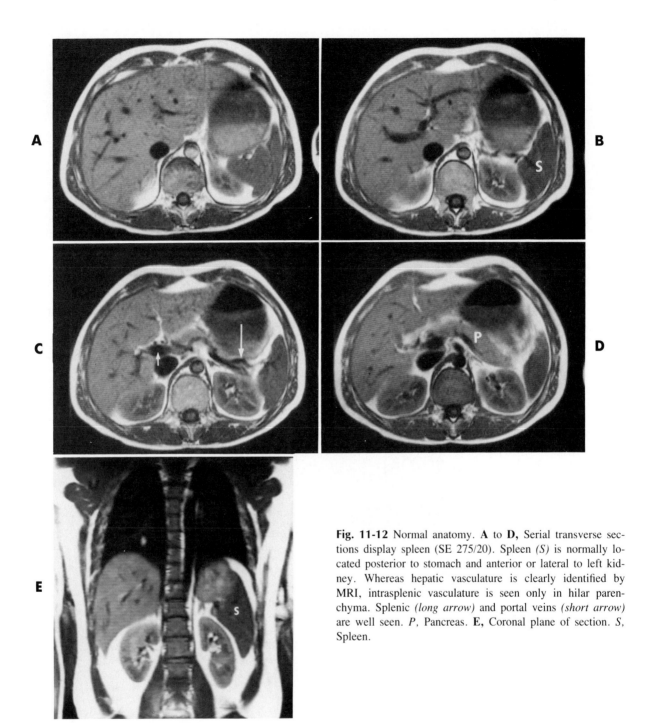

Fig. 11-12 Normal anatomy. **A** to **D,** Serial transverse sections display spleen (SE 275/20). Spleen *(S)* is normally located posterior to stomach and anterior or lateral to left kidney. Whereas hepatic vasculature is clearly identified by MRI, intrasplenic vasculature is seen only in hilar parenchyma. Splenic *(long arrow)* and portal veins *(short arrow)* are well seen. *P,* Pancreas. **E,** Coronal plane of section. *S,* Spleen.

strates abnormally low signal intensity on T_1- and T_2-weighted pulse sequences.

The MR appearance of *splenic infarcts* has been described only in sickle cell disease and lymphoma. In all cases iron overload was present and probably facilitated detection by MR imaging. On both T_1- and T_2-weighted images, infarcts appeared as structures of high signal intensity against the abnormally reduced signal from the iron-overloaded splenic parenchyma.

In *splenomegaly,* the MR signal intensity of congested spleens is similar to that of normal spleens. It is not possible with MR to differentiate the various forms of benign splenomegaly or even to differentiate benign from malignant splenomegaly.

SPLENIC TUMORS

Detection of focal spleen tumors by MR imaging has been disappointing for many reasons. Normal splenic

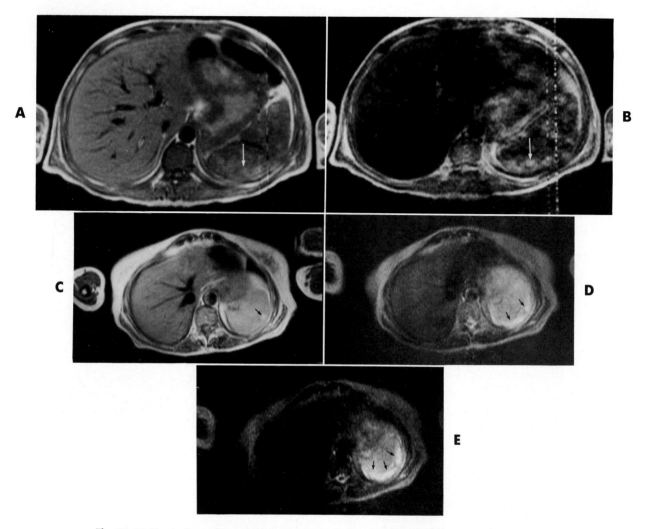

Fig. 11-13 Hemorrhage. Intrasplenic hemorrhage occurs most frequently in hematopoietic disorders (increased clotting times) or after trauma. **A** and **B,** Patient with lymphoma, multiple blood transfusions, and increased clotting time (**A** = SE 500/28, **B** = SE 2000/84/2). Multiple blood transfusions have led to iron overload with decrease in hepatic and splenic MRI signal intensity. Multiple intrasplenic areas of hyperintensity are seen on both T_1- and T_2-weighted images. **C** through **E,** T_1-weighted images (**C** = SE 300/20) show small zone of splenic hyperintensity. T_2-weighted images (**D** = SE 2000/120; **E** = SE 2000/180) display subcapsular hematoma *(arrows)* as linear region of hyperintensity. Electronic image windowing is optimized to differentiate spleen and hematoma.

parenchyma and tumor tissue have similar relaxation times and similar proton densities, resulting in low tumor–spleen contrast. Second, motion from the stomach, bowel, or heart frequently blurs anatomic boundaries of the spleen and casts ghost artifacts onto the spleen.

Despite the insensitivity of MR imaging in diagnosing splenic tumors, detection is possible under certain circumstances. In necrotic tumors, T_1 and T_2 relaxation times are longer than those for spleen, and these lesions are best detected on either heavily T_1-weighted or T_2-weighted pulse sequences (Fig. 11-14). Tumor-induced hemorrhage can also be detected by MR imaging and appears as areas of high signal intensity on both T_1- and T_2-weighted pulse sequences.

Relatively few patients with *splenic lymphoma* (Fig. 11-15) have been studied by MR, and reported sensitivity for detection varies from 10% to 87% (Table 11-5). Unless the spleen is greatly enlarged, splenic size correlates poorly as a diagnostic criterion of splenic lymphoma. Focal splenic lesions are seen more commonly in Hodgkin's disease than in non-Hodgkin's lymphoma.

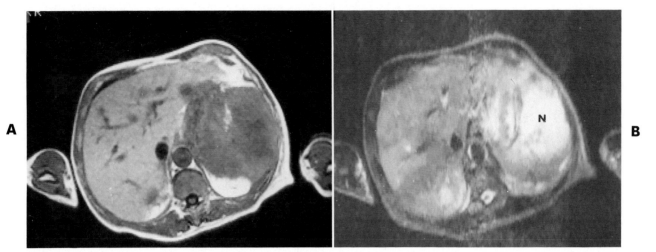

Fig. 11-14 Tumor necrosis. Tumor hemorrhage and necrosis are readily detectable with MRI. Central foci of hemorrhage or necrosis are often only clue to presence of splenic neoplasm. **A,** Gastric adenocarcinoma with hepatosplenic metastases. Entire spleen is replaced by inhomogeneous low-intensity tumor. Hilar vessels are displaced (SE 300/14). **B,** Corresponding SE 2350/180 image. Splenic tumor necrosis *(N)* is now identified as irregular zone of hyperintensity. Intrahepatic infiltration is appreciated. Note multiple hepatic metastases.

Fig. 11-15 Diffuse splenic lymphoma. Lymphoma presents as diffuse enlargement of splenic parenchyma in approximately half of all cases. Since many patients with splenic lymphoma have spleens of normal size and many patients without splenic lymphoma have splenomegaly, sensitivity of splenomegaly as diagnostic criterion of lymphoma is only 35%. **A,** SE 275/14 of diffusely enlarged spleen in patients with stage IV lymphoma. No focal abnormality is seen. Signal intensity of spleen appears normal. **B** and **C,** Corresponding SE 2350/60 **(B)** and SE 2350/180 **(C).**

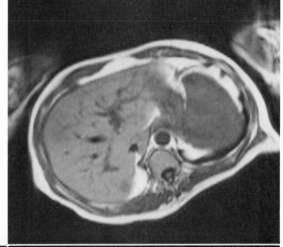

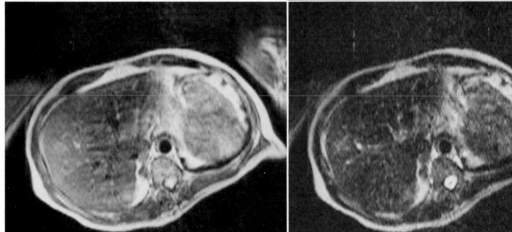

☐ **TABLE 11-5**

MRI of splenic lymphoma

Type	Reference	MRI technique	Sensitivity (%)	Specificity (%)
Hodgkin's lymphoma	31	T_1-weighted, T_2-weighted SE	71	100
	30	T_1-weighted, T_2-weighted SE	67	
Non-Hodgkin's lymphoma	31	T_1-weighted, T_2-weighted SE	10	
Combined	31	T_1-weighted, T_2-weighted SE	35	50
	32	T_1-weighted, T_2-weighted SE	38	50
	10	T_1-weighted, T_2-weighted GR	87	
	29	T_1-weighted, T_2-weighted SE	81	

MRI techniques: 52: SE 500/30, SE 900/30, SE 1500/30, 60, 90, SE 2000/120; 53: SE 275/14, SE 2350/60, 120, 180; 39: SE 800/30, 60, 90, 120; 5*: flash 80/16/60°, flash 80/16/30°; 40: SE 300/20, SE 800/25, SE 2000/40, 80.

Focal splenic lymphoma can appear as lesions of low or high signal intensity on T_1- or T_2-weighted pulse sequences.

In cases of *leukemia,* only massively infiltrated spleens demonstrate increased signal intensity.

Despite the insensitivity of MR, four distinct patterns of *metastases* can be detected by MR imaging: necrotic tumors (long T_2), hemorrhagic tumors (short T_1), tumors that cause gross splenic deformity, and focal splenic tumors in the presence of transfusional iron overload.

Benign splenic tumors are most commonly incidental findings detected on routine MR scans. *Cysts* are the most common. The T_1 and T_2 relaxation times of benign cysts are longer (because of increased water content) than those of solid splenic tumors. As a result, cysts are well visualized on both T_1-weighted images (on which they are hypointense relative to normal spleen) and T_2-weighted images (on which they are hyperintense relative to normal spleen). *Splenic hemangiomas,* like hemangiomas elsewhere in the body, are characterized by apparent long T_2 relaxation times.

FUTURE DEVELOPMENTS IN MR IMAGING OF THE SPLEEN

The most important clinical applications of splenic imaging are detection of splenic involvement in patients with lymphoma, differential diagnosis of splenomegaly, and staging of metastatic cancer. Preliminary clinical and experimental experience suggests that two major advances, the implementation of motion artifact suppression techniques and the use of tissue-specific contrast agents, will greatly modify the role of MR imaging for diagnosing splenic disease.

Contrast agents

MR imaging enhanced by polycrystalline and monocrystalline iron oxides shows great promise in MR of the spleen. As a particulate contrast agent, iron oxide exploits the reticuloendothelial function of the spleen and therefore acts as a tissue-specific, rather than a nonspecific, contrast agent. Iron oxide particles are phagocytosed by macrophages located in the red pulp, but not by splenic tumor. As a result, relaxation times and MR signal intensity of spleen decrease profoundly, whereas tumor remains unaffected.

Nuclear medicine
DAVID C PRICE

The spleen must be enlarged two to three times before it can be palpated clinically below the left anterior costal margin. As a result, noninvasive methods for quantitating spleen size can be useful in the evaluation of diseases such as polycythemia vera. The ability of the spleen to phagocytose intravascular foreign particles and to recognize and destroy damaged erythrocytes is the basis for the current use of radiopharmaceuticals in spleen scintigraphy.

RADIOPHARMACEUTICALS
Radiolabeled damaged erythrocytes

Following the initial description of erythrocyte labeling with chromium-51 by Gray and Sterling in 1950, Johnson and co-workers imaged the spleen using chromium 51–labeled erythrocytes "damaged" with incomplete anti-D antibodies. Winkelman and co-workers extended this principle to the now traditional method of damaging erythrocyte membranes by heating them. Since image quality with chromium-51 scintigraphy is considerably compromised by its 320-keV gamma emission and 9% gamma abundance, technetium-99m (^{99m}Tc) is now being used to label autologous erythrocytes with cell membranes damaged either by heat or by an excess of tin. The recommended degree of heat damage to labeled erythrocytes for effective splenic scintigraphy is 49° to 50° C for 15 to 45 minutes. Before reinfusion and imaging, however, autologous erythrocytes must still be labeled, sensitized, and washed, a relatively complex procedure. Even though in vitro labeling and damaging of erythrocytes is not necessary with mercury-203 or mercury 197–labeled MHP (1-mercury-2-hydroxypropane), it is usually not used because of the considerable radiation dose to the spleen.

Radiocolloids

Since the original description of its production by Harper and co-workers in 1965, ^{99m}Tc-sulfur colloid has been the most widely used radiopharmaceutical for spleen scintigraphy. In fact, the routine use of this radiopharmaceutical for hepatic scintigraphy has led to the incidental scintigraphic evaluation of thousands of spleens, with relatively few splenic pathologic conditions other than mild splenomegaly being uncovered in the process. The infrequency of incidental splenic pathologic conditions is also reflected by the relative rarity with which a nuclear medicine laboratory is asked to image the spleen as a routine clinical procedure.

[99m]Tc-sulfur colloid leaves the circulation with a rapid disappearance half-time of 1.5 to 4.2 minutes. In normal humans approximately 80% to 90% of the radiopharmaceutical goes to the liver, 5% to 10% to the spleen, and 3% to 5% to the bone marrow. Imaging can begin 10 to 15 minutes after the injection of 2 to 5 mCi of the radiocolloid. Routine spleen scans consist of an anterior and posterior view of the left upper quadrant and a lateral view of the spleen and left lobe of the liver. When the liver is enlarged, a left anterior oblique view is often important to separate the spleen from the left lobe of the liver for proper evaluation.

CLINICAL INDICATIONS FOR SPLEEN SCINTIGRAPHY
Spleen size

There are very few clinical situations in which the accurate determination of spleen size influences the diagnosis or management of a given patient. The simplest single measurement correlated with spleen weight is the posterior spleen length, normally 10.7 ± 1.7 cm with a maximum normal length of 14 cm. Spleen weight can be approximated by the following formula:

$$W = 71L - 537$$

where "W" is the spleen weight in grams and "L" is the posterior length in centimeters. Highly accurate estimates of spleen (and liver) volume may also be obtained by single photon-emission computerized tomography (SPECT).

Splenomegaly

Table 11-6 lists the common causes of splenomegaly according to degree.

Left upper quadrant mass

Left upper quadrant masses may be well characterized by combining the spleen scan with renal scintigraphy, an intravenous pyelogram, or abdominal CT scanning or ultrasound. The combination of a spleen scan, gallium scan, and abdominal CT scan has proved to be very effective in characterizing subphrenic abscesses.

SCINTIGRAPHIC EXAMINATION OF BENIGN LESIONS

On scintigraphy, *splenic cysts* are seen as clearly defined focal defects associated with an absence of perfusion when a flow study is performed. *Splenic abscesses,*

□ **TABLE 11-6**
Causes of splenomegaly

Massive splenomegaly (over 1000 g)	Moderate splenomegaly (500-1000 g)	Mild splenomegaly (150-500 g)
Malaria	Early stages of those at left	Acute febrile disorders (infection, toxemia)
Chronic myelogenous leukemia	Portal vein thrombosis	
Myelofibrosis with myeloid metaplasia	Chronic liver disease, portal hypertension	Malignancy (involving or not involving spleen)
Kala-azar, schistosomiasis	Infectious mononucleosis	
Gaucher's and Niemann-Pick diseases	Polycythemia vera	Collagen-vascular disorders
Thalassemia major	Malignant lymphomas	Chronic infections
Some spleen cysts	Chronic hemolytic anemias	Idiopathic thrombocytopenic purpura
	Acute leukemias	
	Early sickle cell anemia (childhood)	
	Tuberculosis, sarcoid	

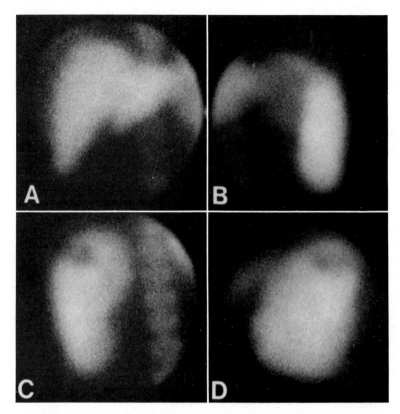

Fig. 11-16 Splenic abscess (septic infarct) in acute bacterial endocarditis leading to mycotic aneurysm (^{99m}Tc–sulfur colloid). Patient was young heroin addict with recurrent history of fever and left upper quadrant pain. **A,** Right anterior; **B,** left anterior; **C,** left posterior; **D,** left lateral.

if sufficiently large, also appear as focal defects, although multiple small abscesses may be below the resolution limits of the scintillation camera (2 to 2.5 cm in vivo). With small splenic abscesses, a ^{67}Ga scan will probably be more useful. Dual radionuclide subtraction imaging of ^{99m}Tc-sulfur colloid with ^{111}In-WBC or ^{67}Ga may be essential for proper identification of intrasplenic or subphrenic abscesses (Fig. 11-16).

On occasion, *splenic infarcts* occur in patients with bacterial endocarditis and are generally seen as peripheral defects in the spleen image. They frequently occur concomitantly with massive splenomegaly.

Spleen scintigraphy is a sensitive technique for the diagnosis of subcapsular and intrasplenic *hematomas*. The accurate diagnosis of splenic hematomas is essential because of the substantial risk of a delayed rupture (20%) and the increased risk of mortality with a delayed rupture. A focal lesion is seen generally within or adjacent to the spleen image, at times even transecting the spleen. The greatest difficulty occurs with subcapsular hematomas that may have little effect on the overall spleen image but may displace the entire spleen medially or anteriorly.

A combination of the radiocolloid study with either lung scintigraphy or a flow study may convincingly demonstrate a negative space between the spleen and left lateral body wall. In a prospective comparison of scintigraphy with ultrasound in 32 patients, the two modalities were essentially identical in sensitivity and specificity for subcapsular hematoma after trauma, although a substantial proportion of the patients could not be properly studied by ultrasound because of injuries or pain. For this reason, scintigraphy is recommended as the primary screening procedure.

ACCESSORY SPLEENS

Accessory spleens are stated to occur in approximately 10% of the normal population, although two studies of nontraumatic postsplenectomy patients have demonstrated the incidence of accessory spleens in this setting to be as high as 43%. Accessory spleens ordinarily remain small. Their presence may be of great importance in patients with autoimmune hemolytic anemias, idiopathic thrombocytopenic purpura, or hereditary spherocytosis who initially respond well to splenectomy but then relapse. The presence and growth of accessory spleens must be ruled out in such patients. The simplest technique is ^{99m}Tc-sulfur colloid scintigraphy, including views of the entire abdomen and pelvis. If clinical suspicion is high and this study is negative, the clinician should repeat the study using autologous tin- or heat-damaged red blood cells labeled with ^{99m}Tc, which has been demonstrated to be more sensitive for the identification of small accessory spleens.

FUNCTIONAL ASPLENIA

Functional asplenia is the presence of palpable splenomegaly associated with absence of radiocolloid spleen labeling in young patients with sickle cell disease. The peripheral blood smear in these patients shows the red cell changes characteristic of absence of the spleen. In adult patients the spleen autoinfarcts to a small fibrous remnant, and the term "functional asplenia" is no longer applicable. It is characteristic of this condition that the failure of labeling with radiocolloids is reversible by transfusion with normal (hemoglobin A) blood. Although the entity is seen predominantly in young sickle cell patients, it has been described in patients with other diseases.

BORN-AGAIN SPLEEN

It has been known for many years that children who undergo splenectomy for traumatic rupture of the spleen do not have the same high risk of infection as children whose spleen is removed for other reasons. In the former there is markedly reduced evidence of splenic hypofunction in the form of red blood cell "pitting." A liver-spleen scan performed in several patients demonstrated splenosis, a condition of multiple small loci of splenic tissue scattered throughout the abdominal and pelvic cavities, which apparently originate from seeding throughout these spaces by scattered spleen cells released at the time of splenic rupture. This regrowth of scattered spleen cells into functionally effective splenic nodules has been called *"born-again spleen."* Spleen scanning in such patients can be an effective way of estimating the risk of infection after posttraumatic splenectomy.

Fig. 11-17 illustrates the typical findings on ^{99m}Tc-sulfur colloid imaging. As might be expected, spleen scintigraphy can be equally useful in evaluating patients who have undergone spleen autotransplantation to minimize long-term risk of overwhelming postsplenectomy infection.

NONIMAGING RADIONUCLIDE STUDIES

There are several probe-counting techniques for the evaluation of the role of the spleen in the production and destruction of circulating blood elements. This can be very important in evaluating the splenic contribution

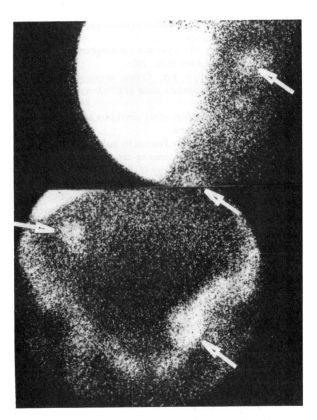

Fig. 11-17 Multiple splenic foci, the "born-again spleen," in 29-year-old man following posttraumatic splenic rupture and splenectomy 7 years previously. Splenic tissue released at time of rupture has settled throughout abdominal and pelvic cavities *(arrows)* and then grown into discrete nodules.

(From Price DC: The hematopoietic system. In Harbert J, DaRocha AFG, editors: *Textbook of nuclear medicine,* ed 2, vol 2 (Clinical applications), Philadelphia, 1984, Lea & Febiger.)

to extramedullary hematopoiesis (myeloid metaplasia) and, to a lesser extent, the destruction of in vivo–labeled erythrocytes. In centers where the positron emitter iron-52 and a positron camera are available, scintigraphic imaging of splenic, as well as marrow, erythropoiesis can be effectively achieved. Probe counting of chromium-51 kinetics over the spleen is a routine procedure in the evaluation of red cell and platelet survival.

RECOMMENDED READING

1. Adler DD et al: MRI of the spleen: normal appearance and findings in sickle cell anemia, *Am J Roentgenol* 147:843, 1986.
2. Armas RR: Clinical studies with spleen-specific radiolabeled agents, *Semin Nucl Med* 15:260, 1985.
3. Burke JS: Surgical pathology of the spleen: an approach to the differential diagnosis of splenic lymphomas and leukemias, *Am J Surg Pathol* 5:551, 1981.
4. Cohen MD et al: Magnetic resonance imaging of lymphomas in children, *Pediatr Radiol* 15:179, 1985.
5. Desai AG, Thakur ML: Radiopharmaceuticals for spleen and bone marrow studies, *Semin Nucl Med* 15:229, 1985.

bances because of severe diarrhea, or possibly by enterotoxin release by offending bacteria.

The colon is often greatly distended with an irregular contour. In severe advanced disease, air in the bowel wall may be seen.

Barium enema is contraindicated if there is a markedly dilated colon with an severe contour in a febrile patient with bloody diarrhea. Histologic and radiographic findings are similar to those of ischemic colitis.

The small bowel may also be affected, and involvement is indicated by edema of the valvulae conniventes and of the bowel wall, with thickening and separation of loops. Ulceration and complete loss of the fold pattern may be seen in more severely involved areas.

Differential diagnosis

Any form of ulcerating colitis (Crohn's disease, amebiasis, *Salmonella-Shigella* colitis, and particularly ischemic colitis), may produce radiographs similar to those in cases of pseudomembranous enterocolitis. When the small bowel is involved, ischemia, radiation enteritis, regional enteritis, periarteritis nodosa, and lymphoma should be considered in the differential diagnosis.

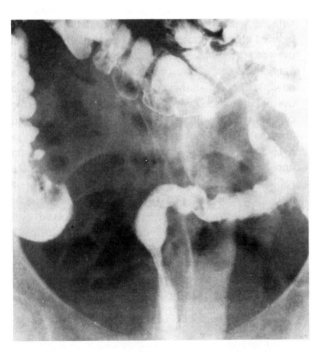

Fig. 12-5 LGV in black man from South Africa. There is marked narrowing of entire rectum and irregular ulcerated contour of moderately narrowed and shortened sigmoid colon. Rectal wall is considerably thickened, rigid, and fibrotic.

(From Reeder MM, Palmer PES: *The radiology of tropical diseases.* Baltimore, 1981, Williams & Wilkins.)

ACUTE GASTROENTERITIS

Acute nonspecific gastroenteritis is the most frequently occurring gastrointestinal disease, yet a cause is rarely, if ever, proved. So-called *traveler's diarrhea, acute epidemic gastroenteritis,* or *mal de turista* may be caused by enteropathic *E. coli* (EEC), by intestinal viruses such as enteric cytopathogenic human orphan (ECHO) and coxsackie A and B viruses, or by mixed flora.

Radiographic findings are nearly always confined to plain radiographs of the abdomen. Air-fluid levels may be seen in dilated loops of small and large bowel. When prominent, dilatation and fluid may simulate mechanical obstruction of the large bowel. Electrolyte loss may also produce an adynamic ileus pattern. No specific radiographic findings are noted. The small bowel is dilated, but the mucosal pattern is normal.

LYMPHOGRANULOMA VENEREUM

Lymphogranuloma venereum (LGV) is caused by a species of the genus *Chlamydia*.

The pathologic changes in the rectum are the result of invasion and blockage of the rectal lymphatics by *Chlamydia*. There is subsequent lymphangitis, lymphatic stasis, rectal edema, cellular infiltration in the submucosa and muscularis, endarteritis and phlebitis, and eventual mucosal destruction (Fig. 12-5).

Radiographic findings

In the prestenotic phase, there is narrowing of the rectal ampulla and spasm, with loss of the normal haustral and mucosal pattern in the rectum and on occasion in the sigmoid colon. The contour of the narrowed rectum is irregular and ulcerated. Fistulous tracts and perirectal abscesses may be present, as well as widening of the presacral space and anterior displacement of the rectosigmoid colon.

As the disease progresses to fibrosis, strictures of varied lengths may develop. LGV strictures are usually long (strictures as long as 25 cm have been noted) and tubular with a tapering proximal (and sometimes distal) edge. They may affect the anorectal area, the entire rectum and sigmoid colon, and, on occasion, areas higher in the colon. Lateral and oblique radiographs of the rectum are necessary to best demonstrate rectovaginal fistulas and retrorectal sinuses when present.

Differential diagnosis

Many inflammatory diseases of the colon must be considered when there is a radiographic finding of rectal stricture, including idiopathic chronic ulcerative colitis and, especially, granulomatous diseases such as Crohn's disease, tuberculosis, schistosomiasis, amebiasis, and actinomycosis.

SPRUE

Depending largely on the geographic area in which the patient is encountered, there are two varieties of sprue. Little differentiates the *nontropical* from the *tropical* variety. Both are usually classified as *idiopathic steatorrhea.*

Malabsorption through the small bowel can occur in many different diseases. The clinical symptoms are similar and the radiologic findings almost identical. The main difference between nontropical and tropical sprue is that the latter is almost megaloblastic and responds to antibiotics and vitamin therapy. Nontropical sprue, however, is difficult to treat and seldom shows a megaloblastic bone marrow. In tropical sprue a chronic inflammatory reaction almost always occurs in the lamina propria with varying degrees of edema; this may be followed by atrophy. All layers of the small bowel may eventually become atrophic and thin. In both varieties of sprue there may be some regeneration, but it is most marked in tropical sprue, in which there often occurs a dramatic response to antibiotic therapy with folate and vitamin B_{12} replacement.

Diarrhea is almost always present, accompanied by fatigue and lassitude. Remissions and exacerbations are frequent, with progressive ill health, steatorrhea, and eventually, abdominal pain with explosive defecation of bulky, foul-smelling stools.

Radiologic findings

The radiologic evidence of sprue depends largely on the duration of the disease. Barium studies must be carried out with micropulverized, nonflocculating barium. The diagnosis of a "sprue" pattern is invalid unless this type of barium is used. In the early stages of sprue a significant difference is seen between various small bowel segments because of a difference in tone. Because there is also some inflammatory reaction, edema, and therefore thickening of the mucosal folds, occurs. None of these early changes are appreciated accurately unless sequential fluoroscopy is used with manual palpation to separate the various loops of the small bowel.

The increase in saturated fatty acids in the lumen of the gut is accompanied by increased secretion of mucin, one of the main causes of the irritation and diarrhea seen in sprue and also of the flocculation that occurs during barium studies. As the edema progresses and the mucosa becomes more swollen, dilatation of the small bowel also occurs (Fig. 12-6).

Segmentation is one of the hallmarks of the sprue syndrome. This may be seen as bowel segments in which peristalsis is diminished to the extent that it is almost absent, or as segments in which rapid passage of contents occurs.

The transverse mucosal folds thicken, and may mea-

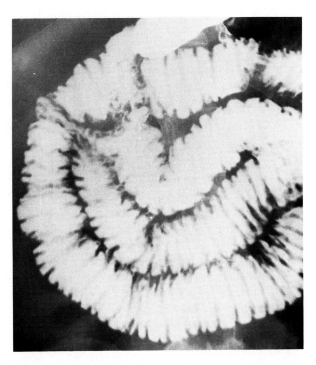

Fig. 12-6 Tropical sprue. Thickening of valvulae conniventes (primary and secondary mucosal folds, valves of Kerckring) produces cogwheel mucosal appearance of proximal small bowel. There is also increase in caliber of these loops caused by loss of tone and slowing of peristalsis.

(From Reeder MM, Palmer PES: *The radiology of tropical diseases,* Baltimore, 1981, Williams & Wilkins.)

sure 4 to 5 mm in thickness. Later, atrophy may occur and the mucosal folds may disappear altogether.

Excess secretion is shown by the presence of *flocculation,* particularly if standard barium sulfate is used. In the lower small bowel there is often coarse clumping of the barium column, which fragments into various sections. This segmentation may be quite marked, particularly in tropical sprue, and some of the segments show considerable stasis. Because of the mucosal changes, the normally clear outline of the mucosal pattern may be smudged and may be made worse if excess bowel secretions cause dilution of the barium mixture. In extreme cases this leads to the *moulage sign,* resulting in a faint outline to that specific segment.

It is impossible to determine the specific cause of the malabsorption pattern by radiographic means. The diagnosis of tropical sprue may be suggested by the combination of the findings as described, along with their very inconstancy.

Differential diagnosis

The radiologic appearance of sprue may also be produced by abnormalities of the pancreas or of biliary flow or by changes in the bowel wall or mesentery caused by amyloidosis, scleroderma, mesenteric thrombosis, various poisons such as arsenic, and some antibiotics. Many intestinal parasites, particularly *Giardia, Ancylostoma, Capillaria,* and *Strongyloides,* produce a similar appearance.

GASTROINTESTINAL CANDIDIASIS

Gastrointestinal candidiasis or *moniliasis* is caused by the fungus *Candida albicans.* This commensal organism is found in the mouth and upper respiratory and gastrointestinal tracts of many normal persons. It nearly always becomes pathogenic as a result of an underlying debilitating state (such as may be caused by prolonged antibiotic therapy that alters the gastrointestinal flora), a malignancy, or chemotherapy for neoplastic disease (immunosuppressive agents, steroids, and antimetabolites). Candidal infections of the gastrointestinal tract are frequently accompanied by oral infection *(thrush).* Dysphagia is the most common presenting symptom.

Radiographic findings

Radiographic abnormalities resulting from *C. albicans* are seen most frequently in the esophagus. *Candidal esophagitis* usually affects a long segment, particularly the lower half of the esophagus, although short plaquelike lesions have also been seen. The esophageal lumen may be wide and remain distended because of involvement of the deeper layers (Fig. 12-7).

Because of granulomas and ulceration, the mucous membrane seen on barium studies is irregular, ragged, and shaggy, like a carpet. This appearance is produced by mucosal ulceration and by a pseudomembrane covering areas of ulceration.

GASTROINTESTINAL HISTOPLASMOSIS

Gastrointestinal involvement by the fungus *Histoplasma capsulatum* produces clinical and radiographic findings similar to those of tuberculosis.

HELMINTHOMA

A helminthoma is an inflammatory tumor of the bowel wall caused by penetration of the wall of the cecum or colon by an intestinal worm. Penetration of the gut occurs occasionally, particularly in *Ascaris* infections, and the usual result is peritonitis.

The essential finding on barium enema is a mass within the wall of the bowel (Fig. 12-8). The helminthoma seldom encircles the bowel lumen, but narrows it eccentrically, since the mass is partially intramural and largely extramural. Distortion is caused by extrinsic pressure and by the mass within the bowel wall. The most common localization is in the region of the cecum or ascending colon.

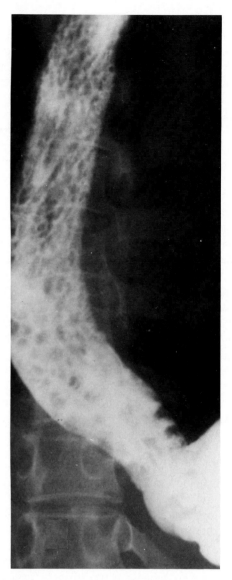

Fig. 12-7 Small nodular contour defects from candidal invasion without ulceration (cobblestone esophagus). (From Goldberg HI, Dodds, WJ: *Am J Roentgenol* 104:608, 1968.)

The tumor is most likely to be mistaken for a colon carcinoma, partially encircling the bowel wall. The helminthoma differs in that it seldom produces mucosal ulceration or destruction. In more acute cases the most likely differential diagnosis is an appendiceal abscess or even an amebic abscess.

CHAGAS' DISEASE

Chagas' disease *(American trypanosomiasis)* occurs only in the central and southern half of the American continent from Texas to Argentina. In rural eastern Brazil, more than 30% of all adults with clinical evidence

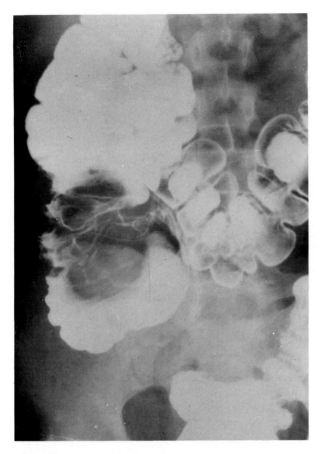

Fig. 12-8 Helminthoma of cecum. This large granulomatous tumor caused by worm burrowing into wall of cecum must be distinguished from ameboma, tuberculosis, and carcinoma in patients from the tropics.

(From Reeder MM, Palmer PES: *The radiology of tropical diseases,* Baltimore, 1981, Williams & Wilkins.)

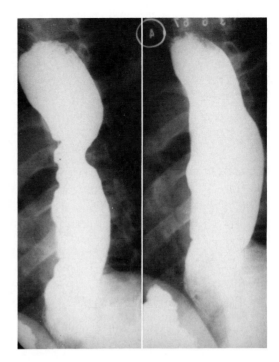

Fig. 12-9 Megaesophagus in Brazilian patient with chronic Chagas' disease. Considerable esophageal dilatation and altered peristalsis denote advanced disease. Local, incoordinate, nonpropulsive contractions are present.

(From Reeder MM, Hamilton LC: *Semin Roentgenol* 3:62, 1968.)

of chronic Chagas' disease die as a result of their infection.

The causative organism, *Trypanosoma cruzi,* is a tiny pleomorphic protozoan that inhabits the blood and tissues of humans and animals. Liberated organisms either invade adjacent cells or are destroyed by macrophages, causing them to release a neurotoxin that attacks and, over a period of time, destroys the ganglion cells in the myenteric plexi of the affected organ.

Radiographic findings

The earliest radiographic manifestations of Chagas' disease in the esophagus relate only to motor dysfunction. As denervation progresses, hypotonia, aperistalsis, stasis, and dilatation occur (Fig. 12-9). The transverse diameter of the flaccid esophagus may reach 7 cm or more.

The appearance of advanced megaesophagus on plain film radiographs of the chest and on barium swal-

low is remarkably similar to that of achalasia (Fig. 12-10). There may be a delay in passage of food or barium at the level of the distal sphincter, as well as a lack of propulsive peristalsis throughout the esophagus. Carcinoma develops in 7% of patients with megaesophagus.

In patients with megacolon, sigmoid volvulus, which occurs in 10% of cases, is often the presenting manifestation. A less distended, short segment of the colon, where loss of ganglia and subsequent dilatation are less pronounced when compared with the dilated adjacent bowel, may predispose to sigmoid volvulus.

TRICHURIASIS

Trichuriasis is an infection of the human cecum and colon, and rarely the distal ileum, that is caused by the whipworm *Trichuris trichiura.* The parasites are attached to the cecum and colon by means of their slender anterior ends, and they lie embedded beneath the surface epithelium between intestinal villi amid considerable mucus.

The worms may be found during barium enema as part of an investigation for rectal bleeding or other colon disease. A routine barium enema may be unremarkable or may show a granular mucosal pattern throughout the colon. The excess mucus surrounding hundreds

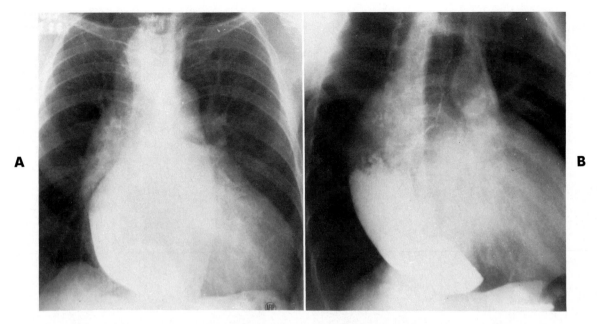

Fig. 12-10 Megaesophagus and myocardiopathy in 58-year-old Brazilian black man with Chagas' disease. **A,** Posteroanterior view shows prominent soft tissue density along entire right mediastinal border caused by greatly dilated esophagus partially filled with barium. Convexities of right and left sides of heart are prominent because of enlargement of both sides of heart. Left atrial enlargement produces bulge along left upper cardiac border and upward displacement of left main bronchus. No pulmonary vascular congestion is noted. **B,** Right oblique view shows posterior displacement of megaesophagus by grossly dilated left atrium.

(From Reeder MM, Simão C: *Semin Roentgenol* 4:374, 1969.)

of small whipworms may occasionally cause flocculation of the barium. An air-contrast barium enema is definitive and clearly demonstrates the wavy radiolucent outlines of numerous small trichurids against the air-barium background of the colon and rectum.

GIARDIASIS

Giardia lamblia is one of the most common intestinal parasites of humans and is worldwide in distribution.

Radiographic findings

Radiographic evidence of a deficiency pattern consists of pronounced segmentation, a moderate degree of dilatation of small bowel loops, coarsening of the mucosal folds in the midportion of the small bowel, and prolonged transit time. Inflammatory changes are usually localized to the duodenum and jejunum (Fig 12–11). The proximal ileum is rarely involved; the lower ileum and the colon appear normal.

The incidence of giardiasis is unusually great in patients with diseases such as dysgammaglobulinemia, nodular lymphoid hyperplasia, recurrent respiratory and urinary tract infections, chronic spruelike diarrhea, and other clinical and radiographic evidence of malabsorption. The innumerable, tiny, uniform, 2 to 3 mm nodular lesions found throughout the small intestine are not related to giardiasis, but represent hypertrophy of the lymphoid follicles in an effort to produce as much gamma globulin as possible.

Localization of the pathologic and radiologic changes in giardiasis to the duodenum and jejunum is of great importance in differential diagnosis, since many other gastrointestinal diseases are thereby excluded.

PARASITIC INFECTIONS

Parasites vary as widely as the human primates and the other animals in which they live. They are found worldwide and are not confined to the tropics or to the poor. They flourish where sanitation and hygiene are inadequate and may easily be acquired by even fastidious travelers. Knowledge of where a patient lived or traveled is as important in diagnosis as are laboratory tests and radiographic images.

The number of people infected with parasites throughout the world is almost unimaginable, but a few examples suffice. Perhaps 25% of the world's population harbors roundworms, and in many parts of the

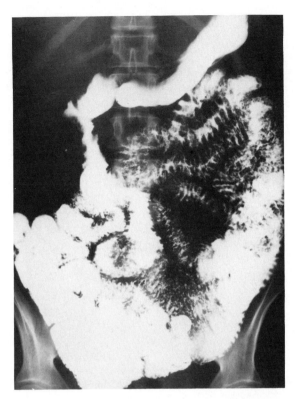

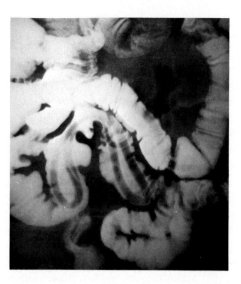

Fig. 12-12 *Ascaris* in mid small bowel outlined with barium.
(Courtesy Dr. JP Balikian.)

Fig. 12-11 Giardiasis. Second portion of duodenum is markedly irregular, and considerable spasm is noted within duodenal sweep and proximal jejunum. These loops are poorly filled because of irritability and are separated from each other. Mucosal folds are thickened, and secretions are increased. Lumen of bowel is slightly rigid and narrowed. Changes suggest actual inflammatory reaction rather than malabsorption pattern. They disappeared after quinacrine hydrochloride therapy for giardiasis.
(Courtesy Dr. Richard H. Marshak.)

tropics the incidence may well be greater than 90%. In 1968 it was estimated that 10% of the world's population harbored the ameba; by 1978 the estimate was increased to 20%. The number of patients with schistosomiasis is difficult to assess, but in 1981 it was thought that 600 million were infected. Figures for ancylostomiasis (hookworm) suggest that 900 million people, almost one quarter of the world's population, are infected. Prevalence varies widely among countries, particularly in the tropics.

Helminthic infections: roundworms (nematodes)
Ascariasis

Ascaris lumbricoides is the most common roundworm, particularly in children. *Ascaris* infection is acquired by ingesting food, water, or soil that has been contaminated with embryonated eggs.

When ova are swallowed, the outer shell is digested by gastric juices, and they hatch in the small bowel to become free tiny larvae, which then penetrate the epithelium of the intestinal mucosa. They mature as worms within the lumen of the small intestine, reaching 35 cm in about 2 months.

As the worm population grows, there may be partial or complete intestinal obstruction. Children may harbor more than 2000 worms, which can be entwined and form a large bolus; this is not an uncommon complication. The most common site of obstruction is the ileocecal region. The laboratory diagnosis depends on the identification of adult worms or eggs in the stool.

The radiologic appearance is characteristic. Large collections of worms are often identifiable on a plain film of the abdomen, contrasted against the gas in the bowel and resembling a tangled group of thick cords. After the patient swallows barium, the outline of the individual worms is shown, most commonly in the jejunum and ileum (Fig. 12-12).

The differential diagnosis is not difficult; the appearances in the gastrointestinal and biliary tracts are so characteristic, either on barium examination or by ultrasonography, that they are not likely to be misinterpreted.

Ancylostomiasis (hookworm disease)

Ancylostomiasis is caused by infection with one or more species of the ancylostomidae. *Ancylostoma duodenale* and *Necator americanus* are the most common. *N. americanus* is predominant in the tropics (in the United States it occurs in the South and in Puerto Rico) and *A. duodenale* in more temperate climates.

In humans, the small hookworms, measured in millimeters, firmly attach themselves to the intestinal mucosa, sucking blood, tissue, and intestinal juices to obtain nourishment.

On intestinal biopsy there is a marked eosinophilia with other findings resembling sprue. Laboratory diagnosis is made by identification of the eggs in a fresh sample of feces. Associated blood loss may result in anemia, usually hypochromic and microcytic. Peripheral eosinophilia is often found.

In most patients the results of barium examinations are normal. In others, there may be some abnormality of the small intestine pattern, resembling a deficiency pattern with coarsening and irregularity of the mucosa. With radiologic studies, attention should be focused on the jejunum. The differentiation between hookworm disease and steatorrhea of another cause may be very difficult.

Strongyloidiasis

Immunosuppression is of particular importance when considering *Strongyloides* parasites. Until recently strongyloidiasis was considered to be a disease of the small bowel, but in severe cases, especially in immunosuppressed patients, very acute ulcerating colitis can occur.

Barium studies show prominent mucosal folds with an irritable, tender duodenum; this allows the correct diagnosis to be suspected radiologically in patients who are referred with a clinical diagnosis of peptic ulceration or other gastrointestinal disease. There may also be excess mucus secretion, with rapid peristalsis and irritability, and such rapid transit time that the proximal small intestine may be difficult to evaluate. The ileum may be widened and show a coarse mucosal pattern. In more severe cases the inflammatory process is widely spread in the duodenum and jejunum, with a malabsorption (Fig. 12-13) or spruelike pattern, delayed gastric emptying, and hypomotility with slow transit times. Peristalsis in the duodenum and proximal jejunum may be absent. There is eventual complete loss of the mucosa and development of a narrow pipe-stem segment, with thickening of the bowel wall and mesenteric lymphadenopathy.

Oesophagostomum (helminthoma)

There are three strongyli in this group of nematode worms: *O. apiostomum, O. stephanostomum,* and the rare *O. brumpti.* These parasites, which are common in sheep, goats, pigs, and cattle, as well as in primates, cause severe illness.

Inflammatory granulomas and sterile abscesses enlarge and extend into the mesocolon but usually do not obstruct the bowel. The worm may calcify within the

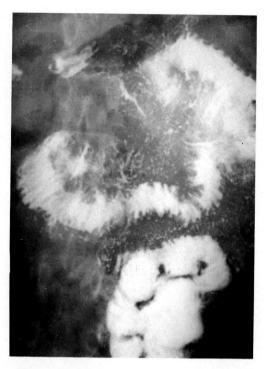

Fig. 12-13 Malabsorption pattern in upper jejunum in strongyloidiasis.
(Courtesy Prof. P. Cockshott.)

mass and may be visible on plain film studies. The essential radiologic finding is a mass of variable size in the wall of the bowel. The mass is most common in the cecum and ascending colon but can be found elsewhere.

Anisakiasis

Anisakis marina is found in the adult stage in whales and dolphins, whereas the larvae are found in many species of fish, including herring, mackerel, cod, salmon, and squid. Humans become infected by eating raw fish, and symptoms may occur within 24 hours. Manifestations usually resemble subacute peptic ulceration, but when the small bowel is infected the complaints suggest gastroenteritis or even appendicitis. In some patients there may be severe pain and evidence of ileus.

A careful double-contrast barium study of the stomach may show a submucosal mass, and the worm may be seen (Fig. 12-14).

Trichuriasis (whipworm infection)

Radiologic demonstration is extremely rare (Fig. 12-15).

In severe *Trichuris* infections the entire colon, including the rectum and appendix, may be infected, but the organism is uncommon in the ileum and may be to-

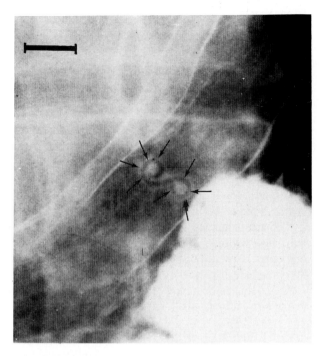

Fig. 12-14 *Anisakis* worm outlined in double-contrast barium meal in stomach of adult patient.
(Courtesy Dr. Masayoshi Namiki.)

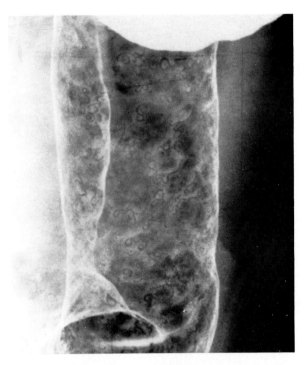

Fig. 12-15 Double-contrast enema shows *Trichuris trichiura* worms outlined in descending colon.
(Courtesy Prof. BJ Cremin.)

tally unsuspected by the clinician. Only in severe infections is there bleeding, ulceration, and inflammatory reaction, which seldom extend beyond the muscularis mucosa. The laboratory diagnosis depends on the identification of the worms during sigmoidoscopy or on stool concentration studies. Eosinophilia is common with a severe whipworm infection, and there may be an iron-deficiency anemia. Double-contrast studies show the wavy outlines of the numerous small "whips," often amid considerable mucus.

Helminthic infections: tapeworms (cestodes)

Tapeworms are among humankind's oldest companions; they may grow to 30 feet in length. The two most common are *Taenia saginata* and *Taenia solium*. *Diphyllobothrium latum* (found in freshwater fish and crustaceans) may cause mechanical intestinal obstruction and a background eosinophilia and anemia.

The beef tapeworm, *T. saginata,* occurs throughout the world. The pork tapeworm, *T. solium,* although widespread, is much less common. The adult worm lives in the alimentary tract of humans, attached by its scolex to the mucosa, usually in the middle small bowel. The eggs pass in the feces and are ingested by grazing cattle or pigs, where they hatch in the intestine of the intermediate host. If the meat is eaten insufficiently cooked or raw, the life cycle in humans starts

again. Laboratory diagnosis depends on recognition of the ova or proglottids in the stools. Eosinophilia is common.

The adult *T. saginata* is very seldom demonstrated by radiologic means. When seen, a long and gradually widening radiolucent line within the barium pattern occurs, usually in the jejunum or ileum. At its neck the tapeworm may be 1 to 2 mm wide, but distally it may be 12 mm or more.

Armillifer (tongue worm)

Two tongue worms infect humans, gaining entry through the alimentary tract, but causing no gastrointestinal symptoms. When dead, they often become calcified within the peritoneum (Fig. 12-16), liver, or spleen, and should be easily recognized and differentiated from calculi or calcified lymph nodes.

The radiographic findings of curved calcified nymphs scattered throughout the peritoneum, pleura, liver, and spleen are characteristic. They are not found in muscle and should be easily distinguished from cysticercosis (which is predominantly in peripheral muscles).

Liver flukes (trematodes)

Of the flukes that infect the biliary tract, three are most important. The Oriental liver fluke, *Clonorchis*

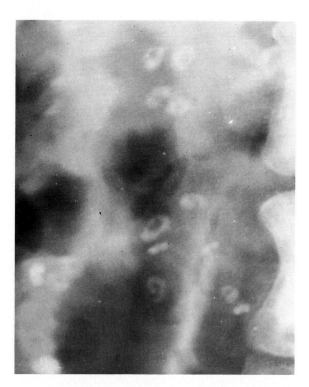

Fig. 12-16 Calcified *Armillifer armillatus* in peritoneum.

sinensis, occurs throughout East Asia, Japan, Korea, coastal China, Taiwan, and Southeast Asia. The liver fluke *Fasciola hepatica* is found in Europe, the former Soviet Union, the Middle East, Asia, Africa, Australia, and Central and South America. *Opisthorchis felineus* occurs in man in central, eastern, and southern Europe, with isolated cases in India, Vietnam, North Korea, Japan, and the Philippines. *O. viverrini* is important in northeast Thailand and in Laos, where it is surprisingly common.

Clonorchiasis

The *Clonorchis* parasite inhabits the bile ducts of humans, mammals, and birds. It is about 10 to 20 mm long, flat, and somewhat pointed. Acute suppurative cholangitis, recurrent pyogenic cholangitis, and acute pancreatitis can be associated; clonorchiasis is probably significant in the causation of carcinoma of the liver. Multiple abscesses that start in the biliary system may progress and cause a severe febrile illness with jaundice.

The flukes can be demonstrated by operative or transhepatic cholangiography and on occasion by intravenous cholangiography. They appear as 1 to 2 cm curved or crescentic filling defects within dilated bile ducts.

Fascioliasis

Another liver fluke, *Fasciola,* although it is common and causes clinical symptoms, cannot be reliably recognized on radiologic examination. With CT, however, characteristic changes in the liver (nodular intrahepatic lesions of diminished attenuation, ranging in size from 4 to 10 mm but sometimes as large as 2 cm) have been described.

Opisthorchiasis

Humans are an accidental host to two additional liver flukes, *O. felineus* and *O. viverrini,* probably by way of eating infected pigs or fish.

Cholangiography, ultrasonography, and CT scanning may show multiple small dilatations of the intrahepatic bile ducts, with diffuse saccular changes as the condition progresses. Marked cystic dilatation eventually occurs, and this combination of large areas of cystic dilatation with multiple small cysts is pathognomonic.

Vascular flukes (schistosomes)

Four species of *Schistosoma* cause significant infection in humans; *S. haematobium, S. mansoni,* and *S. japonicum* are the most common; *S. intercalatum* is less frequently found.

Schistosomiasis, or *bilharziasis,* infects about 200 million persons worldwide.

The pattern of development is similar in all varieties. The flukes may live for 10 to 15 years. Liver flukes seldom cause radiologic findings unless they embolize during treatment and cause an inflammatory reaction when dead.

S. mansoni and *S. japonicum* mainly affect the alimentary tract. The discharge of hundreds of eggs through the intestinal mucosa causes a marked fibrotic reaction.

The earliest radiographic findings in the colon are an edematous mucosa with mural spicules and tiny ulcers. There is often marked spasm and then loss of haustration, particular in the descending and sigmoid colon (Fig. 12-17).

CT scanning has occasionally demonstrated calcification around the rectum and presacral tissues. It is important to remember that this calcification is within the ova and not in the fibrous tissue or granulomas.

Amebic dysentery (amebiasis)

Amebiasis is infection by the pathogenic protozoan *Entamoeba histolytica.* Infection occurs when contaminated food or water is swallowed; it is usually transmitted by human cyst carriers. Because the amebas spread either directly or by embolism, liver abscesses are common and often spread through the diaphragm and pleura

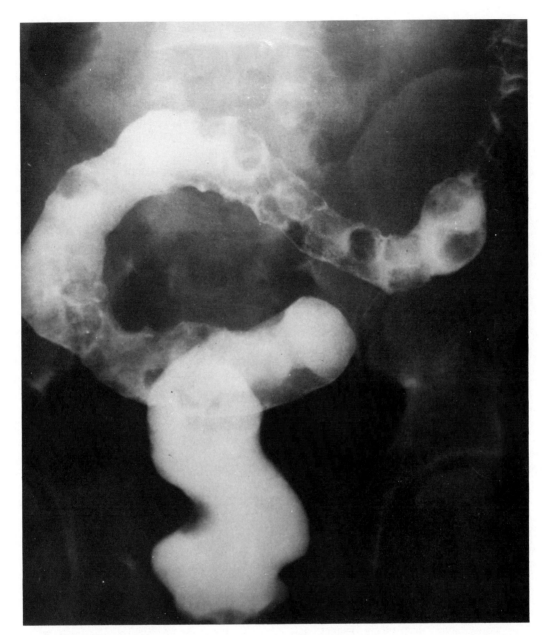

Fig. 12-17 Multiple small filling defects in rectum and sigmoid colon in patient infected with *Schistosoma mansoni*.

to the lungs. Hematogenous spread may cause pulmonary or brain abscesses. When there is direct extension through the wall of the large bowel with associated bacterial infection, a large and sometimes hard tumor (an *amoeboma*) may develop in or adjacent to the bowel (Fig. 12-18).

The earliest radiologic findings occur around the cecum and ascending colon and are due to edema and ulceration of the bowel. There is rigidity and thickening of the bowel wall with an irregular mucosa and multiple tiny ulcers. As the ulcers deepen, the edges become undermined and the characteristic flask-shaped ulcer can be demonstrated radiologically. If the edema is severe, there will be "thumb printing." The entire colon may be involved and may resemble the appearance of acute ulcerative colitis. In very severe and often fatal cases, an acute toxic megacolon may be seen. When the disease is chronic, the picture is that of contraction and rigidity with fixed deformity.

Solitary or multiple abscesses occur anywhere in the

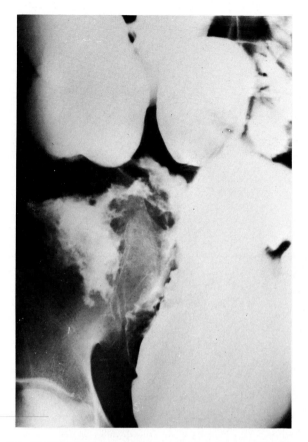

Fig. 12-18 Ameboma adjacent to cecum having cavity connecting with lumen of bowel.

liver, although most frequently in the right lobe. The liver abscesses are best demonstrated by CT, ultrasonography, or MRI, and are frequently peripheral (Figs. 12-19, 12-20).

Amebiasis mimics many diseases, including ulcerative colitis, with or without megacolon; Crohn's disease, with its narrow areas, deep ulcers, fistulas, and skip areas; or the tight stricture mass of malignancy. A serologic check is easy and may not only avoid surgery but may also literally be life saving.

Echinococcosis (hydatid disease)

There are two types of *Echinococcus* infections: *E. granulosus* infection, the most common, and *E. multilocularis* infection, less common but much more invasive and frequently resembling malignancy.

E. granulosus infection

E. granulosus infection results in large cysts and is found worldwide, but is more common in temperate climates. The life cycle requires two hosts: a dog and a grazing animal, usually sheep, cattle, or pigs. It can also be found in wolves and some deer. The adult parasite is a tiny tapeworm, usually found by the hundreds or thousands in the small intestine of dogs. Excreted in the feces, the eggs contaminate wide areas of pasture and are subsequently ingested by grazing animals. Humans become accidently infected either by contact with infected dogs or by ingesting food, water, or soil containing the eggs.

In humans the external layers of the eggs are digested and the larvae migrate through the intestinal mucosa into the mesenteric veins and lymphatics. They are then carried to many different parts of the body. Because it acts as an effective filter, the liver is the most common site for cysts; incidence exceeds 90% in some series. However, the larvae may lodge anywhere in the body and have been found in the peritoneum, spleen, kidneys, brain, bones, heart, and muscles.

On plain radiograph (Fig. 12-21) the cysts may cause generalized enlargement of the liver or a localized bulge in the hepatic outline, with a hump in the diaphragm in some cases. They are usually spheric and sometimes distorted by the rib cage. In more than 50% of cases, partial or crescentic calcification occurs in the cyst wall, or, if the cyst has been damaged, the calcification may show that it is collapsed and amorphous. Ultrasonography, CT scanning, and MRI have made it possible to recognize small cysts and show that they are usually multiple. Their appearance on ultrasound has been divided into the following categories:

1. *pure fluid* (the cyst is sonolucent with marked enhancement of back wall echoes)
2. *fluid with a split wall* (the cyst is less well rounded and sags, and a very characteristic floating membrane may be seen internally)
3. *both fluid and septa* (the cyst is usually well defined but divided into sections of varying shapes, usually oval or rounded)
4. *irregular shape* (irregular cysts with a variable echo pattern, usually round but rough in outline)
5. *hyperechoic* (only the thick reflecting front wall may be seen)

The CT findings are diagnostically very accurate. The attenuation is similar to that of water, and about 80% of the cysts have marginal calcification and more than half have daughter cysts within them. The endocystic membrane can usually be recognized.

Cysts are also clearly demonstrated on MRI with spin-echo pulse sequences and are equally well seen with either T_1- or T_2-weighting, so it is probably best to use both. A thin, low-intensity rim may be seen surrounding the hydatid cysts and can be helpful in the differential diagnosis.

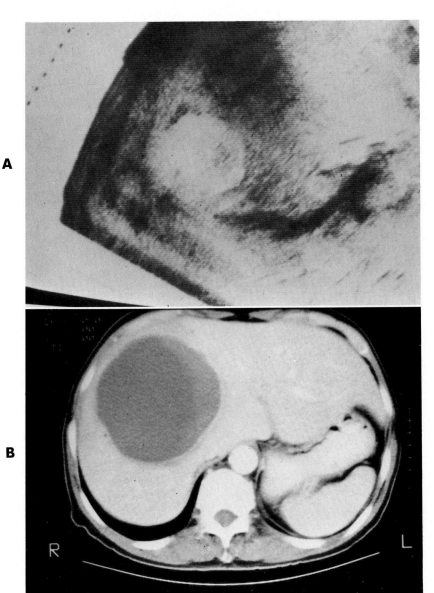

Fig. 12-19 Ultrasonographic appearance, **A,** and computed tomography scan, **B,** of amebic abscesses in liver. Findings are very nonspecific, and amebic abscess cannot be distinguished from any other liver abscess.

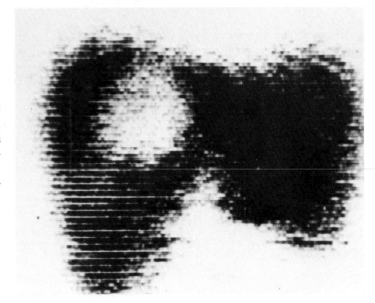

Fig. 12-20 Radionuclide scan (^{99m}Tc-sulfur colloid) shows large amebic abscess in right lobe of liver, spreading upward toward upper surface. Diaphragm was involved, and there was right-sided pleural effusion with edema in right lower lobe.

(From Reeder MM, Palmer PES: *The radiology of tropical diseases.* Baltimore, 1981, Williams & Wilkins.)

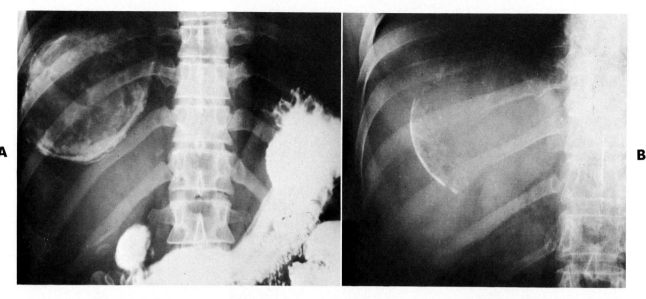

Fig. 12-21 Calcified *Echinococcus* cysts in liver. **A,** Calcified cyst containing multiple daughter cysts in 37-year-old Basque woman. **B,** Segmentally calcified *Echinococcus* cyst in young Greek woman.

E. multilocularis infection

E. multilocularis presents as a very different disease. It is probably most common in eastern Europe and Turkey, but is also found in Canada, Alaska, and parts of China and central Asia. It is particularly prevalent in areas of cold and high altitude. The life cycle is much the same as that of *E. granulosus,* with dogs, cats, or foxes usually being involved. Although it is a benign and afebrile infection at first, the outcome is usually fatal. Multiple cystic spaces, about 0.5 cm in size, produce a honeycomb or spongy appearance *(alveolar echinococcosis).*

The radiologic appearance of the chronic granulomatous reaction and the multiple small cysts is characteristic. In nearly 70% of infections there are numerous small calcified spheres with radiolucent centers, ranging from 2 to 4 mm in size. On CT scanning they may demonstrate great variation in attenuation, from +5 to +60 Hounsfield units. Calcification is demonstrated around the edge of the cysts, but sometimes there is an amorphous, plaque-like, racemose pattern throughout. This combination of clustered microcalcification with necrosis is very suggestive of *E. multilocularis.*

GASTROINTESTINAL MANIFESTATIONS OF AIDS

SUSAN D WALL

Since 1981 the acquired immunodeficiency syndrome (AIDS) epidemic has had an unparalleled impact on the well-being of the people in the United States and the world. As of 1991, more than 160,000 persons in the United States alone were diagnosed with this highly morbid epidemic illness, and it has killed more than 100,000 of them. Radiology often plays a pivotal role in elucidating the early and frequently enigmatic symptomatology of patients with this syndrome.

AIDS is caused by a retrovirus known as human immunodeficiency virus (HIV). Replication of this virus causes a profound and unrelenting depression of the immune system that predisposes the patient to opportunistic tumors and infections. The virus is transmitted largely by intimate sexual contact, but also by exposure to contaminated blood or some body secretions. The disease affects mainly homosexual men, IV drug users, and recipients of previously unscreened blood or blood products.

Gastrointestinal manifestations and barium radiography

The GI tract is one of the most frequently involved organ systems in AIDS patients. Opportunistic tumors (such as Kaposi's sarcoma and lymphoma) and opportunistic pathogens (such as *Candida albicans,* cytomegalovirus, *Cryptosporidium,* and atypical mycobacteria) account for most of the recognized gastrointestinal morbidity in AIDS.

Multifocal gastrointestinal abnormalities (three or more sites) are seen in 65% to 75% of homosexual men with AIDS who are referred for barium examination. Double-contrast examination is the preferred technique;

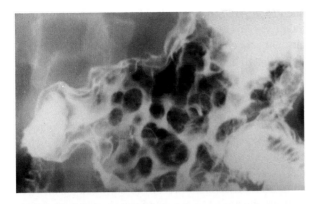

Fig. 12-22 Advanced Kaposi's sarcoma. Multiple, coalescent nodular lesions of advanced Kaposi's sarcoma are present throughout stomach in this AIDS patient.
(From Wall SD: *Contemp Diag Rad* 9(20):1, 1986.)

it can be directive when diagnosis requires visual inspection by endoscopy or colonoscopy with associated biopsy and/or culture. The cause of multifocal abnormalities can be multiple foci of Kaposi's sarcoma, widespread opportunistic infection, multiple opportunistic infections, coexistent tumor and infection, or, less commonly, coexistent Kaposi's sarcoma and lymphoma.

Gastrointestinal Kaposi's sarcoma

The GI tract is a major target organ of Kaposi's sarcoma (Fig. 12-22), and it may be involved at the time of diagnosis or early thereafter in patients with cutaneous disease. Visceral involvement is considered a manifestation of the multicentric nature of this tumor, not metastatic disease.

Early gastrointestinal Kaposi's sarcoma is not detected on barium radiograph because lesions at this stage are macular and therefore not evident even with air-contrast technique. However, the appearance on endoscopy is characteristic, and diagnosis is made by visual inspection. In most cases there are multiple flat, red-purple (violaceous) lesions varying in size from a few millimeters to 1 to 2 cm. With progression of disease the lesions become nodular and then are well demonstrated on barium radiograph. With air-contrast technique central umbilication may be seen, but "bull's eye" or "target" lesions are not present in the majority of cases. Tumor nodules have been seen in all segments of the GI tract, and their radiographic appearance is similar throughout.

Early gastrointestinal Kaposi's sarcoma generally is asymptomatic. However, even small lesions can cause symptoms when they are present in the oropharynx or hypopharynx (Fig. 12-23). Tumor nodules may be seen

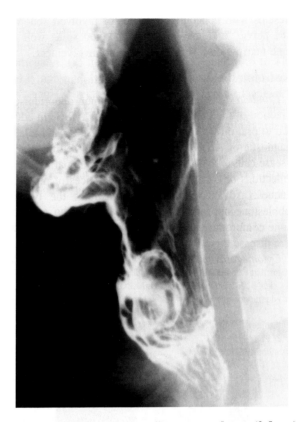

Fig. 12-23 Pharyngeal Kaposi's sarcoma. Large (2.5 cm) nodular lesion of Kaposi's sarcoma is present in pyriform sinus in this man with AIDS. Smaller lesions are present in valleculae and at base of tongue.
(Reprinted from Emeru CD et al: *Am J Roentgenol* 147:919, 1986.)

at the base of the tongue, the posterior oropharynx or hypopharynx, the valleculae, and/or the pyriform sinuses. Barium pharyngography sometimes demonstrates the full extent of disease better than direct visualization at larynoscopy. Furthermore, concurrent examination of the remainder of the upper GI tract can be performed readily with pharyngography.

The barium radiographic findings of gastrointestinal AIDS-related Kaposi's sarcoma are not specific, and the differential diagnosis includes lymphoma, metastatic tumor, opportunistic infection, and Crohn's disease.

AIDS-related lymphoma

Gastrointestinal lymphoma seen in AIDS patients is usually the non-Hodgkin's type. The natural history of AIDS-related *non-Hodgkin's lymphoma* is unusual, since it frequently occurs in extranodal sites including abdominal viscera, mucocutaneous surfaces, bone marrow, and brain. *Hodgkin's disease* is seen less frequently in AIDS patients than is non-Hodgkin's lymphoma, but its natural history is also atypical. It often

13 *Postoperative Radiology*

H JOACHIM BURHENNE

POSTOPERATIVE EVALUATION OF THE ESOPHAGUS

POSTOPERATIVE EVALUATION OF THE STOMACH AND DUODENUM

POSTOPERATIVE EVALUATION OF THE SMALL BOWEL

POSTOPERATIVE EVALUATION OF THE COLON

POSTOPERATIVE EVALUATION OF THE BILIARY TRACT

POSTOPERATIVE EVALUATION OF THE LIVER

POSTOPERATIVE EVALUATION OF THE PANCREAS

Plain abdominal radiography is helpful in the diagnosis of retained foreign bodies and the evaluation of postoperative obstruction and perforation. Barium sulfate remains the most useful diagnostic contrast medium, especially when biphasic technique is used. With barium contrast studies it is possible to evaluate postoperative mucosal detail and to readily demonstrate obstruction. When searching for a postoperative leak or a fistula formation, however, iodinated contrast material is the agent of choice. If there is no evidence of free air on multiple radiographic projections, proceeding with barium sulfate is recommended.

Pulmonary complications (primarily atelectasis, pneumonia, thromboembolism, and aspiration) continue to constitute the most frequent postoperative problems. *Abscesses,* most often subphrenic, are also a common occurrence after surgery on the alimentary tract. Patients with pleural effusion, diaphragmatic elevation, or both, require further examination, ideally with one of the cross-sectional imaging modalities such as ultrasonography or computed tomographic (CT) scanning.

Retained surgical sponges (Fig. 13-1) may result in encapsulated abscesses, chronic sinus tracts, fecal fistulas, and erosion into neighboring viscera. CT scanning may be of help in detecting retained sponges, particularly if they do not contain radiopaque markers.

POSTOPERATIVE EVALUATION OF THE ESOPHAGUS
Instrumentation

Perforation of the esophagus is the most serious complication of esophagoscopy, gastroscopy, dilatation of the esophagus, tamponade for esophageal varices, or simple intubation of the esophagus for any reason. The incidence and the location of perforations are similar with the fiberscope and rigid esophagoscope. Early diagnosis of perforation of the esophagus is most important (Fig. 13-2), because this injury represents a surgical emergency demanding immediate treatment to de-

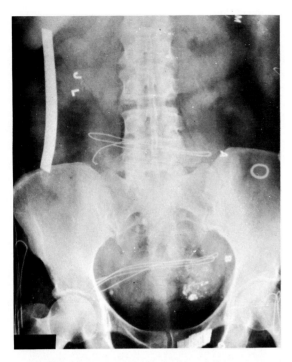

Fig. 13-1 Samples of indicators used for sponges of various sizes made by different manufacturers. Sample radiograph, obtained by draping material over abdomen, is kept in radiology department for reference.

crease mortality. Contrast studies with water-soluble media should identify the point of perforation.

Correction of hiatus hernia and gastroesophageal reflux

The objectives of surgery for a hiatus hernia or gastroesophageal reflux involve restoration of normal anatomic relationships at the esophagogastric junction, with additional construction of a valve or closing mechanism. Surgical results, postoperative complications, and the radiologic appearance vary for the different operations.

Posterior gastropexy

The key to the formation of a sliding hiatus hernia is failure or attenuation of the posterior attachment of the esophagus to the preaortic fascia. Corrective surgical procedure involves transabdominal reduction of the hernia, closure of the hiatus posterior to the esophagus, and anchoring of the gastroesophageal junction to the preaortic fascia and median arcuate ligament, resulting in posterior gastropexy.

Fundoplication

In fundoplication the posterior aspect of the fundus is placed behind the abdominal esophagus from left to

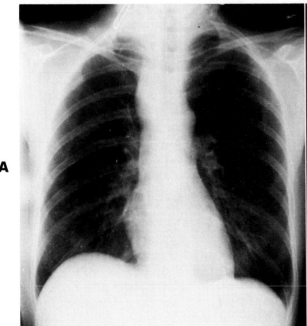

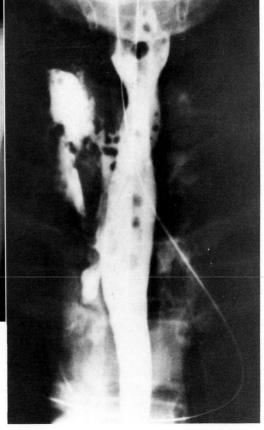

A   **B**

Fig. 13-2 Esophageal perforation and mediastinal abscess 24 hours after esophagoscopy. **A,** Right superior mediastinal widening. **B,** Gastrografin study demonstrates point of esophageal perforation.

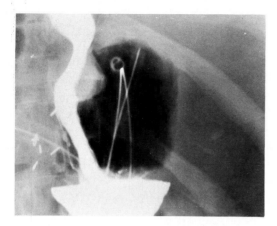

Fig. 13-3 Pseudotumor after fundoplication.

right and wrapped around it to form a cuff that is sutured together anteriorly for about 5 cm. A wide-bore esophageal tube is in place throughout the procedure to ensure an adequate esophageal diameter. The cuff of the gastric fundus narrows the distal esophagus to prevent reflux. Narrowing may be so pronounced that an inability to belch results, and permanent gaseous distention of the fundus is present on abdominal radiographs. The masslike deformity of the fundus must be differentiated from a neoplasm (Fig. 13-3). All types of fundoplication may give the radiographic appearance of a pseudotumor.

Mark VI procedure

In this procedure, the esophagogastric junction and cardia are mobilized, and the acute esophagogastric angle is restored by plicating the stomach to the esophagus. This restores the abdominal segment of the esophagus. A snug closure of the esophageal hiatus of the diaphragm behind the esophagus is then accomplished by approximation of the separated right crus.

Stricture repair

The procedure by Thal was designed for patients with a fibrous stricture in the distal esophagus caused by reflux esophagitis. A left thoracotomy approach is used, and the strictured area is incised. The incision is extended into the upper portion of the stomach, and the defect is covered by the serosal surface of the proximal stomach, which is wrapped over it, enlarging the previous stricture.

Esophagomyotomy

The most common complication noted after Heller esophagomyotomy is reflux esophagitis. Eccentric ballooning at the site of myotomy should be recognized as a normal and frequent postoperative finding.

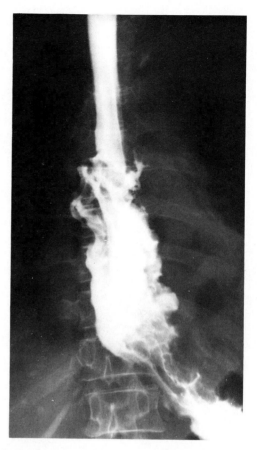

Fig. 13-4 Gastric interposition after resection of small distal esophageal carcinoma.

Esophageal resection and reconstruction

Malignant lesions of the esophagus may require resection or a bypass. Reconstruction with jejunum, colon, stomach (Fig. 13-4), or tubes formed from the stomach are procedures currently in use. Common early postoperative complications include fistula or stricture formation at the cervical anastomosis, transplant gangrene, and gastric stasis. Late complications include reflux, stricture at the distal anastomosis, gastric stasis, and recurrent carcinoma. Radiologic studies with an iodinated contrast medium are most helpful in investigating postoperative problems (Fig. 13-5).

Mobilization of the entire stomach for total esophageal replacement has recently gained renewed interest. Arteriographic studies have demonstrated that the viability of the fundus is not dependent on anastomotic circulation.

POSTOPERATIVE EVALUATION OF THE STOMACH AND DUODENUM

Surgical procedures for peptic disease may be divided into three groups or combinations: gastrectomy, vagotomy, and added drainage operations. The gastrec-

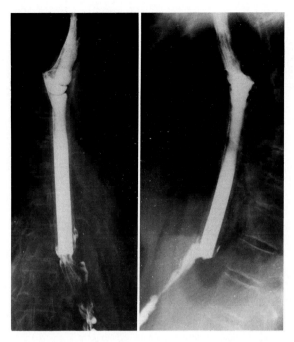

Fig. 13-5 Permanent esophageal intubation. There is partial obstruction at distal end that is due to relative stiffness of Celestin tube. Mechanical difficulty is not apparent on anteroposterior projection.

tomy may be distal, pylorus-preserving, proximal, or total. Vagotomy may be truncal, total gastric, proximal gastric, or selective. Added drainage operations include pyloroplasty and gastrojejunostomy.

Contrast-enhanced radiologic examination (Figs. 13-6, 13-7) remains the most important tool in the diagnosis of both early and late complications of operations on the stomach and duodenum. It is important to assess the preference of emptying from the gastric pouch in either the proximal or the distal jejunum. Radiographs may be obtained with the patient semierect or recumbent. If this does not clarify the layout of the anastomosis, the patient is turned through a complete circle in the erect position while drinking contrast agent in order to separate the two anastomotic loops.

Patients with gastric retention after vagotomy or pyloroplasty must be examined in the right lateral decubitus position. Contrast material retained in the aperistaltic stomach with the patient supine may simulate pyloric obstruction.

The complete radiographic evaluation of any patient after gastrectomy includes the identification of the following 12 basic variants of gastric surgery:

1. extent of gastric resection
2. end or side anastomosis
3. anterior or posterior anastomosis
4. superior or inferior anastomosis
5. large or small stomal diameter

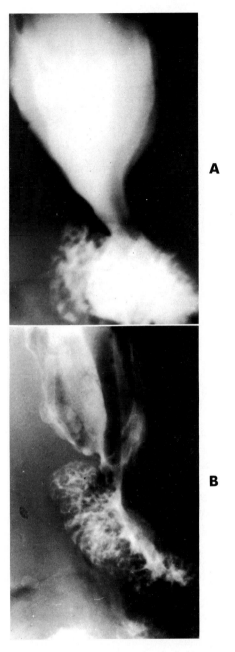

Fig. 13-6 Routine technique for postoperative examination includes full-column films, **A,** and mucosal air contrast studies of gastric pouch, stoma, and anastomotic loop, **B.**

6. slow or rapid gastric emptying
7. antecolic or retrocolic gastrojejunostomy
8. right-to-left or left-to-right direction of anastomosis
9. short or long proximal jejunal limb
10. horizontal or oblique plane of anastomosis
11. direction of gastric emptying
12. evidence of previous vagotomy

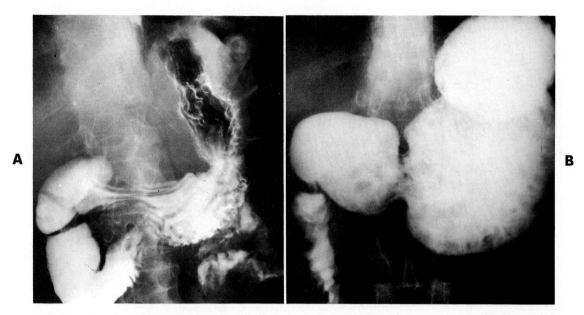

Fig. 13-7 A, Patient with history of previous duodenostomy presenting symptoms of intermittent obstruction. Slight narrowing resulting from scarring, but no obstruction, is seen in descending duodenum. **B,** Partial obstruction is demonstrated with use of mixture of food and barium on same day subsequent to routine upper gastrointestinal contrast investigation.

The identification of these variants is the key to post-gastrectomy diagnosis and enables the radiologist to reconstruct the operative procedure performed.

The eponyms used to designate various operative procedures on the stomach differ, and no uniformity exists. Eponyms therefore serve a limited purpose in the patient's record. In radiology of the postoperative alimentary tract, descriptive terminology is best for all purposes (Fig. 13-8). It is precise and may be applied to any existing or further operative modification.

Sequelae of gastric surgery
Pneumoperitoneum

The usual pneumoperitoneum after laparotomy makes it difficult to make a radiologic diagnosis of a postoperative air leak from an insufficient suture, duodenal stump blowout, or other perforation. There is little diagnostic difficulty if serial films demonstrate an increase in the amount of peritoneal air. Such progression indicates a leak from the gut, except in cases where air continues to enter the abdominal cavity through an indwelling drain.

Gas in the hepatic portal venous system has a distinctive radiologic appearance. It usually indicates bowel infarction, but may be present in cases of ulcerative colitis, intraabdominal abscess, small bowel obstruction, peritoneoscopy with accidental air insufflation into a mesenteric vein, and gastric ulcer.

Acute gastric dilatation

Acute gastric dilatation is a serious postoperative complication. It is a sudden and excessive distention of the stomach by fluid and gas and is often accompanied by vomiting, dehydration, and peripheral vascular collapse. It is often associated with immobilization of the patient or extensive postoperative ileus. The *body cast syndrome* consists of acute gastric dilatation associated with the application of a plaster hip spica cast or body jacket. Rupture of the stomach has been reported in eight cases after the administration of oxygen by nasal catheter.

Rupture, leakage, fistula, and abscess

Rupture of the duodenal stump is one of the most grave complications of gastric surgery and may occur without warning as soon as the first or as late as the nineteenth day after gastrojejunostomy. It causes death in about half of the cases, and has been reported in as many as 5% of cases after gastrojejunostomy and partial gastrectomy.

Radiographic examination with an iodinated contrast medium is the procedure of choice. A leak of the anastomotic suture line is probably related to an area of ischemia. Such leakage usually results in left subdiaphragmatic sinuses and abscess formation. Leakage from the duodenal stump, however, usually causes the

Operation	Roentgen-anatomy		Terminology

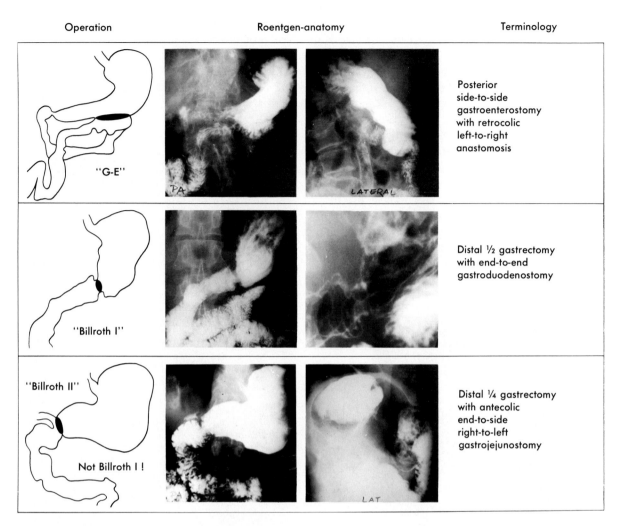

"G-E"   PA   LATERAL

Posterior
side-to-side
gastroenterostomy
with retrocolic
left-to-right
anastomosis

"Billroth I"

Distal ½ gastrectomy
with end-to-end
gastroduodenostomy

"Billroth II"   Not Billroth I !   LAT

Distal ¼ gastrectomy
with antecolic
end-to-side
right-to-left
gastrojejunostomy

Fig. 13-8 Examples of descriptive terminology as compared with eponyms for operative procedures of stomach.

(From Burhenne HJ: *Am J Roentgenol* 91:731, 1964. © 1964, American Roentgen Ray Society.)

same conditions in the right subdiaphragmatic region. Catheter trauma plays an important part in neonatal gastric perforations, and in one study was the cause in 11 of 143 cases reviewed.

Plain, erect, and decubitus radiographs readily show air-fluid levels below the diaphragm or in the lesser sac. These may be the result of leakage from the anastomosis or duodenal stump.

Hemorrhage

The incidence of postgastrectomy hemorrhage is 3%, but may be as high as 12% in emergency surgery or 30% in patients operated on for hemorrhage. Postoperative hemorrhage may be caused by any of the following:

1. inflammation or infection
2. intussusception
3. gastrojejunal prolapse
4. misplaced or slipped sutures
5. artery buttressed to the duodenal stump
6. thrombocytopenia from extensive replacement transfusions during surgery
7. erosions of plication defects
8. neoplasm
9. second ulcer overlooked at the time of operation
10. ulcer recurrence or marginal ulcer
11. hemorrhagic gastritis

Splenic injury during gastrectomy, or as a complication of vagotomy, is not infrequent and is usually caused by injury of the gastrosplenic or phrenosplenic attachment.

Obstruction

Stomal obstructions are caused by edema, submucosal hematoma, mechanical fault at the stoma, stricture after anastomotic ulcer, peristomal fat thickening caused by necrosis after anastomotic leakage or ligation of omental vessels, bezoar, intussusception, or internal hernia. They are best diagnosed by contrast-enhanced radiologic examination, which readily distinguishes between obstruction at the stoma and gastric atony with a patent anastomosis. Anastomotic strictures of the upper gastrointestinal tract are amenable to fluoroscopically guided balloon dilatation. Vagotomy without pyloroplasty often results in obstruction of the gastric outlet. Gastric bezoars (Fig. 13-9) have been described after gastroduodenostomy alone, but in most cases the pyloroplasty or partial gastrectomy had been performed in association with vagotomy. In addition, yeast bezoars have been reported after gastrectomy combined with vagotomy. Prolapse of the gastric mucosa into the anastomotic opening may cause partial obstruction.

Intussusceptions must be considered in the differential diagnosis of stomach obstruction. Intussusceptions

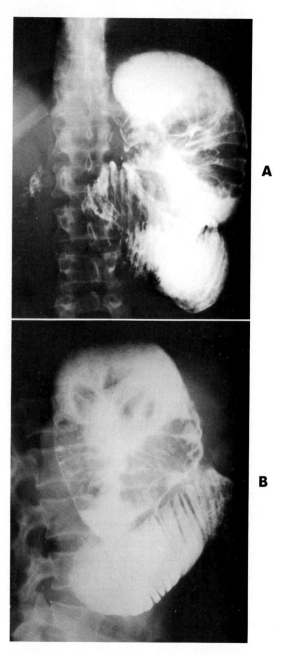

Fig. 13-10 Retrograde jejunogastric intussusception with obstruction, necessitating surgical intervention. Stretched and enlarged valvulae conniventes of intussuscepted jejunum are visualized within dilated gastric pouch and indicate impaired circulation.

(Courtesy Dr. R Rousseau.)

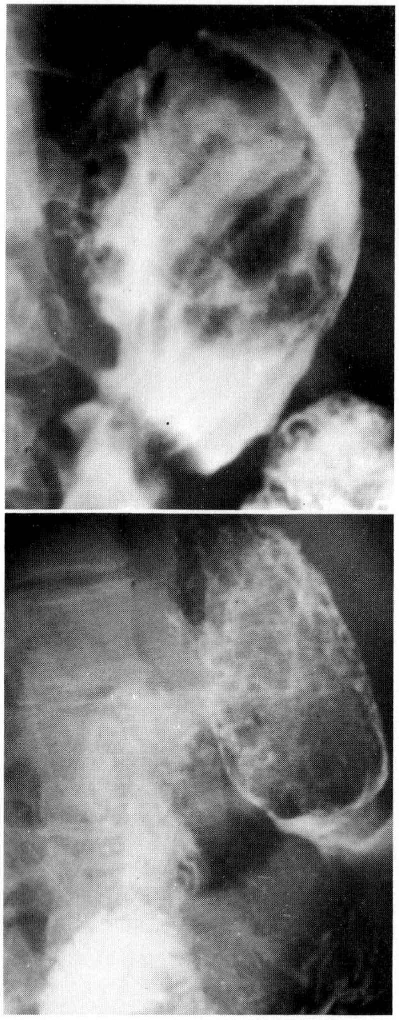

Fig. 13-9 Phytobezoar proximal to gastroduodenostomy, assuming shape of gastric pouch.

(Courtesy Dr. W Gaines.)

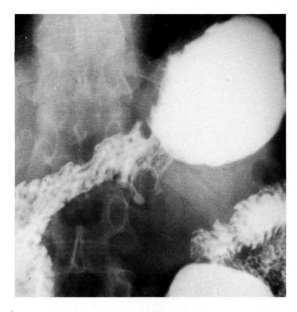

Fig. 13-11 Plication defects at gastroduodenostomy caused by inversion of mucosal margin at anastomosis.

may be either antegrade or retrograde. In retrograde jejunogastric intussusception, the jejunum invaginates into the gastric pouch (Fig. 13-10). The acute type presents with a clinical triad consisting of (1) high intestinal obstruction, (2) left hypochondriac mass, and (3) hematemesis. In addition to the obstruction, a striated filling defect in the stomach is seen on radiographic examination and is considered pathognomonic. The valvulae conniventes seen radiographically within the gastric pouch are stretched and enlarged because of pressure edema or strangulation. The intuscipiens is the distal (efferent) loop in 75% of cases, the proximal (afferent) loop in most other cases, and, in rare cases, both loops.

Plication defects

Temporary or permanent distortion of the mucosal pattern (plication defect) may occur after gastrostomy, gastrotomy, or any other type of surgical intervention with suturing or inversion (Figs. 13-11, 13-12). A char-

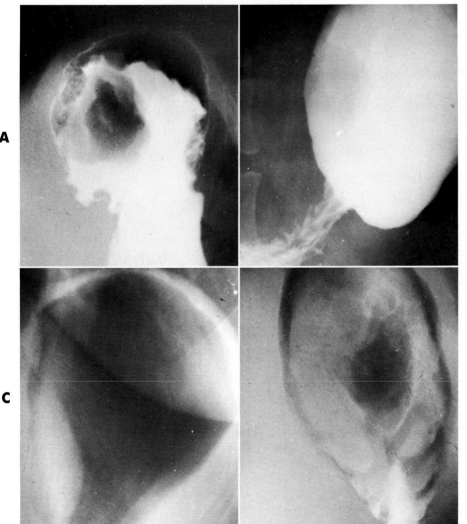

Fig. 13-12 Plication defect on high lesser curvature in typical location just above anastomosis in patient with gastroduodenostomy. **A** and **B,** Plication defect resembling tumor. **C,** Plication stretched and elongated with patient in erect position. **D,** Mucosal conversion resulting from suturing and plication on lesser curvature, seen in lateral projection.

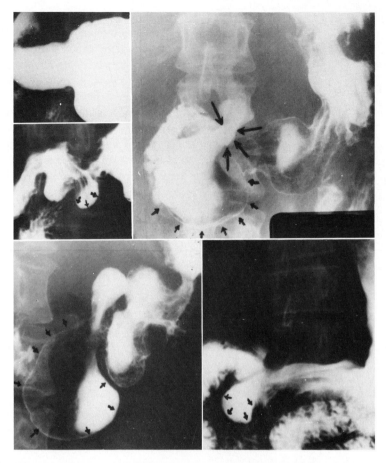

Fig. 13-13 Beagle-ear sign, or pseudodiverticulum *(small arrows)*, at site of Heineke-Mikulicz pyloroplasty, illustrated in four different patients. Normal preoperative greater curvature is demonstrated in first patient. Recurrent duodenal ulcer is present in second patient *(large arrows)*. (Modified from Burhenne HJ: *Semin Radiol* 6:182, 1971.)

acteristic pseudodiverticulum deformity sometimes occurs after the Heineke-Mikulicz pyloroplasty (Fig. 13-13).

Retained gastric antrum

Surgical retention of the endocrinologically active gastric antrum gives poor results. After antral exclusion operations (with transection of the stomach, end-to-side gastrojejunostomy, and retention of the gastric antrum in continuity with the pylorus and duodenum) the incidence of marginal ulcers is 30% to 50%. Resection of the retained antrum is mandatory and results in relief of symptoms. Serum gastrin determinations may identify three causes of recurrent ulcer: incomplete vagotomy, retained antrum, and Zollinger-Ellison tumor.

Postoperative ulcer disease

Esophagitis after gastric surgery has been related to bile reflux. *Gastritis,* which commonly occurs early after surgery and usually subsides within a few weeks, may also be caused by reflux of bile salts. *Jejunitis* in the anastomotic loop is found in 38% of cases after partial gastric resection.

A *recurrent ulcer* may been seen on radiographic studies at the original ulcer site after simple excision or wedge resection. Recurrence of gastric ulcer is also seen after gastroenterostomy alone (Fig. 13-14).

Marginal ulcers, which have also been called postoperative ulcers, jejunal ulcers, stomal ulcers, anastomotic ulcers, gastrojejunal ulcers, and recurrent ulcers, are not recurrent lesions, but new ulcerations occurring after gastric surgery in the jejunum just distal to the anastomosis. Marginal ulcers almost never originate in the gastric mucosa or at the anastomotic margin. Most occur in the first 2 cm of an anastomotic jejunum, usually in the distal jejunal loop. The radiographic diagnosis of marginal ulcer is possible in about 50% of cases, but at least some suggestive abnormality is seen in 80%

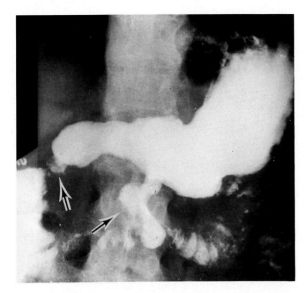

Fig. 13-14 Patient with gastroenterostomy for duodenal ulcer disease. Duodenal ulcer recurred within 1 year *(left arrow),* and marginal ulcer at gastroenterostomy *(right arrow)* is present.

of cases. The ulcer crater is not demonstrated if it is superficial, but concentrically arranged mucosal folds may be present (Fig. 13-15). The double-contrast barium examination is advocated as the radiologic technique of choice to evaluate mucosal detail in the gastric remnant and in the anastomosis. The use of intravenous glucagon (0.5 to 1 mg) usually further improves visualization of the anastomosis and the immediate postanastomotic segment of the jejunum.

Gastrojejunocolic fistula

This fistula between the jejunum and the colon represents a grave complication of marginal ulcers and gastric surgery. Radiologic techniques provide the most accurate means of diagnosis, and diagnoses are correct in 90% of cases. The barium enema is more accurate than an upper gastrointestinal study.

Ulcerogenic tumors

Marginal ulcers associated with ulcerogenic tumors are particularly resistant to medical therapy. The mechanism of ulcerogenesis in these tumors is a gastrinlike substance excreted by tumors of the pancreas (Zollinger-Ellison syndrome) or by polyglandular adenomas, and which is similar to the gastrin produced by a retained gastric antrum after gastrectomy.

The radiographic finding of large or multiple marginal ulcers, which may occur in unusual locations, should alert the radiologist to the diagnostic possibility of ulcerogenic tumors or a retained antrum. The lacy or

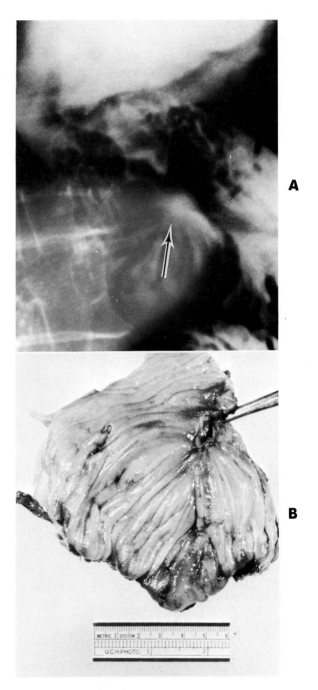

Fig. 13-15 A, Concentrically arranged jejunal folds point to marginal ulcer *(arrow).* **B,** Specimen of resected jejunum.

cobweblike small bowel pattern caused by hypersecretion is an additional radiologic indication of the correct diagnosis.

Postgastrectomy carcinoma

The radiologic diagnosis of malignancy in the postgastrectomy state is difficult, in particular if a postoperative baseline study is not available for comparison. Postgastrectomy gastric carcinoma may be recurrent or primary. The incidence of cancer after surgery for a gastric ulcer exceeds the expected rate, but appears to be less than that expected after surgery for a duodenal ulcer. If postoperative deformities make the radiologic differential diagnosis uncertain, direct visualization by fiberendoscopy and biopsy is recommended.

Postgastrectomy syndromes
Dumping

It is important to differentiate between mechanical dumping, the early postprandial dumping syndrome, and late postprandial hypoglycemia.

MECHANICAL DUMPING

Mechanical dumping merely refers to rapid emptying of contrast medium or food from the stomach into the small bowel. The reservoir capacity of the gastric pouch is somewhat better demonstrated when food rather than barium is used. Jejunal interposition has been used to improve reservoir function after gastrectomy.

DUMPING SYNDROME

The dumping syndrome causes early postprandial vascular symptoms of sweating, flushing, palpitation, and feelings of weakness and dizziness. The symptoms are relieved when the patient lies down.

The mechanism of the dumping syndrome is not clearly understood, but it may be related to that fact that with mechanical dumping a hypertonic solution rapidly enters the jejunum. This osmotically active solution causes a fluid shift from the blood compartment into the small bowel, and absorption of the contents does not take place until isotonicity is established. The resulting drop in plasma volume results in the accompanying vasomotor symptoms.

MALABSORPTION

Malabsorption states after gastric resection may occur with deficient production of extrinsic factor, decreased vitamin B_{12} absorption, increased fat content in the stool, or iron deficiency anemia. Calcium metabolism is sometimes altered, with a decrease in calcium levels, particularly after Polya's gastrectomy in older patients. Radiologic changes resemble osteoporosis or osteomalacia or a combination of the two, with rarefaction, accentuated bony trabeculae, wedging, biconcavity, multiple rib fractures, and Looser's zones in the scapulae and pubic rami.

POSTVAGOTOMY FUNCTIONAL CHANGES

Functional changes after vagotomy include diarrhea and an increase in the incidence of gallstones.

Gastric operation for morbid obesity

Complications of *gastric bypass surgery*, including leakage at the anastomosis, anastomotic stenosis, and abscess formation, can be treated with interventional radiologic procedures. Radiographic examination with Gastrografin is recommended in the investigation of early postoperative changes.

POSTOPERATIVE EVALUATION OF THE SMALL BOWEL
Obstruction in the anastomotic jejunal loop

Obstruction in the anastomotic jejunal loop may result from postgastrectomy internal hernia. There are three potential locations for hernial rings after gastrojejunostomy: (1) the postcolic retroanastomotic space, (2) the antecolic retroanastomotic space, and (3) the defect in the transverse mesocolon. The last of these is usually closed after retrocolic gastrojejunostomy, and the omentum is sutured to the stomach pouch. Kinking, fibrosis, tumor recurrence, or pressure by the mesentery of one anastomotic loop on the other may result in anastomotic obstruction.

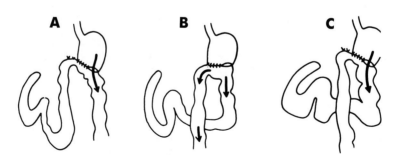

Fig. 13-16 A, Desirable emptying in forward direction in right-to-left anastomosis with oblique cut end of stomach. **B,** Bidirectional emptying with horizontal plane of left-to-right anastomosis. **C,** Undesirable preferential filling of proximal jejunal loop with left-to-right anastomosis and oblique plane of anastomosis resulting in proximal loop stasis.

Small bowel obstruction

Obstructions in the small bowel are readily diagnosed by radiographs. The usual causes of obstruction are adhesions, internal hernias, and intussusceptions. After gastrectomy, patients should avoid whole oranges or similar foods containing fibers that may cause phytobezoars.

Distal gastroenterostomy

Inadvertent gastroileostomy is a surgical emergency. The principal radiologic finding is a proximal loop crossing to the right iliac fossa, with rapid appearance of barium in the colon. If the proximal (afferent) jejunal loop does not lead to the ligament of Treitz and if the distal (efferent) jejunal loop can be traced over a relatively short distance to the ileocecal valve, the diagnosis is not difficult. Upper gastrointestinal studies are more helpful than barium enema.

Dysfunction of the proximal jejunal loop

If the proximal loop is attached to the greater curvature instead of the lesser curvature, this left-to-right anastomosis results in preferential emptying of the stomach into the proximal loop (Fig. 13-16), leading to regurgitation and proximal loop stasis and possibly resulting in the so-called *proximal (afferent) loop syndrome* or *blind loop syndrome,* with vitamin B$_{12}$ deficiency and resulting anemia.

Afferent loop syndrome

The afferent loop syndrome is characterized by postprandial epigastric fullness relieved by bilious vomiting, and radiologic examination plays an important part in its diagnosis. Once the point of obstruction in either the proximal or distal jejunum has been demonstrated, identification of the direction of gastric emptying is important. Serial films or cinefluorograms may be obtained with the patient in the erect position. It is impor-

tant to remember that filling of the proximal loop is not in itself considered abnormal.

Blind pouch syndrome

Stagnant dilated segments of small intestine may be demonstrated radiologically after side-to-side anastomosis of the small intestine. The blind pouch syndrome is characterized by gas-filled structures on plain films.

Ileostomy and ileal pouches

Necrosis, ileostomy prolapse, fistula formation, peristomal hernia, ileostomy stenosis, and bleeding are the complications of conventional ileostomies. The ileostomy segment should be examined in an oblique or tangential position during contrast studies to identify abnormalities, particularly hernia and stenosis. This is best done at the end of the reflux examination without a catheter in place.

The continent ileostomy by Kock is commonly performed (Figs. 13-17, 13-18). Radiologic studies may be of particular value in follow-up by demonstrating postoperative nipple valve extrusion and inflammatory changes in the pouch.

POSTOPERATIVE EVALUATION OF THE COLON

Complications after colonic surgery include anastomotic failure; ileus; fistula formation; hemorrhage; and

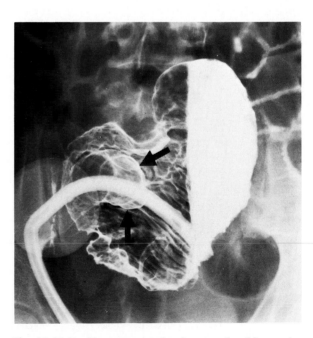

Fig. 13-18 Double-contrast study of a normal and intact nipple valve.

(From Stephens D, Mantell B, Kelly K: *Am J Roentgenol* 132:717, 1979. © 1979, American Roentgen Ray Society.)

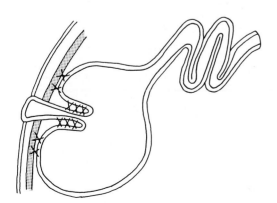

Fig. 13-17 Kock's continent ileostomy with distal ileal pouch and nipple valve.

sepsis such as wound infection, peritonitis, abscess formation, and enteritis. Radiologic studies are useful in identifying free air or abscess formation on plain films, anastomotic leakage and fistula formation with Gastrografin studies, and bowel obstruction with barium contrast examination.

Obstruction is less common after colonic surgery than it is after surgery of the small intestine, but the rate of *anastomotic breakdown* after large bowel surgery is high. Contrast studies may demonstrate more than one fistula, or the internal fistula may go to the small bowel or bladder. Tumor recurrence at the site of the colonic anastomosis can be identified by barium enema examination. Some narrowing at the colon anastomosis is usually present after surgery.

Radiation effects

Radiation effects on the colon may be seen after treatment of malignant lesions of the female pelvic organs, the bladder, and the prostate. Early changes after radiation include proctocolitis with edematous and sometimes ulcerated mucosa. Radiographic identification of segmental stricture is usually a later effect.

POSTOPERATIVE EVALUATION OF THE BILIARY TRACT

Calculous disease accounts for most surgical procedures on the biliary tract. If elective cholecystectomy has been scheduled for cholelithiasis, a recent radio-

graphic study must be available, because it has been shown that stones up to 1 cm in size and up to 30 in number can be evacuated spontaneously (Fig. 13-19).

The contrast medium used for direct injection during *operative cholangiography* must be opaque enough for marginal delineation of the bile duct, yet dilute enough to permit visualization of stones through the contrast medium. Television monitors in the surgical suite are convenient, but do not match the detail seen on radiographs.

Interpretation, pitfalls, and mistakes
Air bubbles

The differentiation between air bubbles and stones in the duct system may be made by placing the patient in the Trendelenburg and semierect positions. However, not everything that is round and rises in fluid is an air bubble; gallstones do not have to be faceted, and cholesterol stones may float in contrast medium. Blockage at Oddi's sphincter may be caused by spasm, particularly after manipulation of the common duct or instrumentation of Oddi's sphincter. This contraction may simulate stones in the distal duct (Fig. 13-20).

Pneumocholangiogram

The presence of gas in the biliary tract may be caused by previous surgical anastomoses; by fistula from a gallstone; by inflammation; by peptic or malignant disease; by gas-forming organisms; or by incompe-

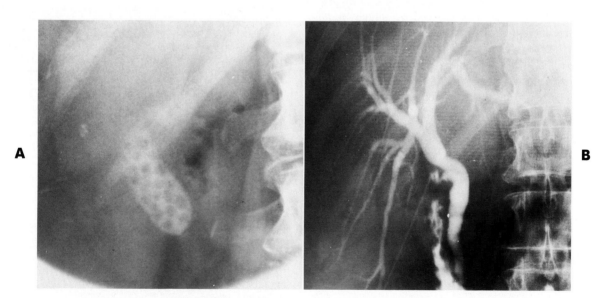

A **B**

Fig. 13-19 A, Oral cholecystogram obtained 4 months before elective cholecystectomy reveals numerous small gallstones. **B,** At time of surgery, gallbladder contained no stones and primary operative cholangiograms were normal. Surgery could have been avoided in this case of "disappearing gallstones," with repeat oral cholecystogram obtained before surgery. Stones of this size may readily pass through ampulla of Vater.

tence of Oddi's sphincter from medication, tumor, adhesions, or paralytic intestinal ileus. Incompetence of Oddi's sphincter with reflux gas and barium has also been seen in newborn infants with duodenal atresia. Reflux of gas and barium also occurs in cases in which the common duct enters the wall of the duodenal diverticulum. An air cholangiogram may also be a sequela of trauma or a complication of attempted thoracocentesis.

Anatomic variations

Compensatory dilatation of the common bile duct after cholecystectomy is not a normal occurrence, and an increase in diameter after surgery is indicative of biliary tract disease. In patients without symptoms, the common duct usually retains its size after surgery, as compared with evidence on preoperative films. Normal common bile ducts do, however, show a slight but definite increase in both outer and inner circumferences with age in men and women.

Anomalies of the major ducts of the biliary tree are relatively common (Fig. 13-21). Schulenburg found anatomic variations of the biliary tract in 230 of 1093 surgical patients, an incidence of 21% (Fig. 13-22).

Postcholecystectomy syndrome

If symptoms occur or persist after cholecystectomy, several of the entities under the heading "postcholecystectomy syndrome" must be considered. These include retained duct stones; cystic duct remnants; duct strictures and injuries; Oddi's sphincter spasm and fibrosis; neoplastic disease, including neuroma of the cystic duct; pancreatitis; and bile peritonitis. Persistent symptoms also have been ascribed to disorders outside the biliary tract, such as hiatus hernia, peptic ulcerations, abdominal angina, coronary artery disease, and spastic colon.

By far the most common cause of postcholecystectomy symptoms is *retained stones in the biliary tract;* intrahepatic stones overlooked at the time of surgery may move distally to cause symptoms. Other abnormalities causing the postcholecystectomy syndrome are quite rare. *Cystic duct remnant* per se is highly unlikely

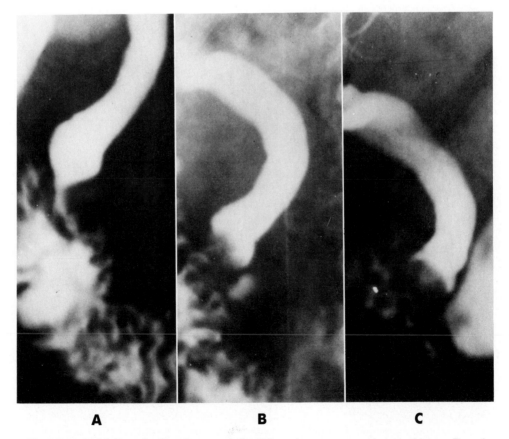

A   **B**   **C**

Fig. 13-20 Serial films showing the normal distal duct, **A,** some contraction at sphincter, **B,** and prominent contraction at sphincter simulating common duct stone, **C.** This "pseudocalculus sign" is frequently seen in secondary operative cholangiography following duct instrumentation.

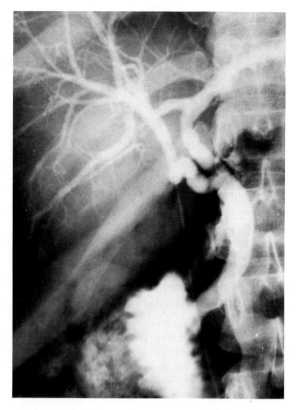

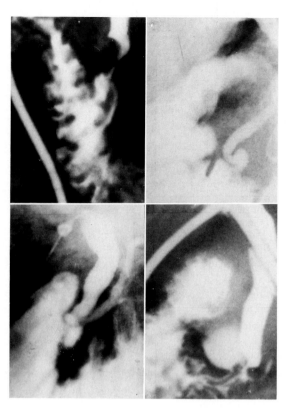

Fig. 13-21 Right hepatic duct joins cystic duct. If this information is available from primary operative cholangiogram, duct transection close to common duct can be avoided.

Fig. 13-22 Four different patients with entrance of biliary tract into wall or neck of duodenal diverticulum. Reflux is common.

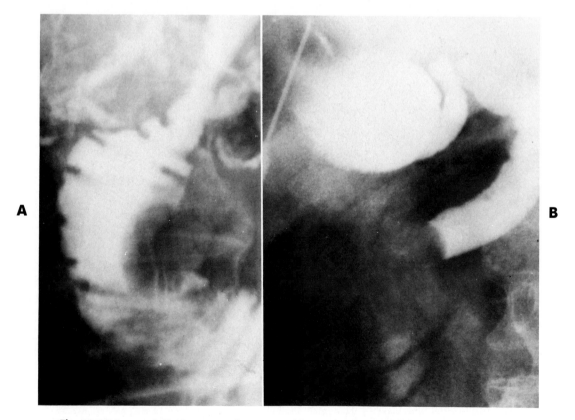

A   B

Fig. 13-23 Impacted distal common duct stone with associated surrounding edema may result in prominent filling defect in descending duodenum on barium examination.

to produce symptoms. However, a cystic duct remnant may be associated with tumors or inflammation, or it may contain stones, in which cases symptoms are more likely to occur.

Fibrosis and *inflammation of Oddi's sphincter* may also give rise to postoperative symptoms. This probably accounts for the majority of cases previously labeled *biliary dyskinesia.*

The initial radiologic imaging procedure for patients with postcholecystectomy symptoms is ultrasonography, with which the caliber of the intrahepatic and extrahepatic bile ducts can be assessed readily. The easiest duct to evaluate is the common hepatic duct above the portal vein. Normally it should measure no more than 4 mm in diameter on ultrasonography. Distention may indicate persistence of preoperative distention, or partial obstruction may be present. If baseline measurements are not available, further investigation, such as

upper GI study, transhepatic cholangiography, or endoscopic retrograde contrast studies may be required (Fig. 13-23).

POSTOPERATIVE EVALUATION OF THE LIVER

Complications are not infrequent after partial *hepatectomy.* Radiologic imaging procedures assist in the diagnosis of subphrenic and subhepatic abscesses, pleural effusion, postoperative bleeding, wound infection, and biliary fistulas. Nuclear medicine HIDA scans are particularly helpful in delineating the anatomy of persistent fistula drainage.

Radiologic techniques are also helpful in evaluating patients with an abnormal course after *liver transplantation.* Biliary obstruction and bile leaks can be detected with direct cholangiography, and stricture at the site of surgical anastomosis in the common bile duct may be

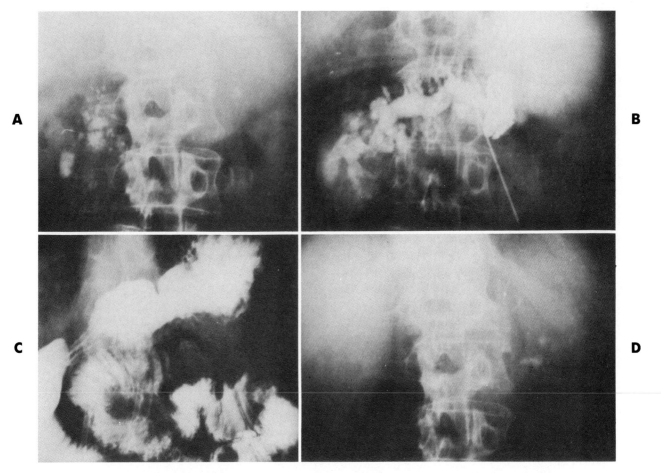

Fig. 13-24 A, Extensive pancreatic calcification in chronic pancreatitis. **B,** Direct pancreatography into dilated duct in same patient. **C,** Puestow's pancreaticojejunostomy was performed. **D,** Radiograph obtained 6 months later shows that most of pancreatic calcification has been passed through anastomosis between pancreatic duct and jejunum.

associated with bile sludge deposition. Cholangiography is also useful in the evaluation of liver abscesses, stones, and problems associated with internal biliary stents. Because the hepatic artery provides the only blood supply to the biliary tree of the liver allograft, posttransplantation arterial occlusion may result in a biliary complication. Patients with transplants who have nonanastomotic contrast leakage or nonanastomotic strictures on cholangiography should be evaluated for occlusion of the hepatic artery as the probable cause.

On CT scans a region of low attenuation around the peripheral portal tracts, the *periportal collar sign,* suggests acute *liver rejection* after liver transplantation. The sign corresponds histopathologically with lymphocytic portal infiltration, but can also be caused by dilated lymphatic vessels as a consequence of total interruption at the time of surgery. Angiography is not advocated as a test for transplant rejection. Hematoma, bilomas, and seromas are best localized by CT scanning.

POSTOPERATIVE EVALUATION OF THE PANCREAS

Pancreatic pseudocysts can be anastomosed to stomach and duodenum, or to the small intestine by a Roux-en-Y drainage procedure. Pancreatic fistulas follow external drainage in 20% to 30% of cases, and endoscopic retrograde cholangiopancreatography is often indicated to evaluate communication with major pancreatic ducts. If caudal pancreaticojejunostomy fails to relieve symptoms in patients with multiple points of ductal obstruction, the Puestow procedure (Fig. 13-24), which involves longitudinal opening of the pancreatic duct and invagination of the pancreas into the Roux-en-Y jejunal loop, may be undertaken. Complications encountered after operation include pancreatic fistula, abscesses, and pneumonia. Percutaneous drainage of pancreatic and peripancreatic fluid collections can be achieved with radiographically guided catheter insertion. This interventional radiographic procedure can help to stabilize patients until surgical intervention is possible.

RECOMMENDED READING

1. Bartow JH, Rao BR: Simplified barium enema examination via colostomy, *Am J Roentgenol* 135:1302, 1980.
2. Becker CD et al: Patterns of recurrence of esophageal carcinoma after transhiatal esophagectomy and gastric interposition, *Am J Roentgenol* 148:273, 1987.
3. Bockus HL: *Gastroenterology,* ed 2, vol 1, Philadelphia, 1963, WB Saunders.
4. Burhenne HJ: Roentgen anatomy and terminology of gastric surgery, *Am J Roentgenol* 91:731, 1964.
5. Chisholm RJ et al: Radiologic dilatation preceding surgical tube placement for esophageal cancer, *Am J Surg* 151:397, 1986.
6. de Lange EE, Shaffer HA Jr: Anastomotic strictures of the upper gastrointestinal tract: results of balloon dilation, *Radiology* 167:45, 1988.
7. Diner WC, Cockrick HH: The continent ileostomy (Kock pouch) roentgenologic features, *Gastrointest Radiol* 4:65, 1979.
8. Fleshman JW et al: The ileal reservoir and ileoanal anastomosis procedure: factors affecting technical and functional outcome, *Dis Colon Rectum* 31:10, 1988.
9. Foley WD et al: Treatment of blunt hepatic injuries: role of CT, *Radiology* 164:635, 1987.
10. Ghahremani GG: Complications of gastrointestinal intubation. In Meyers MA, Ghahremani GG, editors: *Iatrogenic gastrointestinal complications,* New York, 1981, Springer-Verlag.
11. Jolly PC et al: Operative cholangiography. *Ann Surg* 168:551, 1968.
12. Klein J et al: The forgotten surgical foreign body, *Gastrointest Radiol* 13:173, 1988.
13. Kokubo T et al: Retained surgical sponges: CT and US appearance, *Radiology* 165:415, 1987.
14. Letourneau JG et al: Liver allograft transplantation: postoperative CT findings, *Am J Roentgenol* 148:1099, 1987.
15. Meyers MA, Ghahremani GG, editors: *Iatrogenic gastrointestinal complications,* New York, 1981, Springer-Verlag.
16. Mishlin JD et al: Interventional radiologic treatment of complications following gastric bypass surgery for morbid obesity, *Gastrointest Radiol* 13:9, 1988.
17. Nelson JA, Burhenne HJ: Anomalous biliary and pancreatic duct insertion into duodenal diverticula, *Radiology* 120:49, 1976.
18. Payne WS, Ellis FH Jr: Complications of esophageal and diaphragmatic surgery. In Artz CP, Hardy JD, editors: *Management of surgical complications,* ed 3, Philadelphia, 1975, WB Saunders.
19. Schulenburg CA: *Operative cholangiography,* London, 1966, Butterworth.
20. Stammers FA, Williams JA: *Partial gastrectomy: complications and metabolic consequences,* London, 1963, Butterworth.
21. Turner MA et al: Pitfalls in cholangiographic interpretation. *RadioGraphics* 7:1067, 1987.
22. Zaino C, Beneventano TC, editors: *Radiologic examination of the orohypopharynx and esophagus,* New York, 1977, Springer-Verlag.
23. Zajko AB et al: Cholangiography and interventional biliary radiology in adult liver transplantation, *Am J Roentgenol* 144:127, 1985.

14 *Retroperitoneal Space*

RONALD A CASTELLINO
PETER L COOPERBERG
BARBARA E DEMAS
HEDVIG HRICAK
MORTON A MEYERS

RADIOLOGIC ANATOMY AND DIAGNOSIS
    Extraperitoneal compartments
    Ultrasonography
    Computed tomography and magnetic resonance
      imaging
    Lymphography

Radiologic anatomy and diagnosis

MORTON A MEYERS

Disease processes that originate within the alimentary tract may extend and affect extraperitoneal spaces, and abnormalities that arise primarily in extraperitoneal sites may affect the bowel.

The retroperitoneum, an intraabdominal compartment located dorsal to the parietal peritoneum, extends from the diaphragm to the pelvis. Its anterior boundaries consist of the liver, spleen, and luminal gastrointestinal tract in the abdomen, and the bladder in the pelvis. Its posterior boundaries are the spine, ribs, bony pelvis, and erector spinae and quadratus lumborum muscles. The organs normally contained in the retroperitoneal space include the kidneys, adrenal glands, pancreas, great vessels (and adjacent lymph nodes) of the abdomen, and portions of the duodenum and colon.

Basic to an understanding of the pathogenesis of spread of diseases and their radiologic criteria is knowledge of the anatomy of the extraperitoneal fascial planes, compartments, and relationships.

EXTRAPERITONEAL COMPARTMENTS

The retroperitoneal space is bounded anteriorly by the posterior parietal peritoneum and posteriorly by the transversalis fascia and extends from the pelvic brim inferiorly to the diaphragm superiorly. Central to the division of the extraperitoneal region are the conspicuous anterior and posterior layers of renal fascia *(Gerota's fascia)*. These two layers fuse behind the ascending or descending colon to form the single *lateroconal fascia*, which then continues around the flank to blend with the peritoneal reflection. Three distinct extraperitoneal compartments are thus demarcated (Figs. 14-1, 14-2).

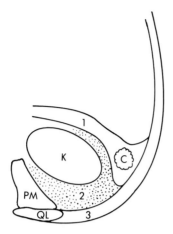

Fig. 14-1 Fascial definitions of three extraperitoneal spaces. Transverse diagram of left flank. *1,* Anterior pararenal space; *2,* perirenal space; *3,* posterior pararenal space. Note their relationships to kidney *(K),* descending colon *(C),* psoas muscle *(PM),* and quadratus lumborum muscle *(QL).*

(Modified from Meyers MA: *Semin Roentgenol* 8:445, 1973.)

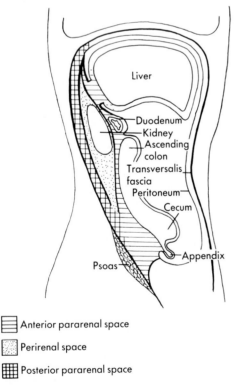

Anterior pararenal space

Perirenal space

Posterior pararenal space

Fig. 14-2 Contents and relationships of three extraperitoneal compartments.

(Modified from Meyers MA: *Semin Roentgenol* 8:445, 1973.)

1. *Anterior pararenal space.* Lying between the posterior parietal peritoneum and anterior renal fascia, this space contains the pancreas and retroperitoneal portions of the alimentary tract. Ventrally the anterior pararenal space is anatomically continuous with the roots of the small bowel mesentery and transverse colon.
2. *Perirenal space.* Lying within the cone of renal fascia, this space contains the kidney and renal vessels, the adrenal gland, the proximal ureter, and a variable amount of fat.
3. *Posterior pararenal space.* Lying between the posterior renal fascia and the transversalis fascia, this space contains no organs; its fat continues laterally as the *properitoneal flank stripe.*

Table 14-1 summarizes the major radiologic criteria of collections localized in each of these three compartments.

Anterior pararenal space

The anterior pararenal compartment is the most common site of extraperitoneal infections. Most arise from primary lesions of the alimentary tract, especially the colon, extraperitoneal appendix, pancreas, and duodenum. Exudates may originate from perforating malignancies, inflammatory conditions, penetrating peptic ulcers, and accidental or iatrogenic trauma. Collections are generally bounded unilaterally on the side of origin.

Perforation of the duodenum

Early recognition of perforation of the duodenum is important. The mortality rate for unrecognized perforation of the duodenum is 65%. In patients who undergo surgery in the first 24 hours after injury, however, the mortality rate is only 1%. Duodenal perforation can be recognized by the characteristic distribution of extraperitoneal gas (Fig. 14-3) with fluid consisting of ex-

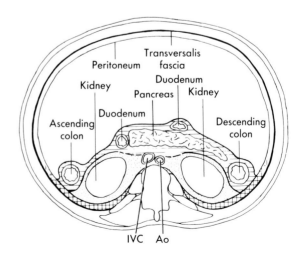

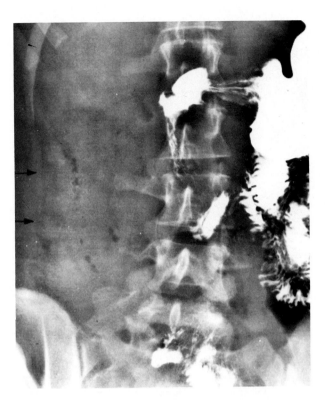

Fig. 14-3 Extraperitoneal perforation of duodenum after blunt trauma. Several gas bubbles associated with fluid soft tissue density are present in right anterior pararenal space. These cause loss of hepatic angle, but flank stripe *(arrows)* is intact. Upper GI series shows medial displacement of the descending duodenum but does not demonstrate site of extravasation.

(From Meyers MA: *Dynamic radiology of the abdomen: normal and pathologic anatomy,* New York, 1976, Springer-Verlag.

travasated bile and pancreatic juices, which is limited to the right anterior pararenal space.

Retroduodenal hematoma

A retroduodenal hematoma resides within the right anterior pararenal space (Fig. 14-4) and almost always displaces the duodenum anteriorly.

Pancreatitis

The extravasated enzymes of pancreatitis, and sequelae such as abscess and pseudocysts, which may become infected, are often confined within the anterior pararenal space (Fig. 14-5). Despite the digestive effects of pancreatic fluid, the renal fascia almost invariably is not transgressed, so that the perirenal fat and kidney retain their integrity. In moderate to severe cases of pancreatitis, retrorenal extension of pancreatic effusion or phlegmon into the potential space between the two laminae of the posterior renal fascia is common (Fig. 14-6).

The mesenteric pathways that are most often involved and that direct the spread of pancreatic enzymes from the anterior pararenal space to remote sites in the intestinal tract are the transverse mesocolon (Fig. 14-7) and the small bowel mesentery. In this way, pancreatic enzymes reach the transverse colon, duodenum, jejunal loops, and ileocecal region. Although involvement of the hepatic flexure, as originally reported by Price when he coined the term *colon cut-off sign,* is rare, the anatomic splenic flexure is the single most common colonic site involved (Fig. 14-8). Splenic flexure involvement is caused by natural drainage from the tail of the pancreas into the phrenicocolic ligament.

☐ **TABLE 14-1**
Radiologic criteria for localizing extraperitoneal fluid and gas collections

Radiologic features	Anterior pararenal space	Perirenal space	Posterior pararenal space
Perirenal fat and renal outline	Preserved	Obliterated	Preserved
Axis of density	Vertical	Vertical (acute) Inferomedial (chronic)	Inferolateral (parallel to psoas margin)
Kidney displacement	Lateral and superior	Anterior, medial, and superior	Anterior, lateral, and superior
Psoas muscle outline	Preserved	Upper half obliterated	Obliterated in lower half or throughout
Flank stripe	Preserved	Preserved	Obliterated
Hepatic and splenic angles	Obliterated	Obliterated	Preserved or obliterated
Displacement of ascending or descending colon	Anterior and lateral	Lateral	Anterior and medial
Displacement of descending duodenum or duodenojejunal junction	Anterior	Anterior	Anterior

From Meyers MA: *Dynamic radiology of the abdomen: normal and pathologic anatomy,* New York, 1982, Springer-Verlag.

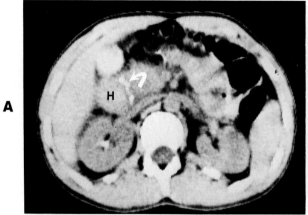

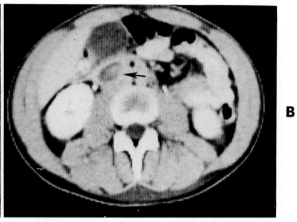

Fig. 14-4 Retroduodenal anterior pararenal hematoma. **A,** CT scan demonstrates prominent hematoma *(H)* within right anterior pararenal space, compressing lateral aspect of contrast-filled descending duodenum *(curved arrow)*. **B,** CT scan 3 weeks later shows partial liquefaction of resolving hematoma *(arrow)* and lateral displacement of proximal right ureter.

(From Love L et al: *Am J Roentgenol* 136:781, 1981. © 1981, American Roentgen Ray Society.)

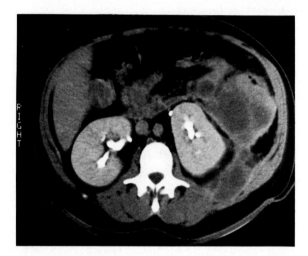

Fig. 14-6 In vivo identification of two layers of posterior renal fascia. **A,** CT demonstrates enlarged left kidney, caused by acute pyelonephritis, abutting posterior renal fascia and presence of double line of posterior renal fascia *(arrows)*. Inner line adjacent to kidney is thickened, and potential space between two leaves of posterior renal fascia is now seen. **B,** Magnetic resonance imaging discretely shows two layers of posterior renal fascia *(arrows)*.

Fig. 14-5 Fluid collection arising from tail of pancreas within left anterior pararenal space continues to widen space between two leaves of posterior renal fascia. Perirenal space is grossly uninvolved.

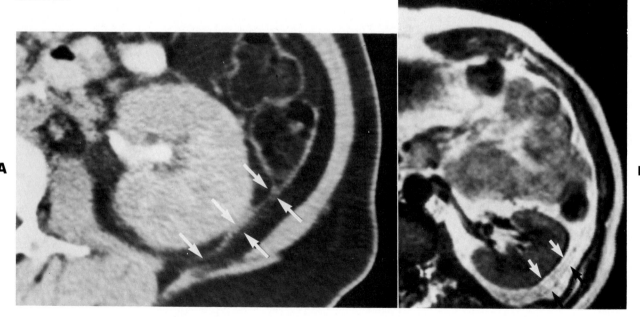

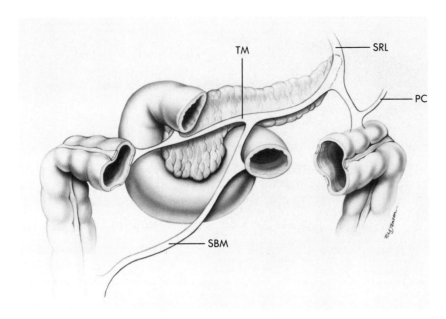

Fig. 14-7 Relationships of pancreas to transverse mesocolon *(TM)* and small bowel mesentery *(SBM)*. Splenorenal *(SRL)* and phrenicocolic *(PCL)* ligaments are shown.

(Modified from Meyers MA, Evans JA: *Am J Roentgenol* 119:151, 1973.)

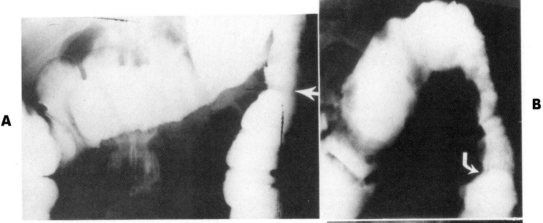

Fig. 14-8 Traumatic pancreatitis. **A,** Flattening of inferior haustral contour of transverse colon is typical evidence of extension from pancreas across anterior pararenal space and through leaves of transverse mesocolon. Pseudosacculations result on uninvolved superior border. Process ends abruptly at level of phrenicocolic ligament at anatomic splenic flexure of colon *(arrows)*. **B,** Spot film documents scalloped narrowing of splenic flexure. Intramural lesions end precisely at level of phrenicocolic ligament *(arrow)*. **C,** Three months later there is marked fibrotic stenosis of splenic flexure, reducing its lumen to diameter of less than 3 mm. Surgical resection of stricture, induced by fat necrosis, was required.

(From Meyers MA, Evans JA: *Am J Roentgenol* 119:151, 1973.)

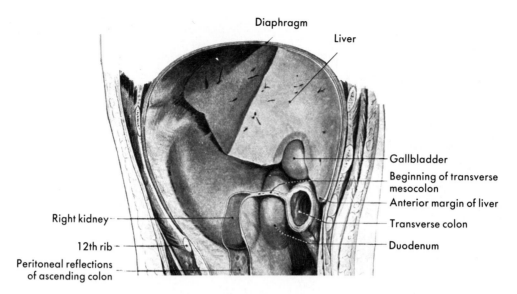

Fig. 14-9 Right parasagittal drawing showing anatomic relationships of right kidney.
(From Meyers MA: *Am J Roentgenol* 123:386, 1975. © 1975, American Roentgenol Ray Society.)

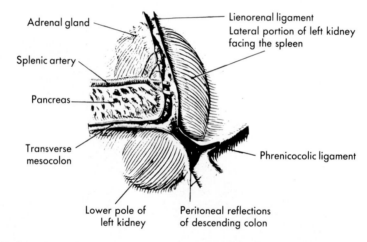

Fig. 14-10 Frontal drawing emphasizing relationship of left kidney to colon by virtue of their peritoneal reflections.
(From Meyers MA: *Am J Roentgenol* 123:386, 1975. © 1975, American Roentgen Ray Society.)

Perirenal space

The *right kidney* is intimately related to two segments of the gastrointestinal tract—the descending duodenum and the hepatic flexure of the colon (Fig. 14-9). The *left kidney* (Fig. 14-10) is intimately related to the distal transverse and proximal descending colon.

Renal masses

Right renal masses typically cause medial and anterior displacement of the descending duodenum, whereas the immediate postbulbar segment tends to be unaffected. The segment of the right colon (Fig. 14-11) most commonly involved is the hepatic flexure, and it usually demonstrates displacement inferiorly, medially, and anteriorly. If the mass originates in the lower pole of the kidney, however, the hepatic flexure is characteristically elevated.

Left renal masses arising in the upper half of the kidney may displace the distal transverse colon inferiorly and anteriorly. Masses projecting from the lower pole displace the descending colon laterally and anteriorly. The anatomic splenic flexure tends to be unaffected.

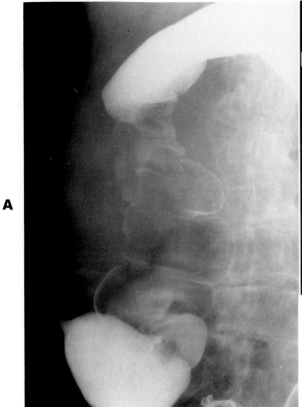

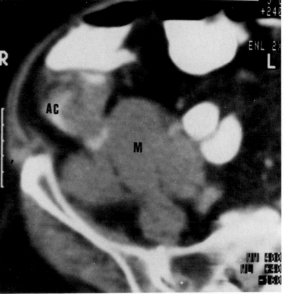

Fig. 14-11 Right hypernephroma invading ascending colon. Barium enema **(A)** and CT scan **(B)** show large lobulated tumor mass *(M)* extending inferiorly from region of right kidney, where it displaces and invades ascending colon *(AC)*.

(Courtesy Dr. Michiel Feldberg, Utrecht, Netherlands.)

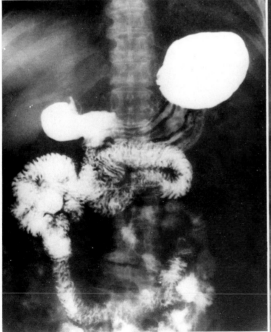

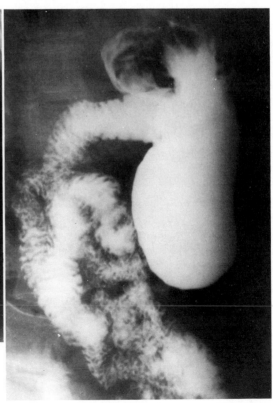

Fig. 14-12 Right renal agenesis with intestinal malposition. Upper GI series demonstrates striking posterior malposition of descending duodenum and proximal jejunal loops in right flank region, simulating some features of right paraduodenal hernia.

(From Meyers MA et al: *Am J Roentgenol* 117:323, 1973. © 1973, American Roentgen Ray Society.)

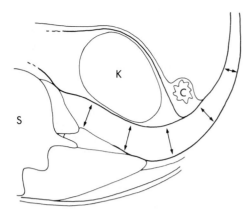

Fig. 14-13 Fluid collection in posterior pararenal space on left, with viscus displacement. There is direct extension into properitoneal fat. *K*, Kidney; *C*, colon; *S*, spine.

(From Meyers MA et al: *Radiology* 104:249, 1972.)

Renal agenesis and ectopia

Agenesis or ectopia of the kidney is frequently accompanied by characteristic malposition of specific portions of the bowel (Fig. 14-12).

Posterior pararenal space

The posterior pararenal space is a common site of spontaneous retroperitoneal hemorrhage in conditions such as bleeding diathesis, overanticoagulation, and hemorrhage from trauma.

Ruptured abdominal aorta or infected graft

Bleeding from a ruptured abdominal aortic aneurysm or infection complicating an aortic graft frequently extend to this compartment. The distinctive complex of findings is evaluated easily (Figs. 14-13, 14-14).

Perforation of the rectum or sigmoid colon

Since the sigmoid colon lies below the limits of the cone of renal fascia and is in anatomic continuity with both the anterior and posterior renal space (Fig. 14-15), gas from a perforation may enter one or both compartments.

ULTRASONOGRAPHY
PETER L COOPERBERG

The ability to produce cross-sectional images with ultrasound and computed tomography has facilitated the demonstration of retroperitoneal anatomy and pathologic conditions.

Abdominal aorta

The abdominal aorta is usually easily visualized by longitudinal scanning just to the left of midline. Real

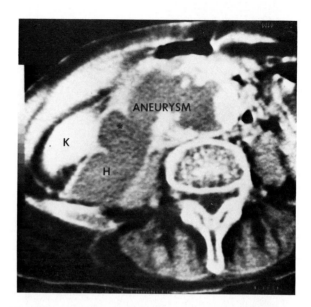

Fig. 14-14 Posterior pararenal hemorrhage from ruptured aneurysm of abdominal aorta. CT demonstrates hemorrhage *(H)* localizing in posterior pararenal space behind kidney *(K)*. Slice level shows precisely the site of leakage *(asterisk)* from large calcified aneurysm.

(Courtesy Dr. Michael Oliphant.)

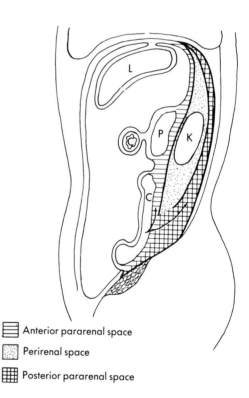

Anterior pararenal space

Perirenal space

Posterior pararenal space

Fig. 14-15 Relationships and structures of three extraperitoneal spaces on left. Sigmoid colon is in continuity with anterior and posterior pararenal compartments. *L*, Liver; *P*, pancreas; *K*, kidney; *C*, colon.

(Modified from Meyers MA: *Semin Roentgenol* 8:445, 1973.)

time transducers make it particularly easy to follow the course of a tortuous aorta. After a longitudinal scan through the long axis of the aorta to its bifurcation, the transducer is angled obliquely to follow the aorta to the common iliac arteries (Figs. 14-16, 14-17). Transverse images of the aorta and iliac arteries are obtained by carefully scanning through the short axis of the vessels.

Normal anatomy

The undulating echo of the anterior border of the lumbar spine is seen deep to the abdominal aorta, and there should be no space or mass between the spine and the abdominal aorta. In most patients the origin of the celiac and superior mesenteric arteries can be seen. Most frequently these arteries arise from the left side of the anterior aspect of the abdominal aorta. Sometimes the superior mesenteric vein is situated anterior to the abdominal aorta rather than toward the right, and it should not be confused with the superior mesenteric artery, which can be traced to its origin from the aorta.

Abnormalities
Abdominal aortic aneurysm

Ultrasonography of the abdominal aorta is the most important clinical factor in detection and measurement of abdominal aortic aneurysms. It is essential to obtain images through the long axis of the aorta to show the longitudinal extent of the aneurysm. In addition to evaluation of size, thrombus within the aneurysm can be detected with ultrasonography (Fig. 14-18). There is generally no difficulty in differentiating periaortic masses from an abdominal aortic aneurysm.

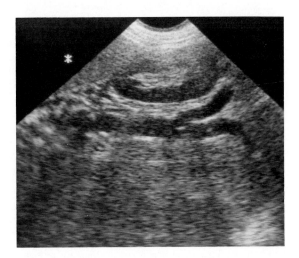

Fig. 14-16 Coronal scan through right lobe of liver and right kidney showing distal abdominal aorta and its bifurcation into common iliac arteries.

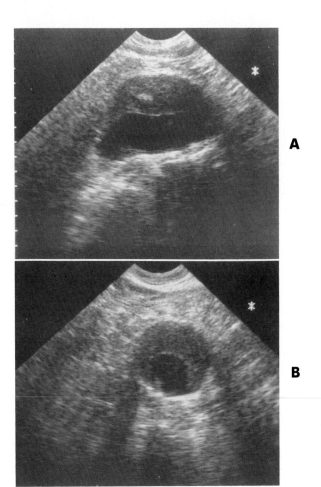

A

B

Fig. 14-18 A, Longitudinal and, **B,** transverse views showing abdominal aortic aneurysm with considerable thrombus in anterior portion.

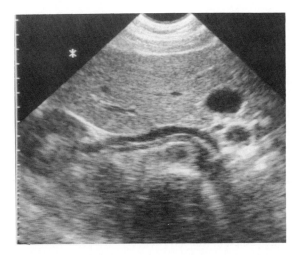

Fig. 14-17 Transverse scan aimed from right anterior axillary line showing right renal artery arising from aorta posterior to right renal vein coursing to IVC. Right kidney can be seen toward left side of image, and gallbladder and portal vein are noted toward right side of image.

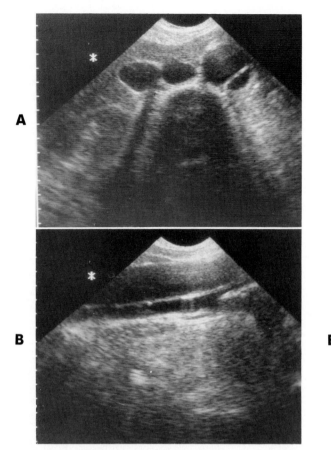

Fig. 14-19 Abdominal aortic dissection. **A,** Transverse scan showing, from right to left, gallbladder, IVC, and abdominal aorta with intimal flap posteriorly and to left. **B,** Longitudinal scan between sagittal and coronal showing intimal flap separating false lumen (toward top of image) from true lumen extending into both right and left iliac arteries (toward right of image).

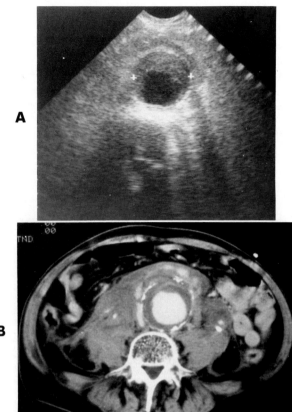

Fig. 14-20 A, Transverse sonogram showing abdominal aortic aneurysm with virtually unappreciated pancake of leaking hematoma. **B,** CT scan at approximately same level showing thin rim of hematoma anteriorly and large collections to both sides.

Aortic dissection

Ultrasonography is also useful in the detection and evaluation of the patient with a dissection involving the abdominal aorta (Fig. 14-19).

Ruptured aortic aneurysm

CT is superior to ultrasound for displaying the site and extent of a retroperitoneal hematoma (Fig. 14-20).

Inferior vena cava

Scanning of the inferior vena cava (IVC) can be performed with the patient in the supine or left lateral decubitus position. Longitudinal scans 2 to 4 cm to the right of midline generally show the long axis of the IVC. Starting at the level of the diaphragm, the IVC is evaluated in longitudinal and transverse views at least to the level of the uncinate process of the pancreas.

Normal anatomy

The IVC is seen at a higher level in the abdomen than is the abdominal aorta, since it enters the liver just after leaving the right atrium. More inferiorly, the caudate lobe of the liver is anterior to the IVC. The right crus of the diaphragm is located medial and posterior to the IVC. The main portal vein in the region of the porta hepatis is intimately related to the anterior aspect of the IVC. Inferior to that level, the common bile duct, in the head of the pancreas, is directly anterior to the IVC. The right renal artery courses obliquely behind (dorsal to) the IVC, and frequently causes a sharp indentation in the posterior wall of the IVC.

Abnormalities
THROMBOSIS

Thrombosis commonly occurs inferiorly, at the level of the renal veins. It is frequently caused by renal cell

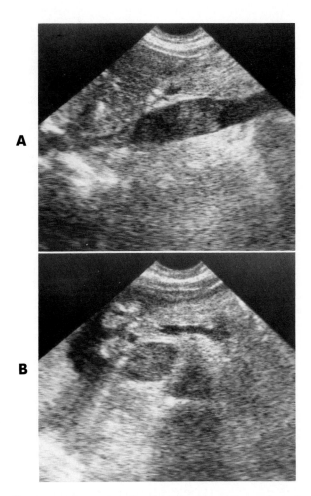

Fig. 14-21 Tumor thrombus in IVC from right renal carcinoma. **A,** Longitudinal and, **B,** transverse scans showing distention of vena cava with tumor thrombus.

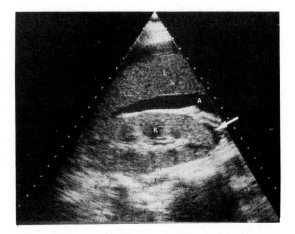

Fig. 14-22 Longitudinal scan showing ascites *(A)* in Morison's pouch separating liver *(L)* from Gerota's fascia around kidney *(K)*. Note small fluid collection in perirenal space *(arrow)*.

carcinomas (Fig. 14-21) that invade the renal vein, and thromboses may extend to the IVC. IVC involvement most commonly arises from large tumors of the right kidney, because of the close proximity to the IVC.

Retroperitoneal masses

Masses that arise in the retroperitoneum can be divided into those that are cystic and those that are solid. *Cystic abnormalities* include *seromas, lymphoceles,* and *urinomas.* Hematomas and abscesses resemble fluid collections (Fig. 14-22) in that they usually have a smooth, deep border and enhance through transmission but always contain some echoes. If there is considerable clot of varying stages within a hematoma, it may appear as an inhomogeneous solid structure. These may all be similar in appearance on ultrasound and cannot be distinguished on the basis of ultrasound alone. However, they can be differentiated from one another with ultrasonographically-guided fine-needle biopsy.

Solid masses are almost always malignant and are usually primary *sarcomas, lymphomas,* or *lymphadenopathy* caused by metastatic involvement of the retrocrural and paraaortic lymph nodes. If the lesion is detected by ultrasound, then fine-needle aspiration biopsy can easily be guided with ultrasonograph. *Retroperitoneal fibrosis* may be similar in ultrasonographic appearance to paraaortic lymph node enlargement.

COMPUTED TOMOGRAPHY AND MAGNETIC RESONANCE IMAGING
HEDVIG HRICAK
BARBARA E DEMAS

The excellent soft tissue–contrast resolution and tomographic image production offered by computed tomography (Fig. 14-23) and magnetic resonance imaging (MRI) have simplified noninvasive evaluation of the retroperitoneal space, advanced our knowledge of retroperitoneal anatomy, facilitated diagnosis of retroperitoneal pathology, guided attempts at therapeutic intervention, and allowed evaluation of therapeutic response.

Computed tomography examination technique

Generous bowel opacification is critical if misdiagnosis of pseudotumors caused by fluid-filled intestinal loops is to be avoided. For routine scanning, intravenous contrast enhancement is of tremendous value. Rapid-sequence scanning with sequential table movement has become increasingly popular in recent years because it can be performed during the intravenous administration of iodinated contrast material by bolus technique. The retroperitoneum is generally examined as a part of a complete abdominal and pelvic CT study, and sequential sections are usually contiguous. When the primary reason for the examination is to search for

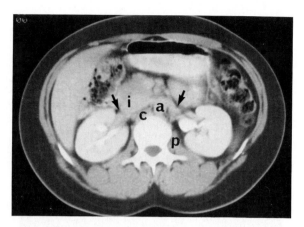

Fig. 14-23 Normal anatomy of retroperitoneum at level of kidneys is demonstrated in this CT image obtained at level of hila during administration of iodinated contrast material. Renal parenchyma is fairly densely enhanced, and contrast material has been excreted into collecting structures. Both left and right renal veins *(arrows)* are clearly delineated as they course medially to enter inferior vena cava *(i)*. Left renal vein crosses midline anterior to aorta *(a)*. Kidneys are surrounded by low-density fat, and intrinsic soft tissue contrast is high. Psoas muscles *(p)* and diaphragmatic crura *(c)* are clearly delineated.

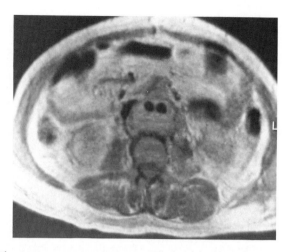

Fig. 14-24 Transverse plane MR image (SE TR is 2000 msec; TE is 30 msec) of aortic prosthesis. Graft limbs are tubular and free of internal signal. Fluid- or thrombus-filled native aorta surrounds prosthetic graft.

retroperitoneal adenopathy, the use of 5 to 10 mm interslice gaps does not greatly degrade information content.

Magnetic resonance imaging examination technique

Clinical examination of the retroperitoneum with MR imaging is undergoing changes as new sequences are developed, some of which are designed to answer specific questions.

Whereas conventional T_1- and T_2-weighted spin echo sequences are still the mainstay of the examination, the sequence is increasingly being replaced by fast T_2-weighted sequences and fat saturation techniques. For increased sensitivity, gadolinium DTPA–enhanced T_1-weighted sequences are often routinely used. Gradient recalled echo approaches are helpful in the study of the vasculature, and MR angiographic techniques are steadily improving. Fast scanning techniques such as turboflash (GRASS) are also improving in spatial resolution, as is the echoplanar approach.

Abdominal aorta
Arteriosclerotic disease

CT scans demonstrate the presence of arteriosclerosis in the aorta and its major branches chiefly by revealing arterial wall calcification and vascular tortuosity. MR images in the presence of arteriosclerosis show in-

creases in the width of the aortic wall, diminution of luminal caliber, and intimal plaques. The plaques themselves are more often visible on MR images than on CT scans.

Aortic aneurysms

CT images demonstrate the external boundaries of the aortic wall and the fusiform or saccular nature of progressive distal aortic dilatation. The distinction of aortic aneurysm from aortic dissection can be accomplished. An aortic dissection produces the appearance of two opacified lumens, with the native lumen deformed in contour with one flat wall. Differential enhancement rates are observed between the true and false lumens. CT scans are more sensitive than arteriograms in the detection of aortic aneurysms, because arteriograms, showing only the patent part of the lumen, may underestimate dilatation. MR, by providing direct imaging of the vasculature in any orthogonal plane, is superior to CT. It also can supply angiography with acceptable spatial resolution.

Prosthetic aortic grafts

When incorporated into the retroperitoneum, prosthetic aortic grafts appear on CT scans as well-defined tubular structures with very high–density walls. Vascular prosthesis infection, which may occur early or late in the postoperative period, is manifested on CT scans as perigraft fluid collections and gas in the surrounding soft tissue. Aortic prosthetic grafts appear on MR images as tubular structures with low intensity walls free of intraluminal signal (Fig. 14-24). MR is generally preferred for detection of graft infection.

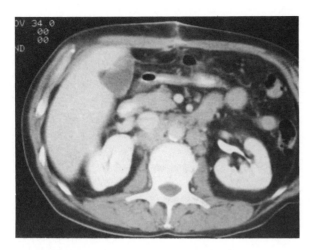

Fig. 14-25 Lobulated soft tissue masses surround the aorta and elevate IVC in this patient with non-Hodgkin's lymphoma involving retroperitoneal lymph nodes.

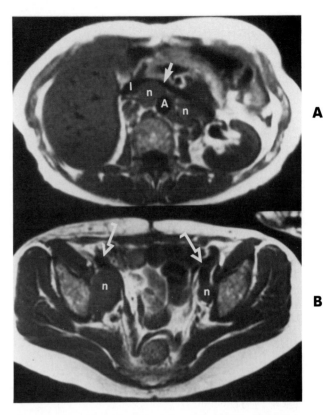

Fig. 14-26 Retroperitoneal and pelvic lymphadenopathy. Transaxial T_1-weighted (550/20) 1.5T MR images at the level of the left renal vein **(A),** and through the pelvis above the acetabulum **(B),** show excellent contrast between the multiple enlarged nodes *(n)* and adjacent vessels and fat. *(A)* aorta, *(I)* inferior vena cava, external iliac vessels *(open arrows),* left renal vein *(arrow).*

Inferior vena cava

On CT and MR scans the IVC appears as a tubular structure in a right paramedian location anterior to the spine. Sites of iliac vessel and renal vein entry are routinely well delineated. The diameter of the IVC varies significantly with inspiration and may be markedly dilated during a Valsalva maneuver.

Venous thrombosis

Thrombosis within the IVC prevents luminal opacification on CT and may partially or totally occlude blood flow. If the IVC lumen is severely compromised, dilated retroperitoneal collateral vessels are apparent. MR imaging shows both tumor thrombus and blood clot as focal sites of intraluminal signal in the IVC. Tumor thrombus may resemble primary tumor in its signal intensity. Advantages of MR imaging in the assessment of venous thrombosis include its multiplanar capability, which facilitates delineation of the cephalad extent of the thrombus, and the fact that exogenous contrast is not necessary.

Lymphatic system

On CT scans lymph nodes are visible as rounded structures of soft tissue attenuation lying in perivascular locations. Nodes are more conspicuous if they are surrounded by fat. Retrocrural lymph nodes are said to be abnormal when they exceed 6 mm in diameter (Fig. 14-25). Abdominal and paraaortic nodes are believed to be enlarged when their diameters are greater than 15 mm. Deep pelvic nodes are considered enlarged if they exceed 12 mm in diameter.

On T_1-weighted MR images lymph nodes appear as rounded structures of medium signal intensity (Fig. 14-26). They are either surrounded by high signal intensity fat or are adjacent to the signal void of retroperitoneal or pelvic vessels. On T_2-weighted images lymph nodes may not be distinguishable from adjacent fat. The contrast between nodes and skeletal muscle is optimal on such scans (Fig. 14-27). Neither MR nor CT can differentiate enlarged hyperplastic from malignant lymph nodes.

Retroperitoneal hemorrhage

CT features of retroperitoneal hematoma include a fairly dense mass lesion that infiltrates retroperitoneal fat, displaces retroperitoneal viscera, enlarges psoas or iliacus muscles, or obscures aortic outlines. Retroperitoneal hematomas initially appear more dense than skeletal muscle, but their CT attenuation decreases, as does their size, during the several-day period of resolution. The MR appearance of hemorrhage in the retroperito-

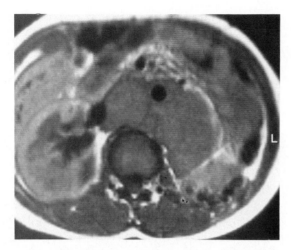

Fig. 14-27 Transverse plane MR image (SE TR is 500 msec; TE is 30 msec) reveals bulky adenopathy surrounding aorta and elevating it from spine. IVC is displaced. Left kidney is absent; patient had undergone radical left nephrectomy for renal cell carcinoma. Adenopathy represents recurrent retroperitoneal tumor.

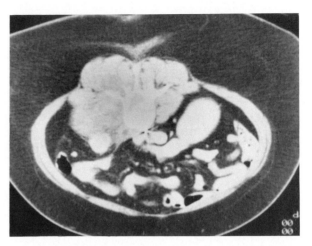

Fig. 14-28 Primary retroperitoneal liposarcoma. Mass of heterogeneous density involves left psoas and quadratus lumborum muscles and invades deep musculature of back. It abuts vertebral body and (at different level) was noted to invade spine. It encases and obstructs left ureter. Although this is most frequently detected of retroperitoneal sarcoma tissue types, one cannot distinguish it on basis of CT criteria from other primary and metastatic soft tissue neoplasms.

neal space varies with TR/TE parameters and with the age of the hematoma.

Retroperitoneal fibrosis

CT images of retroperitoneal fibrosis reveal either a bulky retroperitoneal mass or a plaquelike sheet of tissue that encases the ureters, IVC, and aorta. Fibrotic tissue within the retroperitoneal mass may enhance dramatically during administration of iodinated contrast material. MR is excellent in demonstrating retroperitoneal fibrosis.

Retroperitoneal sarcomas

Poorly differentiated tumors contain little or no visible fatty tissue, and CT scans show a solid mass of soft tissue density. Tumor boundaries are generally indistinct, and invasion of skeletal muscle, retroperitoneal organs, and major vessels is common. Retroperitoneal sarcomas are often greater than 10 cm in diameter at the time of diagnosis, and it is generally impossible to distinguish poorly differentiated or mixed liposarcomas from other types of sarcomas or from metastatic tumors on the basis of radiographic findings (Fig. 14-28). MR imaging provides better delineation of tumor boundaries with skeletal muscle, liver, kidney, and spleen. It demonstrates tumor vascularity and documents major vessel encasement (Fig. 14-29).

Psoas muscles

Psoas abscesses cause enlargement in muscular contour and a decrease in the muscle's density. In the ab-

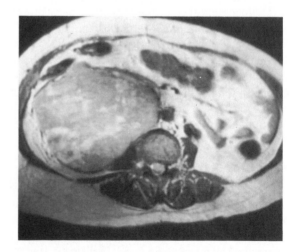

Fig. 14-29 Transverse plane MR image (TR is 2000 msec; TE is 80 msec) of primary retroperitoneal liposarcoma. Large mass lies on right paraspinal location. It emits signal of high but heterogeneous intensity. It displaces and occludes in IVC. Collateral venous drainage from pelvis occurs through dilated gonadal vein.

sence of obvious fluid and air collections, it is not possible to distinguish an abscess from a *phlegmon* within the psoas muscle. A *psoas hematoma* may simulate abscess or tumor.

LYMPHOGRAPHY
RONALD A CASTELLINO

A distinct advantage of lymphography over other imaging techniques such as US, CT, or MRI is that, in addition to demonstrating lymph node size, it displays the internal architecture of the opacified lymph node (Fig. 14-30). This permits detection of lymph node pathologic processes (usually metastasis) prior to nodal enlargement, and consideration of nonmalignant etiologies (usually reactive hyperplasia) in enlarged lymph nodes. Lymphography perhaps finds its most frequent and accepted use in evaluating patients with malignant lymphoma, including Hodgkin's disease.

Technique

With experience, bilateral cannulation of the lymphatics on the dorsum of the feet can be accomplished in almost all patients. Careful attention must be paid to radiographic technique to allow careful assessment of internal architecture. Oblique projections are particularly helpful, since they displace the paraaortic-paracaval lymph nodes from the underlying lumbar spine and open the posteroanterior sweep of iliac lymph nodes for better display.

Indications

In patients with biopsy-proved malignant disease, the lymphogram can provide information on whether the opacified subdiaphragmatic lymph nodes are involved with tumor, and, if so, the anatomic extent of tumor involvement. This information is of obvious value for accurate staging.

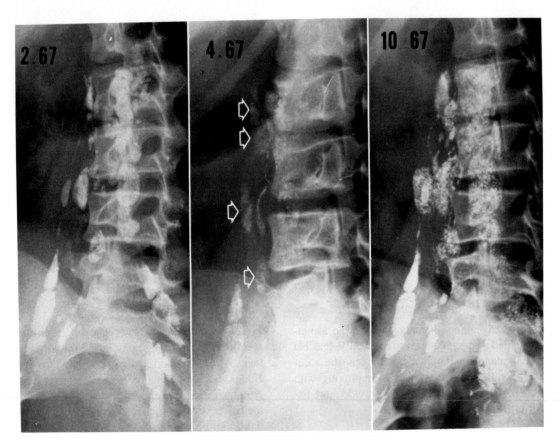

Fig. 14-30 Surveillance abdominal radiographs detecting disease activity. This young girl with non-Hodgkin's lymphoma had staging lymphogram interpreted as being normal. However, surveillance film 2 months later showed interval increase in size of some lymph nodes *(arrows)*, suggesting active disease. Repeat lymphogram performed 6 months later to confirm these findings showed further increase in lymph node size and development of foamy internal architecture, confirming development of disease relapse.
(From Castellino RA et al: *Lymphology* 8:74, 1975.)

barium enema studies are informative. If the entire colon is patent but has an unusually small lumen *(microcolon)*, the obstruction is obviously in the terminal portion of the small bowel. Differential diagnoses include ileal atresia, volvulus, peritoneal bands, meconium ileus, and agangliosis. If the cecum is in an abnormal position, malrotation and volvulus are most likely present. The lumen of the colon is essentially normal in Hirschsprung's disease and in obstruction secondary to volvulus.

Meconium ileus

Meconium ileus deserves special consideration. This is the earliest clinical and radiographic manifestation of *fibrocystic disease*. The absence of air-fluid levels within the small colon and distal small bowel suggests the presence of meconium ileus.

Obstruction of the colon

With obstructions of the colon, distention of the entire small bowel, as well as distention of the colon proximal to the obstruction, is expected. Barium enema studies are of value in confirming this picture.

Meconium plug syndrome

Meconium plug syndrome may be responsible for obstipation during the neonatal period. The majority of cases respond to digital examination or cleansing enemas.

Aganglionosis

Aganglionosis or *Hirschsprung's disease* of the colon may be difficult to diagnose during the neonatal period or early infancy because of insufficient time for *megacolon* to develop. The extent to which the bowel proximal to the aganglionic area is distended with air depends on the severity of the obstruction. In cases of total colonic aganglionosis the small bowel may be markedly distended, far exceeding the diameter of the colon. In the older infant, and sometimes in the neonate, the transition zone between a small rectum and dilated sigmoid can be identified and the diagnosis readily made during fluoroscopy (Fig. 15-7).

Small left colon syndrome

In the small left colon syndrome the barium enema examination shows that the left side of the colon distal to the splenic flexure is small, and that the colon proximal to it is dilated. This condition is probably a variant of the meconium plug syndrome.

Imperforate anus

Imperforate anus and *rectal atresia* are common causes of low alimentary tract obstructions in new-

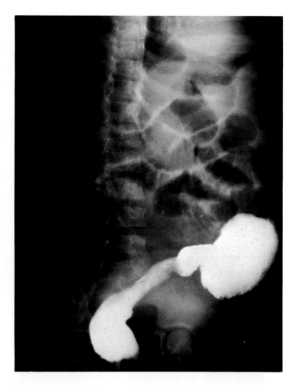

Fig. 15-7 Hirschsprung's disease in 5-year-old child. Rectum is small, and transition zone to dilated sigmoid is identified.

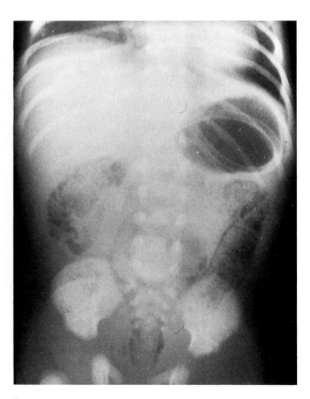

Fig. 15-8 Necrotizing enterocolitis and pneumatosis intestinalis in 1-week-old infant. Gas outlines wall of rectum, sigmoid, and descending portions of colon.

borns. If a perineal fistula is present, the atresia is considered low, (that is, below the levator ani muscle.

MISCELLANEOUS ABNORMALITIES
Necrotizing enterocolitis

Necrotizing enterocolitis is characterized by ischemic changes of the bowel and passage of gas into the ulcerated mucosa producing *pneumatosis cystoides intestinalis,* a pathognomonic finding in necrotizing enterocolitis (Fig. 15-8). If bowel perforation occurs, *pneumoperitoneum* is evident on radiographs.

Duplication of the ileum

The radiologic findings in duplication of the ileum and *Meckel's diverticulum* may be identical, and gastrointestinal bleeding and abdominal pain may be the clinical findings in either case. In duplication, radiographic demonstration is frequently impossible unless barium enters the duplication sac. Meckel's diverticulum occurs on the antimesenteric side of the ileum and duplication is within the mesentery. Technetium nuclide studies provide a more accurate diagnosis because most cases of Meckel's diverticulum and duplications of the ileum contain gastric mucosa (Fig. 15-9).

Hypertrophic pyloric stenosis

Hypertrophic pyloric stenosis is the most common form of acquired alimentary tract obstruction in infants. On ultrasound, which has replaced many of the previously used radiologic examinations, a doughnut configuration is identified in cross-sectional views. If the ultrasound examination is equivocal, radiologic examination is confirmatory. Pathognomonic signs of hypertrophic pyloric stenosis include the *"string sign,"* the *pyloric beak,* and the *"shoulder sign."*

Intussusception

Intussusception offers the radiologist the opportunity for treatment as well as diagnosis. In *hydrostatic or air reduction* of an ileocolic or colocolic intussusception, the advancing column of barium or air should be observed carefully. If an intussusception is present, a convex meniscus defect is observed. With sustained hydrostatic pressure the contrast medium is seen to flow around the intussusception and gradually to displace it proximally.

Inflammatory lesions

Inflammatory lesions of the gastrointestinal tract are rare in infants.

Acute ulcerative colitis

In infants and young children acute ulcerative colitis may be caused by *Shigella, Salmonella,* or other virulent organism. The radiologic examination shows areas of ulceration in the rectosigmoid region and evidence of distinct irritability of the bowel.

Regional enteritis and chronic ulcerative colitis

Radiologic features of regional enteritis, granulomatous colitis, and chronic ulcerative colitis are similar in the adult and pediatric patient.

Ascariasis

The radiologic identification of *Ascaris* species in the bowel is common in many indigent children. *Ascaris* worms may appear as radiolucent filling defects in the bowel.

Acute appendicitis

Acute appendicitis commonly results in rather specific radiographic findings. This is particularly so if per-

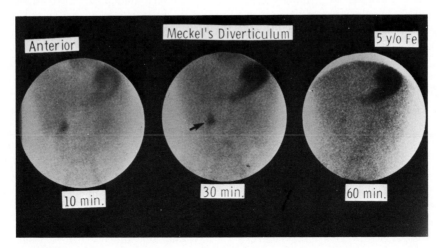

Fig. 15-9 Technetium-99m-pertechnetate nuclide studies demonstrating gastric mucosa in Meckel's diverticulum.

foration of the appendix has occurred. An *appendicolith,* with its characteristic laminated appearance, can commonly be seen. When present, this is pathognomonic evidence of appendicitis. Ultrasound diagnosis of appendicitis is rapidly becoming a popular and accurate method of diagnosis.

Peptic ulcer

A peptic ulcer involving the stomach or duodenum is uncommon in children except in cases of prolonged steroid therapy.

Traumatic lesions

Traumatic lesions of the third portion of the duodenum commonly lead to a *duodenal hematoma* along with distention of the duodenum proximal to the lesion.

Benign polyps

Juvenile polyps of the colon are benign lesions. In most instances the polyp outgrows its blood supply and is passed spontaneously. *Familial polyposis* is a more serious condition in which there is potential malignancy. The *Peutz-Jeghers syndrome* is another form of polyposis involving the small bowel and, on occasion, the stomach and colon. Children with Peutz-Jeghers syndrome show characteristic melanin deposits on their lips as well as on the buccal mucosa.

Neoplasms

Malignant neoplasms of the gastrointestinal tract are extremely rare in infants but become more common during the later years of childhood. Lymphomas of various forms are the most common malignant neoplasms in this age-group.

Malabsorption

There are numerous malabsorption syndromes, and the radiographic findings—coarsening of the mucosal folds of the small bowel along with segmentation and puddling of the barium columns—are similar in all of them.

Chiliaditis syndrome

Chiliaditis syndrome consists of the interposition of the hepatic flexure between the liver and the diaphragm.

Functional constipation

Functional constipation in the young infant is the most common reason for colon examinations in this age-group. Children with functional constipation are well until late infancy or until toilet training begins. In contrast, patients with Hirschsprung's disease have a history of constipation from birth. The child with functional constipation has a very large rectum, and the di-

lated colon is accompanied by marked elongation and redundancy of the rectosigmoid area.

Systemic diseases
J SCOTT DUNBAR

ENDOCRINE DISORDERS
Hypothyroidism

The radiologist asked to perform a barium enema for constipation in an infant should be aware of hypothyroidism as a possible cause. Delayed ossification of the femoral capital epiphyses can be identified in cases of hypothyroidism. The finding of a small rectum and dilatation of the remainder of the colon in a hypothyroid child has been demonstrated to closely mimic the barium enema changes of Hirschsprung's disease.

IMMUNE DISEASES
Acquired immunodeficiency syndrome (AIDS)

The alimentary tract is not as frequently involved in pediatric AIDS as is the respiratory tract, but chronic diarrhea is common. Other gastrointestinal symptoms include oral candidiasis, lymphadenopathy, and parotitis. The most common radiographic manifestation of pediatric gastrointestinal effects of AIDS is lymphadenopathy. Hepatosplenomegaly is second. The aortic, caval, mesenteric, and porta hepatis lymph nodes are typically enlarged, usually forming large, bulky masses. When these are located around mesenteric vessels, pancaking of the celiac axis or superior mesenteric artery may occur, producing the *"sandwich sign,"* seen on ultrasound and/or computed tomography (Fig. 15-10).

Chronic granulomatous disease

Chronic granulomatous disease (CGD) is a syndrome of recurrent bacterial or fungal infections associated with defective microbicidal capacity of phagocytic cells and abnormal oxidative metabolic responses during phagocytosis. About 80% of cases occur in boys, in whom the inheritance is X-linked. In clinical and radiographic terms, hepatosplenomegaly is found in most children with the disease but is nonspecific. Hepatic or perihepatic abscesses have also been found. The organs in which frank infections appear, and reappear, most commonly are the liver, lungs, and bones. The most common, relatively specific, and radiographically identifiable gut lesion in this disease is antral narrowing.

Lymphoid hyperplasia of the gut

Lymphoid follicles may be visible on radiograph in the gut of the normal child. In the terminal ileum, the follicles are aggregated into larger masses *(Peyer's*

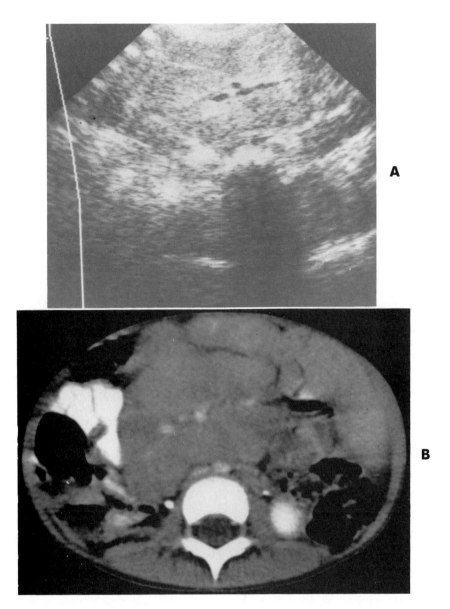

Fig. 15-10 Abdominal ultrasound image of child with AIDS. **A,** Transverse scan shows mesenteric vessels between hyperechoic lymph nodes. **B,** Enhanced CT scan at same level, demonstrating "sandwich sign"—compression of mesenteric vessels between enlarged lymph nodes. Biopsy of nodes revealed Mycobacterium avium intracellulare, and radio findings were confirmed at autopsy.

(From Amodio JB et al: *Roentgenol* 22:66, 1987.)

patches). These masses are easily visualized on standard or compression films. In the normal colon, modular filling defects up to 2 mm in diameter are frequently seen, with or without umbilication. These represent normal lymph follicles. The term *lymphoid hyperplasia* should be reserved for abnormally large follicles. True lymphoid hyperplasia is found in some patients with immune deficiencies.

Pneumatosis intestinalis

Gas may appear in the wall of the bowel, usually the colon, of children with a variety of conditions, most notable of which are immune deficiencies and steroid therapy. There are two conditions in which gas in the gut wall may signal severe or dangerous disease: *typhlitis* and *necrotizing enterocolitis.* The diagnosis is most frequently made by radiographic recognition of gas in the

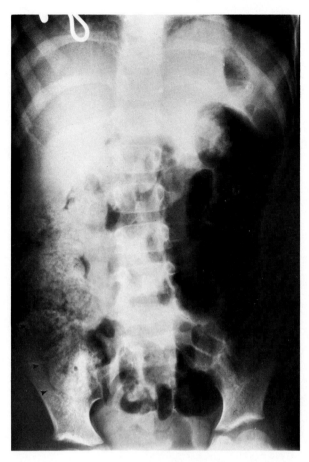

Fig. 15-11 Typhlitis complicating leukemia. Plain film of abdomen shows gas in wall of cecum and proximal ascending colon *(arrowheads)*. This was considered to be characteristic of leukemic typhlitis and to signify poor prognosis. Child died short time after this complication developed.

wall of the cecum, and, variably, the ascending colon (Fig. 15-11), together with the mass effect and inflammatory changes in the involved bowel.

HEMATOLOGIC AND ONCOLOGIC DISEASE
Leukemia

Leukemia may involve any portion of the alimentary tract. Gastrointestinal complications of leukemia should not be considered rare, untreatable, or preterminal. Esophagitis caused by opportunistic organisms is not uncommon in leukemia. Cleansing and diagnostic enemas may be a danger to the leukemia patient because the colonic mucosa is abnormally permeable. Colonic organisms may therefore enter the bloodstream and cause septicemia. If a diagnostic contrast enema is deemed essential, a water-soluble contrast agent should be used.

Lymphoma

Non-Hodgkin's lymphoma, to the degree that it involves the gastrointestinal tract in children, is mostly *Burkitt's lymphoma* (BL), a neoplasm related to African lymphoma, that has distinctive histologic, cytologic, and cytochemical criteria. The tumor consists primarily of large, immature lymphoid cells of B-lymphocyte origin. Enlarging submucosal ileal masses in non-Hodgkin's lymphoma occasionally cause ileocolic intussusception. Gallium-67 scintigraphy is helpful in demonstrating sites of tumor involvement.

Hemophilia and Christmas disease

Hemophilia is a cause of intramural intestinal bleeding. In the duodenum, the resultant intramural mass is sharply marginated and the hematoma may result in intestinal obstruction. Besides in the duodenum, intramural bleeding caused by hemophilia has been demonstrated radiographically in the stomach, jejunum, distal ileum and ileocecal valve area, and the distal descending colon.

Christmas disease (Factor IX deficiency), accounting for about 15% of all hemophiliac patients, causes findings similar to those of hemophilia.

Henoch-Schönlein purpura

Henoch-Schönlein purpura *(nonthrombocytopenic purpura)* is a frequently encountered childhood disorder that is included in the differential diagnosis of spontaneous intramural hemorrhage.

Sickle cell disease

An autosomal recessive gene for homozygous sickle cell disease (SS) is carried by approximately 8% of American blacks, and it is estimated that 1 of 500 black neonates has homozygous sickle cell disease. Plain abdominal films tend to show a small or invisible spleen, presumably because of progressive autoinfarction. Gallstones are present in 17% of sickle cell patients from 10-19 years of age, and routine ultrasound scanning of the biliary tract of sickle cell patients would appear to be justified.

CHROMOSOMAL DISORDERS
Trisomy 21 (Down syndrome)

In patients with Down syndrome there is a high incidence of clinically significant anomalies of the intestine (Fig. 15-12). Duodenal stenosis and duodenal atresia are most frequently encountered. Esophageal atresia and Hirschsprung's disease also have a disproportionately high incidence in patients with trisomy 21. In view of the known association of congenital heart disease with trisomy 21, the heart and lungs of such patients should be examined on chest films.

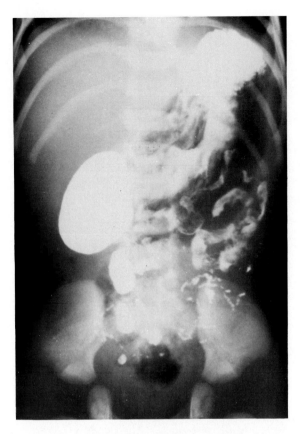

Fig. 15-12 Partial duodenal obstruction is present in this newborn infant with trisomy 21. Pelvis shows widening of iliac wings and horizontally disposed acetabular roofs, characteristic of Down's syndrome.

Turner syndrome (ovarian dysgenesis)

An increased incidence of inflammatory bowel disease has been reported in patients with Turner syndrome. The inflammatory bowel disease may take the form of ulcerative colitis or Crohn's disease.

Disorders associated with pharyngeal and esophageal abnormalities

FAMILIAL DYSAUTONOMIA (RILEY-DAY SYNDROME)

The Riley-Day syndrome (RDS), a familial autosomal recessive disturbance in autonomic and peripheral sensory functions, usually has gastrointestinal manifestations. There is almost always impaired pharyngeal and esophageal coordination, which leads to chronic aspiration of ingested liquid and can be demonstrated by barium swallow. Improper relaxation of the lower esophageal sphincter is also often present.

Epidermolysis bullosa

Epidermolysis bullosa (EB) is a rare hereditary skin disease in which slight trauma disrupts the cohesion between the epidermis and dermis, resulting in the formation of vesicles, bullae, and ulcers. These changes also occur in the esophagus, and may result in esophageal stenosis or webs.

COLLAGEN VASCULAR DISEASES
Scleroderma (progressive systemic sclerosis)

Scleroderma is rare in children, and gut disturbances are less common than in adults with the disease. Loss of haustration in the colon is a characteristic finding, and in pediatric patients dilatation of the duodenum also occurs.

Dermatomyositis

Dermatomyositis is a nonsuppurative inflammation of striated muscle. The pharynx, esophagus, and duodenum are most often shown to be abnormal in function and structure by radiographic studies.

CHILD ABUSE

Battered infants may sustain trauma to many organs, including those of the gastrointestinal tract. Rupture of the liver, pneumoperitoneum, chylous ascites, mesenteric tear, and pancreatic disruption have all been described as being caused by trauma, as has secondary celiac syndrome. One of the most common lesions found is a duodenal or duodenojejunal hematoma (Fig. 15-13). Plain films of the abdomen demonstrate rib fractures. Ultrasound is of great value in demonstrating an abdominal mass.

MISCELLANEOUS DISORDERS
Neurofibromatosis

The protean manifestations of neurofibromatosis occasionally include intraabdominal masses and gastrointestinal abnormalities, but pediatric gut lesions caused by this disease are very uncommon.

Multiple endocrine neoplasia IIB syndrome (mucosal neuroma syndrome)

Multiple endocrine neoplasia (MEN) IIB is now recognized as a clinically characteristic constellation of findings. The radiologist confronted with a child who is suspected of having chronic constipation or Hirschsprung's disease must remember that if the colonic mucosa appears unduly rich, nodular, and redundant, the possibility of MEN IIB syndrome should be considered.

Blue rubber bleb nevus syndrome

Gastrointestinal cutaneous angiomatosis, or the blue rubber nevus syndrome, is uncommon. It consists of

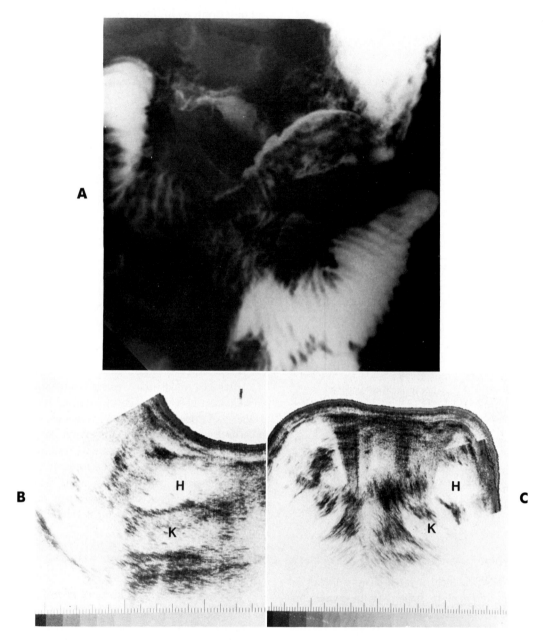

Fig. 15-13 Duodenojejunal hematoma in battered infant. **A,** Barium examination of upper gastrointestinal tract shows long segment of duodenum and proximal jejunum widened, with separation of plicae conniventes, characteristic of duodenojejunal hematoma. **B** and **C,** Ultrasound confirms hematoma *(H)* anterior to left kidney *(K).*

rubbery blue cutaneous nevi and hemangiomatoses, frequently hemorrhagic, in the bowel. The gastrointestinal lesions, which are shown to be polypoid by barium studies, may require surgery.

Pseudomembranous colitis

Pseudomembranous colitis may be caused by recent surgery, debilitation, or broad-spectrum antibiotic therapy. The latter is most likely to occur after administration of clindamycin, with overgrowth of *Clostridium difficile,* which produces a powerful toxin. The radiographic findings on barium enema consist of edema, inflammation, and discrete or confluent plaques. In most cases the child's condition is so grave that radiographic procedures are contraindicated. Endoscopy, with membrane and culture material obtained for laboratory examination, is the procedure of choice.

Familial Mediterranean fever

Familial Mediterranean fever is a form of *amyloidosis*. It is characterized by recurrent episodes of fever and inflammation. Plain films show adynamic ileus of the small gut, and barium examination shows discontinuity of the small bowel column, with dilatation and delayed transit.

Liver and biliary system
RONALD A COHEN
HOOSHANG TAYBI

LIVER

The liver is relatively large in newborns. As the child grows, liver size becomes less prominent. Scintigraphy and sonographic measurements of liver size have shown a high correlation. Plain film evaluation of liver size is difficult, particularly if there is a prominent Riedel's lobe.

Congenital anomalies

Infantile polycystic kidney disease is an autosomal recessive disorder that is most often fatal. Some patients develop hepatic fibrosis and portal hypertension. In others, multiple hepatic cysts have been found at autopsy. In adult-type (autosomal dominant) polycystic disease, hepatic cysts develop in about one third of patients.

Many inherited *metabolic diseases* may affect the liver in children. These include glycogen storage diseases, mucopolysaccharidoses, Gaucher's disease, other storage diseases, cystic fibrosis, Wilson's disease, α_1-antitrypsin deficiency, galactosemia, fructose intolerance, tyrosinemia, and others. Variable degrees of hepatic enlargement or cirrhosis occur with these disorders. Some conditions are associated with development of hepatic tumors, such as glycogen storage disease type I (von Gierke's disease), tyrosinemia, galactosemia, and anabolic steroid therapy.

Acquired diseases

Pyogenic liver abscesses in children often occur when there is a compromise in immune defense mechanisms, as in chronic granulomatous disease or childhood malignancies. The abscesses may be single or multiple. Percutaneous drainage is recommended for large pyogenic abscesses. *Amebic abscesses* are uncommon complications of intestinal amebiasis in children.

Tumors, cysts, and tumorlike lesions

Hepatoblastomas are the most common primary liver tumors in children, followed by hepatocellular carcinoma. Hemangiomas, mesenchymal hamartomas, and infantile hemangioendotheliomas are the most common benign tumors.

Hepatoblastoma, the third most common malignant intraabdominal neoplasm in children less than 3 years of age, most often presents as a single lesion, frequently containing amorphous or punctate calcifications. *Hepatocellular carcinoma*, on the other hand, usually appears in children over 3 years of age, calcifies infrequently, and is often multifocal.

Ultrasonography is generally the first imaging examination in patients with a suspected mass. Simple *hepatic cysts* require no further imaging unless cysts in other organs are suspected. If a solid or complex mass is detected, CT and/or magnetic resonance imaging (MRI) are recommended. Calcification, best detected on CT, is found most often in hepatoblastomas, vascular tumors, metastatic neuroblastoma, and teratomas.

Fatty liver

Fatty liver has been noted in patients with cystic fibrosis, Reye's syndrome, acute starvation, kwashiorkor, malabsorption syndromes, high-dose steroid therapy, glycogen storage disease, exposure to toxins, acute hepatitis, and cholesterol ester storage disease (Fig. 15-14). The radiolucent fatty densities of the liver and properitoneal fat produces a distinct interface with the more radiodense abdominal musculature. Blurring of the medial margin of the right properitoneal fat stripe is probably the earliest plain film radiographic change. On non-contrast CT, the vessels are more dense than the hepatic parenchyma.

Hepatic calcifications

Hepatic calcification in neonates has been reported in cases of intrauterine infections (herpes simplex, cyto-

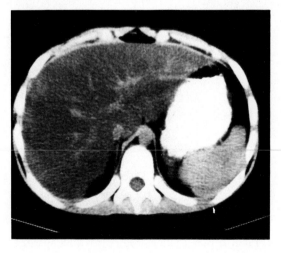

Fig. 15-14 Fatty liver in 10-year-old boy undergoing chemotherapy for leukemia. On noncontrast CT, hepatic parenchyma has lower attenuation than blood vessels.

megalovirus, varicella, and toxoplasmosis), tumors (hemangioendotheliomas, hamartomas, and metastatic neuroblastomas), postumbilical catheterization (parenchymal and intravascular calcification), and ischemic necrosis. Subcapsular calcification in premature and stillborn infants probably represents a manifestation of portal venous thrombosis.

Hepatic calcification in children occurs in cases of chronic granulomatous disease of childhood, tuberculosis, fungal infections, parasitic diseases, cholesterol ester storage disease, intrahepatic lithiasis, amebic and pyogenic abscesses, primary and secondary neoplasms, and after trauma.

Hemosiderosis and hemachromatosis

In children, hemosiderosis and hemachromatosis usually result from multiple blood transfusions. CT may show increased attenuation in the liver. MRI demonstrates decreased signal in the liver from the ferromagnetic effect of excess iron and is more sensitive than CT in detecting early stages of hemosiderosis and hemachromatosis.

Intrahepatic gas

Gas in the liver is in the portal veins, biliary tract, hepatic veins, or hepatic parenchyma. *Portal venous gas* usually results from bowel injury with collection of intramural gas and subsequent passage of gas through mesenteric veins to the portal system. In the newborn this is usually associated with necrotizing enterocolitis or is related to injection of air through an umbilical venous catheter. *Biliary tract gas* is seen in postoperative biliary-enteric anastomosis; duodenal obstruction, such as duodenal atresia; or penetrating duodenal ulcer. Portal venous gas generally extends more peripherally than does biliary gas, which tends to be more central in location.

Liver trauma

Most injuries involve the right lobe of the liver, particularly the posterior segment (Fig. 15-15).

BILIARY SYSTEM
Congenital anomalies
Biliary atresia and neonatal hepatitis

Considerable overlap exists between the clinical picture and the liver biopsy findings in cases of biliary atresia and neonatal hepatitis. Ultrasound is performed to rule out biliary obstruction and to assess the size of the bile ducts and gallbladder. The gallbladder is usually small or nonvisualized in biliary atresia.

Biliary scintigraphy is very important in the differentiation of biliary atresia and neonatal hepatitis. In neonatal hepatitis, hepatic uptake and excretion may be reduced, but the radionuclide should eventually pass into the intestines in all except the most severe cases. In biliary atresia, the radionuclide stays in the liver and existing bile ducts but is not found in the intestines.

Biliary tract stenosis or hypoplasia

Excluding the various forms of biliary atresia, there are other less common obstructive lesions of the bile ducts. These include stenosis, compression by anoma-

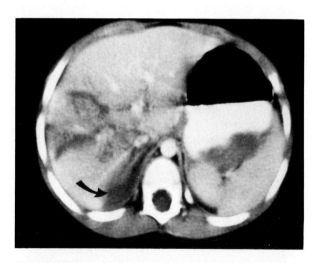

Fig. 15-15 Hepatic injury in 6-year-old boy hit by car. Complex injury is noted in right lobe of liver on this contrast-enhanced CT. Also note associated periadrenal hematoma (arrow).

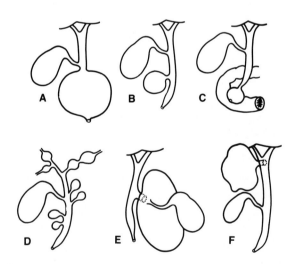

Fig. 15-16 Types of cystic dilatation of bile ducts. **A,** Choledochal cyst. **B,** Diverticulum cyst. **C,** Choledochocele. **D,** Multiple hepatocholedochal cysts. **E,** Cystic duct cyst. **F,** Hepatic duct cyst, diverticulum type.

(Redrawn from Arthur GW, Stewart JO: *Br J Surg* 51:671, 1964; Eisen HB et al: *Radiology* 81:276, 1963; Silberman EL, Glaessner TS: *Radiology* 82:470, 1964; Weinstein C: *Arch Intern Med* 115:339, 1965.)

lous vessels, congenital diaphragm, and stenosis of Vater's ampulla.

Cystic dilatation of bile ducts

There are many types of cystic dilatation of the biliary tract (Fig. 15-16). The most common is globular dilatation of the distal common bile duct *(choledochal cyst)* (Fig. 15-17). The classic triad of abdominal pain, a mass, and jaundice is present in about two thirds of patients with a choledochal cyst. Ultrasound should be the initial imaging technique. Choledochal cysts are generally anechoic masses (some low-level echoes may be present) that are contiguous with the common bile duct and separate from the gallbladder. The entire biliary ductal system should be examined for evidence of duct dilatation or diverticula.

A *choledochocele* is a filling defect in the duodenum. Percutaneous cholangiography or endoscopic retrograde cholangiopancreatography can be used in selected cases.

Caroli's disease

Caroli's disease is characterized by segmental saccular ectasia of the intrahepatic bile ducts. These patients have a marked predisposition to biliary calculi, cholangitis, and liver abscesses. Percutaneous transhepatic cholangiography is an excellent method for the demonstration of the anomalous biliary tract.

Miscellaneous anomalies

The *aberrant gallbladder* location may be intrahepatic, left-sided, transverse, suprahepatic, or retrodisplaced.

Acquired diseases
Cholecystitis

Cholecystitis is relatively rare in children and is often mistaken for either appendicitis or urinary tract infection. Unlike with adults, acalculous inflammation makes up most cases of cholecystitis in infants and children. Ultrasonographic findings are variable. A thickened gallbladder wall (3 mm or greater) is sometimes seen but is not specific. Ascites, hypoproteinemia, congestive failure, hepatitis, and other conditions also cause gallbladder wall thickening (Fig. 15-18).

Cholelithiasis

Cholelithiasis is also relatively uncommon in infancy and childhood. However, an increasing number of cases are being reported in premature infants and other children who receive long-term parenteral nutrition. About 20% of children with gallstones have hemolytic disease. In patients with sickle cell disease, ultrasonographic studies revealed a 27% incidence of gallstones.

Inspissated bile syndrome

Inspissated bile syndrome (or *bile-plug syndrome*) is an uncommon condition seen in young infants with signs and symptoms of biliary obstruction. There is generally an identifiable etiologic factor, such as hemolytic anemia, dehydration, or sepsis.

Rupture

In early infancy a spontaneous rupture may occur on the anterior aspect of the common bile duct or at the junction of the gallbladder and the cystic duct. The cause of the spontaneous rupture in infants and children remains unsettled in most cases.

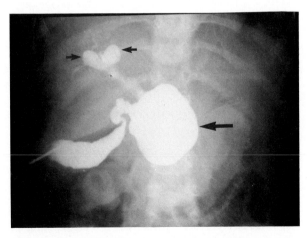

Fig. 15-17 Choledochal cyst in 3½-year-old girl. Operative cholangiogram demonstrates cystic dilatation of common bile duct *(large arrow)* and dilatation of some intrahepatic ducts *(small arrows)*.

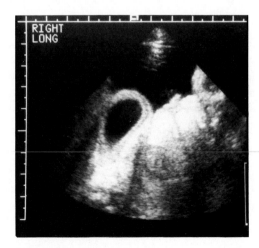

Fig. 15-18 Thick gallbladder wall in 4½-year-old girl with ascites from portal hypertension and cavernous transformation of portal veins.

Tumors

Primary tumors of the gallbladder and bile ducts are rare. Reported cases include rhabdomyosarcoma, hamartoma, carcinoma, cholangiosarcoma, and papilloma.

Sclerosing cholangitis

Sclerosing cholangitis is rare in childhood.

Other causes of duct obstruction

Other acquired causes of obstructive jaundice include pancreatitis, pancreatic pseudocysts, posttraumatic or postsurgical strictures, and parasitic infestations. Biliary ascariasis in children may be associated with abdominal pain, tenderness, vomiting, and/or jaundice.

PANCREAS

Plain radiographs and contrast studies of the alimentary tract can demonstrate localized ileus from inflammation, a mass suggesting a pseudocyst, mucosal thickening, or pancreatic calcifications. Generally, when pancreatic disease is suspected, cross-sectional imaging techniques such as ultrasonography and CT are used. Endoscopic retrograde cholangiopancreatography has been used in children in selected cases to evaluate the pancreatic ducts.

Congenital diseases

Annular pancreas is caused by abnormal rotation of the ventral pancreatic bud, which forms a ring of tissue surrounding the second portion of the duodenum. This malformation sometimes results in symptoms of upper gastrointestinal obstruction.

Ectopic pancreatic tissue (pancreatic rests) is found in various parts of the gastrointestinal tract, particularly in the duodenum, gastric antrum, jejunum, or Meckel's diverticulum.

Pancreatitis and pancreatic injuries

In children acute pancreatitis is more common than chronic forms (Fig. 15-19). The most common cause is blunt abdominal trauma. Pseudocyst formation may occur rapidly after traumatic pancreatitis. Mumps infection is also known to cause pancreatitis.

Tumors

Cysts of the pancreas are uncommon in children, but are occasionally seen in cystic diseases that affect the kidney and liver. *Insulinoma* is a β islet cell tumor that causes hypoglycemia in newborns, infants, and children. The small tumors are sometimes difficult to identify on ultrasound or CT. Arteriography may demonstrate a prominent, persistent vascular blush in the region of the tumor.

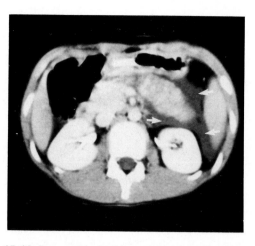

Fig. 15-19 Pancreatitis in 11-year-old girl with abdominal pain. CT scan demonstrates fluid in anterior pararenal space *(arrows)* and mild swelling of pancreatic body and tail. Scans at other levels revealed peritoneal fluid in lesser sac and pelvis.

Other primary pancreatic tumors include adenoma, carcinoma, cystadenocarcinoma, hemangioendothelioma, and sarcomas, including rhabdomyosarcomas. All of these tumors are very rare in childhood.

Imaging techniques in pediatric disease

SONOGRAPHY
HENRIETTA KOTLUS ROSENBERG
BARRY B GOLDBERG

As a nonionizing imaging modality with no known biologic effects, high resolution real-time sonography is ideal for examining infants and children.

Technique

To reduce the amount of gas in the gastrointestinal tract, patients fast before the sonogram. Babies younger than 1 year old are studied at the time they are due for a feeding. Toddlers and older children fast for at least 8 hours before the examination. If the pelvis is to be examined as well as the abdomen, the distended bladder is used as a sonic window.

Esophagus

The proximal and distal ends of the esophagus are the more easily imaged portions of this tubular structure because of the lack of interposed air between the transducer and the esophagus. Since the degree of esophageal reflux cannot be quantified with ultrasound, this problem is better evaluated with radionuclide and bar-

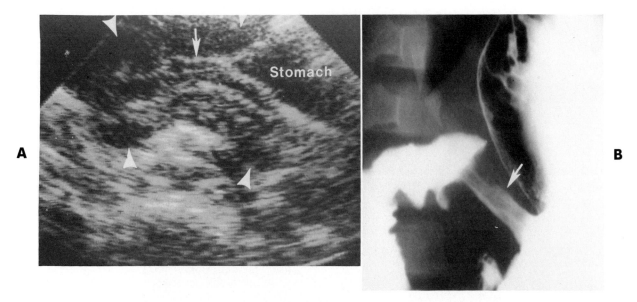

Fig. 15-20 Chronic granulomatous disease of childhood. Two-year-old boy presented with vomiting and known chronic granulomatous disease of childhood. **A,** Water contrast sonography showed narrowing of gastric antrum *(arrows)* caused by significant thickening of antral wall *(arrowheads).* **B,** Upper GI series showing narrowed antrum and pyloric channel *(arrow).*

ium studies. Sonography is quite reliable for the evaluation of masses related to the esophagus, such as esophageal duplications and neurenteric canal cysts. These lesions may be purely cystic, but may contain echogenic material (mucus).

Stomach

The normal gastric wall should be less than 4 mm thick. A diameter greater than 5 mm may be an indication of abnormalities such as gastroenteritis, ulceration, lymphoid hyperplasia, Henoch-Schönlein purpura, Crohn's disease, chronic granulomatous disease of childhood (Fig. 15-20), or ectopic pancreas. Cystic anechoic benign masses include duplication cysts and teratomas. *Gastric duplications* are usually located on the greater curvature in the region of the gastric antrum and account for 4% of gastrointestinal duplications. *Teratomas* are likely to contain calcifications. *Leiomyomas* are solid, hypoechoic masses that may protrude into the gastric lumen.

Pylorus

A previously healthy baby with rapid onset of progressive nonbilious projectile vomiting should be studied with sonography to more specifically evaluate the pyloric channel and muscle for evidence of *hypertrophic pyloric stenosis (HPS)*. This entity is more common in first-born male infants ages 3 to 6 weeks. Nor-

mal pyloric muscle thickness is approximately 2 to 2.5 mm; for the diagnosis of HPS the muscle should measure 4 mm or more. The normal pyloric channel length is less than 1.4 cm, but with HPS the channel is longer, often greater than 1.7 cm (Fig. 15-21). It is imperative that the findings are reproducible and not a transient abnormality, such as may be seen with pylorospasm.

Duodenum

Sonography plays an especially important role in cases of esophageal atresia and *duodenal atresia without a tracheoesophageal fistula* by identifying the fluid-filled portions of the gastrointestinal tract that contain no air for visualization on plain films. In addition, sonography can demonstrate the fluid-filled dilated distal esophageal pouch.

The ultrasound appearance of *hematomas* varies depending on the age of the bleeding. Although hematomas may initially be anechoic, they are more likely to be of mixed echogenicity and gradually become sonolucent following liquefaction.

There are several causes of localized thickening of the duodenal wall in children. *Retroperitoneal hemangiomas* may be associated with *Rendu-Osler-Weber syndrome*. With cavernous transformation of the portal vein, small clustered or discrete grapelike anechoic areas may be identified in the duodenal wall and confirmed with duplex or Doppler. Although rare in chil-

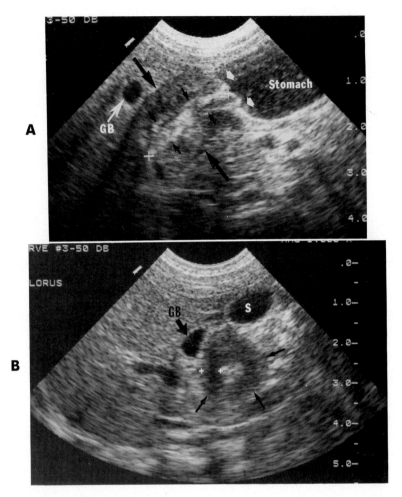

Fig. 15-21 Hypertrophic pyloric stenosis; 5-week-old healthy male infant with sudden onset of nonbilious projectile vomiting. **A,** Long-axis view of pylorus ("cervix sign") demonstrating elongated pyloric channel *(small arrows)* and thickened pyloric muscle *(large arrows).* **S,** Stomach filled with sugar water; *GB,* gall bladder. **B,** Short-axis view of pylorus ("target sign"). Cross-sectional image of hypertrophied pyloric muscle *(arrows). S,* Stomach; *GB,* gallbladder.

dren, anechoic, focal duodenal masses without good through transmission may be seen with *lymphoma.* Another predominantly anechoic mass that may be contiguous with the duodenum or pyloroduodenal region is the *duplication cyst.* Serial sonograms may show that duplication cysts can change in size.

Jejunum and ileum

Sonography plays an important role in evaluation of children with abdominal distention. Elucidation of the underlying cause based on plain film radiography alone may be difficult, whereas sonography rapidly demonstrates ascites, dilatation of the bowel, closed loop obstruction, thickened bowel wall, and underlying masses.

The sonographic criteria for *acute terminal ileitis* and *mesenteric adenitis* are nonvisualization of an inflamed appendix; visualization of mural thickening (4 to 6 mm) of the terminal ileum and cecum with diminished peristalsis; and visualization of multiple, round, enlarged, echolucent mesenteric lymph nodes.

In *necrotizing enterocolitis* the abnormal bowel can be shown to have a thickened hypoechoic rim with a central echogenic focus *(pseudokidney sign* or *target sign),* a nonspecific sign of abnormal bowel infiltrated by blood, pus, edema or tumor. In an infant with necrotizing colitis, however, this picture is diagnostic for gangrene with or without perforation. In addition, bright areas of echogenicity may be demonstrated in the thickened bowel wall because of *pneumatosis intestina-*

lis. Perforation may be suspected in the presence of an extraluminal collection and free intraabdominal fluid. Microbubbles of gas in the portal venous system appear as dramatically mobile, highly echogenic particles in the hepatic parenchyma because of air flowing through the portal venous vasculature.

The diagnosis of *meconium ileus* can be confirmed when ultrasound demonstrates echogenic, thick meconium filling the dilated distal bowel lumen.

The most common gastrointestinal masses in the neonate are *bowel duplications (enteric cysts),* which may appear late in the first decade with symptoms of obstruction. Although they may involve any part of the gastrointestinal tract, they are most frequently encountered on the mesenteric border of the terminal ileum.

Although the most common clinical manifestation of a *Meckel's diverticulum* is gastrointestinal bleeding, it has the potential for small bowel obstruction by causing volvulus or intussusception, or solely because of its

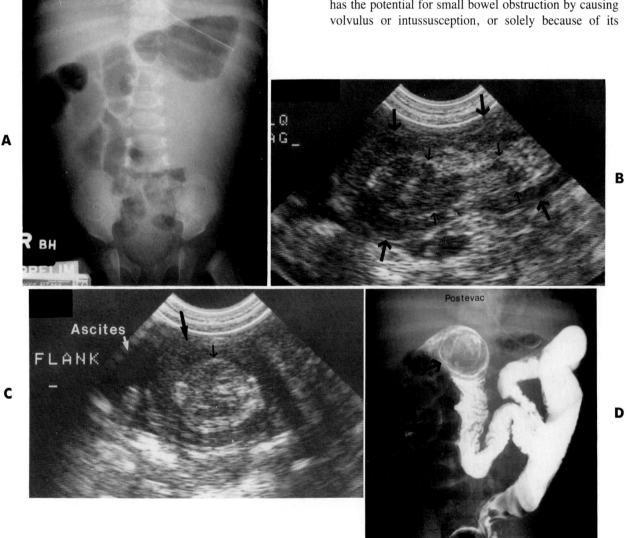

Fig. 15-22 Intussusception; 4-month-old boy with left lower quadrant mass. Plain radiograph showing paucity of gas in left middle and lower abdomen, dilated right-sided bowel loops, bulging flanks, and poor soft tissue landmarks, suggesting ascites. **A,** Kidney, ureter, and bladder film shows paucity of gas in left abdomen with several dilated bowel loops occupying right abdomen and pelvis. Bowel loops are separate, suggesting ascites. **B,** Sagittal scan of left lower quadrant demonstrating "pseudo-kidney" sign due to edematous intussuscepiens *(large arrows)* and edematous intussusceptum *(small arrows).* **C,** Sector scan of left flank showing "double doughnut" sign, indicating bowel wall edema of both the intussusceptum *(small black arrow)* and intussuscepiens *(large black arrow).* **D,** Postevacuation film demonstrating irreducible intussusception *(arrow).*

large size. The cystic nature of the mass and the well-defined muscular wall may be shown by ultrasound. ^{99m}Tc pertechnetate radionuclide scans can be used to detect ectopic gastric mucosa in a Meckel's diverticulum when bleeding is the initial symptom. Sonography can establish the diagnosis of intussusception (Fig. 15-22). The thickened hypoechoic rim represents the edematous wall of the intussusceptum, surrounding the hyperechoic center, because of the interfaces of the compressed mucosa.

Colon

Acute *appendicitis* is the most common cause of emergency surgery in children. High-resolution real-time sonography can be very sensitive for identifying the inflamed appendix, particularly when the graded compression technique is used. The appendix appears as a tubular structure with a blind end. The most central portion is hypoechoic, whereas the inner lining of the appendiceal wall is echogenic and the outer wall is hypoechoic. When the appendix is inflamed, it appears on longitudinal imaging as a sausage-shaped, blind-ending structure with rigid hypoechoic thick walls; it lacks peristalsis; and it does not compress when the examiner gently compresses the abdominal wall with the transducer. On transverse imaging it appears as a target lesion. Ultrasound plays an important role in demonstrating complications of perforated appendix, such as abscess formation and pus accumulation in the pelvis, along the psoas muscle, in Morrison's pouch, and in the subphrenic spaces.

Hypoechoic *thickening of the colonic wall* may be identified in necrotizing enterocolitis, amebiasis, antibiotic-induced pseudomembranous colitis, and Behçet's syndrome. Marked bowel wall thickening is seen with toxic megacolon. Pronounced concentric bowel wall thickening and lumenal narrowing may be seen on sonograph in the presence of adenocarcinoma, whereas lymphomatous infiltration is quite anechoic with asymmetric thickening.

Miscellaneous conditions

Sonography can be useful in evaluating abnormalities of the mesentery. A *congenital mesenteric cyst* or *retroperitoneal lymphangioma* represents a benign neoplasm of the lymphatic system. Because of the thin wall surrounding the cyst, it may mimic ascites.

Cystic teratomas may also arise in the mesentery and omentum and demonstrate peripheral calcification and floating echogenic debris suggesting fat. Other rare mesenteric tumors include benign fibromatosis, neurofibroma, mesenchymoma, lipoma, mesothelioma, and metastatic deposits.

ANGIOGRAPHY

Angiography, or digital subtraction angiography, has a role in the diagnosis of pediatric, as well as adult, disease. The exact vascular anatomy is demonstrated by angiography in children and is often needed before surgical resection of primary liver tumors. Angiography should differentiate benign from malignant tumors in a

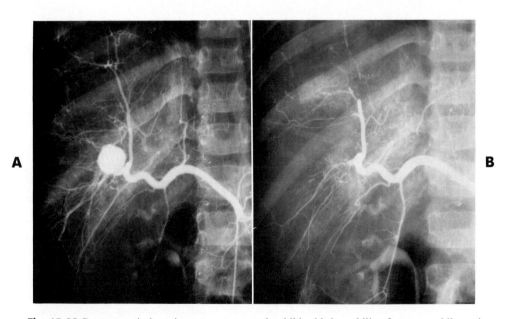

Fig. 15-23 Posttraumatic hepatic artery aneurysm in child with hemobilia after automobile accident. **A,** Before embolization, angiography demonstrates aneurysm. **B,** After embolization, aneurysm is occluded.

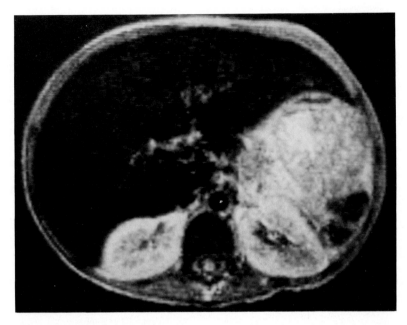

Fig. 15-24 MRI demonstrates hemochromatosis in child resulting from transfusional hemosiderosis. Liver has very low signal intensity because iron deposition (Fe^{+3}) produces long T_1 relaxation time.

high percentage of patients. After the diagnosis of vascular intrahepatic abnormalities, such as tumor or aneurysm, has been established, ablation of the abnormal vessels may be achieved by therapeutic transcatheter embolization (Fig. 15-23).

PERCUTANEOUS FINE-NEEDLE BIOPSY

Percutaneous fine-needle biopsy (PFNB) has received increasing acceptance in recent years. The major indication for PFNB is suspected metastatic disease or diagnosis of primary malignancy when radiation or chemotherapy is planned before surgical resection. No significant morbidity results from this procedure. Some PFNB procedures have been performed on an outpatient basis, yielding considerable cost savings.

MAGNETIC RESONANCE IMAGING

Magnetic resonance imaging (MRI) provides higher contrast resolution than CT, and offers the opportunity to image the abdomen in the coronal and sagittal planes as well as the axial plane. No ionizing radiation is required, and use of intravenous or oral contrast media is not necessary. On T_1-weighted sequences, the liver parenchyma, the common bile duct, and the origin of the celiac axis and superior mesenteric artery, as well as the portal vein, can be evaluated. Generalized liver diseases in children, such as hemochromatosis (Fig. 15-24) or cirrhosis, are well evaluated by MRI. The ability to depict portal venous anatomy with MRI is especially use-

ful in children. MRI can potentially obviate the need for angiography by demonstrating detailed vascular anatomy. MRI also has a role in the diagnosis of intrahepatic lesions such as cysts, abscesses, and tumors. The most common hepatic neoplasms in children are hepatomas, hepatoblastomas, and lymphomas. These lesions usually have low signal intensity on T_1-weighted images. On T_2-weighted images, lymphomas usually show only a slight increase in signal intensity, whereas hepatomas and hepatoblastomas usually demonstrate higher signal intensity.

RECOMMENDED READING

1. Abramson SJ et al: Gastrointestinal manifestations of cystic fibrosis, *Semin Roentgenol* 22:97, 1987.
2. Amman AJ. In Behrman RE et al, editors: *Nelson textbook of pediatrics,* ed 13, Philadelphia, 1987, WB Saunders.
3. Baker DE et al: Postappendectomy fluid collections in children: incidence, nature, and evolution evaluated using US, *Radiology* 161:341, 1986.
4. Ball TI et al: Ultrasound diagnosis of hypertrophic pyloric stenosis: real-time application and the demonstration of a new sonographic sign, *Radiology* 147:499, 1983.
5. Berdon WE, Baker DH: Roentgenographic diagnosis of Hirschsprung's disease in infancy, *Am J Roentgenol* 93:432, 1965.
6. Blumhagen JD, Weinberger E: Pediatric gastrointestinal ultrasonography. In Sanders RC, Hills M, editors: *Ultrasound annual,* New York, 1986, Raven Press.
7. Cammerer RC et al: Clinical spectrum of pseudomembranous colitis, *JAMA* 235:2502, 1976.
8. Diament MJ et al: Interventional radiology in infants and children: clinical and technical aspects, *Radiology* 154:359, 1985.

9. Dodds WJ et al: Gastrointestinal roentgenographic manifestations of hemophilia, *Am J Roentgenol* 110:413, 1970.
10. Dominguez R et al: Pediatric liver transplantation. II. Diagnostic imaging in postoperative management, *Radiology* 157:339, 1985.
11. Franken EA Jr: *Gastrointestinal imaging in pediatrics,* ed 2, New York 1982, Harper & Row.
12. Garel L et al: US in infancy and childhood, *Clin Gastroenterol* 13:161, 1984.
13. Gross RE: *The surgery of infancy and childhood,* Philadelphia, 1953, WB Saunders.
14. Hayden CK, Swischuk LE: The gastrointestinal tract. In Hayden CK, Swischuk LE, editors: *Pediatric ultrasonography,* Baltimore, 1987, Williams & Wilkins.
15. Jeffrey RB et al: Acute appendicitis: high resolution real-time ultrasound findings, *Radiology* 163:11, 1987.
16. Kass DA, et al: ^{31}P Magnetic resonance spectroscopy of mesenteric ischemia, *Magn Reson Med* 4:83, 1987.
17. Kopen PA, McAlister WH: Upper gastrointestinal and ultrasound examinations of gastric antral involvement in chronic granulomatous disease, *Pediatr Radiol* 14:91, 1984.
18. Magid D et al: Computed tomography of the spleen and liver in sickle cell disease, *Am J Roentgenol* 143:245, 1984.
19. McGahan JP et al: Sonography of the normal pediatric gallbladder and biliary tract, *Radiology* 144:873, 1982.
20. Miller JH, Greenspan BS: Integrated imaging of hepatic tumors in childhood. I. Malignant lesions (primary and metastatic), *Radiology* 154:83, 1985.
21. Miller JH, Greenspan BS: Integrated imaging of hepatic tumors in childhood. II. Benign lesions (congenital, reparative, and inflammatory), *Radiology* 154:91, 1985.
22. Miller JH, Kemberling CR: Ultrasound scanning of the gastrointestinal tract in children: subject review, *Radiology* 152:671, 1984.
23. Miller JH, Kemberling CR: Ultrasound of the pediatric gastrointestinal tract, *Semin Ultrasound* 8:349, 1987.
24. Patriquin H et al: Surgical portosystemic shunts in children: assessment with Duplex Doppler US, *Radiology* 165:25, 1987.
25. Siegel MJ et al: Normal and abnormal pancreas in children: US studies, *Radiology* 165:15, 1987.
26. Silverman FN: *Caffey's pediatric x-ray diagnosis,* ed 8, Chicago, 1985, Mosby–Year Book.
27. Singleton EB: Radiologic evaluation of intestinal obstruction in the newborn, *Radiol Clin North Am* 1:571, 1963.
28. Singleton EB et al: *Radiology of the alimentary tract in infants and children,* Philadelphia, 1977, WB Saunders.
29. Stunden RJ et al: The improved ultrasound diagnosis of hypertrophic pyloric stenosis, *Pediatr Radiol* 16:200, 1986.
30. Weinreb JC et al: Imaging the pediatric liver: MRI and CT, *Am J Roentgenol* 147:785, 1986.

16 *Special Procedures*

PATRICK C FREENY
FREDERICK S KELLER
JOSEF RÖSCH

ANGIOGRAPHY OF THE ALIMENTARY TRACT
　Techniques
　Complications
　Acute gastrointestinal hemorrhage
　Chronic gastrointestinal hemorrhage
　Vascular diseases of the gastrointestinal tract
　Alimentary tract tumors
　Pancreatic angiography
　Hepatic angiography
　Splenic angiography

VENOGRAPHY
　Portal venography
　Liver
　Pancreas and spleen
　Small bowel and duodenum

Angiography of the alimentary tract

FREDERICK S KELLER
JOSEF RÖSCH

Visceral angiography is requested to localize and treat bleeding, to palliate tumors, to delineate vascular lesions, and to precisely demonstrate arterial anatomy before contemplated surgery.

TECHNIQUES

The basic technique in arteriography of the alimentary tract is *selective* catheterization and injection into the primary visceral branches of the aorta—the celiac, superior mesenteric, and inferior mesenteric arteries. When detailed evaluation of specific vascular beds is required, *superselective* studies, with advancement of the catheter into secondary to tertiary branches of the visceral arteries, are necessary (Fig. 16-1). Pharmacologic vasoactive drugs, both arterial dilators and constrictors, can be injected through the angiographic catheter immediately before injection of contrast material, either increasing or decreasing blood flow to the vascular bed under study.

COMPLICATIONS

In experienced hands, the complication rate of visceral angiography should be less than 0.5%. Potential complications include hematoma, vascular spasm, occlusion, pseudoaneurysm, arteriovenous fistula, embolism, and subintimal dissection. The radiologist must be prepared to treat vasovagal episodes, which are a common occurrence, as well as serious, life-threatening contrast reactions, which are unusual with intraarterial contrast administration.

ACUTE GASTROINTESTINAL HEMORRHAGE

The endoscope is now the primary diagnostic modality for *upper gastrointestinal bleeding,* and if varices

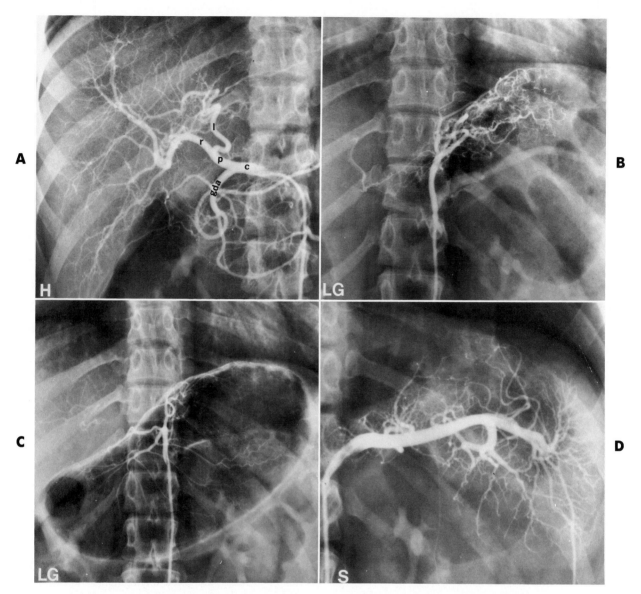

Fig. 16-1 Superselective angiograms of celiac artery branches. **A,** Normal common hepatic arteriogram. Catheter is in common hepatic artery *(c)*. Proper hepatic *(p)*, right hepatic *(r)*, left hepatic *(l)*, and gastroduodenal *(gda)* arteries are demonstrated. **B,** Normal left gastric angiogram. **C,** Left gastric angiogram following gastric insufflation. **D,** Normal splenic angiogram.

are found, sclerotherapy can be initiated. Arteriography is required only if medical therapy is unsuccessful in controlling hemorrhage. Endoscopy is less effective in diagnosis of lesions responsible for acute *lower gastrointestinal hemorrhage*, especially during an episode of active bleeding, and angiography is performed to localize, as well as treat, the bleeding lesion. The angiographic diagnosis of *acute arterial bleeding* rests on the visualization of direct extravasation of contrast material into the gastrointestinal lumen (Fig. 16-2).

Angiographic control of acute gastrointestinal hemorrhage

Precise localization of the bleeding artery is the first step in catheter therapy of acute gastrointestinal hemorrhage. In patients with gastric hemorrhage, supply to the bleeding lesion is from the left gastric artery in 85% of cases. Duodenal bleeding may be supplied by either the gastroduodenal or inferior pancreaticoduodenal artery or a combination of the two. Small bowel and colonic hemorrhage originate from the various branches of

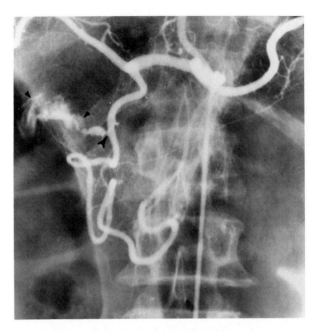

Fig. 16-2 Acute gastrointestinal bleeding from peptic ulcer. The ulcer has eroded into gastroduodenal artery *(large arrowhead)* causing extravasation of contrast material into lumen of duodenum *(small arrowheads).*

the superior and inferior mesenteric arteries that supply the area of the bleeding lesion. Distal rectal or anal bleeding may have a dual supply: superior hemorrhoidal branches of the inferior mesenteric artery and/or middle hemorrhoidal branches of the internal iliac arteries.

Vasoconstrictive infusion therapy

Vasopressin is most important for its use in controlling gastrointestinal bleeding. The mechanism for control of bleeding is vasopressin-induced smooth muscle contraction in the walls of arterioles, which causes vasoconstriction. Vasopressin infusion is frequently successful in controlling bleeding from superficial gastric lesions such as Mallory-Weiss tears, hemorrhagic gastritis, and stress ulcers. Diverticula and angiodysplasias, the lesions most commonly responsible for massive acute colonic hemorrhage, are both quite responsive to vasopressin infusion, and surgery can often be avoided (Fig. 16-3). Vasoconstrictive infusion therapy is substantially less effective in controlling hemorrhage from the duodenum than from the stomach, small bowel, or colon.

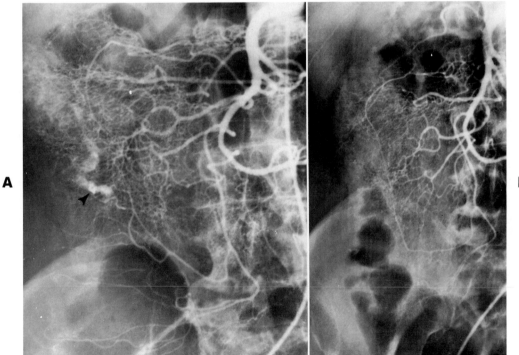

Fig. 16-3 Bleeding diverticulum of ascending colon controlled with vasopressin infusion. **A,** Active hemorrhage is present on initial arteriogram *(arrowhead).* **B,** Following infusion of 0.3 units of vasopressin for 20 minutes, no hemorrhage is evident. Branches of superior mesenteric artery are constricted.

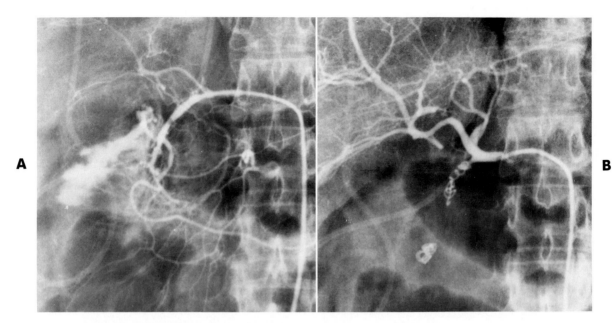

Fig. 16-4 Control of acute hemorrhage from duodenal ulcer. **A,** Marked extravasation caused by massive bleeding is present on initial gastroduodenal arteriogram. Patient is in hypovolemic shock as evidenced by intense vasoconstriction of common hepatic artery. **B,** Follow-up arteriogram after placement of coilspring occluders both distal and proximal to the peptic erosion of gastroduodenal artery reveals control of hemorrhage. Bleeding had ceased, and caliber of hepatic artery is now normal.

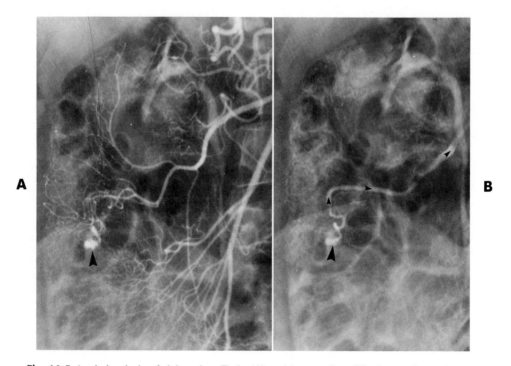

Fig. 16-5 Angiodysplasia of right colon. Early **(A)** and intermediate **(B)** phases of superior mesenteric arteriogram reveal vascular tuft *(large arrowhead)* of angiodysplasia. Prominent and intense venous drainage *(small arrowheads)* is present from angiodysplasia, while remainder of colon is still in late arterial phase of angiogram.

Embolotherapy

Embolization without an initial trial of vasoconstrictive therapy is now preferred by many radiologists. The goal of embolotherapy is to decrease the blood pressure at the site of the bleeding lesion and to allow a stable clot to form without causing tissue ischemia or necrosis. Embolic materials vary, but *surgical gelatin* or *Gelfoam*, a temporary vasoocclusive agent, is widely used. Recanalization usually occurs in 1 to 3 weeks. Cut into small pieces and mixed with contrast medium, the Gelfoam is slowly injected under fluoroscopic control. Permanent embolic materials are usually reserved for hemorrhage from invasion of the gastrointestinal tract by primary or secondary malignancies. When peptic erosion has caused large defects in the gastroduodenal artery, small particles of Gelfoam are frequently ineffective, because they pass directly through the hole in the artery into the duodenal lumen. When this occurs, placement of *coil springs* distal and proximal to the arterial defect or sealing it with *cyanoacrylate* often can be successful in stopping the hemorrhage (Fig. 16-4).

CHRONIC GASTROINTESTINAL HEMORRHAGE
Angiodysplasia

Known variously as *telangiectasias, vascular ectasias, angiodysplasias,* and *arteriovenous malformations,* these lesions are commonly responsible for lower gastrointestinal bleeding, especially in the elderly. They are seen more frequently in patients with aortic and mitral valvular disease or with hereditary hemorrhagic telangiectasia. Angiodysplasias are clusters of ectatic submucosal vascular spaces. Precise preoperative localization of angiodysplasias is required, because these lesions can neither be seen or palpated at surgery (Fig. 16-5). Although acute bleeding episodes can almost always be controlled with vasopressin infusion, rebleeding usually occurs, and surgical resection is the primary form of therapy for angiodysplasias causing recurrent gastrointestinal bleeding.

Meckel's diverticulum

Meckel's diverticulum is a common cause of both acute and chronic lower gastrointestinal bleeding in

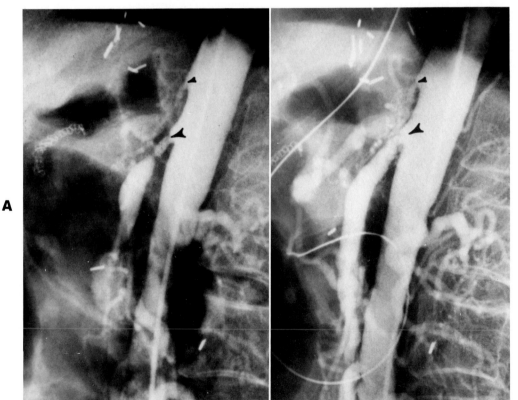

Fig. 16-6 Abdominal angina treated by transluminal angioplasty. **A,** Control lateral aortography demonstrated occlusion of celiac artery *(small arrowhead,* also in **B**) with very tight stenosis of superior mesenteric artery *(large arrowhead).* **B,** Following percutaneous transluminal angioplasty, stenosis of superior mesenteric artery is considerably reduced *(large arrowhead).*

young patients. Because ectopic gastric mucosa is found in many Meckel's diverticula, patients frequently present with melena, even though the lesion is located in the distal ileum. Arteriography performed during an episode of acute hemorrhage from Meckel's diverticulum demonstrates extravasation of contrast material.

VASCULAR DISEASES OF THE GASTROINTESTINAL TRACT
Atherosclerosis

Stenoses or occlusions of individual visceral arteries can result from atherosclerotic plaque developing in the artery itself, by aortic plaque encroaching on the arterial ostia, or from involvement of the arterial origins by an abdominal aortic aneurysm. Because of excellent collateral circulation, occlusion of any single visceral vessel is not likely to cause ischemia as long as the others remain free from obstruction.

Abdominal angina

The syndrome of abdominal angina is characterized by abdominal pain after eating that is often relieved by nitroglycerine. It is characterized by weight loss, anorexia, diarrhea, and occasionally by nausea and vomiting. It occurs when increased postprandial visceral blood flow requirements cannot be met because of fixed obstructions (light stenoses or occlusions) of two or more visceral arteries. On occasion it can signal imminent bowel infarction. Treatment for abdominal angina has traditionally been surgical endarterectomy of the celiac or superior mesenteric arteries or bypass to the superior mesenteric and occasionally to the hepatic arteries. Recently, however, transluminal angioplasty of stenotic visceral branches has been successfully used to treat patients with abdominal angina (Fig. 16-6).

Visceral embolism

Most acute emboli to the visceral circulation originate from cardiac sources, either mural thrombi or diseased prosthetic valves. Angiographic findings of emboli include an abrupt cutoff of the column of contrast material or a filling defect in the lumen of the artery with contrast streaming around it (Fig. 16-7).

Aneurysms

Dissections of the aorta that originate in the aortic arch and extend distally to involve the distal aorta may occlude visceral artery origins.

Arteritis

Involvement of the gastrointestinal tract arteries by autoimmune vasculitis is usually part of a generalized systemic process. In *polyarteritis nodosa,* aneurysms are seen in medium-sized and small arterial branches. Arterial occlusions may result from the inflammatory component of the arteritis, causing ischemia or even infarction of the involved organs.

Unlike the small and medium-sized arterial changes seen in polyarteritis nodosa, *Takayasu's arteritis* affects major aortic branches, usually at or close to their ori-

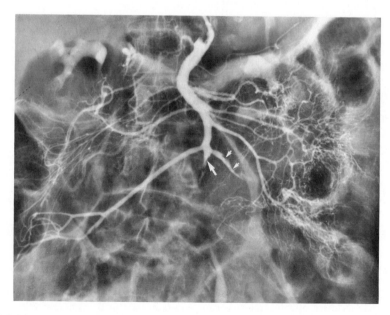

Fig. 16-7 Mesenteric embolus. There is abrupt occlusion of ileocolic branch of superior mesenteric artery *(large arrow).* Occlusion of large ileal branch is also present *(small arrows).*

gin. Known as *"pulseless disease,"* it was originally thought to be limited to aortic arch branches, but it is now evident that the abdominal aorta and its major branches may also be affected.

ALIMENTARY TRACT TUMORS
Angiographic characteristics of gastrointestinal neoplasia

Both benign and malignant gastrointestinal neoplasms demonstrate characteristic changes in the angiographic appearance of the involved arteries and veins. These angiographic changes include vascular invasion or encasement, vascular displacement, neovascularity or formation of new tumor vessels, and increased accumulation of contrast material within the tumor (tumor blush).

Vascular encasement is a reliable sign of malignant neoplasia. Encasement of vessels results from the scirrhous nature of many gastrointestinal tumors and their ability to evoke a desmoplastic reaction in the tissues they invade (Fig. 16-8).

Angiogenesis, or new vessel formation, is characteristic of many nonscirrhous malignant and sometimes benign tumors.

Tumor blush is usually seen with vascular neoplasms and occasionally with infiltrating, scirrhous tumors. Tumor blush is not a specific finding for neoplasm, because it is frequently present in inflammatory processes as well.

PANCREATIC ANGIOGRAPHY

With the introduction of and rapid technological improvement in noninvasive imaging, predominantly ultrasound and computed tomography (CT), the role of pancreatic angiography has changed considerably. Once used as a primary method of screening patients with suspected pancreatic disease, pancreatic arteriography is now reserved for cases in which the results of noninvasive imaging studies and percutaneous needle biopsy are inconclusive or negative despite clinical evidence of pancreatic disease, especially pancreatic carcinoma (Fig. 16-9).

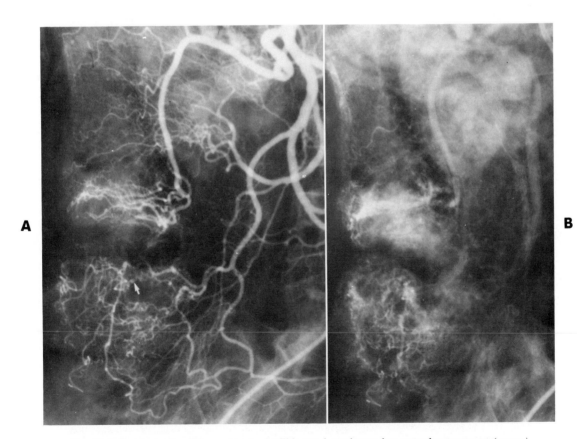

Fig. 16-8 Encasement and tumor blush. **A,** This cecal carcinoma has caused encasement *(arrow)* of individual branches of ileocolic artery. **B,** Late phase shows increased accumulation of contrast material within tumor *(tumor blush)* and prominent draining vein.

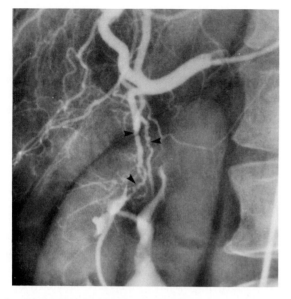

Fig. 16-9 Small unresectable pancreatic carcinoma. Encasement of gastroduodenal artery and superior pancreatico-duodenal artery *(arrowheads)* is present. Encasement of gastroduodenal artery indicates tumor extension beyond confines of pancreas. This lesion was unresectable.

Islet cell tumors

Most islet cell tumors have a typical arteriographic appearance regardless of their cell type or hormonal activity. They are usually hypervascular, well-circumscribed lesions that opacify early in the arterial phase, blush densely, and stay opacified into the venous phase (Fig. 16-10).

HEPATIC ANGIOGRAPHY

Angiographic demonstration of the entire liver can be achieved by common hepatic arteriography in approximately 60% of patients. In the remainder, variations in hepatic arterial anatomy require injections of the left gastric artery, which supplies all or part of the left hepatic lobe in about 20% of cases, and/or the right hepatic artery, whose origin is partially or completely replaced to the superior mesenteric artery in approximately 25% of cases.

Cirrhosis

The angiographic findings in cirrhotic patients vary with the stage of the disease and the degree of hepatic atrophy (Fig. 16-11). Usually the liver is hypervascular, with enlargement and occasionally with tortuosity of the hepatic artery.

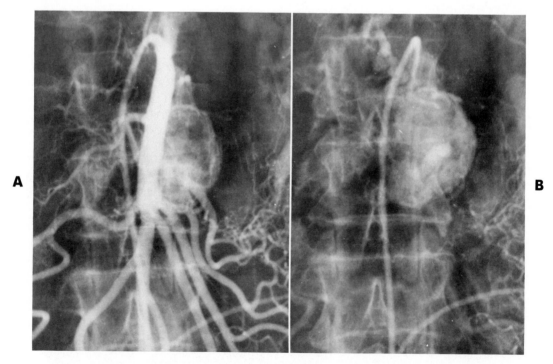

Fig. 16-10 Large islet cell adenoma. Superior mesenteric arteriography shows islet cell adenoma, 3 cm in diameter, in uncinate process of pancreas. It is hypervascular, with blush that starts in early arterial phase **(A)** and persists into late venous phase **(B).**

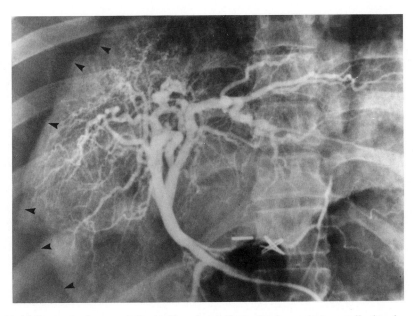

Fig. 16-11 Severe, end-stage cirrhosis. Hepatic arteriography demonstrates small, shrunken, atrophic liver with marked tortuousity and "corkscrewing" of intrahepatic arteries. Liver edge is nodular *(arrowheads)* and separated from lateral abdominal wall by large amount of ascitic fluid.

Hepatic neoplasms
Cavernous hemangioma

The angiographic characteristics of cavernous hemangioma, the most common benign hepatic tumor, are very distinctive. The feeding arteries are normal in caliber. Groups of irregular dilated spaces inside the hemangioma begin to fill with contrast material during the middle arterial phase of the angiogram. Contrast material is retained undiluted in these spaces and persists there, appearing like "cotton wool," late into the venous phase.

Hepatocellular carcinoma

Arteriography is very useful in determining the resectability of hepatocellular carcinoma and should be performed on all patients before the contemplated resection. Because the tumor is usually hypervascular, small satellite lesions are frequently detected by angiography in a lobe or segment that was previously found to be tumor free by CT and ultrasound.

Cholangiocarcinoma

Cholangiocarcinoma, or *primary bile duct carcinoma,* is scirrhous and infiltrating in nature. Generally less vascular than hepatoma, primary bile duct carcinomas usually encase rather than displace hepatic artery branches. Because cholangiocarcinoma grows by infiltration rather than by creating a mass effect, CT and ultrasound are usually not very sensitive in determining its extent (Fig. 16-12).

Hepatic metastases

Hypervascular metastases are very noticeable against the relatively homogeneous background of liver parenchyma during the capillary phase of the angiogram and can thus be detected when quite small. In contrast, hypovascular metastases are more difficult to diagnose by conventional angiography.

Hepatic trauma

Though rarely indicated for initial evaluation of patients with liver trauma, angiography is useful whenever vascular complications are suspected or hemorrhage persists following hepatic injury. With liver contusion the arteriogram reveals stretching and straightening of intrahepatic arterial branches with slow flow through them. If active bleeding is present in the contused area, extravasation of contrast material is visualized.

SPLENIC ANGIOGRAPHY
Splenic trauma

Of all intraabdominal organs, the spleen is the most commonly injured in blunt abdominal trauma. CT is usually the initial radiologic examination performed in evaluation of the patient with blunt abdominal trauma,

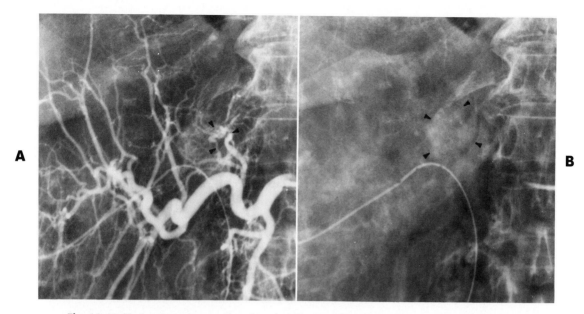

Fig. 16-12 Cholangiocarcinoma. Transhepatic biliary drainage has been established. Arteriogram was requested to determine whether cholangiocarcinoma extended outside biliary ductal system into hepatic parenchyma. **A,** Multiple encased vessels are present in region of tumor, indicating extension into hepatic parenchyma. **B,** Moderate tumor blush *(arrowheads).*

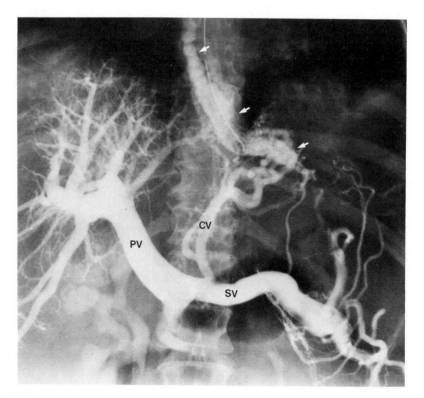

Fig. 16-13 Transhepatic portal venogram. Transhepatic portal venogram shows good filling of splenic vein *(SV)* and portal vein *(PV)* and retrograde flow into network of gastroesophageal varices *(arrows)* by way of coronary vein *(CV).*

and angiography is commonly reserved for patients in whom serious vascular injury is suspected.

Venography
PATRICK C FREENY

The venous system of the upper abdominal visceral organs and gastrointestinal tract is important in both diagnostic and interventional radiology. It may be studied by a variety of techniques, including direct percutaneous venography, indirect arterial portography, computed tomography, ultrasonography, and magnetic resonance.

PORTAL VENOGRAPHY

Portal venography may be performed by the techniques of splenoportography, transhepatic or transjugular portography, indirect arterial portography, umbilical portography, and wedged hepatic venography, with retrograde filling of the portal vein. *Indirect arterial portography* and *transhepatic portography* (Fig. 16-13) are currently the most widely used methods. Transhepatic portography is performed by percutaneous catheterization of a right portal vein branch through a right lateral intercostal approach. Selective splenic and superior and inferior mesenteric angiography provides excellent opacification of the main tributaries and intrahepatic branches of the portal vein.

LIVER
Portal hypertension

Since pressure is the product of flow and resistance, portal hypertension may develop as a result of increased portal flow *(hyperkinetic portal hypertension)* or increased resistance within the portal venous system (Fig. 16-14). Radiologic evaluation of patients with known or suspected cirrhosis and portal hypertension may be used to (1) establish the diagnosis, (2) define the portal vascular anatomy for surgical portosystemic shunts or other therapeutic maneuvers, and (3) evaluate the patency of surgical portosystemic shunts. In addition, interventional angiographic techniques, such as transhepatic embolization of gastroesophageal varices, may be efficacious for nonsurgical management of patients with portal hypertension. The measurement of *wedged hepatic venous pressure* is a reliable indication of portal venous pressure. The most clinically useful determination is *corrected sinusoidal pressure* (CSP), which is the wedged hepatic venous pressure minus the inferior vena caval pressure.

Interventional radiologic techniques for variceal hemorrhage and portal hypertension

Vasopressin infusion controls variceal hemorrhage by lowering portal venous pressure. Comparisons of

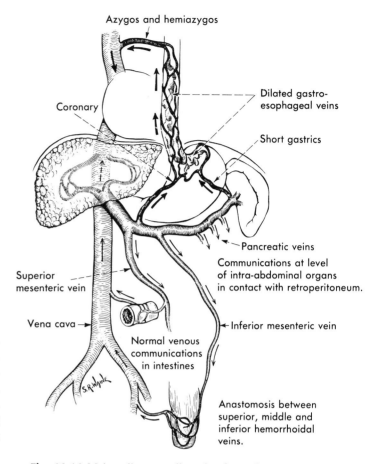

Fig. 16-14 Major tributary collaterals of portal venous system.

(Modified from Rousselot LM et al: *Ann Surg* 150:384, 1959.)

systemic and intraarterial infusion showed both techniques to be similarly efficacious in controlling variceal hemorrhage. It is now well accepted that variceal hemorrhage can be controlled effectively by systemic venous infusion.

Transhepatic variceal obliteration, by transhepatic catheterization of the portal vein and selective obliteration of gastroesophageal varices by sclerosing agents plus embolic agents, is an appropriate technique for acute control of hemorrhage if conservative therapeutic modalities fail and the patient is not considered an acceptable risk for immediate portosystemic shunt surgery.

Endoscopic sclerotherapy consists of the direct injection of a sclerosing agent (sodium norrhuate) into distal esophageal varices using a fiberoptic endoscope. The success rate for control of acute hemorrhage is approximately 90%.

PANCREAS AND SPLEEN
Pancreatic islet cell tumors

The technique of transhepatic pancreatic vein catheterization has permitted endocrine tumor localization by

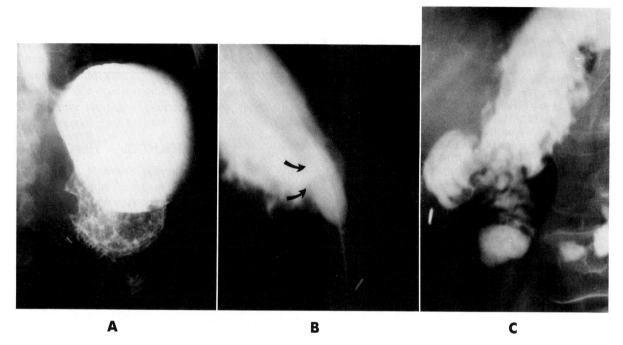

A **B** **C**

Fig. 17-1 Dilatation of gastroenterostomy anastomosis. **A,** Upper GI series demonstrates dilatation of gastric remnant and poor gastric emptying. **B,** A 20 mm balloon *(arrows)* is inflated in anastomosis. **C,** Follow-up upper GI series 2 days later shows widely patent anastomosis and free gastric emptying.

low-compliance balloon catheters developed for angioplasty now offer a much safer alternative for esophageal dilatation. With this technique the force of dilatation is perpendicular to the stricture, and several studies have confirmed its safety and efficacy. Because of its simplicity and safety, *balloon dilatation therapy* has also been employed for strictures elsewhere in the gastrointestinal tract. For example, strictures at anastomotic sites in the colon and at gastroenterostomy anastomoses (Fig. 17-1) can be effectively dilated.

MANAGEMENT OF ENTEROCUTANEOUS FISTULAS

The evolution of various interventional radiologic catheterization techniques has made safe and detailed exploration of fistulous tracts possible and has allowed a new nonsurgical option to accomplish these goals (Fig. 17-2).

PERCUTANEOUS PUNCTURE OF THE ALIMENTARY TRACT
Percutaneous gastrostomy

Nutritional support by gastrostomy feeding is an important therapeutic adjunct for patients with swallowing difficulty secondary to neurologic problems or obstructive pharyngeal or esophageal tumors. Although nutrition can often be provided for these patients by nasoenteric tubes, transnasal tubes are uncomfortable and not usually well tolerated for long periods. Gastrostomy feeding is therefore usually preferred, and although surgical gastrostomy is a relatively minor procedure, it usually requires general anesthesia and has a mortality rate of 1% to 6%. Percutaneous gastrostomy is a safe and relatively simple alternative. Not only can a feeding tube be placed directly into the stomach by percutaneous methods, but it can also be readily advanced through the pylorus and into the proximal jejunum, where feeding can begin immediately in the most optimal location.

Percutaneous transjejunal puncture of Roux-en-Y choledochojejunostomies

Patients with complex biliary tract pathology are often treated surgically by construction of a Roux-en-Y biliary jejunal anastomosis. Recent reports have documented the usefulness of constructing the Roux-en-Y loop with an extraperitoneal segment that is marked with metal clips. The extraperitoneal segment can then be punctured percutaneously, and catheterization into the biliary tree can be readily accomplished.

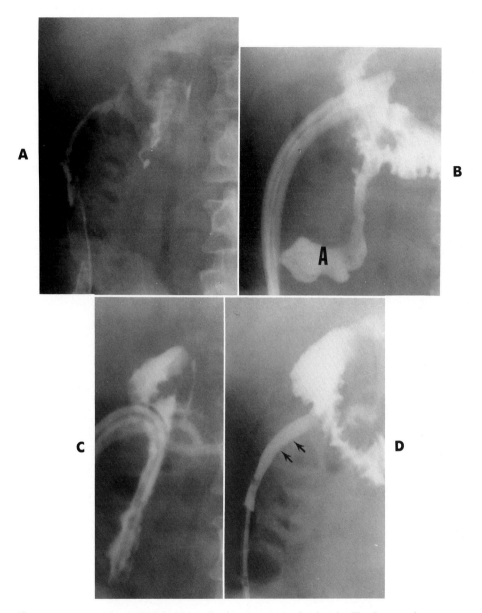

Fig. 17-2 Management of high-output duodenocutaneous fistula. **A,** Fistulagram demonstrates tract with minimal contrast entering duodenum. **B,** Steerable catheter is manipulated through tract. Injection of contrast close to fistula shows open communication to duodenum and dependent abscess *(A)*. **C,** Large-bore sump tube is positioned in abscess, and drain is placed into duodenum to control flow of duodenal contents. **D,** Drains are removed after abscess has cleared and mature fibrous tract has formed *(arrows)*.

The vascular system
ANDERS LUNDERQUIST

Over the past 3 decades angiographers have become even more occupied with the treatment of patients, leading to a wide spectrum of interventional vascular procedures.

LIVER
Trauma

Surgeons who favor conservative treatment of trauma to the liver are satisfied with contrast-enhanced CT of the abdomen to map the damage. If there are clinical signs of continuing hemorrhage, however, and

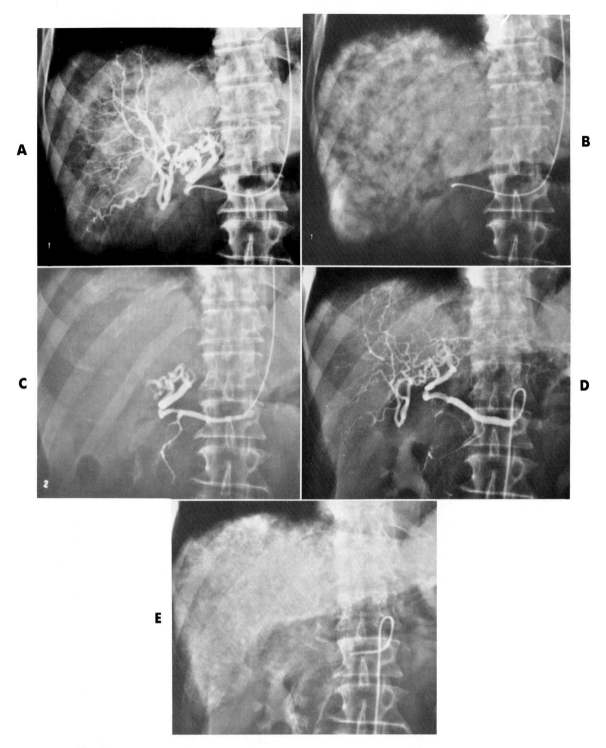

Fig. 17-3 Patient with liver metastases from carcinoid tumor and carcinoid syndrome. **A,** Selective catheterization of proper hepatic artery, arterial phase. **B,** In parenchymal phase whole liver is filled with hypervascular metastases. **C,** After embolization with Gelfoam powder, blood flow to liver is obliterated. **D,** One month later vessels are recanalized and, **E,** metastases are less vascular. Patient became free from carcinoid syndrome 2 days after embolization and remained symptom free for 9 months.

the patient's condition does not necessitate immediate laparotomy, angiography should be performed. With angiography, the bleeding can be localized and selective embolization performed. In many cases laparotomy can be prevented and the patient treated conservatively. The most elegant way to obliterate the bleeding vessel is to introduce a detachable balloon, which does not need to be detached until its position is correct. The high cost of balloon catheters has prevented their extensive use, however, and other embolization materials, such as Gelfoam, Ivalon, and Gianturco coils, are often used. The ability to control hemorrhage in the traumatized liver by hepatic artery embolization has been well documented.

Tumors

Although introduced with high expectations, treatment of primary liver tumors and metastatic tumors from colorectal carcinoma by hepatic arterial infusion of cytotoxic drugs through either percutaneously placed catheters or surgically placed catheters connected with subcutaneous infusion chambers has not produced the expected dramatic improvement. On the other hand, patients with carcinoid syndrome associated with liver metastases have been successfully treated with hepatic artery embolization (Fig. 17-3).

Portal hypertension

Bleeding from esophagogastric varices in patients with portal hypertension has for many years been treated with the Sengstaken-Blakemore tube and intravenous vasopressin infusion. *Transhepatic embolization* of the left and short gastric veins was first introduced in the treatment of patients whose bleeding could not be managed otherwise, and acute variceal bleeding was controlled in 43% to 95% of patients for varying periods. When this method is successfully employed, the patient is no longer in the situation of needing emergency surgery and can be considered a candidate for elective surgery. Transhepatic obliteration of esophageal varices has now been replaced by *endoscopic sclerosing injections* into the varices.

PANCREAS

Pancreatitis with pseudocyst or abscess formation sometimes produces erosion of the splenic or pancreatic arteries with hemorrhage into the pseudocyst or into the pancreatic duct. If the main stem of the splenic artery is eroded, a catheter is advanced to the place of erosion, and that part of the vessel is obliterated (Fig. 17-4).

SPLEEN

During the last few years, partial splenic infarction in patients with hypersplenism has been treated with transcatheter splenic artery embolization to improve tolerance to immunosuppressive drugs in renal transplant candidates and in patients with hematologic disorders. *Partial splenic embolization* causes a marked increase in the platelet and white blood cell counts within a few days.

GASTROINTESTINAL HEMORRHAGE
Stomach

Hemorrhage into the stomach from peptic ulcers, Mallory-Weiss tears, gastric erosions, or surgical anastomoses are best treated with intraarterial infusion of

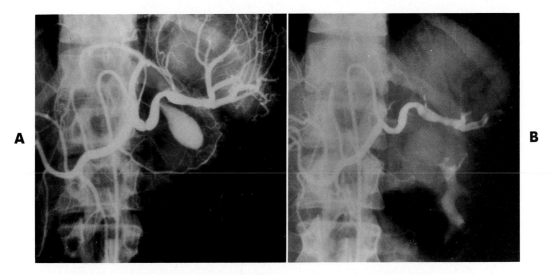

Fig. 17-4 Pancreatitis and intestinal hemorrhage in 38-year-old woman. **A,** Celiac angiography demonstrates large pseudoaneurysm extending into pancreas. **B,** Splenic artery obliterated with bucrylate mixed with Ethiodol. Hemorrhage was stopped.

vasopressin. If vasopressin cannot control the hemorrhage, the bleeding artery can be embolized.

Small bowel and colon

Hemorrhage is the most common indication for interventional radiology in the small bowel and colon. After the site of hemorrhage has been identified, bleeding can frequently be stopped by selective intraarterial vasopressin infusion. Some patients do not respond to vasopressin infusion, however, and their clinical conditions are too poor for surgical intervention. In these selected cases, embolization of the bleeding artery may be performed, with the knowledge that bowel necrosis may ensue. For embolization, the catheter should be as close to the bleeding vessel as possible for two reasons. First, if embolization with particles of Gelfoam is started too far from the source of bleeding, too many vessels are obliterated and the risk of bowel infarction increases. Second, if embolization is performed with coils, a localized obliteration of the vessel may be too far from the bleeding point and hemorrhage may continue, fed by collaterals.

ARTERIOVENOUS FISTULA

Trauma to the abdomen may cause arteriovenous fistulas. After an arteriovenous fistula has been angiographically localized, it can be obliterated either with a detachable balloon or with coils.

MESENTERIC ISCHEMIA

It has been suggested that mesenteric ischemia does not develop unless two of the three large intestinal arterial branches—the celiac artery, the superior mesenteric artery, and the inferior mesenteric artery—are occluded and the one left is stenosed. Arteriosclerotic stenosis or occlusion of the first part of the superior mesenteric artery can be treated by percutaneous transluminal angioplasty and the blood flow restored. Collateral blood flow over the middle colic artery is almost always enough to supply the branches of the inferior mesenteric artery.

The biliary tract
H JOACHIM BURHENNE

Access to the biliary tract for interventional procedures can be gained through three different routes: retrograde with gastrointestinal endoscopy, antegrade through the liver or gallbladder, or through the T-tube tract. Retrograde procedures were developed by gastroenterologists, and the majority of endoscopic procedures are still performed by these specialists. The trans-

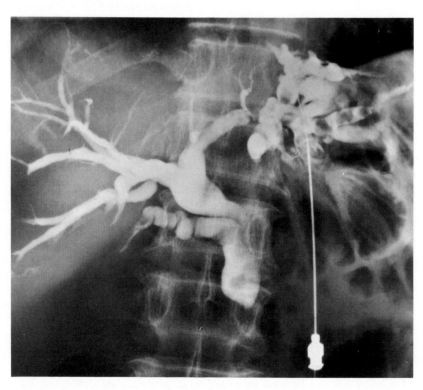

Fig. 17-5 Selective puncture of left intrahepatic bile duct using real-time scanner demonstrates intrahepatic gallstones.

hepatic approach was pioneered by radiologists as a further development of percutaneous needle cholangiography.

PERCUTANEOUS TRANSHEPATIC CHOLANGIOGRAPHY

Percutaneous transhepatic cholangiography (PTC) with a thin needle has now been documented as a safe approach to evaluating patients with jaundice and biliary tract disorders.

Technique

A puncture site is usually selected at the level of the seventh or eighth intercostal space. A fine needle with a stylet is introduced horizontally and parallel to the tabletop. Under fluoroscopic control the needle is advanced in a relatively cephalic direction during apnea. As the needle is withdrawn slowly, a small amount of contrast medium is continuously injected. When the biliary tree is punctured, contrast medium remains and outlines the intrahepatic ducts, the common hepatic duct, and then the common bile duct.

Success rate

The overall success rate of PTC is 99% for dilated bile ducts and 85% for nondilated ducts.

Complications

Serious complications of PTC include bile leakage, hemorrhage, and endotoxic shock caused by biliary venous reflux.

Indications

The relative indications for PTC and endoscopic retrograde cholangiopancreatography (ERCP) are becoming better defined (Fig. 17-5). PTC is less costly and relatively simple, whereas ERCP is less invasive and enables opacification of both the biliary tract and pancreatic ducts.

Mirizzi syndrome

Impaction of a gallstone in the cystic duct or neck of the gallbladder may cause common hepatic duct stenosis or obstruction. This is known as the Mirizzi syndrome. PTC demonstrates the stenosis and displacement of the common hepatic duct.

Biliary tract carcinoma

PTC is useful in the preoperative diagnosis of bile duct carcinoma (Fig. 17-6).

BILIARY DRAINAGE

Biliary drainage can be accomplished via the transhepatic or subhepatic route, and in the vast majority of

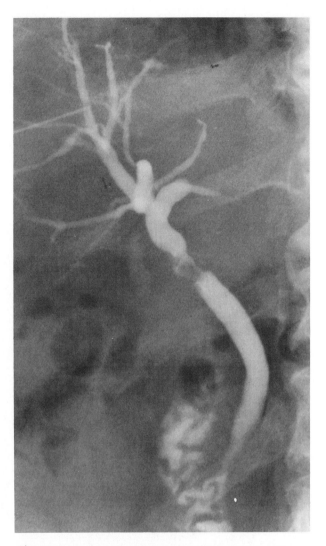

Fig. 17-6 Early cancer of bile duct. PTC shows polypoid carcinoma of common hepatic duct. Histology of resected specimen disclosed mucosal cancer. Five-year survival rate after resection of mucosal bile duct cancers is 100%.

cases is performed in patients with malignant obstruction of the extrahepatic bile ducts. Interventional relief of biliary tract obstruction allows bile to pass normally from the liver through the ducts into the gut via a catheter or stent.

External bile drainage

The extension of transhepatic cholangiography from a diagnostic modality to a therapeutic method for external bile drainage was initiated in Argentina. The transhepatic needle was left in place 7 days for drainage, and small catheters were used in subsequent patients to provide an external bile fistula. Pruritus and jaundice usually improved within a few days.

Preoperative bile drainage

Randomized studies to determine the effect of preoperative bile drainage on operative mortality, morbidity, hospital stay, and hospital cost have shown no reduced operative risk but an increase in hospital cost. Preoperative drainage diminishes serum bilirubin levels but does not reduce perioperative morbidity.

Internal bile drainage

Percutaneous decompression of obstructive jaundice for internal bile drainage is a logical extension of percutaneous transhepatic cholangiography and external drainage. A catheter is advanced through the obstructing lesion in the bile duct over a guidewire to act as a conduit. Side holes are placed above, and an end hole is placed below the lesion (Fig. 17-7). Drainage catheters can also be placed for intrahepatic biliary obstruction caused by cholangiocarcinoma or sclerosing cholangitis. When the obstruction is at the porta hepatis, the procedure for drainage through the left hepatic duct system involves a 45-degree angle approach under the left costal margin toward the area of the porta hepatis.

Percutaneous transhepatic or endoscopic internal biliary drainage is the treatment of choice for patients with

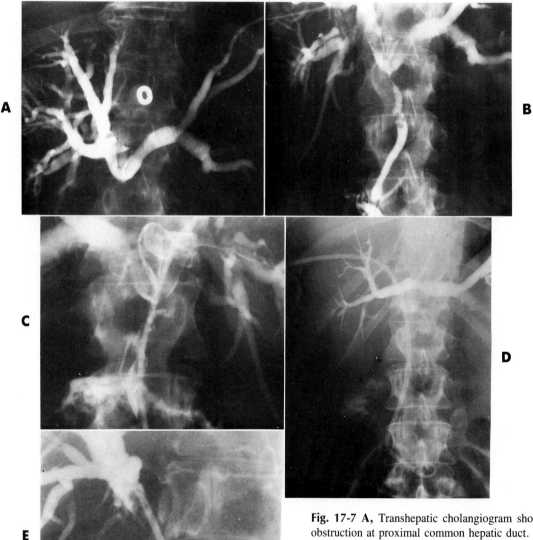

Fig. 17-7 A, Transhepatic cholangiogram showing complete obstruction at proximal common hepatic duct. B, Small catheter has been wedged into rattail of Klatzkin tumor. Forceful injection of undiluted contrast medium now results in demonstration of malignant stricture extent. C, Filling defect in hepatic ducts on day of instrumentation demonstrates hemobilia. Follow-up study 3 days later showed blood clots resolved. D, Pigtail catheter in place for internal bile drainage. E, Follow-up cholangiogram 3 months after internal drainage procedure shows tumor extension into right hepatic duct.

a malignant bile duct obstruction caused by unresectable lesions originating in the pancreas or common duct or with an obstruction caused by metastatic disease surrounding the porta hepatis. It is particularly useful in the large number of patients in whom surgical bypass is not possible because of technical difficulties.

Reports on complications from percutaneous biliary drainage vary greatly. Major complications have been reported to be as low as 5% and as high as 35%. The incidence of complications appears to depend greatly on the experience of the interventional radiologist. Endoscopically performed biliary drainage has been reported to carry a lower mortality than percutaneous transhepatic catheter placement.

Biliary endoprosthesis

The placement of an internal biliary drainage prosthesis avoids some of the problems of bile leakage, infection, catheter displacement, and patient intolerance often associated with catheter drainage. Insertion of a plastic or metallic endoprosthesis is performed with the help of an introducer of the same diameter as the catheter needle. The endoprosthesis is centered in the obstruction with sufficient extension for drainage both above and below. An anterior subcostal approach from the left may also be employed to place an endoprosthesis through the left main hepatic radicle. Obstruction and migration (Fig. 17-8) of the endoprosthesis, as well as duodenal perforation, may occur. Overall, however,

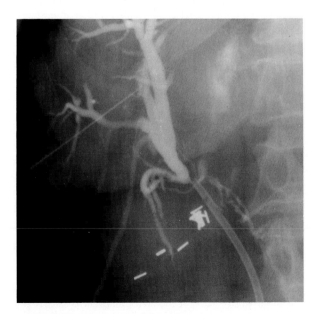

Fig. 17-8 Transhepatic cholangiogram demonstrating distal migration of endoprosthesis 3 weeks after initial placement. Note filling of lymphatics. Prosthesis was extracted by endoscopy and replaced.

clinical satisfaction is better with an endoprosthesis than with catheter drainage.

Placement of an internal stent via a percutaneous transhepatic route is now less commonly used because of the advances that have occurred in endoscopic approaches. The advent of the larger duodenoscope allows placement of a large-bore prosthesis. Expandable stents constructed of stainless steel wire are a more recent innovation that holds promise for use in the biliary tract.

Local radiotherapy

With widespread acceptance of percutaneous transhepatic drainage as an established technique, localized internal radiotherapy using iridium-192 wire by means of transhepatic catheter has been advocated. Patients may receive internal radiation alone or in combination with external irradiation. An increase in mean survival time with this technique has been reported.

CHOLELITHIASIS
Stone extraction

The retention of biliary tract stones after what the experienced surgeon considers to be a thorough removal, as seen with postoperative T-tube cholangiography, continues to be a problem. The incidence is still at least 5% of patients after common duct exploration, amounting to 3000 patients in the United States annually. Retained stones can be treated by radiologic or endoscopic nonoperative extraction, by irrigation techniques, by chemical dissolution, or by surgical removal. The radiologic interventional technique of percutaneous removal through the T-tube tract is the method of choice at present.

Percutaneous extraction of retained stones via T-tube tract from the common duct is widely practiced, and its success rate is 95% (Fig. 17-9). The majority of patients are ambulatory at the time of the procedure and receive no premedication. Small stones and fragments, about 3 mm in diameter, frequently pass spontaneously through the ampullary part of the common duct into the duodenum. Large stones, greater than 6 to 8 mm in diameter, cannot be extracted through the sinus tract with a No. 14 French T-tube, and fragmentation is then indicated (Fig. 17-10). Steady pull on the stone basket results in the stone being cut by the basket wires. No common duct injury has been reported.

Impacted stones in hepatic radicles or in the distal common duct may be difficult to engage in the wire basket because their position does not permit complete opening of the basket distal to them. Impacted stones must therefore be moved, which may be accomplished with a variety of maneuvers. Sometimes waiting is beneficial; at a second session the stone may have moved. Suction through the catheter or a strong contrast injec-

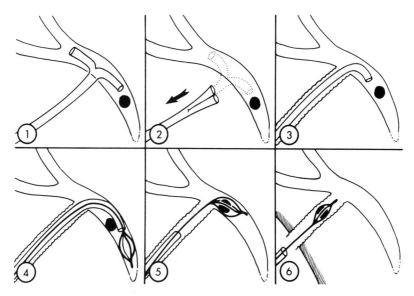

Fig. 17-9 Technical steps of subhepatic stone extraction. *1,* T-tube cholangiogram shows retained common duct stone. *2,* Catheter is extracted. *3,* Steerable catheter is manipulated through sinus tract into common duct. *4,* Tip of steerable catheter is advanced beyond stone, and wire stone basket is opened distally to stone. *5,* After partial withdrawal of steerable catheter, retained stone is snared in open basket. *6,* Stone is withdrawn through sinus tract.

tion distal to the stone is occasionally of help. If the stone cannot be moved, a vascular Fogarty balloon catheter may be used.

In one survey of 612 patients undergoing nonoperative extraction of retained common duct stones in 39 institutions, morbidity was 5%, and there were no deaths. It must be remembered that reexploration for retained stones, the previous method of choice for stone removal, carries a mortality of about 3%. At this time nonsurgical removal by radiologic interventional techniques through the sinus tract remains the procedure of choice. Other techniques such as stone dissolution or endoscopic removal have a significantly lower success rate.

Endoscopic sphincterotomy for retained common bile duct stones in patients with T-tube in situ can be effective in the early postoperative period, but this procedure carries at least a 7.7% complication rate, sometimes requiring reoperation. Endoscopic sphincterotomy and basket removal of common duct stones is the method of choice if no T-tube access is available.

Shockwave lithotripsy

In 1975 electrohydrolytic shockwaves were shown to fragment gallstones in vitro and in vivo. *Intracorporeal lithotripsy* provided 80% calculi fragmentation and was successfully used by radiologists via a percutaneous transhepatic approach. The first work on *extracorporeal*

fragmentation of gallbladder stones with shockwaves was reported in 1986. Oral chemolitholysis was used as an adjuvant litholytic therapy. Clearance of stone fragments requires 12 to 18 months.

The experience with lithotripsy of *bile duct stones* is more encouraging, particularly when interventional access to the biliary tract is available transhepatically, endoscopically, or via a T-tube tract or cholecystostomy (Fig. 17-11). As opposed to fragment passage after cholecystolithotripsy, stone fragments readily pass through a sphincterotomy or may be amenable to fragment clearing by basket extraction.

CHOLECYSTOSTOMY PROCEDURES

As with interventional access through a postoperative T-tube tract, instrumentation through cholecystostomy tracts or percutaneous gallbladder puncture may be used to gain access to the gallbladder and common duct (Fig. 17-12).

Gallbladder stones

Instrumentation through the cholecystostomy tract following drainage or acute cholecystitis is indicated for patients whose general medical condition does not permit subsequent surgical gallbladder removal. Gallbladder stones of any size may be crushed and removed through the cholecystostomy tract.

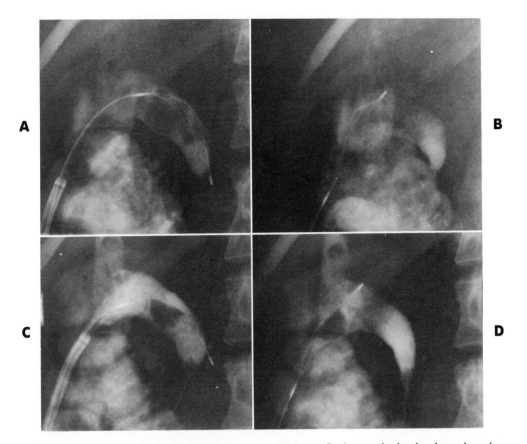

Fig. 17-10 Fragmentation of large retained stone. **A,** Large Cook stone basket has been draped over stone on greater curvature aspect of common duct. Steerable catheter has been withdrawn to sinus tract. **B,** Stone has been ensnared and brought to junction of common duct and sinus tract. Continuous strong traction has been applied to wire of basket. Note deformity of basket during traction, but there is no deviation of bile duct. **C,** Basket has been repositioned after strong fragmentation. Note clean-cut margin of stone produced by basket wire. There is another fragment in common hepatic duct and another in distal end of common duct. **D,** Large fragment has been engaged in basket for further fragmentation. After extraction of some fragments, straight catheter was placed through sinus tract into duct, and all remaining fragments were removed in second session.

Bile duct stones

The same subhepatic interventional approach through a cholecystostomy tract may be used to gain access to the bile ducts. Patients with acute gallbladder disease who are considered high operative risks or who are unsuitable for cholecystectomy can be treated with cholecystostomy catheter insertion using local anesthesia. The gallbladder is sutured to the abdominal wall, and stones from the gallbladder and biliary tract are removed subsequently by interventional radiologic techniques (Figs. 17-13, 17-14). The overall success rate for this combined surgical and radiologic technique for complicated cholelithiasis in high-risk patients has been reported to be 86%, with better results for gallbladder

stones than for cystic duct stones or common bile duct stones.

STRICTURE DILATATION

Interventional dilatation of benign *bile duct strictures* is indicated if biliary stones are retained proximal to the strictures (which usually result from cholangitis or previous surgery). Coaxial arterial catheters, ureteral dilators, and specially designed balloon catheters may be used, but the Grüntzig *arterial balloon catheters* are best suited for this purpose. Even malignant strictures are readily dilated to accommodate a No. 14 French catheter for internal bile drainage.

It has been suggested that indwelling splint catheters

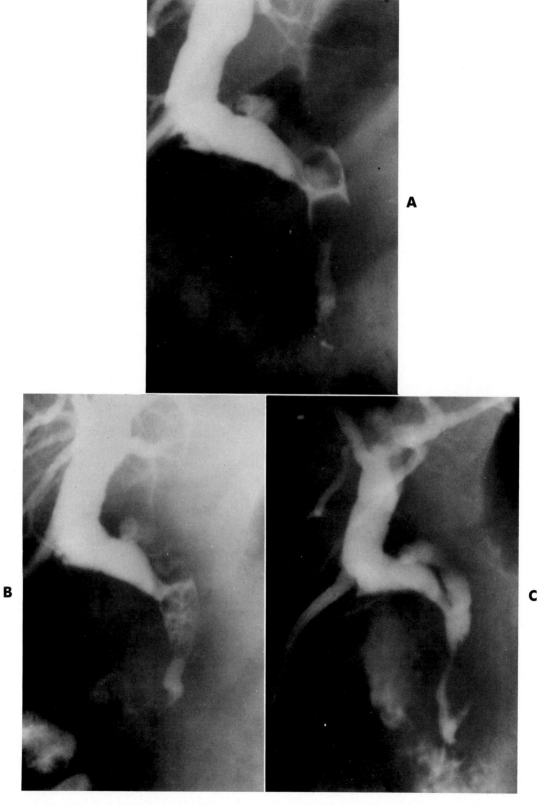

Fig. 17-11 A, Two retained stones impacted in cystic duct remnant are not accessible by interventional technique via T-tube tract. **B,** Extracorporeal shock-wave lithotripsy resulted in stone fragmentation, which permitted subsequent basket extraction. **C,** Duct system is clear of retained material.

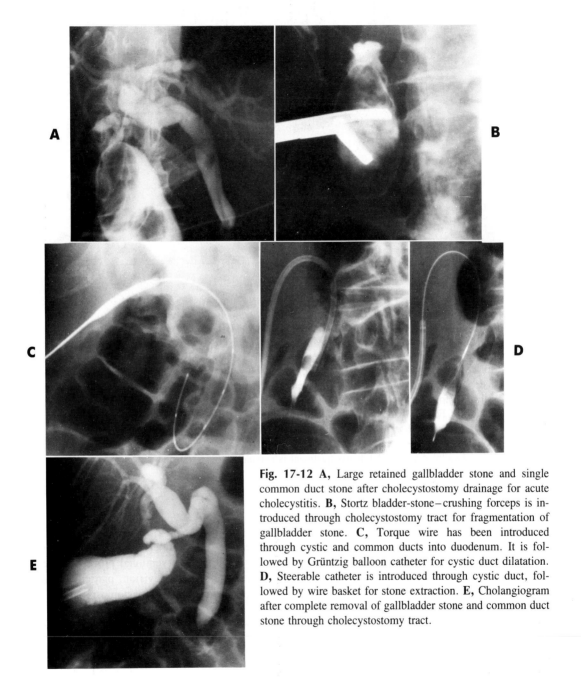

Fig. 17-12 A, Large retained gallbladder stone and single common duct stone after cholecystostomy drainage for acute cholecystitis. **B,** Stortz bladder-stone–crushing forceps is introduced through cholecystostomy tract for fragmentation of gallbladder stone. **C,** Torque wire has been introduced through cystic and common ducts into duodenum. It is followed by Grüntzig balloon catheter for cystic duct dilatation. **D,** Steerable catheter is introduced through cystic duct, followed by wire basket for stone extraction. **E,** Cholangiogram after complete removal of gallbladder stone and common duct stone through cholecystostomy tract.

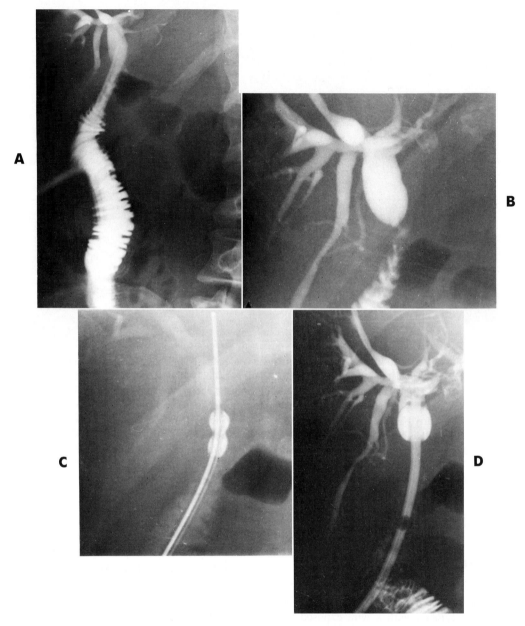

Fig. 17-15 A, T-tube in place after hepatojejunostomy. **B,** Stricture at anastomosis site with patients jaundiced 3 weeks after short arm of T-tube slipped back into jejunum. **C,** Balloon catheter placed over guide wire through jejunostomy is seen distended with contrast medium during stricture dilatation. **D,** Retention catheter in place after stricture dilatation with retention balloon inflated in common hepatic duct above hepatojejunostomy. Side hole in Silastic catheter provides for internal drainage with catheter closed at skin. Note narrowing of intrahepatic ducts from previous cholangitis. Stones ratained in left hepatic duct were removed in subsequent session. Catheter remained in place for 2½ years to maintain and splint previous stricture. This 1974 case was first instance of interventional radiology for nonoperative stricture dilatation and internal drainage.

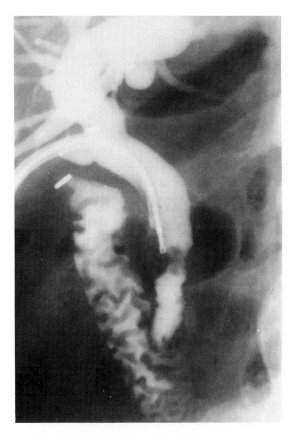

Fig. 17-16 Postoperative cholangiogram demonstrated defect in common duct. Subhepatic biopsy access through T-tube tract with flexible biopsy forceps revealed carcinoma.

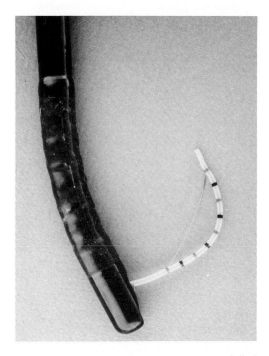

Fig. 17-17 Typical side-viewing duodenoscope and diathermy sphincterotome.

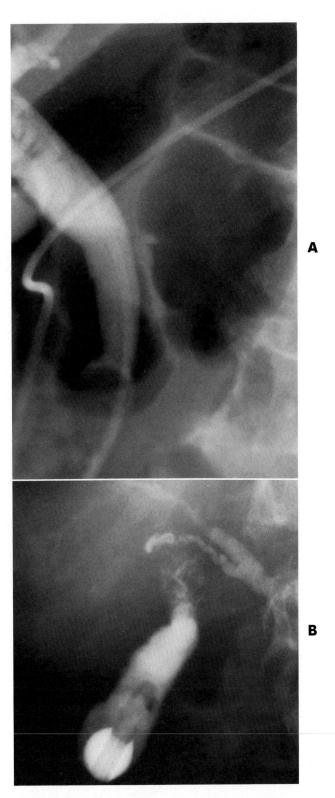

A

B

Fig. 17-18 A, Large impacted distal common duct stone. Nasobiliary catheter placed for decompression. **B,** Cholangiography after lithotripsy with external shockwave application shows fragmentation of large impacted stone in gallbladder neck.

using injection of contrast through a nasobiliary tube (or other drainage tube) for focusing.

Complications

Endoscopic sphincterotomy carries the usual rare risks of ERCP. Specific complications occur in about 10% of patients; 2% to 3% require urgent surgery for these complications, and 1% die. Bleeding is the most common problem.

INDICATIONS FOR ENDOSCOPIC TREATMENT
Postcholecystectomy

The most common indication for sphincterotomy is removal of stones from the duct of a patient who has previously undergone cholecystectomy (and who does not have a T-tube drain). Surgical exploration of the duct is relatively safe in young and fit patients, but the mortality rises to 5% to 10% with increasing age and frailty. The endoscopic approach must therefore be considered as the treatment of choice in high-risk patients.

Patients with gallbladders

Endoscopic treatment is increasingly used as an emergency procedure in patients with acute symptoms caused by duct stones—such as acute cholangitis and gallstone-related pancreatitis—even when the gallbladder is in place. The clinical results are usually dramatic.

Benign papillary stenosis

Many experts now perform endoscopic sphincterotomy for "papillary stenosis" despite diagnostic and conceptual difficulties.

Bile duct strictures

ERCP is an accurate method for detecting and delineating traumatic strictures of the bile duct. Angioplasty-type balloons are used for dilatation. The recurrence rate is high after a single dilatation, and most experts now leave a splinting stent in place for 3 to 12 months.

Malignant obstructive jaundice

Jaundice caused by malignant obstruction above the papilla can be managed by endoscopic stenting, using a three-layer system of guide-wire, catheter, and stent. Larger instruments now allow placement of No. 12 and 15 French stents (Figs. 17-19 and 17-20).

Endoscopic biliary stents provide excellent palliation in patients with tumors of the distal bile duct and pancreas, but hilar lesions are more difficult to manage,

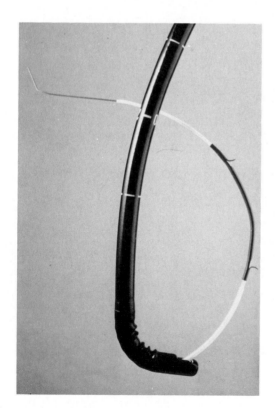

Fig. 17-19 Three-layer system for endoscopic insertion of No. 11.5 French stents—guidewire, inner catheter, and stent with terminal barbs.

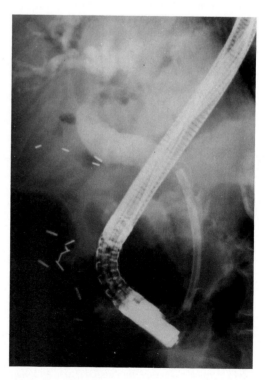

Fig. 17-20 Endoscopic placement of No. 15 French stent with experimental duodenoscope.

and a combined percutaneous–endoscopic approach may be necessary. In these cases the radiologist passes a guidewire percutaneously through the appropriate segment of the liver and into the duodenum. The large-channel duodenoscope is then passed and the guidewire grasped and withdrawn through the endoscope. A standard stent can then be passed through the endoscope over this guidewire. The same percutaneous assistance can be given to an endoscopist who has difficulties in cannulating the papilla for sphincterotomy, for example, in a patient with a large papillary diverticulum.

PANCREATIC DISEASE

Sphincterotomy is used in patients with acute gallstone *pancreatitis,* and endoscopic stenting is now established in the management of jaundice caused by tumors of the pancreatic head. *Pancreatic pseudocysts* have been drained by endoscopic puncture through the stomach or duodenal wall with use of diathermy or laser probes. Pseudocyst resolution has also been facilitated by temporary placement of an endoscopic stent or drain.

The widespread use of ERCP has highlighted the congenital anomaly of *pancreas divisum,* in which the main pancreatic drainage from the dorsal pancreas is through Santorini's duct and the accessory papilla. This anomaly occurs in about 7% of the population and is usually clinically irrelevant. However, there is now clear evidence that the orifice of the accessory papilla may be inadequate in some patients, resulting in recurrent pain and pancreatitis. Endoscopic sphincterotomy at the accessory papilla has been largely abandoned because of rapid restenosis, but the results of temporary insertion of a stent appear encouraging.

Percutaneous abdominal biopsy and drainage

GARY M ONIK
ROBERT KERLAN

Percutaneous biopsy and drainage of abdominal fluid collections are now routine procedures in most hospitals and are accepted as standard care. They have been shown to be both safe and effective and are preferred to open laparotomy for diagnosis and treatment.

PERCUTANEOUS BIOPSY

Using ultrasound, CT, and now even magnetic resonance imaging, percutaneous fine-needle biopsy has become a common practice (Fig. 17-21).

Ultrasound

Real-time ultrasound is fast, inexpensive, and therefore the most cost-effective means of guiding a biopsy. It is ideal for liver and pancreatic biopsies; however, it may not be useful in the lower abdomen if gas obscures the pathologic condition.

Computed tomography

With the traditional method of CT-guided biopsy, the path to the lesion is calculated, and the level of the scan slice of interest is marked on the patient using the laser localization lights of the CT scanner. The reference point on the patient is found, and the distance to the entry point is measured. Even if the entry point for the biopsy or drainage is correctly found, however, major problems with accuracy can occur because of inaccurate angulation of the needle. To solve these problems, much work has recently been done on *body stereotaxis.* With body stereotaxis methods, although they

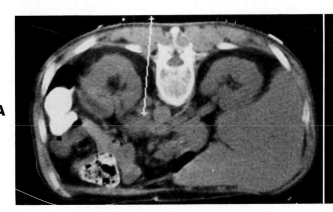
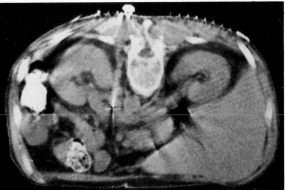

A   **B**

Fig. 17-21 A, Calculated path to small 1.5 cm retroperitoneal lymph node. Note that path goes just underneath transverse process and just medial to rib and kidney. **B,** Needle is noted to have followed path exactly, and biopsy was positive for lymphoma.
(From Onik G et al: *Radiology* 166:389, 1988.)

have some limitations, accuracy of placement is clearly superior to that with hand guidance.

Results of percutaneous biopsy

The expected sensitivity for malignancy is 85% to 95%. Of great importance is that false-positive diagnoses for malignancy are extremely rare.

Complications

The most important advantage of percutaneous fine-needle biopsy is that its morbidity is extremely low. This makes it the procedure of choice for obtaining pathologic confirmation of intraabdominal lesions.

DRAINAGE OF ABDOMINAL FLUID COLLECTIONS

CT-guided percutaneous drainage of abdominal fluid collections has become a commonly performed, safe, and effective procedure. Since parenchymal organs, bowel, and major vascular structures are clearly depicted on CT, a safe percutaneous approach can be identified. The procedure can be performed on critically ill individuals and avoids the morbidity of a major operation. Most abdominal and pelvic fluid collections can be managed with percutaneous techniques. Operative management should be reserved for patients without safe percutaneous access routes, for patients in whom an adjunctive surgical procedure must be performed, or when the debris is so viscous that percutaneous aspiration is ineffective.

Guidance and catheter insertion

CT provides the best depiction of abdominal fluid collections and clearly demonstrates adjacent organs, bowel, and major vascular structures. For these reasons, CT is the best available modality for planning percutaneous drainage. Subsequent catheter manipulations are better controlled with fluoroscopic imaging.

Some investigators have advocated real-time ultrasound imaging for abdominal abscess drainage. Ultrasound may be a useful adjunct, but it is clearly more operator dependent than CT or fluoroscopy.

After the fluid is aspirated, the patient is rescanned to check for undrained loculations and to confirm appropriate tube position. The tube is then externally secured.

Special considerations
Pancreas

Pseudocysts may be approached anteriorly if no intervening loops of bowel are present. Sinograms performed 3 to 5 days after pseudocyst drainage often opacify the pancreatic duct. If the duct is obstructed, the pseudocyst will not resolve without adjunctive therapy to relieve the obstruction. When the sinogram opacifies an unobstructed pancreatic duct, rapid resolution may be anticipated.

Thick-walled *pancreatic abscesses* can also be managed percutaneously (Fig. 17-22), however, pancreatic phlegmons cannot be managed with existing percutaneous techniques.

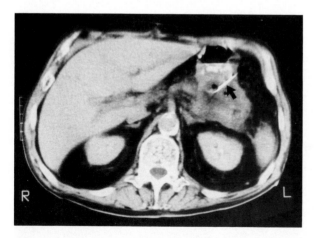

Fig. 17-22 Sixty-year-old man with abdominal distention and sepsis. Thick-walled pancreatic abscess is punctured from anterolateral approach between stomach and spleen. Subsequently No. 16 French drainage tube was placed, yielding 50 ml of thick, purulent fluid. Patient's condition improved, and elective surgical debridement was performed.

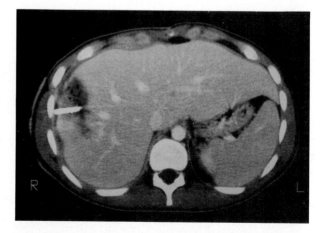

Fig. 17-23 Thirty-eight-year-old man with right upper quadrant pain and fever. No. 12 French sump tube has been inserted to drain pyogenic abscess in right lobe. Abscess resolved after 3 weeks of drainage.

Spleen

Fluid collections in the spleen can be safely drained percutaneously.

Liver

Hepatic abscesses are well suited for percutaneous drainage (Fig. 17-23). Both pyogenic and amebic abscesses can be successfully treated.

Patient management and follow-up

All patients return to the fluoroscopic suite 3 to 5 days after abscess drainage for sinography. Tubes are routinely replaced and repositioned in the dependent portion of the cavity at that time. If significant retained debris is present in the cavity, the tract is dilated and a larger drainage tube inserted.

Not infrequently, sinography reveals communications to the alimentary canal, biliary tract, or pancreatic ductal system. In this case, a drainage tube may be positioned adjacent to the fistulous tract, evacuating the cavity more effectively. Patients without fistulous communications generally require 2 to 3 weeks of drainage; patients with fistulous communications may require 4 to 6 weeks for complete healing.

RECOMMENDED READING

1. Alzate GD et al: Percutaneous gastrostomy for jejunal feeding: new technique, *Am J Roentgenol* 147:822, 1986.
2. Ariyama J et al: Experience with percutaneous transhepatic cholangiography using Japanese needle, *Gastrointest Radiol* 2:359, 1978.
3. Bengmark S et al: Arterial ligation and temporary dearterialization. In Blumgart LH, editor: *Surgery of the liver and biliary tract,* vol 2, Edinburgh, 1988, Churchill Livingstone.
4. Berk RN et al: Radiology of the bile ducts, *Radiology* 145:1, 1982.
5. Bret P et al: Abdominal lesions: a prospective study of clinical efficacy of percutaneous fine needle biopsy, *Radiology* 159:345, 1986.
6. Burhenne HJ: Nonoperative roentgenologic instrumentation technics of the postoperative biliary tract, *Am J Surg* 128:111, 1974.
7. Burhenne HJ: Percutaneous extraction of retained biliary tract stones: 661 patients, *Am J Roentgenol* 134:888, 1980.
8. Burhenne HJ, Li DK: Needle orientation for transhepatic cholangiography, *Gastrointest Radiol* 5:143, 1980.
9. Burhenne HJ et al: Biliary lithotripsy: an integrated approach of nonoperative intervention, *Am J Roentgenol* 150:1279, 1988.
10. Classen M, Demling L: Endoskopische sphincterotomoie der papilla vateri und steinextraktion aus dem ductus choledochus, *Dtsch Med Wochenschr* 99:496, 1974.
11. Cotton PB: Endoscopic methods for relief of malignant obstructive jaundice, *World J Surg* 8:854, 1984.
12. Cotton PB, Williams CB: *Practical gastrointestinal endoscopy,* ed 2, Oxford, England, 1982, Blackwell Scientific Publications.
13. Eggermont AM et al: Ultrasound-guided percutaneous transhepatic cholecystostomy for acute acalculous cholecystitis, *Arch Surg* 120:1354, 1985.
14. Ferrucci JT Jr et al: Advance in the radiology of jaundice: a symposium and review, *Am J Roentgenol* 141:1, 1983.
15. Ferrucci JT Jr et al: Biliary stone removal. In Ferrucci JT Jr et al, editors: *Interventional radiology of the abdomen,* ed 2, Baltimore, 1984, Williams & Wilkins.
16. Gerzof SG et al: Percutaneous catheter drainage of abdominal abscesses guided by ultrasound and computed tomography, *Am J Roentgenol* 133:1, 1979.
17. Gibney RG et al: Combined surgical and radiologic intervention for complicated cholelithiasis in high-risk patients, *Radiology* 165:715, 1987.
18. Gray R et al: Percutaneous abscess drainage, *Gastrointest Radiol* 10:79, 1985.
19. Hamlin JA et al: Percutaneous biliary drainage: complications of 118 consecutive catheterizations, *Radiology* 158:199, 1986.
20. Harbin WP et al: Transhepatic cholangiography: complications and use patterns of the fine-needle technique: a multi-institutional survey, *Radiology* 135:15, 1980.
21. Hoevels J et al: Percutaneous transhepatic intubation of bile ducts for combined internal-external drainage in preoperative and palliative treatment of obstructive jaundice, *Gastrointest Radiol* 3:23, 1978.
22. Kerlan RK et al: Abdominal abscess with low-output fistula: successful percutaneous drainage, *Radiology* 155(1):73, 1985.
23. Kerlan RK Jr et al: Radiologic management of abdominal abscesses, *Am J Roentgenol* 144:145, 1985.
24. Kerlan RK Jr et al: Percutaneous cholecystolithotomy: preliminary experience, *Radiology* 157:653, 1985.
25. Lind LJ, Mushlin PS: Sedation, analgesia, and anesthesia for radiologic procedures, *Cardiovasc Intervent Radiol* 10:247, 1987.
26. Lunderquist A, Vang J: Transhepatic catheterization and obliteration of the coronary vein in patients with portal hypertension and esophageal varices, *N Engl J Med* 291:646, 1974.
27. Lunderquist A et al: Gelfoam powder embolization of the hepatic artery in liver metastases of carcinoid tumors, *Radiologe* 22:65, 1982.
28. Margulis AR: Interventional diagnostic radiology: a new subspecialty, *Am J Roentgenol* 99:761, 1967.
29. May GR et al: Nonoperative dilatation of dominant strictures in primary sclerosing cholangitis, *Am J Roentgenol* 145:1061, 1985.
30. McGahan JP: A new catheter design for percutaneous cholecystostomy, *Radiology* 166:49, 1988.
31. McLean GK et al: Miscellaneous interventional procedures. In Ring EJ, McLean GK, editors: *Interventional radiology: principles and techniques,* Boston, 1981, Little, Brown.
32. McLean GK et al: Radiologically guided balloon dilation of gastrointestinal strictures. Part I. Technique and factors influencing procedural success, *Radiology* 165:35, 1987.
33. Molnar W, Stockum AE: Relief of obstructive jaundice through percutaneous transhepatic catheter: a new therapeutic method, *Am J Roentgenol* 122:356, 1974.
34. Mueller PR et al: Percutaneous drainage of 250 abdominal abscesses and fluid collections. II. Current procedural concepts, *Radiology* 151:343, 1984.
35. Mueller PR et al: Biliary stricture dilatation: multicenter review of clinical management in 73 patients, *Radiology* 160:17, 1986.
36. Nordentoft JM, Hansen H: Treatment of intussusception in children: brief survey based on 1,838 Danish cases, *Surgery* 38:311, 1955.
37. Olak J et al: Operative versus percutaneous drainage of intraabdominal abscesses: comparison of morbidity and mortality, *Arch Surg* 121:141, 1986.
38. Onik G et al: CT guided aspirations for the body: comparison of hand guidance with stereotaxis, *Radiology* 166:389, 1988.
39. Palmaz JC et al: Normal and stenotic renal arteries: experimental balloon-expandable intraluminal stenting, *Radiology* 164:705, 1987.

40. Pereiras R et al: The role of interventional radiology in diseases of the hepatobiliary system and the pancreas, *Radiol Clin North Am* 17:555, 1979.

41. Ring EJ, Kerlan RK Jr: Inpatient management: a new role for interventional radiologists, *Radiology* 154:543, 1985.

42. Sackmann M et al: Shock-wave lithotripsy of gallbladder stones: the first 175 patients, *N Engl J Med* 318:393, 1988.

43. Teplick SK et al: Common bile duct obstruction: assessment by transcholecystic cholangiography, *Radiology* 161:135, 1986.

44. Uflacker R: Transcatheter embolization for treatment of lower gastrointestinal bleeding, *Acta Radiol* 28:425, 1987.

45. vanSonnenberg E et al: Diagnostic and therapeutic percutaneous gallbladder procedures, *Radiology* 160:23, 1986.

46. vanSonnenberg E et al: Periappendiceal abscesses: percutaneous drainage, *Radiology* 163:23, 1987.

47. White RJ et al: Therapeutic embolization with detachable balloon, *Cardiovasc Intervent Radiol* 3:299, 1980.

48. Zajko AB et al: Percutaneous transhepatic cholangiography and biliary drainage after liver transplantation: a five-year experience, *Gastrointest Radiol* 12:137, 1987.

18 *Clinical Overview*

DAVID C CARTER
MICHAEL COLLIER
HARVEY V FINEBERG
THEODORE L PHILLIPS
VERNON SMITH
JACK WITTENBERG

CLINICIAN'S PERSPECTIVE ON ABDOMINAL IMAGING
    Appropriate use of diagnostic methods
    Histologic confirmation of diagnosis
    Interventional techniques as an alternative to surgery
    Developments in liver surgery

ONCOLOGY
    Imaging needs in oncology
    Radiotherapy treatment planning and imaging

COST EFFECTIVENESS
    Principles of cost-effective analysis
    Cost-effective radiologic practice

Clinician's perspective on abdominal imaging

DAVID C CARTER

The last 20 years have brought a dramatic increase in the number and variety of techniques available for the diagnosis of alimentary tract disorders. In addition, nonoperative management by interventional radiology and endoscopy now offers a real alternative to surgery in the treatment of a number of important alimentary disorders. More than ever before there is a pressing and continuing need for the clinician and radiologist to work in close collaboration, to maintain detailed mutual feedback, and for each to be fully aware of the other's strengths and limitations. In this context it cannot be overemphasized that not all radiologists have equal diagnostic and intervention skills, and likewise, not all surgeons have equal operative ability.

APPROPRIATE USE OF DIAGNOSTIC METHODS

Obstructive jaundice is an excellent example of a diagnostic problem that can usually be resolved safely and efficiently by the careful selection of a few key investigations. Before even considering radiologic investigation, the clinician must confirm that the patient indeed has jaundice and that the jaundice is likely to be obstructive. Dark urine, pale stool, and pruritus (caused by inability to excrete bile salts) all favor a diagnosis of obstructive jaundice. Bilirubin in the urine and hyperbilirubinemia associated with significant elevation in serum alkaline phosphatase levels are confirmatory findings.

Once the clinical and biochemical diagnoses of obstructive jaundice are secure, appropriate imaging evaluation must be determined. Ultrasonography and computed tomography (CT) are now the accepted preliminary noninvasive investigations. The first objective is to determine whether distension of the biliary tree is present. Once the site of blockage is defined, much can be inferred about the nature of the blockage. For example, obstruction at the confluence of the right and left hepatic ducts is much more likely to be due to neoplasia than to calculous obstruction. Blockage at the lower end of the common bile duct, however, is more often caused by neoplasia or gallstones. The examiner must remember that although ultrasonography is a reliable means of diagnosing the presence of stones in the gallbladder, it is much less reliable in the detection of stones in the lower reaches of the common bile duct.

If major duct obstruction is confirmed by ultrasonography, judgment must now be exercised in the choice of subsequent investigations. In the years following its introduction, percutaneous transhepatic cholangiography (PTC) was used widely as the next procedure. A cholangiogram was virtually always obtained for patients with distended ducts; the use of slim flexible needles markedly reduced the risk of bleeding or bile leak-

age, and the avoidance of overdistension minimized the risk of precipitating bacteremia and septicemia.

Once the likely cause of obstruction has been defined by cholangiography, the diagnostic pathways diverge. For example, if gallstones are shown on endoscopic retrograde cholangiopancreatography (ERCP), most endoscopists relieve the obstruction at that time by endoscopic papillotomy and stone retrieval. If, on the other hand, the obstruction is due to neoplasia, the help of the radiologist is invaluable, first to facilitate target biopsy or fine-needle aspiration cytology under ultrasonographic or radiologic control, and then to assess resectability. CT, which can provide useful information on tumor size, local invasion, and dissemination, is particularly useful in definition of tumor resectability.

HISTOLOGIC CONFIRMATION OF DIAGNOSIS

Although radiologic detection of a lesion may sometimes be sufficient to guide clinical management, in many cases histologic confirmation is necessary to determine appropriate treatment options (Fig. 18-1). For example, biliary obstruction from chronic pancreatitis

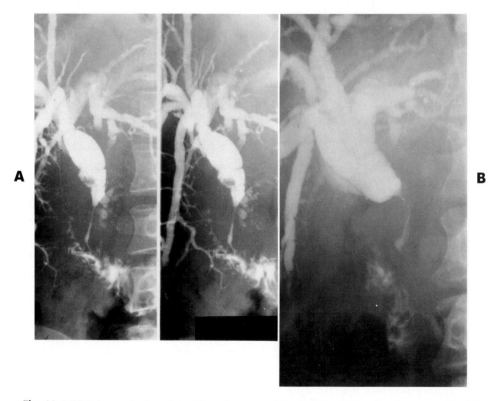

Fig. 18-1 PTC demonstrating obstruction of common bile duct caused by chronic pancreatitis (**A**) and pancreatic carcinoma (**B**). Although pancreatic calcification may help to differentiate between two lesions, configuraton of stricture may pose major difficulties in diagnosis. Note elevation of distended bile duct from tumor mass in **B**.

remains a source of real diagnostic uncertainty. Other benign conditions that can cause confusion include sclerosing cholangitis, benign inflammatory bile duct tumors, compression of the bile ducts by an inflamed gallbladder, and the Mirizzi syndrome.

A preoperative diagnosis of pancreatic cancer can now be obtained safely by percutaneous fine-needle aspiration cytology of lesions targeted by US, CT, or ERCP.

INTERVENTIONAL TECHNIQUES AS AN ALTERNATIVE TO SURGERY

The vast majority of patients who have surgery for pancreatic or biliary cancer are elderly, have extensive disease, or are so ill that resection for attempted cure is seldom feasible. Jaundice is the main indication for palliation, and cholecystojejunostomy is the operation usually performed. Although the issue is debated, many surgeons add gastroenterostomy on the grounds that otherwise approximately 15% of patients will have trouble with duodenal obstruction. Collected reviews indicate that mean duration of survival following operative biliary bypass is only 5.4 months, and that the mean operative mortality is almost 20%.

It is hardly surprising that these poor statistics have prompted the assessment of alternative methods of pal-

liation, and percutaneous internal drainage has provided encouraging results. It seems reasonable to attempt endoscopic stenting in the first instance. If this fails, it may be possible to use the percutaneous route to pass a guidewire through the obstructing lesion and to retrieve the end of the guidewire from the duodenum with an endoscope and to introduce a stent from below.

In patients with choledocholithiasis, and in whom T-tube access is no longer available, endoscopic papillotomy with stone retrieval now offers a valid alternative to surgery. Collected reviews suggest that stones can be retrieved in 80% to 90% of cases, with an estimated complication rate of 10% and a mortality rate of approximately 1%. Extracorporeal shock wave lithotripsy is now being applied to the destruction of gallstones.

DEVELOPMENTS IN LIVER SURGERY

Recent years have seen a growing awareness of the importance of a thorough understanding of hepatic surgical anatomy. Each side of the liver can be divided into two sectors, and further subdivision allows the description of eight segments (Fig. 18-2). The right and left sides of the liver are independent in their portal and arterial blood supplies. Resections may consist of hepatectomy (left or right), sectoriectomy, or segmentectomy.

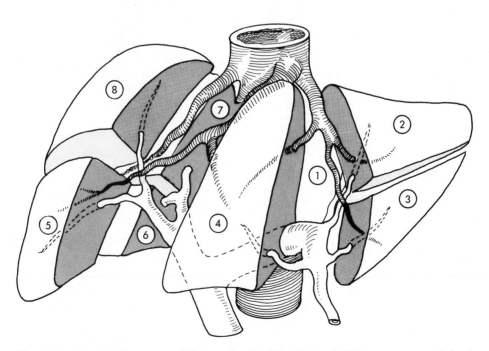

Fig. 18-2 Segmental anatomy of liver as described by Couinaud. Eight segments are defined. Segment *1* is caudate lobe; segments *2* and *3* constitute left lobe; and segment *4,* also part of left hemiliver, contains quadrate lobe. Segments *5* to *8* comprise right side of liver, which can be divided into anterior and posterior portions.

(Redrawn from Bismuth H, Castaing D: *Operative ultrasound of the liver and biliary ducts,* Berlin, 1987, Springer-Verlag.)

Intraoperative ultrasonography is being used increasingly to supplement the information obtained by preoperative ultrasonography, CT, and selective angiography. It may be particularly useful in cirrhotic patients who develop hepatocellular carcinoma, because it may detect small tumors and minimize the amount of liver that must be resected to remove them.

There is also growing interest in the use of liver resection for the treatment of hepatic metastases from colorectal cancer. It is now recognized that occult hepatic metastases may be detected with CT in approximately one fourth of patients thought not to have such metastases at the time of surgery. In this context intraoperative ultrasonography may prove useful as a means of detection of secondary liver tumors at operation.

Oncology

Gastrointestinal cancer represents about 35% of all cancer diagnosed in the United States. Approximately 20% of all cancers occur in the colon—accounting for 100,000 cases per year in the United States. At 5% of cases, carcinoma of the rectum is the next most frequently occurring, representing approximately 25,000 cases per year. Both stomach and pancreatic cancers account for about 3% of tumors.

The treatment of gastrointestinal cancers is extremely complex and involves a thorough integration of surgery, radiotherapy, and chemotherapy.

IMAGING NEEDS IN ONCOLOGY

Staging of a neoplasm in the gastrointestinal tract is extremely important in predicting prognosis. Thus imaging needs are often more demanding for staging than for initial diagnosis; sometimes additional studies are required. Accurate imaging, especially with CT and magnetic resonance imaging (MRI), is required for modern treatment by radiotherapy. Evaluation of response to treatment is another function of imaging in gastrointestinal oncology.

RADIOTHERAPY TREATMENT PLANNING AND IMAGING

CT and MR imaging play increasingly important roles in radiotherapy planning (Fig. 18-3). Their ade-

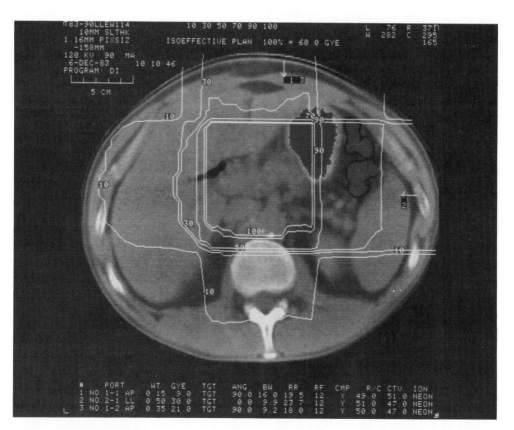

Fig. 18-3 CT-based treatment plan for carcinoma of pancreas using neon ions with three beams, or portals. Correction for density on pixel-by-pixel basis is included. Because of day-to-day changes, air density in bowel has been converted to water density.

quate use requires a method of indexing the CT to films taken on the radiotherapy simulator, as well as to portal films taken on the treatment delivery machine. To employ CT and MRI data, the CT or MR images must be taken with the patient in the exact treatment position. Optimal treatment planning, therefore, is conducted using computer systems, many of which display the CT and MRI data on a high-resolution device, which allows overlays of radiation isodose curves. With two-dimensional CT-based planning, the image is generally displayed, and the isodose distributions calculated for the treatment device in use are superimposed on it.

Cost effectiveness
HARVEY V FINEBERG
JACK WITTENBERG

Analysis of cost effectiveness attempts to measure and compare the costs, risks, and benefits of medical care. Many cost-effectiveness analyses in radiology focus on a particular procedure (such as upper gastrointestinal series or arteriography), or a particular piece of equipment (such as CT or ultrasound scanner). In either case, it is essential to also specify the range of patients to be included in the analysis.

PRINCIPLES OF COST-EFFECTIVE ANALYSIS
Alternative approaches

Every cost-effectiveness assessment is relative to some alternative use of available resources. A clinical procedure or piece of machinery is more or less cost effective in comparison with specified alternatives.

Measurement of benefits

Most discussions of cost-effectiveness analysis tend to determine health benefits in terms of ultimate health effects, usually measured in terms of mortality and morbidity. Several combined measures of mortality and morbidity have been used, such as the number of quality-adjusted life years or the number of well years.

A useful, if still inconclusive, cost-effectiveness analysis could adopt a measure of effect, such as the impact on therapeutic decision making, which is more immediate than the ultimate health benefit, such as mortality. For example, the results of one diagnostic test can influence the choice of further tests, either prompting or discouraging their selection. The advantage of such measures is their accessibility to be studied; the limitation is their tenuous connection with the ultimate benefits. The discovery of an unresectable pancreatic carcinoma by CT, for instance, may not alter the mortality, but it can avoid the need for exploratory laparotomy. As to the level of effect on treatment, an analyst seeks to identify the changes in the treatment plan con-

sequent to the test. When the radiologist directly performs a therapeutic maneuver, as in percutaneous abscess drainage, its cost effectiveness can be compared directly with that of alternative treatments.

Benefits of CT

An example of an evaluation of clinical efficacy is a study of computed body tomography that was conducted at Massachusetts General Hospital from 1976 to 1982. Patients were prospectively classified into 1 of 12 protocols according to the principal clinical problem and anatomic region to be examined. Before the CT examination, referring physicians completed questionnaires that prospectively indicated their diagnostic considerations and treatment plans. After performance of the CT examination, the radiologist provided the usual formal report, as well as a written estimate of the probabilities of each possible diagnosis, to facilitate later review of the examinations's contribution.

At the time of discharge, or approximately 4 weeks after examination of outpatients, the physician completed a follow-up questionnaire on the overall contribution of CT. These ratings of diagnostic and therapeutic contributions of CT were reviewed independently by the investigators and checked for consistency against the patient's record. Overall, 53% of CT examinations produced a substantial or unique contribution to diagnostic understanding. The proportion of patients in whom CT contributed to a change in treatment was 15% overall. Performance among the 12 different protocols varied considerably. Lymphoma and disorders of the pancreas, retroperitoneum, lung, and liver ranked in the top half for both diagnosis and therapeutic efficacy, whereas urinary tract conditions and disorders of the pelvis and colon fell in the bottom third.

The effect of CT on proposed therapeutic measures such as surgery was determined by comparing procedures actually performed with those initially proposed, and the results showed a net reduction of 14%. Significant decreases in the frequency of angiographic, sonographic, and lymphangiographic examinations were also observed.

Factors affecting cost-effectiveness

Any cost-effectiveness study applies to the equipment and technique of a particular technologic capability. As advances occur, for example with successive generations of faster and more versatile CT scanners or with improved interventional techniques, the initial findings may no longer apply. Evolution of the pattern of a disease also affects the projected cost effectiveness of a diagnostic test or clinical intervention. For example, the incidence of ulcer disease and carcinomas of the stomach has been declining. The incidence of pancreatic cancer, in contrast, has been increasing, and the cost-effectiveness of tests to detect this disease would be expected to improve even without any further technologic advances.

COST-EFFECTIVE RADIOLOGIC PRACTICE

A number of radiologists have advocated an orderly, integrated approach to diagnostic imaging through the use of algorithms. The many radiologic alternatives in both diagnostic and therapeutic procedures have created the potential for more expeditious and safer patient care.

Clinical algorithms have been developed and tested for a variety of common ambulatory medical problems. Some evaluations of widely used conventional imaging procedures have yielded more efficient selection criteria for patients. In general the radiologic algorithm is a responsible attempt to foster more cost-effective and time-efficient solutions to diagnostic problems. The algorithm should represent an institution's consensus for a uniform diagnostic approach to common clinical problems. The strategy represented by the algorithm must take into account factors such as technologic availability, patient endurance, and risks, as well as the accuracy and purpose of alternative tests in different patient populations. An algorithm cannot be a rigid dictator; it merely generates guidelines for effective patient care that may be altered by either the clinician or the radiologist. Every radiologist can introduce cost-effective principles into daily practice by establishing examination criteria and monitoring their implementation.

RECOMMENDED READING

1. Bismuth H: Surgical anatomy and anatomical surgery of the liver, *World J Surg* 6:3, 1982.
2. Bismuth H, Castaing D: *Operative ultrasound of the liver and biliary ducts,* Berlin, 1987, Springer-Verlag.
3. Dahlin H et al: User requirements on CT-based computed dose planning systems in radiation therapy, *Acta Radiol (Oncol)* 22:397, 1983.
4. Ferrucci JT Jr, Wittenberg J: *Interventional radiology of the abdomen,* Baltimore, 1981, Williams & Wilkins.
5. Gastrointestinal Tumor Study Group: Further evidence of effective adjuvant combined radiation and chemotherapy following curative resection of pancreatic cancer, *Cancer* 59(12):2006, 1987.
6. Margulis AR: Radiologic imaging, changing costs, greater benefits, *Am J Roentgenol* 136:657, 1981.
7. Martin DF, Tweedle DEF: Endoscopic management of common duct stones without cholecystectomy, *Br J Surg* 74:209, 1987.
8. McPherson GAD et al: Pre-operative percutaneous transhepatic biliary drainage: the results of a controlled trial, *Br J Surg* 71:371, 1984.
9. Office of Technology Assessment, United States Congress: *The implication of cost-effectiveness analysis of medical technology,* Washington, DC, Sept 1980, US Government Printing Office.
10. Pitt HA et al: Does preoperative percutaneous biliary drainage reduce operative risk or increase hospital cost? *Ann Surg* 201:545, 1985.
11. Sarr MG, Cameron JL: Surgical management of unresectable carcinoma of the pancreas, *Surgery* 91:123, 1982.
12. Weinstein MC, Fineberg HV: *Clinical decision analysis,* Philadelphia, 1980, WB Saunders.
13. Wittenberg J et al: Clinical efficacy of computed body tomography, *Am J Roentgenol* 154:1111, 1980.
14. Yamamoto R et al: Histocytologic diagnosis of pancreatic cancer by percutaneous aspiration biopsy under ultrasonic guidance, *Am J Clin Pathol* 83:409, 1985.

Index

A

A cells of endocrine pancreas, 39
Abdomen
  acute, 42-65
    from acute cholecystitis, 46-48
    from acute diverticulitis, 49
    from acute intestinal ischemia, 50
    from acute pancreatitis, 48
    from acute ulcerative colitis, 49-50
    from amebic colitis, 50
    from appendicitis, 45-46
    from colon obstruction, 58-59
    from duodenal obstruction, 55
    from gastric obstruction, 52-55
    from ileal obstruction, 55-58
    from inflammatory diseases, 45-46
    from intestinal atony and dilatation, 59
    from intestinal tract obstruction, 52
    intramural air in, *44, 45*
    from intraperitoneal abscess, 51-52
    intraperitoneal air in, 42-44
    from jejunal obstruction, 55-58
    nontraumatic, 42-59
    from peritonitis, 50-51
    from pseudomembranous enterocolitis, 50
    from retroperitoneal abscess, 52
    traumatic, 60-65
  preliminary plain radiographs of, 221-222
  trauma to, 60
Abdominal angina, angiography of, *463, 464*
Abdominal aorta
  computed tomography of, 432
  magnetic resonance imaging of, 432
  ruptured, 428
  ultrasonography of, 428-430
Abscess(es)
  after gastric surgery, postoperative evaluation of, 408-409
  amebic, diagnosis of, 331
  diverticular, demonstration of, 242-243
  evaluation of, ultrasonography in, 27-28
  fungal, diagnosis of, 331
  hepatic
    amebic, in pediatric patient, 449
    drainage of, 491
    nuclear medicine of, 351
    pyogenic
      magnetic resonance imaging of, 343
      in pediatric patient, 449
  intraperitoneal, 51-52
  pancreatic, *306,* 307
    drainage of, 490
    in pancreatitis, 301

Abscess(es)—cont'd
  psoas, computed tomography of, 434-435
  pyogenic, diagnosis of, 331
  splenic, 367
    ultrasonography of, 373
  subhepatic, 51-52
  subphrenic, 51-52
Absorption
  colonic, 40
  intestinal, 37
Abuse, child, 447, *448*
Acalculous cholecystitis, acute, 47-48
Accessory spleens, scintigraphy for, 380-381
Acetylcholine, gastric acid secretion and, 36
Achalasia, 85-86
  cricopharyngeal, 72
  in pediatric patient, 440
Acid neutralization in esophagus, 35-36
Acid secretion by stomach, 36
Acinar cell carcinoma of pancreas, 314
Acquired immunodeficiency syndrome (AIDS)
  gastrointestinal manifestations of, 400-403
  in pediatric patient, 444, *445*
Actinomyces israelii, bacterial colitis from, 257
Actinomycosis, small bowel in, 201
Adenocarcinoma(s)
  colonic, 278-280, *281, 282*
  duodenal, 168
    Crohn's disease differentiated from, 198
  pancreatic, 308-314
  small bowel, 213, *214*
Adenoma(s)
  colonic, 270
  gastric, diagnosis of, 145-146
  liver cell, diagnosis of, 336
  small bowel, 205
  villous
    duodenal, 167, 168
    rectal, 280, *283*
Adenomatous polyps, duodenal, 167
Adenomyomatosis, 325, 327
Afferent loop syndrome, postoperative evaluation of, 414
Aganglionosis, 59
  in pediatric patient, 442
Air
  intramural, *44, 45*
  intraperitoneal, 42-44
Air bubbles after biliary tract surgery, postoperative evaluation of, 416, *417*

Alcoholism, esophageal motor dysfunction in, 89
Alimentary tube; *see also* Gastrointestinal tract
  nuclear medicine of, 24-26
  ultrasonography of, 26-32
Amebiasis, 396-398, *399*
  colitis in, 259
Amebic colitis, 50
Amebic dysentery, 396-398, *399*
Amebic liver abscess(es)
  diagnosis of, 331
  nuclear medicine of, 351
  in pediatric patient, 449
Amebic liver disease, magnetic resonance imaging of, *342,* 343
American trypanosomiasis, 390-391
Amine precursor uptake and decarboxylation (APUD) system, 33
Ampulla, phrenic, 82
Amyloidosis
  esophageal motor dysfunction in, 89
  gastric, 137
Anal atresia, prenatal ultrasonic detection of, 32
Anaphylactic changes of colon, 259
Anastomotic jejunal loop, obstruction in, postoperative evaluation of, 414
Ancylostomiasis, 393-394
Aneurysm(s)
  abdominal aortic
    ruptured, ultrasonography of, 430
    ultrasonography of, 429
  aortic
    angiography of, 464
    computed tomography of, 432
    magnetic resonance imaging of, 432
Angina, abdominal, angiography of, *463, 464*
Angiodysplasia in GI tract, angiography of, *462, 463*
Angiogenesis in alimentary tract tumors, 465
Angiography
  of alimentary tract, 459-469
    complications of, 459
    for gastrointestinal hemorrhage
      acute, 459-463
      chronic, 463-464
      hepatic, 466-467
      pancreatic, 465-466
      splenic, 467-469
    techniques of, 459
    for tumors, 465
    for vascular disease of GI tract, 464-465
  of pancreas, *296,* 297

Colon—cont'd
  obstruction of, 58-59
    in pediatric patient, 442
  perforation of
    complicating granulomatous colitis,
      256
    complicating ulcerative colitis, 252
  physiology of, 40
  postoperative evaluation of, 415-416
  radiologic examination of, 221-234
    defecography in, 235-239; see also
      Defecography
    preliminary plain abdominal
      radiographs in, 221-222
    special, 228-234
  reduction of intussusception and volvulus
    in, 228-229
  right, peroral double-contrast
    examination of, terminal ileum
    and, 228, 229
  sigmoid, perforation of, 428
  sonography of, in pediatric patient, 456
  transit in, 40
  tuberculosis of, 385
  water-soluble contrast media for stool
    softening in, 229
Colon cut-off sign in pancreatitis, 297,
  298, 423
Colonoscopy in colonic polyp detection,
  265-266
Colorectal cancer, 277-289
  complications of, 285, 287
  differential diagnosis of, 287-288
  etiology of, 277-278
  histologic tumor types in, 278-284
  metastases of, 284-285
  neoplastic staging of, 288-289, 289-291
  radiographic patterns of, 278-284
Colostomy, double-contrast examination
  through, 226-227
Computed tomography (CT)
  in acute pancreatitis, 298, 299
  benefits of, cost effectiveness and, 497
  of colon, 230-231
  contrast media for, 16-18
  for Crohn's disease, 184, 185
  for esophageal tumors, 111-113
  in gastric cancer diagnosis, 143, 144
  of gastrointestinal manifestations of
    AIDS, 403
  for inflammatory disease of colon, 260,
    261-262
  instrumentation for, 3-4
  of pancreas, 294
    for cancer, 309-310, 310-311, 312
  for percutaneous biopsy, 489-490
  of pharynx, 67, 68, 69
  for small bowel examination, 181,
    182-183
Computed tomography (CT) scanners, 4-5
Computer system for magnetic resonance
  imaging, 14
Connective tissue disorders, esophageal
  motor dysfunction in, 87-88
Constipation, functional, in pediatric
  patient, 444

Contractions, esophageal, nonpropulsive,
  90
Contrast media, 15-23
  barium sulfate as, 15-16
  for biliary disease, 18-20, 21
  for colon examination
    barium as, 222-227
    water-soluble, 227-228
  for computed tomography, 16-18
  filling defects of, in biliary ducts,
    360-361, 363
  for magnetic resonance imaging, 20, 22,
    23
    of liver, 343
  for small bowel radiologic examination
    barium as, 173-179
    water-soluble, 179, 181
  for vascular disease, 18-20
  water-soluble, for stool softening, 229
Contrast range of image intensifier tube, 2
Conventional Bucky radiography, 2-3
Conversion factor of image intensifier tube,
  2
Corrosive gastritis, 54
Corrosive gastropathy, 133
Cost effectiveness, 497-498
Coupling in television viewing system, 2
Cricopharyngeal achalasia, 72
Cricopharyngeal chalasia, 73
Cricopharyngeal sphincter, abnormalities
  of, 72
Crohn's disease, 184-198
  computed tomography of, 184, 185
  differential diagnosis of, 196-198, 199
  of duodenum, 170
  gastric, 132
  imaging findings in, 193, 196
  magnetic resonance imaging of, 185,
    185-186
  radiologic features of, 185, 187,
    192-193, 194-196
  recurrences of, 198
Cronkhite-Canada syndrome, 275-276
  small bowel in, 207-208
Cryptosporidium
  colitis from, 259
  infections from, 402-403
Curling esophagus, 83, 84
Cyst(s)
  choledochal
    diagnosis of, 330
    in pediatric patient, 450, 451
    radiologic diagnosis and differential
      diagnosis of, 360, 361
  duplication, ultrasonography in
    evaluation of, 30, 31
  echinococcal, diagnosis of, 333
  esophageal, 116
  hepatic
    diagnosis of, 334-335
    in pediatric patient, 449
    ultrasonography of, 344
  pancreatic, in pediatric patient, 452
  pulmonary, nuclear medicine techniques
    of evaluation of enterogenous, 24

Cyst(s)—cont'd
  splenic, 367
    ultrasonography of, 373
Cystic neoplasms of pancreas, 314-315
Cytomegalovirus ileitis, 200
Cytoprotection, definition of, 35

D

D cells of endocrine pancreas, 39
Dedicated small bowel follow-through
  examination, 173-174
Defecation, 40-41
Defecography, 235-239
  anatomic landmarks in, 236-238
  normal, 238
  pathologic, 237, 238-239
  procedure for, 236
Deglutition, normal, 70-71
Depth resolution of transducer, 6
Dermatomyositis in pediatric patient, 447
Descending perineum syndrome, 239
Diabetes mellitus, esophageal motor
  dysfunction in, 89
Diaphragm, 117-118
  antral, 128
Diaphragmatic hernias
  congenital, prenatal ultrasonic detection
    of, 32
  in pediatric patient, 440, 441
Diarrhea, traveler's, 388
Diffuse endocrine system, 33
Diffuse esophageal spasm, 86
Digestion, 37
Dilatation and atony, intestinal, 59
Dissection, aortic, ultrasonography of, 430
Disse's space, 39
Diverticulitis, 241-243
  acute, 49
Diverticulum(a)
  classification of, 245
  colonic, 239-245
    complications of, 243
    incidence of, 240
    with neoplasm, 245, 246
    pathogenesis of, 240-241
    technique of examination of, 239-242
  duodenal, 170-171
  esophageal, 92-93
  gastric, 137, 138
  Meckel's
    angiography of, 463-464
    evaluation of, nuclear medicine
      techniques of, 24
    in pediatric patient, 443
    sonography of, 455-456
  pharyngeal, 69-70
Double-contrast examination of esophagus,
  80, 81
Double-contrast pharyngography, 69
Down syndrome in pediatric patient, 446,
  447
Drainage
  of abdominal fluid collections, 490-491
  biliary, percutaneous transhepatic
    cholangiography for, 477-479

Drugs, disorders of small bowel associated with, 204
Dumping, postgastrectomy, postoperative evaluation of, 414
Duodenal atresia, prenatal ultrasonic detection of, 32
Duodenal ileus in acute pancreatitis, 297
Duodenal stump, rupture of, after gastric surgery, postoperative evaluation of, 408
Duodenitis, nonspecific, 170
Duodenum, 161-171
    abnormalities of, pancreatitis from, 301
    anatomy of, 161, *162,* 163
    configuration of, variations in, 171
    congenital stenoses of, 170
    disease of, diffuse intrinsic, 169-170
    diverticula of, 170-171
    duplications of, 171
    erosions of, 169
    examination of, technique of, 163-166
    fistulas of, 171
    indentation of, at aorta and superior mesenteric artery, 161
    intramural hematoma of, 171
    mucosal relief of, *162,* 163
    obstruction of, 55
        congenital, in pediatric patient, 440, *441*
    papilla of, major, enlargement of, 169
    perforation of, 422-423
    physiology of, 37-38
    postoperative evaluation of, 404
    sonography of, in pediatric patient, 453-454
    tuberculosis of, 384
    tumors of, 166-169
    ulcers of, 156, *157*
        healing of, radiographic appearance of, 160
    venography of, 470
Duplex scanning of liver, 321
Duplication cyst, evaluation of, ultrasonography in, *30, 31*
Duplications
    of bowel in pediatric patient, sonography of, 455
    of duodenum, 171
    of esophagus, 92
    of ileum in pediatric patient, 443
Dynamic focusing of transducer, 6
Dynamic recording of barium swallow, 69
Dysautonomia, familial, in pediatric patient, 447
Dysentery
    amebic, 396-398, *399*
    bacillary, 387
Dysphagia
    from cervical osteophytes, 74
    postvagotomy, 89
Dysphagia aortica, 116

E

Echinococcal cyst, diagnosis of, 333
Echinococcosis, 398, 400

Echinococcus granulosus infection, 398, *400*
Echinococcus multilocularis infection, 400
Echogenic bile, ultrasonography of, 347
Ectopic pancreas, 141, *142,* 143
Ectopic spleen, 367
Embolism, visceral, angiography of, 464
Embolization
    splenic, portal, 475
    transhepatic, for portal hypertension, 475
Embolotherapy for acute GI hemorrhage, *462,* 463
Emission tomography, instrumentation for, 10
Emphysema, intramural, 140
Emphysematous cholecystitis, 47, 323
Emphysematous gastritis, 130
Empyema of gallbladder, 47
Endocrine cells, location of, in gut, 35
Endocrine disorders
    esophageal motor dysfunction in, 89
    in pediatric patient, 444
Endocrine pancreas, 39
Endocrine system, diffuse, 33
Endometriomas, 271
Endoprosthesis, biliary, for drainage, 479
Endoscopic retrograde cholangiopancreatography (ERCP), 354-356
    anatomy for, 355
    in chronic pancreatitis, 300-301
    complications of, 355, 357
    diagnostic accuracy and success rate of, 358
    of pancreas, 295, 297
        for cancer, 312
    technique of, 355
Endoscopic sclerosing injections for portal hypertension, 475
Endoscopic sonography of pancreas, 295
Endoscopic sphincterotomy, 480
Endoscopic therapies, 485, *487,* 488-491
    indications for, 488-489
    for pancreatic disease, 489
    sphincterotomy as, 485, *487,* 488
Endoscopic ultrasound, 32
Enema
    barium; *see* Barium enema
    ileostomy, 227
    small bowel, for small bowel radiologic examination, 174-179
Entamoeba histolytica, colitis from, 259
Enteric neuropeptides, 33-35
Enteritis
    pseudomembranous, 204
    radiation, of small bowel, 203-204
    regional, in pediatric patient, 443
    tuberculous, 200-201
Enteroclysis for small bowel radiologic examination, 174-179
Enterocolitis
    necrotizing, in pediatric patient, *442,* 443, 445-446
        sonography of, 454-455
    pseudomembranous, 50, 204, 387-388

Enterocolitis—cont'd
    tuberculous, 200-201
Enterocutaneous fistula management, 472, *473*
Enterogenous pulmonary cysts, evaluation of, nuclear medicine techniques of, 24
Enteroliths, 385
Eosinophilic gastritis, 136-137
Eosinophilic gastroenteritis, 204
Epidermolysis bullosa (EB) in pediatric patient, 447
Equipment, radiographic, 1-3
Erosions, duodenal, 169
Erosive gastritis
    acute, 129
    chronic, 131-132
Erythrocytes, radiolabeled, damaged, for spleen scintigraphy, 378-379
Escherichia coli, bacterial colitis from, 257
Esophagitis, 96-104
    after gastric surgery, postoperative evaluation of, 412
    caustic, 102-103
    cytomegalovirus, 402
    drug-induced, 103
    herpes, 99
    infectious, 97-98, *101*
    radiation, 103
    reflux, 88-89
    in tuberculosis, 102
    viral, 99, 102
Esophagography, 80, *81*
Esophagomyotomy, postoperative evaluation of, 406
Esophagus, 78-117
    abnormalities of, disorders with, in pediatric patient, 447-449
    acquired lesions of, in pediatric patient, 439
    anatomy of, 78-79
    atresia of, in pediatric patient, 438, *439*
    Barrett's, 97, *100-101*
        evaluation of, nuclear medicine techniques of, 24
    congenital anomalies of, 91-92
    congenital lesions of, in pediatric patient, 438-439
    deviation of, 117
    dilatation of, 90
    disorders of, in pediatric patient, 447-449
    distal, 90
    diverticula of, 92-93
    duplication of, 92
    examination of, 79-80, *81*
    fistula of, in pediatric patient, 438
    foreign bodies in, in pediatric patient, 440
    indentations of, 116-117
    metastatic disease of, 114
    motility disorders of, 82-91
        differential diagnosis of, 90-91
        primary, 85-87
        radiographic evaluation of, 82-85
        secondary, 87-90

Esophagus—cont'd
nutcracker, 86-87
perforations of, 94-95
postoperative evaluation of, 404-406
proximal, 90
resection and reconstruction of,
postoperative evaluation of, 406,
407
rings of, 104-105
sonography of, in pediatric patient,
452-453
spasm of, diffuse, 86
strictures of, *105-106,* 107
caustic, in pediatric patient, 440
congenital, in pediatric patient, 438,
439
dilatation of, 471-472
transit and acid neutralization in, 35-36
traumatic lesions of, 93-95
tuberculosis of, 384
tumors of, 109-116
varices of, 108-109
in pediatric patient, 440
webs of, 107
Exocrine pancreas, 40
Extrahepatic bile ducts, ultrasonography of,
349
Extrapyramidal diseases, esophageal motor
dysfunction in, 89

F

Factor IX deficiency in pediatric patient,
446
Familial dysautonomia
in pediatric patient, 447
pharyngeal dysfunction in, 73
Familial Mediterranean fever in pediatric
patient, 449
Familial multiple polyposis, 272, *273*
Familial polyposis coli, small bowel and,
208
Fascioliasis, 396
Fasting
gastric motility during, 37
intestinal motility during, 38
Fatty liver in pediatric patient, 449
Fed state, intestinal motility during, 38
Feeding, gastric motility after, 36
Fetal omphalocele, prenatal ultrasonic
detection of, 32
Fibrosis, retroperitoneal, 434
Fibrous ischemic strictures of small bowel,
202
Fibrovascular polyp, esophageal, 115
Filiform polyposis in Crohn's disease, 187
Filiform polyps in ulcerative colitis, 249,
250
Fine-needle aspiration biopsy of pancreas,
297
Fine-needle fluid aspiration of pancreas,
297
Fistula(s)
after gastric surgery, postoperative
evaluation of, 408-409

Fistula(s)—cont'd
arteriovenous, interventional procedures
for, 476
biliary-enteric, spontaneous, 324
biliary tract, radiologic diagnosis of, 363
bronchoesophageal, congenital, 92
complicating granulomatous colitis, 256
in Crohn's disease, 187, 196
duodenal, 171
duodenobiliary, 171
duodenocolic, 171
duodenorenal, 171
enterocutaneous, management of, 472,
473
esophageal, in pediatric patient, 438
formation of, complicating diverticular
disease, 244
gastrojejunocolic, postoperative
evaluation of, 413
tracheoesophageal, 87
in pediatric patient, 438, *439*
Fixed-focus transducer, 6
Fluid collections complicating pancreatitis,
302-305
Flukes
liver, 395-396
diagnosis of, 333
vascular, 396, *397*
Fluoroscopy of esophagus, 80
Focal nodular hyperplasia of liver,
diagnosis of, 336
Focal spot of x-ray tube, 2
Follicles, lymphoid, in GI tract defense
mechanisms, 38
Foreign bodies in esophagus, 93-94
in pediatric patient, 440
Functional asplenia, scintigraphy for, 381
Fundoplication for hiatus
hernia/gastroesophageal reflux,
405-406
Fungal colitis, 258
Fungal liver abscesses, diagnosis of, 331

G

Gallbladder
aberrant, in pediatric patient, 451
acute inflammation of, 46-48
agenesis of, 327
congenital anomalies of, 327
diseases of, 323-328
duplication of, 327
empyema of, 47
hydrops of, 47
neoplasms of, 328
perforation of, 47
phrygian cap of, 327
porcelain, 324
strawberry, 325
tumors of, in pediatric patient, 452
ultrasonography of, 346-347
Gallstones, 327, *328*
extraction of
cholecystostomy procedures for, 480
interventional procedures for,
479-480, *481, 482*

Gallstones—cont'd
in pediatric patient, 451
radiologic diagnosis of, 360
Gantries, scanning, in computed
tomography, 4
Gardner's syndrome, 272, 274
small bowel and, 208-209
Gas, intrahepatic, in pediatric patient, 450
Gastrectomy, carcinoma after
of gastric stump, 149-150
postoperative evaluation of, 413-414
Gastric accommodation after feeding, 36
Gastric antrum, retained, after gastric
surgery, postoperative evaluation
of, 412
Gastric bezoar, 55
Gastric bypass surgery, postoperative
evaluation of, 414
Gastric cancer
diagnosis of, 143-152
for adenoma, 145-146
advanced, 147-149
for Borrmann types in, 148
for carcinoma of gastric stump after
gastrectomy, 149-150
computed tomography in, 143, *144*
conventional and endoscopic
ultrasonography in, 144-145
differentiation of advanced and type II
cancer in, 149
early, 143-144
depressed, 146, *147*
smaller than 1 cm, 147
for early polypoid cancer, 145
for linitis plastica, 148-149
for malignant lymphoma, 150
radiographic, correlation of, with
endoscopy, 143-144
superficial spreading, 147
for type IIc, type IIc + III and type
III, 146-147
types I and IIA, 146
for types IIa + IIc, 146
Gastric emptying, evaluation of, nuclear
medicine techniques of, 24
Gastric mucosa, nuclear medicine of, 24
Gastric obstruction, 52-55
Gastric stump, postgastrectomy, carcinoma
in, 149-150
Gastrin, 33-34
gastric acid secretion and, 336
Gastrinoma, 315
Gastritis, 128-132
after gastric surgery, postoperative
evaluation of, 412
chronic, 130
corrosive, 54
cytomegalovirus, 402
emphysematous, 130
eosinophilic, 136-137
erosive
acute, 129
chronic, 131-132
granulomatous, 132
hemorrhagic, 130

Gastritis—cont'd
  infectious, 129
  phlegmonous, 129-130
  radiation, 133
Gastroenteritis, 388
  eosinophilic, 204
Gastroenterostomy, distal, postoperative
      evaluation of, 415
Gastroesophageal reflux, 90-91
  correction of hiatus hernia and, 405-406
  evaluation of, nuclear medicine
      techniques of, 24
  in pediatric patient, 438, 440
Gastroesophageal reflux disease (GERD),
      96-97, *98, 99, 100*
Gastrointestinal candidiasis, 390
Gastrointestinal cutaneous angiomatosis in
      pediatric patient, 447-448
Gastrointestinal hemorrhage, evaluation of,
      nuclear medicine techniques of,
      25, 26
Gastrointestinal histoplasmosis, 390
Gastrointestinal manifestations of AIDS,
      400-403
Gastrointestinal propulsion, evaluation of,
      nuclear medicine techniques of,
      24
Gastrointestinal tract
  disorders of, in pediatric patient,
      438-444
  hemorrhage in, interventional procedures
      for, 475-476
  location of endocrine cells in, 35
  nuclear medicine of, 24-26
  physiology of, 33-41
  prostaglandins and, 35
  upper, radiologic study of, 119-127; *see
      also* Upper GI study
Gastrointestinal tuberculosis, 383-386
Gastrojejunocolic fistula after gastric
      surgery, postoperative evaluation
      of, 413
Gastropathy, 128, 132, 136-137
  corrosive, 133
  hypertrophic, 133
  injury, 132-133
Gastropexy, posterior, for hiatus
      hernia/gastroesophageal reflux,
      405
Gastroschisis, prenatal ultrasonic detection
      of, 32
Gastrostomy, percutaneous, 472
Gelfoam for acute GI hemorrhage, 463
Generator, 1-2
Gerpta's fascia, 421
Giardiasis, 392, *393*
Glucagon, 34
  transit time through small bowel and,
      173
Grafts, aortic
  prosthetic, 432
  ruptured, 428
Granularity in ulcerative colitis, 248
Granulomatous colitis, 253-256
Granulomatous disease, chronic, in
      pediatric patient, 444

Granulomatous gastritis, 132
Gut tube neoplasms, evaluation of,
      ultrasonography in, *30, 31*

H

H₂ histamine receptor antagonists for
      peptic ulcer disease, 158
Heat units of x-ray tube, 2
Helminthic infections, 393-395, *396*
Helminthoma, 390, *391, 394*
Helminths, colitis from, 259
Hemangioma(s)
  cavernous, hepatic
      angiography of, 467
      diagnosis of, 335-336
  hepatic, magnetic resonance imaging of,
      341, *342*
  small bowel, 206
Hematologic disease in pediatric patient,
      446
Hematoma(s)
  duodenal, sonography of, in pediatric
      patient, 453
  intramural, duodenal, 171
  retroduodenal, 423, *424*
  subcapsular, 61
Hemobilia, radiologic diagnosis of, 361
Hemophilia in pediatric patient, 446
Hemorrhage
  after gastric surgery, postoperative
      evaluation of, 409
  into colon, interventional procedures for,
      476
  gastrointestinal
      acute, angiography for, 459-463
      chronic, angiography for, 463-464
      evaluation of, nuclear medicine
          techniques of, *25, 26*
      interventional procedures for, 475-476
  retroperitoneal, 433-437
  into small bowel, interventional
      procedures for, 476
  splenic, magnetic resonance imaging of,
      374, *376*
  into stomach, interventional procedures
      for, 475-476
Hemorrhagic gastritis, 130
Hemosiderosis in pediatric patient, 450
Henoch-Schönlein purpura in pediatric
      patient, 446
Hepatectomy, partial, postoperative
      evaluation of, 419
Hepatic metastases, magnetic resonance
      imaging of, 339-340
Hepatitis, neonatal, 450
Hepatoblastoma
  diagnosis of, 336
  in pediatric patient, 449
Hepatocarcinoma, diagnosis of, 336
Hepatocellular carcinoma
  angiography of, 467
  magnetic resonance imaging of, 340
  radiologic diagnosis of, 361
Hepatocellular diseases, ultrasonography
      of, 344

Hepatocytes, 38
Hepatolithiasis, radiologic diagnosis of,
      360-361
Hepatomegaly, diagnosis of, 331
Hepatotropic contrast agents, 19-20
Hernia(s), 58
  Bochdalek's, 117
  diaphragmatic, 117
      congenital, prenatal ultrasonic
          detection of, 32
      in pediatric patient, 440, *441*
  hiatus, 95-96
      correction of gastroesophageal reflux
          and, 405-406
  Morgagni's, 117
Hirschsprung's disease, 59
Histamine, gastric acid secretion and, 36
Histoplasma capsulatum, colitis from, 259
Histoplasmosis
  gastric, 129
  gastrointestinal, 390
  small bowel in, 201
Hodgkin's disease, small bowel findings
      in, 212
Hookworm disease, 393-394
Hormones, enteric, 33-35
Huntington's chorea, esophageal motor
      dysfunction in, 89
Hydatid disease, 398, 400
Hydrops of gallbladder, 47
Hyperplastic cholecystoses, 325
Hyperrugosity, 136
  causes of, *133*
Hypertension, portal
  diagnosis of, 331
  interventional procedures for, 475
  venography of, 469
Hypertensive peristalsis, 86-87
Hyperthyroidism, esophageal motor
      dysfunction in, 89
Hypertrophic gastropathy, 133-136
Hypertrophic pyloric stenosis (HPS), 53
  sonography of, in pediatric patient, 453,
      454
Hypothyroidism in pediatric patient, 444

I

Idiopathic intestinal pseudoobstruction, 87
Ileal pouches, postoperative evaluation of,
      415
Ileitis
  associated with ulcerative colitis, 199
  cytomegalovirus, 200
  terminal, acute, 199
Ileocecum, tuberculosis of, 384-385
Ileostomy, postoperative evaluation of, 415
Ileostomy enema, 227
Ileum
  duplication of, in pediatric patient, 443
  obstruction of, 55, 57-58
  in pediatric patient, 440
  sonography of, in pediatric patient,
      454-456
  terminal

Ileum—cont'd
    terminal—cont'd
        in granulomatous colitis, 256
        lymphoid hyperplasia of, 199-200
        in ulcerative colitis, 250-251
Ileus
    duodenal, in acute pancreatitis, 297
    meconium
        in pediatric patient, 442
        sonography of, 455
Image intensifier tube, 2
Image reconstruction in computed
        tomography, 3-4
Imaging, abdominal
    clinician's perspective on, 493-496
    developments in, in liver surgery,
        495-496
    diagnostic, appropriate use of, 493-494
    histologic confirmation of diagnosis
        from, 494-495
Immune deficiencies, small bowel in,
        219-220
Immune diseases in pediatric patient,
        444-445
Immunoglobulin A (IgA), 38
Immunology, gastrointestinal, 38
Imperforate anus in pediatric patient,
        442-443
Incontinence, fecal, 239
Infarction, bowel, evaluation of, nuclear
        medicine techniques of, 26
Infectious colitis, 257
Infectious diseases, 383-403
    acute gastroenteritis as, 388
    amebic dysentery as, 396-38, *399*
    bacillary dysentery as, 387
    Chagas' disease as, 390-391, *392*
    echinococcosis as, 398, 400
    gastrointestinal candidiasis as, 390
    gastrointestinal histoplasmosis as, 390
    gastrointestinal tuberculosis as, 383-386
    giardiasis as, 392, *393*
    helminthic, 393-395, *396*
    helminthoma as, 390, *391*
    liver flukes as, 395-396
    lymphogranuloma venereum as, 388
    parasitic, 392-400
    pseudomembranous enterocolitis as,
        387-388
    Salmonella infections as, 386
    sprue as, 389-390
    trichuriasis as, 391-392
    typhoid fever as, 386-387
    vascular flukes as, 396, *397*
Infectious gastritis, 129
Inferior vena cava, 430-433
Inflammation, spread of, complicating
        diverticular disease, 244
Inflammatory lesions in pediatric patient,
        443-444
Inflammatory polyp, esophageal, 115-116
Injury gastropathy, 132
Inspissated bile syndrome in pediatric
        patient, 451
Instrumentation, 1-14
    for computed tomography, 3-4

Instrumentation—cont'd
    for emission tomography, 10
    for magnetic resonance imaging, 11-14
    for nuclear medicine, 6-11
    radiographic, 1-3
    for ultrasonography, 5-8
Insulin, 34
Insulinoma, 315, *316*
    in pediatric patient, 452
Interlacing in television viewing system, 2
Interventional radiology, 471-491
    in alimentary canal, 471-472
    as alternative to surgery, 495
    in biliary tract, 476-484; *see also* Biliary
        tract, interventional procedures
        for
    for drainage of abdominal fluid
        collections, 490-491
    for endoscopic therapies, 485-489
    for percutaneous abdominal biopsy,
        489-490
    in vascular system, 473-476
Intestinal atony and dilatation, 59
Intestinal ischemia, acute, 50
Intestinal perforation, prenatal ultrasonic
        detection of, 32
Intestinal permeability, 38
Intestinal tract obstruction, 52
Intestines; *see* Bowel
Intrahepatic bile ducts, ultrasonography of,
        348
Intramural air, *44, 45*
Intramural pneumatosis, 140-141
Intramural pseudodiverticulosis, 93
Intraperitoneal abscess, 51-52
Intraperitoneal air, 42-44
Intraperitoneal bleed, 60-61
Intussusception, 58
    after gastric surgery, postoperative
        evaluation of, 410-411
    complicating colorectal cancer, 285, *286*
    in pediatric patient, 443
    rectal, *237,* 238
    reduction of, 228-229
Ischemia
    mesenteric, interventional procedures
        for, 476
    segmental, Crohn's disease differentiated
        from, 196, 198
Ischemic colitis, 256-257
Islet cell tumors of pancreas, 315-316, *317*
    angiography of, 466
Ivemark's syndrome, 367

J

Jaundice, 319-320
    obstructive, malignant, endoscopic
        treatment for, 488-489
Jejunal loop, proximal, dysfunction of,
        postoperative evaluation of, 415
Jejunum
    obstruction of, 55, 57-58
    in pediatric patient, 440
        sonography of, 454-456
Juvenile polyp, colonic, 270

Juvenile polyposis, 276
Juxtapyloric ulcer, 154, 156

K

Kaposi's sarcoma, gastrointestinal, 400
Kidney(s)
    agenesis of, 428, *427*
    ectopia of, 428
    masses of, in perirenal space, 426, *427*
Killian's dehiscence, 67
Kilowatt rating of x-ray tube, 2
Kinescope in television viewing system, 2

L

Lag of image intensifier tube, 2
Laryngography, 67
Lateral resolution of transducer, 6
Lateroconal fascia, 421
Laxatives, mechanisms of, 40
Leiomatosis, diffuse esophageal, 115
Leiomyomas
    duodenal, 167
    esophageal, 114-115
    gastric, 151
    small bowel, 205-206
Leiomyosarcomas
    duodenal, 168
    gastric, 151
Lesser sac abscess, 52
Leukemia in pediatric patient, 446
Limy blue syndrome, 324
Linear array scanners, 6, *7, 8*
Lipomas
    colonic, 270
    duodenal, 167
    small bowel, 20, *207-208*
Lithotripsy, shockwave, 480, *482*
Liver, 319-363
    abscesses of
        pyogenic, magnetic resonance imaging
            of, 343
        ultrasonography of, 344
    angiography of, 466-467, *468*
    calcifications of, diagnosis of, 331, *332*
    cysts of
        diagnosis of, 334-335
        ultrasonography of, 344
    diseases of
        amebic, magnetic resonance imaging
            of, *342,* 343
        diagnosis of, 328-337
        diffuse, diagnosis of, 331
        vascular, diagnosis of, 331
    disorders of, in pediatric patient,
        449-450
    duplex scanning of, 321
    endoscopy for, 354-363; *see also*
        Endoscopic retrograde
        cholangiopancreatography
        (ERCP)
    fatty, in pediatric patient, 449
    fluid collections in, drainage of, 491
    focal lesions of
        nuclear medicine of, 350

Liver—cont'd
  ultrasonography of, 344
  focal nodular hyperplasia of, diagnosis
      of, 336
  hemangioma of, magnetic resonance
      imaging of, 341, *342*
  inflammatory lesions of, diagnosis of,
      331-333
  injuries to, 61, *62*
  jaundice and, 319-320
  localized imaging defects in, 320-321,
      322
  lymphoma of, magnetic resonance
      imaging of, 341
  magnetic resonance imaging of, 337-343
  magnetic resonance spectroscopy of,
      362, 363
  metastases to, ultrasonography of,
      345-346
  nuclear medicine of, 349-351
  physiology of, 38-39
  postoperative evaluation of, 419-420
  radiology of, in pediatric patient,
      449-450
  secretion in, 39
  synthesis of proteins in, 39
  transplantation of, 321
      postoperative evaluation of, 419-420
  trauma to, 320
  tumors of
      benign, diagnosis of, 335-336
      malignant, diagnosis of, 336, *337*
      ultrasonography of, 344, *345*
  ultrasonography of, 343-346
  vascular system of, interventional
      procedures for, 473-475
  venography of, 469
Liver cell adenoma, diagnosis of, 336
Liver flukes, 395-396
  diagnosis of, 333
Lower esophageal sphincter (LES),
      opening of, abnormal, 90
Lundh test, 40
Lung, pancreatitis, 308
Lymphatic system, 433, *434*
Lymphogranuloma venereum, 388
Lymphography of retroperitoneal space,
      435-436
Lymphoid follicles in GI tract defense
      mechanisms, 38
Lymphoid hyperplasia
  of duodenum, benign, *167,* 168
  of gut in pediatric patient, 444-445
  of terminal ileum, 199-200
Lymphoma(s)
  AIDS-related, 401-402
  colonic, 281, 284
  duodenal, Crohn's disease differentiated
      from, 198
  esophageal, 114
  hepatic, magnetic resonance imaging of,
      341
  malignant
      duodenal, 168
      of stomach, diagnosis of, 150

Lymphoma(s)—cont'd
  pancreatic, 316-317
  in pediatric patient, 446
  small bowel, 210-213
  splenic, magnetic resonance imaging of,
      376-378

M

Magnetic gradients for magnetic resonance
      imaging, 13
Magnetic resonance imaging (MRI)
  of colon, 232-234
  contrast media for, 20, *22,* 23
  for Crohn's disease, 185, *185-186*
  for esophageal tumors, 113
  for inflammatory bowel disease, 263
  instrumentation for, 11-14
  of liver, 321, 323, 337-343; *see also*
      Liver, magnetic resonance
      imaging of
  of pancreas, 295
      for cancer, 312
  in pediatric patient, 457
Magnetic resonance imaging
  of pharynx, 67, *68*
  for small bowel examination, 182
  of spleen, 374-378; *see also* Spleen,
      magnetic resonance imaging of
Magnetic resonance spectroscopy (MRS) of
      liver, *362,* 363
Magnets for magnetic resonance imaging,
      12-13
Mal de turista, 388
Malabsorption, 37
  diseases associated with, 216-219
  in pediatric patient, 444
  postgastrectomy, postoperative
      evaluation of, 414
Malignancy complicating ulcerative colitis,
      252
Mallory-Weiss syndrome, esophageal tears
      in, 95
Mark IV procedure for hiatus
      hernia/gastroesophageal reflux,
      406
Mecholy test of esophageal function,
      83-84, *85*
Meckel's diverticulum
  angiography of, 463-464
  evaluation of, nuclear medicine
      techniques of, 24
  in pediatric patient, 443
  sonography of, 455-456
Meconium ileus
  in pediatric patient, 442
  sonography of, 455
Meconium plug syndrome in pediatric
      patient, 442
Mediastinal masses, esophageal
      indentations from, 117
Mediterranean lymphoma of small bowel,
      212-213
Megacolon, toxic, complicating ulcerative
      colitis, 251, *252*

Meglumine diatrizoate for CT examination,
      16
Ménétrier's disease, *135,* 136
Mercedes-Benz sign in cholelithiasis, 323
Mesenteric abnormalities, evaluation of,
      ultrasonography in, 28, *29*
Mesenteric artery, superior, indentation of
      duodenum at, 166
Mesenteric ischemia, interventional
      procedures for, 476
Mesenteric venous thrombosis, acute, 202,
      203
Mesentery, thickening/retraction of, in
      Crohn's disease, 187, 192, 196
Mesodermal sarcomas of rectum, 281, *283*
Metabolic disorders
  esophageal motor dysfunction in, 89
  in pediatric patient, 449
Metastases
  esophageal, 114
  gastric, 152
  hepatic
      angiography of, 467
      magnetic resonance imaging of,
          339-340
      nuclear medicine of, 350
      ultrasonography of, 345-346
  pancreatic, 317
  small bowel, 214-216
  splenic, magnetic resonance imaging of,
      378
Metoclopramide, oral, for CT examination,
      16-17
Micelles in fat absorption, 337
Microcarcinomas, gastric, diagnosis of,
      147
Microcystic adenoma of pancreas, *314,*
      315
Mid-gut volvulus, 58
Migrating myoelectric complex (MMC), 37
Milk of calcium, bile, 324
Mirizzi syndrome
  percutaneous transhepatic
      cholangiography for, 477
  radiologic diagnosis of, 361
Moniliasis, esophageal, 98-99
Monitor, television, 2
Morgagni's hernia, 117
Motility, 36-38
Mucin-hypersecreting tumor of pancreatic
      duct, 314
Mucinous cystic neoplasms of pancreas,
      315
Mucosa, gastric, heterotopic, 167
Mucosal cytoprotective agents for peptic
      ulcer disease, 158
Mucosal neuroma syndrome in pediatric
      patient, 447
Mucus secretion by stomach, 36
Multiple endocrine neoplasia (MEN) IIB
      syndrome
  in pediatric patient, 447
  small bowel and, 209
Muscle(s)
  psoas, computed tomography of,
      434-435

Muscle(s)—cont'd
  puborectal dyskinetic, 239
Myasthenia gravis
  esophageal motor dysfunction in, *89, 90*
  pharyngeal dysfunction in, 72
Mycobacterium, colitis from, 258
Myobacterium avium-intracellulare (MAI), 403
Myotonia, esophageal motor dysfunction in, 89-90
Myotonic dystrophy, pharyngeal dysfunction in, 73
Myxedema, esophageal motor dysfunction in, 89

N

Necrotizing enterocolitis
  in pediatric patient, *442,* 443, 445-446
  sonography of, in pediatric patient, 454-455
Neisseria gonorrhoeae, colitis from, 258
Nematodes, 393-395
Neoplasm(s); *see also* Tumor(s)
  colonic, in pediatric patient, 444
  complicating in ulcerative colitis, 252
  diverticular disease with, 245, *246*
  gut tube, ultrasonographic evaluation of, *30,* 31
Nephrotropic contrast agents, 18-19
Neurofibromatosis in pediatric patient, 447
Neurogenic tumors, gastric, 152
Neuromuscular disease, esophageal motor dysfunction in, 89-90
Neuromuscular dysfunction of pharynx, 71-72
Neuropeptides, enteric, 33-35
Neuroregulation of swallowing, 67
Newborn, transient pharyngeal incoordination of, 74
Nodular pattern in Crohn's disease, 187
Noninfectious colitis, 259-260
Nuclear medicine, 24-26
  instrumentation for, 8-11
    in gamma ray-photon production, 8-9
    in photon detection, 9
    pulse-height analyzer as, 9
  of spleen, 378-381; *see also* Spleen, nuclear medicine of
Nutcracker esophagus, 86-87

O

Obesity, morbid, gastric bypass for, postoperative evaluation of, 414
Obstruction(s)
  complicating diverticular disease, 243
  gastric outlet, complicating peptic ulceration, 160
  stomal, after gastric surgery, postoperative evaluation of, 410
Oculopharyngeal syndrome, pharyngeal dysfunction in, 73-74
Oesophagostomum, 394

Omental abnormalities, evaluation of, ultrasonography in, 28, *29*
Omphalocele, fetal, prenatal ultrasonic detection of, 32
Oncologic disease in pediatric patient, 446
Oncology, 496-497
Opisthorchiasis, 396
Opportunistic infections, gastrointestinal, 402-403
Oropharynx, swallowing and, 35
Osseous complications of pancreatitis, 308
Osteophytes, cervical, dysphagia from, 74
Ovarian dysgenesis in pediatric patient, 447

P

Pancreas, 292-317
  aberrant, 308
  adenocarcinoma of, 309-310, *310-311,* 312-313
  anatomy of, 292
  angiography of, 297, 465-466
  annular, 308
  carcinomas of, unusual, 314
  computed tomography of, 294
  congenital abnormalities of, 308
  cystic neoplasms of, 314-315
  diagnostic examination of, 292-294
  disease of, endoscopic treatment for, 489
  ectopic, 141, *142,* 143, 308
  endoscopic retrograde cholangiopancreatography of, 295, 297
  fine-needle aspiration biopsy of, 297
  fine-needle fluid aspiration and percutaneous pancreatography of, 297
  fluid collections in, drainage of, 490
  islet cell neoplasms of, 315-316, *317*
  lesions of
    neoplastic, 308-314
    nonneoplastic, 297-308
  magnetic resonance imaging of, 295
  metastatic neoplasms of, 317
  nonepithelial neoplasms of, 316-317
  percutaneous transhepatic cholangiography of, 297
  physiology of, 39-40
  postoperative evaluation of, 414
  radiology of, in pediatric patient, 452
  radionuclide examination of, 295
  transhepatic venography of, 297
  trauma to, 63, 65
  ultrasonography of, 294-295
  vascular system of, interventional procedures for, 475
  venography of, 469-470
Pancreas divisum
  endoscopic treatment for, 489
  pancreatitis from, 301-302, *303*
Pancreatic digestion tests, 40
Pancreatic islet cell tumors, venography of, 469-470

Pancreatic tissue, heterotopic, in duodenum, 168
Pancreatitis, 423, *424-425*
  acute, 48, 297, 299
    radiologic diagnosis of, 297, *298-299,* 299
  chronic, radiologic diagnosis of, 299-301
  clinical and radiologic staging of, 301
  complications of, 302-308
  etiology of, 301-302
  interventional procedures for, 475
  in pediatric patient, 452
  radiologic diagnosis of, 297-299
  traumatic, 63, *64-65,* 302
Papilla, duodenal, 161
  major, enlargement of, 169
Papillary stenosis, benign, endoscopic treatment for, 488
Papillomas, esophageal, 116
Pararenal space
  anterior, 422-423, *424-425*
  posterior, 428
Parasites in biliary tract, radiologic diagnosis of, 361, 363
Parasitic colitis, 259
Parasitic infections, 392-400
Parasympathomimetic agents, transit time through small bowel and, 173
Parenchymal necrosis in pancreatitis, 301, 307
Parkinsonism, esophageal motor dysfunction in, 89
Pediatric radiology, 438-457
  for biliary system, 450-452
  for gastrointestinal tract disorders, 438-444
  imaging techniques in, 452-457
  for liver, 449-450
  for pancreas, 452
  for pharyngeal/esophageal abnormalities, 447-449
  for systemic diseases, 444-447
Pelvic abscesses, 52
Pelvic floor, relation of, to pubococcygeal line, 236
Penetration complicating peptic ulceration, 160-161
Pepsin secretion by stomach, 36
Peptic disease, 152-161; *see also* Peptic ulceration
Peptic ulceration
  complications of, 160-161
  differential diagnosis of, 161
  epidemiology of, 152
  healing and scar formation in, 158-160
  location of, 154-156
  morphologic features of, 156, 158
  pathogenesis of, 152
  in pediatric patient, 444
  perforation of, pneumoperitoneum from, 44
  radiographic appearance of, 152-154, *155*
Percutaneous biopsy, 489-490
  fine-needle, in pediatric patient, 457

Percutaneous biopsy—cont'd
  fine-needle aspiration, of lymph nodes of
      retroperitoneal space, 436
Percutaneous gastrostomy, 472
Percutaneous pancreatography, 297
Percutaneous transhepatic cholangiography
      (PTC), 477
  of pancreas, 297
    for cancer, 313-314
Percutaneous transjejunal puncture of
      Roux-en-Y
      choledochojejunostomies, 472
Perforation
  complicating granulomatous colitis, 256
  complicating peptic ulceration, 160
  complicating ulcerative colitis, 252
  of gallbladder, 47
Pericholecystic fluid, ultrasonography of,
      347
Perirenal space, 426, 427, 428
Perisplenic masses, 368
Peristalsis, esophageal, 82-83
  abnormal, 90
  hypertensive, 86-87
Peritoneal tuberculosis, 385
Peritonitis, 50-51
  barium, 16
Permissible loading of x-ray tube, 2
Peroral pneumocolon (PPC) for small
      bowel radiologic examination,
      179
Peutz-Jeghers syndrome, 274-275
  in pediatric patient, 444
  small bowel in, 207, 209
Peyer's patches, 38
  in pediatric patient, 444-445
Pharyngoesophageal interrelationships, 73
Pharyngography, double-contrast, 69
Pharynx, 66-77
  abnormalities of, disorders with, in
      pediatric patient, 447-449
  anatomy of, 66-67
  disorders of, 69-77
    compensation for, 77
    diverticula as, 69-70
    dysphagia from cervical osteophytes
        as, 74
    familial dysautonomia as, 73
    functional, 70-71
    myotonic dystrophy as, 73
    neuromuscular, 71-72
    oculopharyngeal syndrome as, 73-74
    in pediatric patient, 447-449
    pharyngoesophageal interrelationships
        and, 73
    postoperative, 74-75
    in schizophrenia, 74
    transient pharyngeal incoordination of
        newborn as, 74
    tumors as, 75, 76, 77
    webs as, 74, 75
  palsy of, unilateral, 72
  radiographic anatomy of, 69
  radiographic evaluation of, 67-69
Phase in generator selection, 1-2

Phased array scanners, 6, 7, 8
Phlegmon, pancreatic, 305
Phlegmonous gastritis, 129-130
Phrenic ampulla, 82
Phrygian cap of gallbladder, 327
Phytobezoar, 55, 139
Pleomorphic carcinoma of pancreas, 314
Plication defects after gastric surgery,
      postoperative evaluation of,
      411-412
Plummer-Vinson syndrome, 75
Pneumatosis, intramural, 140-141
Pneumatosis intestinalis, 44, 45
  in pediatric patient, 445-446
Pneumobilia, intrahepatic, ultrasonography
      of, 348
Pneumocholangiogram after biliary tract
      surgery, postoperative evaluation
      of, 416-417
Pneumoperitoneum, 42-44
  after gastric surgery, postoperative
      evaluation of, 408
  causes of, 43
Polyarteritis nodosa, angiography of, 464
Polycystic disease
  of kidney in pediatric patient, 449
  of liver, diagnosis of, 334-335
Polyhydramnios, ultrasonic evaluation of,
      32
Polyp(s)
  adenomatous
    diagnosis of, 145-146
    duodenal, 167
  colonic, 264-276
    adenomatous, 270
    malignant potential of, 269-270
    management of, 272
    pathologic findings in, 264-265
    in pediatric patient, 444
    detection of, 265-266
  fibrovascular, esophageal, 115
  filiform, in ulcerative colitis, 249, 250
  inflammatory
    esophageal, 115-116
    in ulcerative colitis, 249
  postinflammatory, in ulcerative colitis,
      249
  radiologic features of, 266-270
Polypeptide, vasoactive intestinal, 34-35
Polypoid cancer, early, diagnosis of, 145
Polypoid changes in ulcerative colitis,
      249-250
Polyposis
  familial
    multiple, 276
    in pediatric patient, 444
  juvenile, 276
    small bowel and, 209
Polyposis syndromes, 272-276
Polysplenia, 367
Porcelain gallbladder, 324
Portal hypertension
  diagnosis of, 331
  interventional procedures for, 475
  venography of, 469

Portal venography, 468, 469
Portal venous gas in pediatric patient, 450
Positron emission tomography (PET), 10,
      11
Postcholecystectomy syndrome,
      postoperative evaluation of, 417,
      419
Postgastrectomy carcinoma after gastric
      surgery, postoperative evaluation
      of, 413-414
Postgastrectomy syndromes, postoperative
      evaluation of, 414
Postoperative radiology, 404-420
  of biliary tract, 416-419
  of colon, 415-416
  of duodenum, 406
  of esophagus, 404-406
  of liver, 419-420
  of pancreas, 420
  of small bowel, 414-415
  of stomach, 406-414
Postvagotomy dysphagia, 89
Postvagotomy functional changes,
      postoperative evaluation of, 414
Power rating in generator selection, 1
Prenatal ultrasound, 32
Presbyesophagus, 87
Progressive systemic sclerosis in pediatric
      patient, 447
Prostaglandins and gut, 35
Prosthetic aortic grafts, 432
Pseudo-Whipple's disease, 201
Pseudocysts, pancreatic, 63
  complicating pancreatitis, 302-303, 304,
      305
  drainage of, 490
  endoscopic treatment for, 489
Pseudodiverticula, duodenal, 160
Pseudodiverticulosis, intramural, 93
Pseudolymphoma of stomach, 131, 132
Pseudomembranous colitis in pediatric
      patient, 448
Pseudomembranous enteritis, 204
Pseudomembranous enterocolitis, 50,
      387-388
Pseudopolyps in ulcerative colitis, 249
Pseudosarcomas, esophageal, 113-114
Psoas muscles, computed tomography of,
      434-435
Pubococcygeal line, relation of pelvic floor
      to, 236
Puborectal muscle, dyskinetic, 239
Pulmonary complications of pancreatitis,
      308
Pulmonary cysts, enterogenous, evaluation
      of, nuclear medicine techniques
      of, 24
Pulseless disease, angiography of, 465
Purpura, Henoch-Schönlein, in pediatric
      patient, 446
Pyloric hypertrophy, adult, 127-128
Pyloric stenosis, hypertrophic, 53
  idiopathic, evaluation of,
      ultrasonography in, 31
  in pediatric patient, 443

Pylorus, sonography of, in pediatric patient, 453, *454*
Pyogenic liver abscesses
    diagnosis of, 331
    magnetic resonance imaging of, 343
    in pediatric patient, 449
Pyogenic liver disease, nuclear medicine of, 351
Pyriform sinus, 66

R

Radiation
    effects of, on colon, postoperative evaluation of, 416
    esophagitis from, 103
Radiation colitis, 260
Radiation enteritis of small bowel, 203-204
Radiocolloids for spleen scintigraphy, 379
Radiofrequency coil, transmitter, and receiver
        for magnetic resonance imaging, 13-14
Radiographic equipment, 1-3
Radiographic evaluation of pharynx, 67-69
Radiographic instrumentation, 2, 3
Radiology, postoperative, 404-420; *see also* Postoperative radiology
Radionuclide examination of pancreas, 295
Radiopharmaceuticals for spleen scintigraphy, 378-379
Real-time sonography of pancreas, 294-295
Receiver, radiofrequency, for magnetic resonance imaging, 114
Rectocele, 239
Rectum
    intussusception of, *237*, 238
    perforation of, 428
    prolapse of, 238
    transrectal ultrasonography of, 231-232
    tuberculosis of, 385
Reflux
    esophageal, evaluation of, nuclear medicine techniques of, 24
    gastroesophageal, 90-91
        correction of hiatus hernia and, 405-406
        in pediatric patient, 438, 440
Reflux esophagitis, 88-89
Regional enteritis in pediatric patient, 443
Rendu-Osler-Weber syndrome, sonography of, in pediatric patient, 453
Resolution of image intensifier tube, 2
Retroduodenal hematoma, 423, *424*
Retroperitoneal abscess, 52
Retroperitoneal fibrosis, 434
Retroperitoneal hemorrhage, 433-434
Retroperitoneal masses, ultrasonography of, 431
Retroperitoneal sarcomas, 434
Retroperitoneal space, 421-436
    computed tomography of, 431-435
    extraperitoneal compartments of, 421-428
    lymphography of, 435-436

Retroperitoneal space—cont'd
    magnetic resonance imaging of, 431-435
    radiologic anatomy and diagnosis of, 421
    ultrasonography of, 428-431
Riley-Day syndrome
    in pediatric patient, 447
    pharyngeal dysfunction in, 73
Rings, esophageal, 104-105
Rokitansky-Aschoff sinuses in adenomyomatosis, 327
Rotate-rotate systems in computed tomography, 4
Rotate-stationary systems in computed tomography, 4
Roundworms, 393-395
Roux-en-Y choledochojejunostomies, percutaneous transjejunal puncture of, 472
Ruvalcaba-Myhre-Smith syndrome, 275
    small bowel in, 209

S

Salmonella enteritidis, colitis from, 258
Salmonella infections, 386
Salmonellosis, small bowel in, 200
Santorini's papilla, 161
Sarcoma(s)
    esophageal, 113-114
    hepatic, diagnosis of, 336, *337*
    Kaposi's, gastrointestinal, 400
    mesodermal, of rectum, 281, *283*
    retroperitoneal, 434
    small bowel, 213-214
Sarcoma botryoides, diagnosis of, 337
Scan converter in ultrasonography, 8
Scanners, CT, fast, 4
Scanning gantries in computed tomography, 4
Schatzki ring, 104-105
Schistosomes, 396
Schizophrenia, swallowing problems in, 74
Scintigraphy, white-blood cell, for Crohn's disease, 185
Scintillation camera, 9-10
Scleroderma, 218-219
    esophageal motor dysfunction in, 87-88
    in pediatric patient, 447
Sclerosing cholangitis, diagnosis of, 331, 333
Sclerosing injections, endoscopic, for portal hypertension, 475
Sclerotherapy, endoscopic, for portal hypertension, 469
Sedatives, transit time through small bowel and, 173
Segmentation in sprue, 389
Serous cystadenoma of pancreas, *314,* 315
Sessile nodules in ulcerative colitis, 249
Shigella, colitis from, 258
Shigellosis, 387
    small bowel in, 200
Shockwave lithotripsy, 480, *482*
Sickle cell disease in pediatric patient, 446

Sigmoid colon, perforation of, 428
Single-contrast examination of esophagus, 80, *81*
Single photon-emission tomography (SPECT), 10
Sinus(es)
    in Crohn's disease, 187, 196
    Rokitansky-Aschoff, in adenomyomatosis, 327
Sinusoids, 38-39
Skip lesions in Crohn's disease, 192
Sludge, intraluminal, ultrasonography of, 347
Small bowel, 172-220
    anatomy of, 172
    Behçet's syndrome in, 199
    Crohn's disease of, 184-198; *see also* Crohn's disease
    drug-associated disorders of, 204
    eosinophilic gastroenteritis and, 204
    hemorrhage into, interventional procedures for, 476
    ileitis in, 199
    immune deficiencies of, 219-220
    infectious diseases of, 200-201
    inflammatory diseases of, 184-200
    malabsorption in, diseases associated with, 216-219
    neoplastic lesions of, 205-216
    obstruction of, postoperative evaluation of, 415
    physiology of, 37-38
    postoperative evaluation of, 414-415
    radiation enteritis of, 203-204
    radiologic examination of, 172-182
        agents affecting transit time and, 172-173
        barium, 173-179
            indications for, 179, *180-181, 182*
        computed tomography for, 181, *182-183*
        dedicated small bowel follow-through in, 173-174
        enteroclysis in, 174-179
        magnetic resonance imaging for, 182
        peroral pneumocolon in, 179
        preliminary plain radiographs of abdomen in, 173
        retrograde, 179
        small bowel enema in, 174-179
        small bowel follow-through in, 123
        water-soluble contrast material for, 179, 187
    retrograde examination of, 227
    segmental ischemia of, 201-203
    syndromes rarely affecting, 208-209
    transit time through, agents affecting, 172-173
    tuberculosis of, 384
    tumors of
        adenocarcinomas as, 213, *214*
        benign, 205-209
        carcinoid, 209-210
        lymphomas as, 210-213
        metastatic, 214-216

Small bowel—cont'd
tumors of—cont'd
sarcomas as, 213-214
venography of, 470
Small bowel follow-through (SBFT)
examination, 173
Small left colon syndrome in pediatric
patient, 442
Solid and papillary epithelial neoplasm,
314
Somatostatin, 35
South American blastomycosis, small
bowel in, 201
Spectroscopy, magnetic resonance, of
liver, 362, 363
Sphincter(s), esophageal, 78, 79
functional abnormalities of, 84-85
Sphincterotomy, 485, 487, 488
endoscopic, 480
Spleen, 365-403
abnormalities of, 367-370
abscess in, 367
accessory, scintigraphy for, 380-381
angiography of, 467, 469
born-again, scintigraphy for, 381
fluid collections in, drainage of, 491
hemorrhage in, magnetic resonance
imaging of, 374, 376
imaging of, 366
infarcts of, magnetic resonance imaging
of, 375
injuries to, 61
magnetic resonance imaging of, 374-378
normal, 366
nuclear medicine of, 378-381
for accessory spleen, 380-381
for born-again spleen, 381
for functional asplenia, 381
nonimaging, 381
radiopharmaceuticals in, 378-379
scintigraphy in
for benign lesions, 379-380
clinical indications for, 379
tumors of, 375-378
ultrasonography of, 369-374
for consistency, 371-373
for contour, 371
pitfalls in interpretation of, 373-374
for size, 370-371
vascular system of, interventional
procedures for, 475
Splenomegaly, 367, 368t, 371, 375
Sprue, 389-390
and sprue pattern, 216-218
Squamous cell carcinoma of colon, 280
Steatorrhea, idiopathic, 389
Stenosis
biliary tract, in pediatric patient,
450-451
esophageal, in pediatric patient, 438
Stierlin's sign in ileocecal tuberculosis, 384
Stomach, 119-152
abnormalities of
pancreatitis from, 301
in shape and function, 137-140

Stomach—cont'd
anatomy of, 127-128
atony of, 137, 139
cancer of, 143-152; see also Gastric
cancer
dilatation of, acute, after gastric surgery,
postoperative evaluation of, 408
diverticula of, 137
emptying of, barium studies of, 125-126
hemorrhage into, interventional
procedures for, 475-476
inflammation of, 128-132; see also
Gastritis
leiomyomas of, 151
leiomyosarcomas of, 151
motility in, 36-37
neoplastic disorders of, 143-152; see
also Gastric cancer
nonneoplastic lesions of, 127
miscellaneous, 140-143
nuclear medicine of, 24
outlet of, obstruction of, 52-55
physiology of, 36-37
postoperative evaluation of, 404-414
radiation injury of, 133
receptive relaxation of, after feeding, 36
secretion in, 36
sonography of, in pediatric patient, 453
surgery on, sequelae of, postoperative
evaluation of, 408-414
tuberculosis of, 384
tumors of, 151, 152
ulcers of, 154, 156
healing of, radiographic appearance
of, 158-160
upper gastrointestinal radiologic study
of, 119-127; see Upper GI study
varices of, 141
volvulus of, 139-140
Stomal obstructions after gastric surgery,
postoperative evaluation of, 410
Stones
in bile ducts
extraction of, cholecystostomy
procedures for, 481, 483-485
lithotripsy of, 480, 482
in gallbladder; see Gallstones
Stool softening, water-soluble contrast
media for, 229
Strawberry gallbladder, 325
Stricture(s)
bile duct
dilatation of, 481, 484, 486
endoscopic treatment for, 488
complicating in ulcerative colitis, 252
esophageal, 105-106, 107
caustic, in pediatric patient, 440
congenital, in pediatric patient, 438,
439
dilatation of, 471-472
String sign
in Crohn's disease, 187
in granulomatous colitis, 254
Strongyloides stercoralis, colitis from, 259
Strongyloidiasis, 394

Subcapsular hematomas, 61
Subhepatic abscess, 51-52
Subphrenic abscess, 51-52
Superior mesenteric artery, indentation of
duodenum at, 166
Swallowing
neuroregulation of, 67
oropharynx and, 35
Syphilis of GI tract, 129, 130

T

Takayasu's arteritis, angiography of,
464-465
Tapeworm, 395
Technology, future, 3
Television camera pickup tube in television
viewing system, 2
Television viewing system, 2
Terminal ileitis, acute, 199
Terminal ileum
in granulomatous colitis, 256
peroral double-contrast examination of
right colon and, 228
in ulcerative colitis, 250-251
Thrombosis of inferior vena cava, 430-431,
433
Timing control in generator selection, 2
Tomography
computed; see Computed tomography
(CT)
emission, instrumentation for, 10
Tongue worm, 395
Toxic megacolon complicating ulcerative
colitis, 251, 252
Tracheoesophageal fistula, 87, 91-92
in pediatric patient, 438, 439
Tranquilizers, transit time through small
bowel and, 173
Transducer in ultrasonography, 5-8
Transhepatic pancreatic venography of
pancreas, 297
Transit in esophagus, 35-36
Transmitter, radiofrequency, for magnetic
resonance imaging, 14
Transplantation of liver, 321
postoperative evaluation of, 419-420
Transrectal ultrasonography of rectum,
231-232
Trauma
abdominal, 60
hepatic, 61, 62, 320
angiography of, 467
in pediatric patient, 450
intestinal, 63
pancreatic, 63-65
in pediatric patient, 452
splenic, 61, 369
angiography of, 467, 469
ultrasonography of, 373
Traveler's diarrhea, 388
Trematodes, 395-396
Trichobezoar, 55, 139
Trichuriasis, 391-392, 394-395
Trisomy 21 in pediatric patient, 446, 447

Trypanosomiasis, American, 390-391
Tuberculosis
    of colon, 385
    of duodenum, 384
    esophagitis in, 102
    of esophagus, 384
    gastrointestinal, 383-386
    of ileocecum, 384-385
    of peritoneum, 385
    of rectum, 385
    of small bowel, 384
    of stomach, 129, 384
Tuberculous enteritis/enterocolitis, 200-201
Tumor(s)
    alimentary tract, angiography of, 465
    biliary tract, in pediatric patient, 452
    hepatic
        angiography of, 467, *468*
        interventional procedures for, *474,*
            475
        nuclear medicine of, 350
        in pediatric patient, 449
    pancreatic, in pediatric patient, 452
    pharyngeal, 75, 77
    splenic, 367-368
        magnetic resonance imaging of,
            375-378
    ulcerogenic, after gastric surgery,
        postoperative evaluation of, 413
Tumor blush in alimentary tract tumors,
    465
Turcot's syndrome, 275
Turner syndrome in pediatric patient, 447
Typhlitis in pediatric patient, 445-446
Typhoid fever, 386-387

U

Ulcer(s)
    in Crohn's disease, 187, *190-191*
    definition of, 152
    duodenal, 156, *157*
        healing of, radiographic appearance
            of, 160
    gastric, 154, 156
        healing of, radiographic appearance
            of, 158-160
    juxtapyloric, 154, 156
    marginal, after gastric surgery,
        postoperative evaluation of, 412
    peptic; *see* Peptic ulceration
    small bowel, primary nonspecific, 200
    in ulcerative colitis, 248-249
Ulcer disease, postoperative, postoperative
    evaluation of, 412-413
Ulcer scar, 53
Ulcerative colitis, 49-50, 248-253
    clinical features of, 248
    complications of, 251-252

Ulcerative colitis—cont'd
    ileitis associated with, 199
    in pediatric patient, 443
    radiographic findings in, 248-251
    surgical procedures for, 252-253
Ulcerogenic tumors after gastric surgery,
        postoperative evaluation of, 413
Ulceronodular pattern in Crohn's disease,
    187, *188-189*
Ultrafast CT scanners, 4-5
Ultrasonography, 26-32
    in acute pancreatitis, 299
    of alimentary tube, 26-32
    endoscopic, 32
    for inflammatory disease of colon, 260
    instrumentation for, 5-8
    of liver, 343-346
    of pancreas, 294-295
        for cancer, 312
    in pediatric patient, 452-456
    for percutaneous biopsy, 489
    prenatal, 32
    of retroperitoneal space, 428-431
    of spleen, 369-374; *see also* Spleen,
        ultrasonography of
    transrectal, of rectum, 231-232
Upper GI study
    biphasic routine examination in, 122,
        123*t,* 124-125
    double-contrast examination in, 121, *122*
    emergency, 126
    functional, 125-126
    patient preparation and instructions for,
        121
    renal photofluorography and
        videofluorography in, 125|
    second look, 126
    single-contrast examination in, 121, *122*
    techniques of, 121-126

V

Vagotomy
    dysphagia after, 89
    functional changes after, postoperative
        evaluation of, 414
Varices
    esophageal, 108-109
        in pediatric patient, 440
    gastric, 141
Vascular anomalies, esophageal
    indentations from, 117
Vascular complications of pancreatitis,
    307, 308
Vascular diseases
    contrast media for, 18-20
    of GI tract, angiography of, 464-465
    of liver, diagnosis of, 331
    of spleen, 368-369

Vascular flukes, 396, *397*
Vascular system
    of liver, interventional procedures for,
        473-475
    of pancreas, interventional procedures
        for, 475
    of spleen, interventional procedures for,
        475
Vasoactive intestinal polypeptide (VIP),
    34-35
Vasoconstrictive infusion therapy for acute
        GI hemorrhage, 461
Vasopressin infusion
    for acute GI hemorrhage, 461
    for portal hypertension, 469
Vater's papilla, 161
Vena cava, inferior, 430-431, 433
Venography, 469-470
    pancreatic, transhepatic, 297
Vidicon in television viewing system, 2
Villous adenoma
    duodenal, 167, 168
    rectal, 280, *283*
Viral colitis, 258
Visceral embolism, angiography of, 464
Volvulus, 54
    colonic obstruction from, 58-59
    gastric, 139-140
    mid-gut, 558
    reduction of, 228-229

W

Web(s)
    antral, 128
    esophageal, 107
    pharyngeal, *74,* 75
Whipple's disease, 218
    small bowel in, 201
Whipworm infection, 394-395
White-blood cell scintigraphy for Crohn's
        disease, 185
Wilson's disease, esophageal motor
        dysfunction in, 89

X

X-ray tube, 2

Y

Yersinia enterocolitica, colitis from, 258

Z

Zenker's diverticula, 70, *73*
Zollinger-Ellison syndrome
    duodenal changes in, 170
    ulcers in, 161